Gonadotropins

GONADOTROPINS

Edited by

BRIJ B. SAXENA,
Departments of Medicine and Obstetrics and Gynecology

CARL G. BELING
Department of Obstetrics and Gynecology

HORTENSE M. GANDY
Department of Obstetrics and Gynecology

The New York Hospital
and Cornell University Medical College

WILEY-INTERSCIENCE, a Division of John Wiley & Sons, Inc.

New York ● London ● Sydney ● Toronto

Library of Congress Cataloging in Publication Data

International Symposium on Gonadotropins,
    New York Hospital-Cornell Medical Center, 1971.
    Gonadotropins.

    1. Gonadotropin–Congresses. I. Saxena, Brij B.,
ed. II. Beling, Carl G., ed. III. Gandy, Hortense M.,
date, ed.
RM291.2.G6157 1971   612.61   73-38948
ISBN 0-471-75570-2

Preface

The present volume contains papers presented by eminent scholars during the International Symposium on Gonadotropins held in New York City, June 17-19, 1971, on the occasion of the 200th Anniversary celebration of The Society of The New York Hospital. As the second oldest hospital in the United States, The New York Hospital has earned a reputation for excellent medical care and has a record of meritorious accomplishments in biomedical research.

One of the greatest challenges facing humanity today is the population explosion. The Organizing Committee of the symposium felt a need for a meeting designed to integrate recent studies on the hypothalamic-hypophyseal-gonadal axis and its relation to human reproduction. The present volume is highlighted by the latest information on the subunits of gonadotropins, gonadotropin releasing factors, measurement of human gonadotropins and prolactin, and the clinical use of gonadotropins. It is our fond hope that endocrinologists will find this book a valuable reference for evaluation of current hypotheses and development of new approaches in the control of fertility.

It is with a feeling of honor that the Organizing Committee of the symposium dedicates this volume to the memory of a great endocrinologist, Professor Emil Witschi.

Organizing Committee

Fritz Fuchs
Ralph E. Peterson
Brij B. Saxena
Hortense M. Gandy
Carl G. Beling

New York
November 1971

Acknowledgments

The International Symposium on Gonadotropins was made possible by Grant No. 67-455 from The Ford Foundation to the Department of Obstetrics and Gynecology, Cornell University Medical College. We are indebted to the Rockefeller University for the use of Caspary Hall and Abby Aldrich Hall.

The organizing committee is grateful to the contributors and to the many discussants. We are indebted to Om P. Bahl, Solomon A. Berson, Robert M. Blizzard, Piero Donini, Fritz Fuchs, Carl A. Gemzell, Roger Guillemin, Charles W. Lloyd, Bruno Lunenfeld, Luciano Martini, Janet W. McArthur, Samuel McCann, Roland K. Meyer, Francis J. Morgan, Raghuveer N. Moudgal, C. Alvin Paulsen, Leo E. Reichert, Jr., Griff T. Ross, Hilton A. Salhanick, Kenneth Savard, A. Louis Southren, Darrell N. Ward, and Rosalyn S. Yalow for serving as session chairmen. We wish to thank Mina Rano, Mimi Halpern, and Roberta Revell for excellent secretarial assistance.

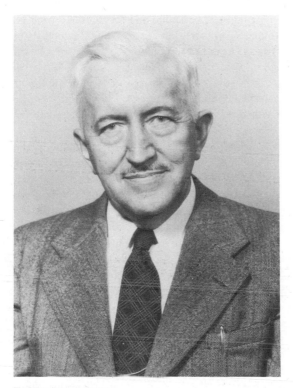

EMIL WITSCHI

February 2, 1890-June 10, 1971

May I tell you about a man who was a pioneer in the field of reproductive biology during the early part of this century and continued as an active contributor to the field until the time of his death last week.

Emil Witschi was born in an Alpine village near Bern, Switzerland. He developed early a fascination for the variety of animals with which he shared his valley. This interest in nature led him to zoology and to the laboratory of the classical embryologist, Richard Hertwig, with whom Professor Witschi prepared for his doctorate, awarded by the University of Munich in 1913. His indoctrination as a naturalist and his recognition of the importance of comparative biology in the understanding of embryologic and physiologic events led him to range broadly in his investigations of gonadal phenomena and other reproductive problems. Contained in his scientific bibliography of 250 titles are studies with more than 30 different animal forms, ranging from invertebrates to human beings, including such unusual creatures as the Western banded gecko, African bishop birds, the nine-banded armadillo and the diamond-back terrapin. Few scientists have achievements so diversified as to include the identification of a subspecies of frog, description of ear development for underwater hearing, the analysis of nuptial plumage in weaver finches, and the study of sex behavior of herring gulls. The broad scope of his work, itself, a tribute to his zealous scientific curiosity, pursued with endless vitality and with the highest degree of competence. It is also, of course, the legacy he leaves to all of us and to future generations.

The name of Witschi is identified most intimately with the inductor theory of sex differentiation, formulated and proposed by him in 1914. In those early years his studies on the process of sex differentiation in *Rana temporaria* led him to the realization that all embryos and primordial germ cells are bipotential and that several factors, both genetic and nongenetic, decide the alternative of male of female differentiation. He demonstrated that the embryonic gonadal cortex is an inductor of female differentiation and the medulla an inductor of male differentiation. These concepts, formulated by Witschi more than 50 years ago serve as the basis for the current understanding of human intersexuality.

In 1926 Professor Witschi left Switzerland and his post as lecturer at the University of Basel to visit the United States as a Rockefeller Foundation Fellow. He spent over a year in the Osborn laboratory at Yale, with Carl Moore at Chicago and with Herbert Evans at California. At each laboratory he found a stimulating environment and a great interest in the field of sex differentiation. With the emphasis on this area of research shifting from Europe to the United States, the decision to return to this country and assume American citizenship was a natural one for Professor Witschi, supported by his faithful wife Martha. That he was forgiven his departure from the Swiss scientific community is evidenced by his appointment, 25 years ago, to the Swiss Academy of Sciences and by the conferring of the honorary Doctor of Medicine degree by the University of Basel on the occasion of the 500th anniversary of that distinguished institution. These are but two of the abundant honors he received during his career.

In America, Professor Witschi chose the beautiful setting of the University of Iowa, located on the gently rolling hills overlooking the Iowa river. A department already prominent in endocrine research under the leadership of W. W. Swingle perpetuated this quality by the appointment of Witschi as Professor of Zoology in 1927. Continuously, Professor Witschi and his growing school of Iowa students broadened the attack on the problem of sex differentiation to include the study of fishes, reptiles, birds and mammals. As a result, Witschi's inductor theory found widespread acceptance as a fundamental principle in the development of all vertebrate gonads. Through the years he developed a truly remarkable laboratory for studies in comparative endocrinology and studied hormonally controlled sexual characteristics in many species. His studies on the comparative aspects of pituitary gonadotropins provide important fundamentals for the current activity in this field. His analysis of hormonal control of feather and bill coloration in birds reveals basic considerations bearing on the evolution of endocrine reaction. His work on temperature effects and overripeness of amphibian eggs has been of considerable importance in the fields of teratogenesis and fetal abnormalities. Among his numerous contributions to the field of genetics is included the discovery of the chromosomal mechanisms for sex inheritance in two different species of amphibia. His place in the history of reproductive science is assured by his monumental study of the migration of the germ cells of human embryos from the yolk sac to the primitive gonadal folds.

Throughout this lifetime of devotion to scientific research, Emil Witschi fulfilled with great conscience his responsibilities as a member of the teaching faculty of a great state university. In 1955 he published his second book, an outstanding textbook, entitled The Development of Vertebrates. Replete with original concepts and data, it represents an important contribution to the teaching of embryology. The first book under Witschi's authorship appeared nearly 40 years earlier, it too was prepared for students. At that time, as a teacher in the Science Gymnasium of Basel, he wrote and illustrated a delightful volume entitled, The Land Animals, which was to inspire in his young students an interest in biology, and was to serve, also, as an outlet for his artistic inclinations. With this volume, Witschi purged himself of a lingering idea to foresake science in favor of a career in the graphic arts. Those who have observed his classroom lectures, which could serve, as well, for sketching lessons in a school of fine arts, recognize that he succeeded in pursuing both courses.

But perhaps his greatest pride derived from his success in inspiring young scientists. He advised and guided more than forty to the Ph.D. degree. Countless other young men whose research bordered on his interests profited from his consultation, encouragement, and suggestions. This boundless fervor to broaden the horizon of scientific understanding characterizes Emil Witschi. It led him into yet another avenue of scientific achievement as project specialist in reproductive physiology to the Ford Foundation, and more recently, The Population Council. In this capacity Emil Witschi provided guidance to investigators throughout the world. He lived a full life.

Sheldon J. Segal

June 18, 1971

Contributors

AMOSS, MAX S.
   The Salk Institute for Biological Studies, La Jolla, California

ANAST, CONSTANTINE S.
   Department of Pediatrics, University Hospital and the Medical School, University of Missouri, Columbia, Missouri

ARIMURA, AKIRA
   Department of Medicine, Tulane University School of Medicine, New Orleans, Louisiana

ARMSTRONG, DAVID T.
   Department of Physiology, The University of Western Ontario, London, Canada

BADAWY, S.
   The Population Council, The Rocefeller University, New York, New York

BAGHDASSARIAN, ALICE
   Department of Pediatrics, Temple University School of Medicine, Philadelphia, Pennsylvania

BAHL, OM P.
   Department of Biochemistry, Faculty of Health Sciences, State University of New York at Buffalo, Buffalo, New York

BAKER, H. W. G.
   Department of Medicine, Prince Henry's Hospital and Monash University, Melbourne, Victoria, Australia

BECKERS, C.
   Laboratory of Nuclear Medicine, University of Louvain, Louvain, Belgium

BEHRMAN, HAROLD R.
   Departments of Physiology and Anatomy, Harvard Medical School, Boston, Massachusetts

BERAULT, ANNETTE
    Equipe de Recherches du C.N.R.S. No. 86, Collège de France, 11, Paris
    France

BERGLAND, RICHARD M.
    Department of Surgery, Milton S. Hershey Medical Center, Hershey,
    Pennsylvania

BERMUDEZ, JOSE A.
    Reproduction Research Branch, National Institute of Child Health and
    Human Development N.I.H., Bethesda, Maryland

BETTENDORF, GERHARD
    Division of Endocrinology, Universitäts-Frauenklinik, Hamburg, Germany

BISHOP, W.
    Department of Physiology, University of Texas Southwestern Medical
    School, Dallas, Texas

BLACKWELL, RICHARD
    The Salk Institute for Biological Studies, La Jolla, California

BLIZZARD, ROBERT M.
    Department of Pediatrics, Johns Hopkins University School of Medicine
    and the John Hopkins Hospital, Baltimore, Maryland

BOCCELLA, LOUISE
    Department of Obstetrics and Gynecology, University of Pittsburgh
    School of Medicine and the Magee-Womens Hospital, Pittsburgh, Pennsylvania

BOILERT, BRITT
    Department of Obstetrics and Gynecology, University Hospital, Uppsala
    14, Sweden

BONGIOVANNI, ALFRED M.
    The Children's Hospital of Philadelphia and the Department of Pediatrics,
    University of Pennsylvania School of Medicine, Philadelphia, Pa.

BRAUNSTEIN, G. D.
    National Institute of Child Health and Human Development, National
    Institutes of Health, Bethesda, Maryland

BRECKWOLDT, M.
    Division of Endocrinology, Universitäts-Frauenklinik, Hamburg, Germany

BRINSON, A.
    Population Council, The Rockefeller University, New York, New York

BRYANT, G. D.
    Department of Biochemistry and Biophysics, University of Hawaii,
    Honolulu, Hawaii

BULAT, GEORGE
    Medical Research Institute of Worcester, Inc., Worcester, Massachusetts

BURGER, HENRY G.

Medical Research Center and the Department of Medicine, Prince Henry's Hospital and Monash University, Melbourne, Australia

BURGUS, ROGER

The Salk Institute for Biological Studies, La Jolla, California

BUTLER, PHILIP S.

Medical Research Institute of Worcester, Inc., Worcester, Massachusetts

CANFIELD, ROBERT E.

Department of Medicine, College of Physicians & Surgeons, Columbia University, New York, New York

CARMEL, PETER

Department of Neurological Surgery, College of Physicians & Surgeons, Columbia University, New York, New York

CHRISTIANSEN, PETER

Hormone Department, Statens Seruminstitut and the University Hospital of Copenhagen, Copenhagen, Denmark

COULSON, PATRICIA

Department of Zoology, University of Tennessee, Knoxville, Tennessee

COWCHOCK, F. SUSAN

Department of Obstetrics & Gynecology, College of Physicians & Surgeons, Columbia University, New York, New York

CRIGLER, JOHN F., JR.

Endocrine Division, The Children's Hospital Medical Center and The Harvard Medical School, Boston, Massachusetts

DAUGHADAY, WILLIAM H.

Department of Medicine, Washington University School of Medicine, St. Louis, Missouri

DE KRETSER, DAVID M.

Departments of Medicine and Anatomy, Monash University, Melbourne, Victoria, Australia

DE LA LLOSA, M. PALOMA

Equipe de Recherches du C.N.R.S. No. 86, College de France, Paris, France

DEN HOLLANDER, F. C.

N. V. Organon, Oss, Holland

DIERSCHKE, D. J.

Department of Physiology, The University of Pittsburgh School of Medicine, Pittsburgh, Pennsylvania

DONOSO, A. O.

Department of Physiology, University of Texas Southwestern Medical School, Dallas, Texas

DYRENFURTH, INGE
Department of Obstetrics and Gynecology, College of Physicians & Surgeons, Columbia University, New York

ELDRIDGE, J. C.
Department of Endocrinology, Medical College of Georgia, Augusta, Georgia

ESHKOL, ALIZA
Institute of Endocrinology, Tel Hashomer Government Hospital Tel-Aviv, Israel

FAWCETT, C. P.
Department of Physiology, University of Texas Southwestern Medical School, Dallas, Texas

FERIN, J.
Physiology of Human Reproduction Research Unit, University Hospital, Louvain, Belgium

FERIN, MICHELLE
International Institute for the Study of Human Reproduction, College of Physicians & Surgeons, Columbia University, New York

FLINT, A. P. F.
Department of Obstetrics and Gynecology, University of Western Ontario, London, Canada

FOLEY, T. P., Jr.
Department of Pediatrics, Johns Hopkins University School of Medicine and the Johns Hopkins Hospital, Baltimore, Maryland

FRANCHIMONT, PAUL
Institut de Medecine, Hopital de Baviere, Liege, Belgium

FRANTZ, ANDREW G.
Department of Medicine, College of Physicians & Surgeons, Columbia University, New York

GABBE, STEVEN G.
Department of Biological Chemistry and Laboratory of Human Reproduction and Reproductive Biology, Harvard Medical School, Boston, Massachusetts

GANDY, HORTENSE M.
Department of Obstetrics and Gynecology, Cornell University Medical College, New York

GEMZELL, CARL A.
Department of Obstetrics and Gynecology, University of Uppsala, Uppsala, Sweden

GORSKI, JACK
Department of Physiology and Biophysics, University of Illinois, Urbana, Illinois

GRAESSLIN, D.
Division of Endocrinology, Universitäts-Frauenklinik, Hamburg, Germany

GREENWOOD, F. C.
Department of Biochemistry and Biophysics, University of Hawaii, Honolulu, Hawaii

GREEP, ROY O.
Laboratory of Human Reproduction and Reproductive Biology and the Department of Anatomy, The Harvard Medical School, Boston, Massachusetts

GRUMBACH, MELVIN M.
Department of Pediatrics, University of California School of Medicine, San Francisco, California

GUILLEMIN, ROGER
The Salk Institute for Biological Studies, La Jolla, California

HARTREE, ANNE STOCKELL
Department of Biochemistry, University of Cambridge, Cambridge, England

HASSOUNA, H.
The Population Council, The Rockefeller University, New York, New York

HENDRICK, J. C.
Departments of Internal Medicine and Pathology, Institute of Medicine, University of Liege, Belgium

HOTCHKISS, J.
Department of Physiology, University of Pittsburgh School of Medicine, Pittsburgh, Pennsylvania

HUDSON, BRYAN
Department of Medicine, Prince Henry's Hospital and Monash University, Melbourne, Victoria, Australia

INSLER, VACLAV
Department of Gynecology and Obstetrics, Tel Hashomer Government Hospital, Tel-Aviv, Israel

JACOBS, HOWARD S.
Division of Endocrinology, Department of Medicine, Harbor General Hospital and the U.C.L.A. School of Medicine, Torrance, California

JACOBS, LAURENCE S.
Department of Medicine, Washington University School of Medicine, St. Louis, Missouri

JAN, WAN F.
Endocrine Division, The Children's Hospital Medical Center and Harvard Medical School, Boston, Massachusetts

JOHANSON, A.
Department of Pediatrics, University of Virginia School of Medicine, Charlottesville, Virginia

JOHANSSON, ELOF D. B.
Department of Obstetrics and Gynecology, University of Uppsala, Akademiska Sjukhuset, Kvinnokliniken, Uppsala, Sweden

JOHNSEN, SVEND G.
Statens Seruminstitut and the University Hospital of Copenhagen, Copenhagen, Denmark

JOHNSON, PALEY
Department of Biochemistry, University of Cambridge, Cambridge, England

JOSIMOVICH, JOHN B.
Department of Obstetrics and Gynecology, University of Pittsburgh School of Medicine and the Magee-Womens Hospital, Pittsburgh, Pennsylvania

JUTISZ, MARIAN
Equipe de Recherches du C.N.R.S. No. 86, College de France, Paris, France

KALRA, P. S.
Department of Physiology, University of Texas Southwestern Medical School, Dallas, Texas

KALRA, S. P.
Department of Physiology, University of Texas Southwestern Medical School, Dallas, Texas

KAMMERMAN, SANDRA
Department of Medicine, College of Physicians & Surgeons, Columbia University, New York, New York

KAPLAN, SELNA L.
Department of Pediatrics, University of California School of Medicine, San Francisco, California

KARSCH, F. J.
Department of Physiology, University of Pittsburgh School of Medicine, Pittsburgh, Pennsylvania

KASTIN, ABBA J.
Endocrinology Section, Veterans Administration Hospital, New Orleans, Louisiana

KELCH, ROBERT P.
Department of Pediatrics, University of California, San Francisco, California

KERDELHUE, BERNARD
Equipe de Recherches du C.N.R.S. No. 86, College de France, Paris, France

KIM, S.
The Population Council, The Rockefeller University, New York, New York

KLEINBERG, DAVID L.
Department of Medicine, College of Physicians & Surgeons, Columbia University, New York, New York

KNOBIL, E.
Department of Physiology, University of Pittsburgh School of Medicine, Pittsburgh, Pennsylvania

KORACH, K. S.
Department of Endocrinology, Medical College of Georgia, Augusta, Georgia

KRULICH, L.
Department of Physiology, South Western Medical Center, University of Texas, Dallas, Texas

LAMKIN, WILLIAM M.
Department of Biochemistry, M. D. Anderson Hospital and Tumor Institute and the University of Texas, Houston, Texas

LAURENCE, KENNETH A.
The Population Council, The Rockefeller University, New York, New York

LEACH, ROBERT B.
Division of Endocrinology, William Beaumont Hospital, Royal Oak, Michigan

LEE, SI G.
Medical Research Institute of Worcester, Inc., Worcester, Massachusetts

LEGROS, J. J.
Departments of Internal Medicine and Pathology, Institute of Medicine, University of Liege, Belgium

LEHMANN, FRANK
Division of Endocrinology, Universitäts-Frauenklinik, Hamburg, Germany

LEONARD, JOHN M.
Section of Endocrinology and Metabolism, The Mason Clinic, Seattle, Washington

LEVITT, MONTE J.
Department of Obstetrics and Gynecology, University of Pittsburgh School of Medicine and the Magee-Womens Hospital, Pittsburgh, Pennsylvania

LEYENDECKER, GERHARD
Endokrinologische Abteilungder Universitäts-Fruenklinik,   Bonn-Venusberg, Germany

LI, CHOH HAO
Hormone Research Laboratory, University of California, School of
Medicine San Francisco, California

LIU, TSUI-CHU
Department of Physiology and Biophysics, University of Illinois, Urbana,
Illinois

LIU, WAN-KYNG
Department of Biochemistry, M. D. Anderson Hospital and Tumor
Institute and University of Texas, Houston, Texas

LLOYD, CHARLES W.
Worcester Foundation for Experimental Biology, Shrewsbury, Massachusetts

LOEWENSTEIN, JOSEPH E.
Department of Medicine, Washington University School of Medicine, St.
Louis, Missouri

LOEWITT, K.
The Population Council, The Rockefeller University, New York, New
York

LUNENFELD, BRUNO
Institute of Endocrinology, Tel Hashomer Government Hospital, Tel-Aviv,
Israel

MAC LEOD, JOHN
Department of Anatomy, Cornell University Medical College, New York,
New York

MAHESH, VIRENDRA B.
Department of Endocrinology, Medical College of Georgia, Augusta,
Georgia

MALARKEY, WILLIAM B.
Department of Medicine, Washington University School of Medicine, St.
Louis, Missouri

MALVA, RUBY
Division of Endocrinology, Department of Medicine, Cornell University
Medical College, New York, New York

MARIZ, IDA K.
Department of Medicine, Washington University School of Medicine, St.
Louis, Missouri

MC ARTHUR, JANET W.
Vincent Memorial Hospital and the Departments of Obstetrics and
Gynecology, Harvard Medical School, Boston, Massachusetts

MC CANN, SAMUEL M.

Department of Physiology, University of Texas Southwestern Medical School, Dallas, Texas

MIDGLEY, A. REESE, JR.

Department of Pathology, The University of Michigan, Ann Arbor, Michigan

MONASTIRSKY, R.

The Population Council, The Rockefeller University, New York, New York

MORGAN, FRANCIS J.

Department of Medicine, College of Physicians & Surgeons, Columbia University, New York, New York

MORRIS, PAUL

Department of Physiology and Biophysics, University of Illinois, Urbana, Illinois

MOUDGAL, N. RAGHUVEER

Departments of Physiology and Anatomy, Harvard Medical School, Boston, Massachusetts

MULDOON, T. G.

Department of Endocrinology, Medical College of Georgia, Augusta, Georgia

NAIIM, HYUN S.

Department of Biochemistry, M. D. Anderson Hospital and Tumor Institute and the University of Texas, Houston, Texas

NEALE, C.

Division of Endocrinology, Universitats-Frauenklinik, Hamburg, Germany

NEW, MARIA I.

Department of Pediatrics, Cornell University Medical College, New York, New York

NEY, ROBERT L.

Department of Medicine, University of North Carolina, Chapel Hill, North Carolina

NOCKE, WOLFGANG

Endokrinologische Abteilung der Universitäts-Frauenklinik, Bonn-Venusberg, Germany

NOEL, GORDON L.

Department of Medicine, College of Physicians & Surgeons, Columbia University, New York, New York

NUREDDIN, AIDA

Department of Biochemistry, University of Cambridge, Cambridge, England

ODELL, WILLIAM D.
Division of Endocrinology, Department of Medicine, Harbor General Hospital and the U.C.L.A. School of Medicine, Torrance, California

PAPKOFF, HAROLD
Hormone Research Laboratory, University of California Medical School, San Francisco, California

PARKS, GARY A.
Department of Pediatrics, University of California Irvine College of Medicine, Irvine, California

PAULSEN, C. ALVIN
Department of Medicine, University of Washington School of Medicine and the USPHS Hospital, Seattle, Washington

PENNY, ROBERT
Department of Pediatrics, Johns Hopkins University School of Medicine and the Johns Hopkins Hospital, Baltimore, Maryland

PHIFER, R. F.
Department of Pathology, The Medical University of South Carolina, Charleston, South Carolina

RAO, CH. V.
Department of Obstetrics and Gynecology, Cornell University Medical College, New York, New York

RATHNAM, PREMILA
Department of Medicine, Cornell University Medical College, New York, New York

RAYFORD, P. L.
National Institute of Child Health and Human Development, National Institutes of Health, Beshesda, Maryland

REICHERT, LEO E., JR.
Department of Biochemistry, Division of Basic Health Sciences, Emory University, Atlanta, Georgia

REUTER, A.
Departments of Internal Medicine and Pathology, Institute of Medicine, University of Liege, Belgium

ROSEMBERG, EUGENIA
Medical Research Institute of Worcester, Inc., Worcester, Massachusetts

ROOS, PAUL
Institute of Biochemistry, University of Uppsala, Uppsala 1, Sweden

ROSS, GRIFF T.
National Institute of Child Health and Human Development, Reproduction Research Branch, National Institutes of Health, Bethesda, Maryland

SAIRAM, M. R.
> Hormone Research Laboratory, University of California Medical School, San Francisco, California

SAXENA, BRIJ B.
> Department of Medicine, Cornell University Medical College, New York, New York

SCHALLY, ANDREW V.
> Department of Medicine, Tulane University School of Medicine, and the Veterans Administration Hospital, New Orleans, Louisiana

SCHNEIDER, H. P. G.
> Department of Physiology, University of Texas Southwestern Medical College, Dallas, Texas

SCHORR, IMMANUEL
> Department of Medicine, University of North Carolina, Chapel Hill, North Carolina

SCHUURS, A. H. W. M.
> N.V. Organon, Oss, Holland

SILER, T. M.
> Department of Biochemistry and Biophysics, University of Hawaii, Honolulu, Hawaii

SNYDER, MITCHELL
> Computer Center, Bar Ilan University, Tel-Aviv, Israel

SPICER, S. S.
> Department of Pathology, Medical University of South Carolina, Charleston, South Carolina

SULIMOVICI, SOREL
> Institute of Endocrinology, Tel Hashomer Government Hospital, Tel-Aviv, Israel

SWERDLOFF, RONALD S.
> Division of Endocrinology, Department of Medicine, Harbor General Hospital and the U.C.L.A. School of Medicine, Torrance, California

TAFT, H. PINCUS
> Ewen Downie Metabolic Unit, Alfred Hospital, Melbourne, Victoria, Australia

THOMAS, K.
> Department of Obstetrics and Gynecology, University Hospital, Louvain, Belgium

VAITUKAITIS, JUDITH L.
> National Institute of Child Health and Human Development, National Institutes of Health, Bethesda, Maryland

VALE, WYLIE
> The Salk Institute for Biological Studies, La Jolla, California

VANDE WIELE, RAYMOND
Department of Obstetrics and Gynecology, College of Physicians & Surgeons, Columbia University, New York, New York

VAN HALL, E. V.
Department of Obstetrics and Gynecology University of Nymegen, Nymegen, Holland

VAN HELL, H.
N. V. Organon, Oss, Holland

VILLEE, CLAUDE A.
Department of Biological Chemistry and Laboratory of Human Reproduction and Reproductive Biology, Harvard Medical School, Boston, Massachusetts

WARD, DARRELL N.
Department of Biochemistry, M. D. Anderson Hospital and Tumor Institute and the University of Texas, Houston, Texas

WARDLAW, SHARON
Endokrinologische Abteilung der Universitäts-Frauenklinik, Bonn-Venusberg, Germany

WEICK, R. F.
Department of Physiology, University of Pittsburgh School of Medicine, Pittsburgh, Pennsylvania

WEISE, H. CHR.
Division of Endocrinology, Universitäts-Frauenklinik, Hamburg, Germany

WEISZ, JUDITH
Worcester Foundation for Experimental Biology, Shrewsbury, Massachusetts

YAMAJI, T.
Department of Physiology, University of Pittsburgh School of Medicine, Pittsburgh, Pennsylvania

YEN, S. S. C.
Department of Reproductive Biology, Case Western Reserve School of Medicine, Cleveland, Ohio

ZIMMERMAN, EARL
Department of Neurology, College of Physicians & Surgeons, Columbia University, New York, New York

CONTENTS

ISOLATION, CHEMISTRY, AND STRUCTURE OF GONADOTROPINS

SEXUAL MATURATION

PITUITARY-TESTICULAR AXIS

Control of Secretion
of Gonadotropins

1. An Electronmicroscopic Study of the Human Median Eminence

Richard M. Bergland

The neurosecretory materials which control anterior pituitary function leave the central nervous system within the median eminence (1). The median eminence is immediately adjacent to the pituitary in most lower species; in the human, the pituitary stalk, or infundibulum, intervenes. There are few functional, vascular or microscopical distinctions between the median eminence and infundibulum; in both areas neurosecretory material is released into the capillary beds that are the beginning of the pituitary portal system.

The vascular anatomy of the pituitary is distinctive (2). The main portion of the pituitary portal system, the so-called long portal system, is derived from the several superior hypophyseal arteries within the subarachnoid space. These vessels penetrate the pars tuberalis to form capillary coils within the neural elements of the infundibulum and median eminence. Here these capillaries receive neurosecretory material which is conveyed to the pituitary by the long portal vessels which lie chiefly in the pars tuberalis. About 80 to 85% of the human pituitary is nourished by this vascular system.

The other 15 to 20% of the gland derives its blood supply from the short portal system. This takes its origin from the paired inferior hypophyseal arteries within the cavernous sinus. These vessels break up into capillaries within the pars nervosa and, after receiving neurosecretory material, extend directly to the posterior and medial part of the anterior pituitary. There is no significant arterial supply directly to the anterior pituitary.

The present study includes the electronmicroscopic analysis of the human pituitary stalk; within this area are found the neurovascular connections between

3

the neurons originating in the hypothalamus and the beginning capillaries of the long portal system.

MATERIALS AND METHODS

Biopsies were taken of the midportion of the infundibulum in five patients undergoing hypophysectomy for advanced cancer. These were cross-sectional full-thickness biopsies measuring 2 to 3 mm in thickness. The tissues were routinely prepared for electronmicroscopy.

RESULTS AND DISCUSSION

Capillaries

The isolated vessels within the neural tissue, presumably either the beginning or the end of capillary coils, are regularly surrounded by a small and uniform perivascular space. The axons in these areas are further separated from the vascular spaces by a cuff of supporting cells, similar to the astrocytes of the central nervous system. These supporting cells have traditionally been called pituicytes. However, in areas where capillaries are found in abundance, presumably within the capillary coils, the perivascular space becomes greatly enlarged. Axons, free nerve endings, and smooth muscle are commonly found within this enlarged perivascular space.

Pituicytes

The supporting cells, the so-called pituicytes, are of two types. The first is relatively small with scant, dark cytoplasm. It provides a myelin sheath for some axons and resembles the oligodendrocyte of the central nervous system. The second and more frequent cell possesses a more abundant, clear cytoplasm and its long processes intermingle with the surrounding axons much like the astrocyte of the central nervous system. The axons themselves are generally unmyelinated and have conspicuous neurotubules and neurofilaments.

Herring Bodies

With light microscopy, enlarged axons are often found which are readily stained with aldehyde fuchsin, the commonly employed stain used to identify neurosecretory material (Fig. 1). By tradition these structures have been called Herring bodies (3). Similar axonal enlargements are found with electronmicroscopy (Fig. 1), most of which are filled with dense core vesicles, the ultrastructural organelle that has been equated to neurosecretory material (4). However, it is important to note that some Herring bodies are more readily stained with PAS than with aldehyde fuchsin (5), and with electronmicroscopy many axonal enlargements are composed of mitochondria or dense bodies

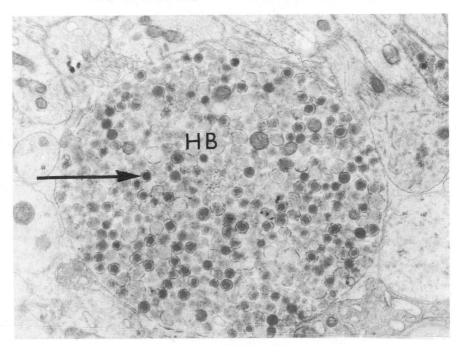

FIG. 1. A dilated axon (Herring body) filled with type A dense core vesicles (arrow) is shown (X9500).

instead of dense core vesicles. The function of Herring bodies is not clear. Presumably they result from the transient arrest of the flow of organelles down the axon.

Dense Core Vesicles

The dense core vesicles within axons are of two sizes. The larger measure 1500 to 3000Å and the smaller from 500 to 1000Å. These two types of vesicles do not coexist in the same axon and, as has been done in other species (6), the axons can be separated into two groups or systems by the size of their dense core vesicles. Axons containing the larger vesicles have been called type A; those with the smaller vesicles, type B.

Nerve Endings

Within the dilated perivascular space surrounding the capillary coils free nerve endings are found, often devoid of basement membrane. Again the nerves can be separated by the size of their dense core vesicles; the type B dense core vesicles measure 500 to 1000Å (Fig. 2.) and the type A dense core vesicles measure 1500 to 3000Å (Fig. 3.). In addition to the dense core vesicles the nerve endings have an abundance of mitochondria, dense bodies, and clear vesicles. It should be reemphasized that type A and type B vesicles are not found in the same nerve ending.

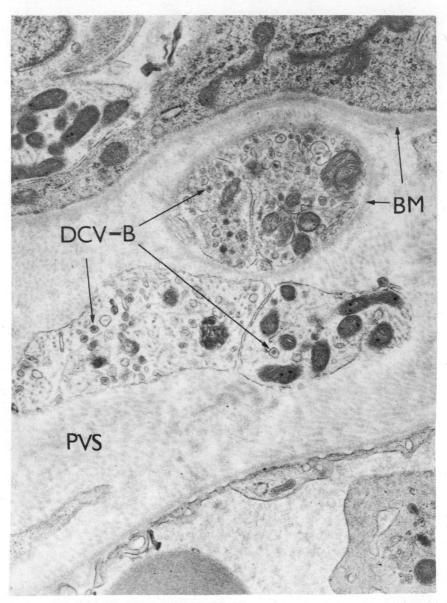

FIG. 2. Several nerve endings are shown within the perivascular space (PVS) near a portal capillary. The basement membrane (BM) is incomplete around some nerve endings. Type B dense-core vesicles (DCV-B) are noted (X20,000).

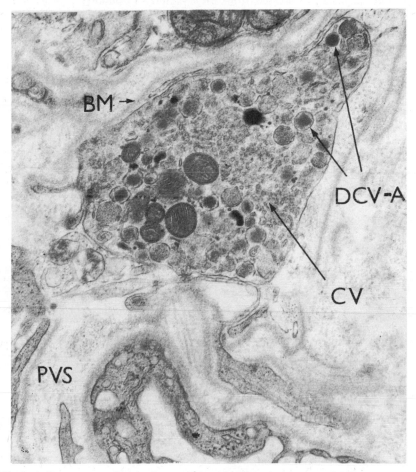

FIG. 3. A free nerve ending is shown within the perivascular space (PVS) near a portal capillary. The basement membrane (BM) is incomplete. Type A dense-core vesicles (DCV-A) and clear vesicles (CV) are noted (X20,000).

Since the function of the median eminence is to transfer neurosecretory material from axons to the portal system it is appropriate to focus on the characteristics of the dense-core vesicles.

Type B vesicles are similar to catecholamines as they exist elsewhere in the nervous system; catecholamines are found in great quantity within the median eminence (7) and may function to control release of other neurotransmitters or to control vascular flow and permeability within the portal system. Type A vesicles are morphologically similar to polypeptides as they are found within the posterior pituitary (8). It is tempting to speculate that type A vesicles are small packets of releasing factor destined for the anterior pituitary but such speculation cannot be justified from these simple morphological observations. The termination of both type A and type B axons within the perivascular space of the portal system supports the thesis that the portal system is the final common pathway of the neural control of the pituitary.

REFERENCES

1. Harris, G. W., in Neural Control of the Pituitary Gland, Arnold, London, 1955, p. 298.
2. Landsmeer, J. M. F., in A. V. Nalbandov (Ed.) Advances in Neuroendocrinology, Univ of Illinois Press, Urbana, Illinois, 1963, p. 29.
3. Herring, P. T., Quart J Exp Physiol 1:121, 1908.
4. Bergmann, W., Int Rev Cytol 19:183, 1966.
5. Unpublished data.
6. Knowles, F., Arch Anat Micro 54:343, 1965.
7. Fuxe, K., Z Zellforsch 61:710, 1964.
8. Dean, C. R., and D. B. Hope, Biochem J 104:1082, 1967.

2. Histology of the Human Hypophyseal Gonadotropin Secreting Cells

R. F. Phifer, A. Reese Midgley, Jr., and S. S. Spicer

For decades histological staining has been utilized by pituitary cytologists to identify cells responsible for the production of adenohypophyseal hormones. Limitations in the tinctorial methods, however, led many cytologists to seek other approaches. Thus several immunohistological studies have been undertaken to delineate the human hypophyseal cell types responsible for the secretion of FSH and LH (1-9).

Earlier investigators did not entirely exclude the possibility that antisera to gonadotropins might cross-react with human TSH. The importance of such documentation is illustrated by our observation that human TSH cells (10) react with antibodies to the HCG preparation distributed by the National Pituitary Agency for radioimmunoassay purposes. The biochemical basis for the cross-reactions has recently been elucidated by the demonstration that glycoprotein hormones are composed of two nonidentical α and β subunits. The α subunits of the pituitary gonadotropin hormones and HCG are homologous, whereas the β subunits are hormone specific (11-15). Further evidence in this direction is provided by the finding that antiserum to the α subunit of HCG[1] reacts with both TSH and gonadotropin-producing cells, whereas an antiserum to the β subunit of HCG reacts only with gonadotrophs (9). The present investigation was undertaken to delineate human FSH and LH cells immunohistologically using antisera characterized by their cross-reactivities.

---

[1] Antisera to the α and β chains of HCG were generously provided by Drs. J. Vaitukaitis and G. T. Ross.

IMMUNOHISTOLOGIC STAINING

The immunoglobulin-peroxidase bridge procedure (16) was employed to localize the hormonal antigens in tissue sections. This technique involves the attachment of peroxidase to antigenic sites and subsequent histochemical demonstration of the enzyme. The primary advantage of this procedure is the production of an enzymatic reaction product which is visible in ordinary light microscope. By utilizing serial tissue sections thin enough to give more than one section of the same cell, immunostaining could be compared cell for cell with histologic staining.

CHARACTERIZATION OF ANTISERA

Antisera to FSH and LH from various species were assessed as to their relative binding affinities to radioactively labeled glycoprotein hormones. An antiserum to human FSH and to porcine LH were selected for immunohistologic identification of cells producing human FSH and LH (17). Prior to use, the FSH antiserum was absorbed with HCG and human LH (LER-960)[2]. The antiserum to human TSH[3] was absorbed with HCG. It did not react with the gonadotrophs and was used in the present study (Fig. 1).

The specificity of the different antisera was studied in two steps. The first entailed the use of radioactively labeled FSH, LH, and TSH to determine the amount bound by each antiserum. Highly purified human FSH, LH, and TSH labeled with radioactive iodine and purified by electrophoresis (17) were used for this purpose. The percentage of labeled hormone bound by each is shown in Table I. It was found that each antiserum reacted almost exclusively with its own antigen.

TABLE I.

Antiserum	Initial dilution	Percent of total labeled hormone bound to antiserum		
		Human FSH	Human LH	Human TSH
Human TSH antiserum[a]	1:400	1.8	1.6	52.9
Human FSH antiserum[b]	1:800	73.3	1.9	5.9
Porcine LH antiserum	1:400	0.8	67.8	2.0

[a] 130 IU/ml HCG initial dilution.

[b] 1050 IU HCG and 7 IU LH/ml initial dilution.

[2] LER-960, LER-869-2, LER-1456-1, and LER-1112-2 were generously supplied by Dr. L. E. Reichert.

[3] This TSH antiserum and TSH(DEAE-4-III) were kindly made available by Drs. B. Shome and J. G. Pierce.

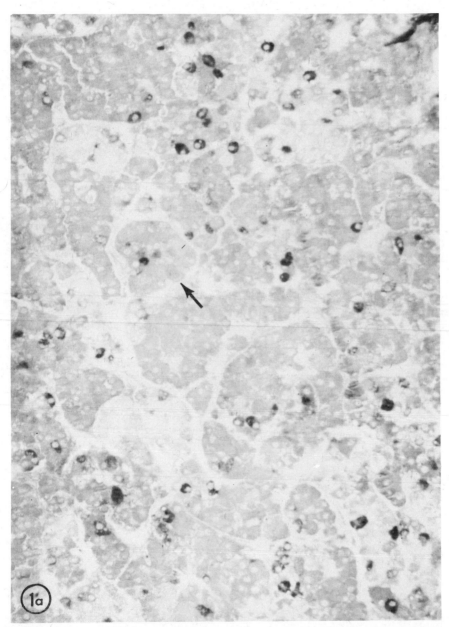

FIG. 1. Three serial sections of the same area of a human hypophysis. Black reaction product throughout cytoplasm of cells indicates site where enzyme peroxidase is linked to glycoprotein hormones by the immunoglobulin peroxidase bridge procedure (1a) Immunostained with antisera to human FSH; (1b) human TSH; and (1c) porcine LH. Small intense black deposits shown in (1c) represent areas of nonimmunologic precipitation of reaction products. Arrow indicates acinus. Note that cells reacting with FSH antiserum in (1a) and cells reacting with LH antiserum in (1c) are not the same as those reacting with TSH antiserum in (1b) (X 130).

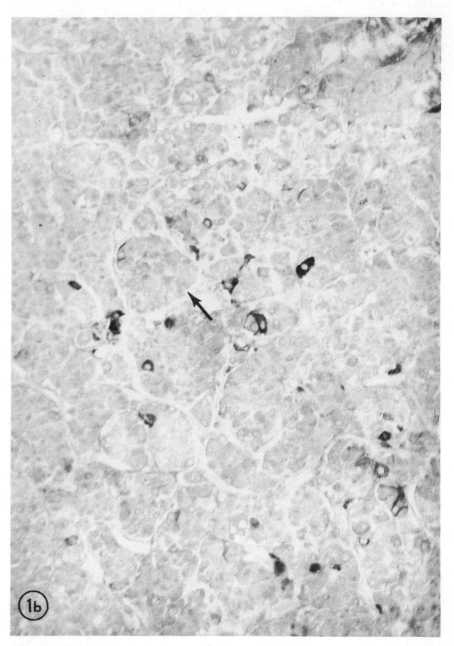

FIG. 1. (continued)

12

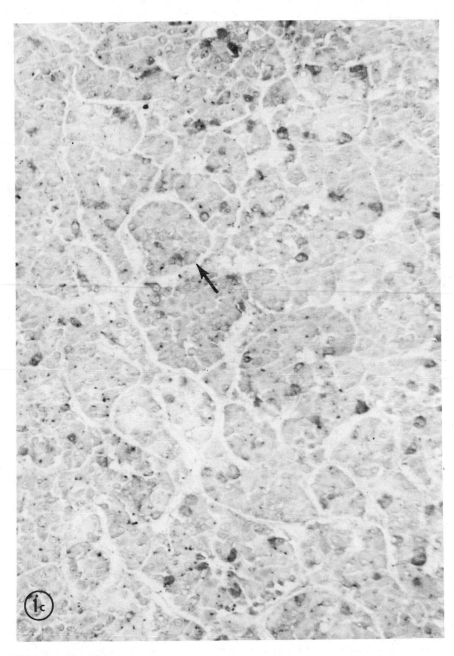

FIG. 1. (continued)

13

The second step, documenting the specificity of the antisera, involved selective immunostaining of their own antigens in tissue sections. The FSH, LH, and TSH antisera showed no reactivity with cells secreting growth hormone (GH) (18) or adrenocorticotropic hormone (ACTH) (19). Reactivity with melanocyte-stimulating hormone was not tested since it is probably secreted by ACTH cells (19). Reactivity with prolactin was considered unlikely since the pituitaries used in this investigation were obtained from patients whose glands supposedly contained only very small amounts of prolactin (20, 21). Demonstration that the FSH and LH antisera did not cross-react with TSH could theoretically be achieved by showing that absorption with purified TSH does not abolish immunostaining. Preliminary studies in this direction indicated that available TSH preparations contained too much gonadotropin to allow definitive characterization by TSH absorption.

An alternative approach would involve demonstrating that absorption with FSH and LH did not abolish immunostaining with TSH antiserum. Such documentation could substantiate that the FSH and LH antisera were not reacting with TSH, since the TSH antiserum and the gonadotropin antisera reacted with different cell types. When human LH (LER-960)[2] and human FSH (LER-869-2)[2] were added in varying amounts to the TSH antiserum, slightly more than 10 μg/ml each had the same effect in eliminating immunostaining with TSH antiserum as had 1 μg of TSH (DEAE-4-III)[3] (Fig. 2). Absorption of the second human TSH antiserum distributed by the National Pituitary Agency yielded identical results. The abolishment of the immunostaining of two TSH antisera following absorption with LH (LER-960) and FSH (LER-869-2) suggested that both hormone preparations contained too much TSH to be used in absorption studies. The equal elimination of immunostaining for TSH after absorption with both gonadotropins might be explained by previous findings that LER-960 and LER-869-2 contained approximately the same amount of immunoreactive TSH (22) (Fig. 2).

Further attempts were made to document the specificity of the TSH antiserum absorbed with gonadotropin preparations containing little TSH. The TSH antiserum was absorbed with a human LH preparation (LER-1456-1)[2] containing 81% of the LH activity but only 3% of the TSH activity of LER-960. This LH preparation, when added in amounts up to at least 40 μg/ml did not abolish immunostaining with TSH antiserum (Fig. 2). Since an FSH preparation with a purity greater than LER-869-2 was not available, a different preparation of FSH (LER-1112-2)[2], which had 84% of the FSH activity of LER-869-2, was further purified by polyacrylamide gel electrophoresis in the hope of minimizing TSH contamination. As shown in Fig. 2, immunostaining was not abolished by

[2]LER-960, LER-869-2, LER-1456-1, and LER-1112-2 were generously supplied by Dr. L. E. Reichert.

[3]This TSH antiserum and TSH(DEAE-4-III) were kindly made available by Drs. B. Shome and J. G. Pierce.

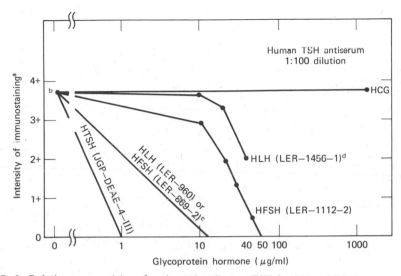

FIG. 2. Relative nonreactivity of antiserum to human TSH for LH and FSH in sections of human hypophyses. Human TSH cells were not immunostained with the TSH antiserum after the addition of 1 mg of TSH, but 40 and 50 times as much highly purified human LH (LER-1456-1) and human FSH (LER-1112-2) respectively, failed to abolish immunostaining. Absorption with LH (LER-960) and FSH (LER-869-2) was much less effective in demonstrating the relative specificity of the TSH antiserum. Addition of LER-960 or LER-869-2 was equally effective in abolishing immunostaining with the TSH antiserum probably because each contains approximately the same amount of immunoreactive TSH (22). Addition of much more HCG than that required to prevent immunostaining of gonadotropin cells with the TSH antiserum had no effect on the intensity of immunostaining of TSH cells. [a] Only thyrotropin cells were immunostained. [b] Antiserum already contained 520 IU HCG/ml at this point [c] LER-960 and LER-869-2 contain, respectively, 85 and 90 ml IU TSH/mg. [d] 1 mg of LER-1456-1 has 81% of the LH activity and 3% of the TSH activity of 1 mg of LER-960.

the addition of up to 50 μg/ml of the electrophoretically purified LER-1112-2. Thus, since as little as 1 μg/ml of TSH (DEAE-4-III) abolished immunostaining with TSH antiserum the latter serum seemed to be reacting selectively with TSH alone in the tissue section. Inasmuch as the TSH antiserum selectively stained TSH and did not react with the cells stained by gonadotropin antisera, it can be concluded that neither gonadotropin antiserum was reacting with TSH in the tissue section.

To determine whether the gonadotropin antisera were reacting specifically with their respective antigen in the tissue sections, each antiserum was absorbed with varying amounts of FSH and LH. The relative lack of reactivity of the FSH antiserum with LH was established by the finding that as much as 80 μg/ml of FSH (LER-869-2) abolished all immunostaining (Fig. 3). Specificity of the porcine LH antiserum for human LH could not be established by absorption with FSH (LER-869-2), probably because of its known content of LH (17).

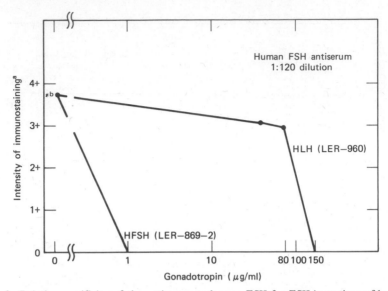

FIG. 3. Relative specificity of the antiserum to human FSH for FSH in sections of human hypophysis. One μg of human FSH abolished all immunostaining of gonadotropin cells whereas 80 times more human LH did not. [a] Only gonadotropin cells were immunostained. [b] Antiserum already contained 3500 IU HCG and 230 IU HLH/ml at this point.

However, the FSH obtained from LER-1112-2 by electrophoresis did not eliminate immunostaining in any of the reactive cells when added to the LH antiserum in amounts up to 125 μg/ml. Thus, the LH antiserum proved relatively selective for human LH, since as little as 1.5 μg/ml LH (LER-960) abolished immunostaining (Fig. 4). The specificity of each gonadotropin antiserum was further substantiated by the results of absorption with isolated α and β subunits of human FSH and LH (13, 14)[4]. Absorption with these subunits indicated that the antiserum to porcine LH predominantly reacted with the β chain of human LH whereas the antiserum to human FSH mainly reacted with the β chain of human FSH. These results of absorption might be expected with antisera specific for human FSH and LH, if, as in other species, the β chains of the glycoprotein hormones are found to be the dissimilar portions of the molecules.

Results of Immunostaining

The same cells (Figs. 5a and b) were found to react with FSH and LH antisera in serial immunostained sections. It seems, therefore, that human FSH and LH are produced in the same adenohypophyseal cell.

Most of the immunostained gonadotrophs are rounded, small cells with an

---

[4]α and β subunits of human FSH and LH were kindly provided by Dr. B. B. Saxena.

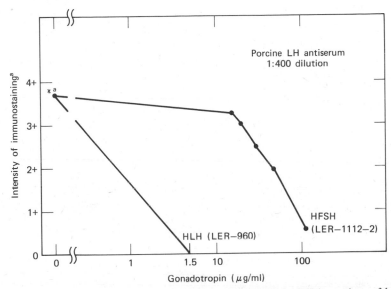

FIG. 4. Relative specificity of the antiserum to porcine LH for LH in sections of human hypophysis. 1.5 μg of human LH abolished all immunostaining of gonadotropin cells whereas 83 times more human FSH did not. [a] Only gonadotropin cells were immunostained.

eccentrically placed nucleus. The cells were found to be distributed uniformly throughout the gland in horizontal sections as illustrated diagramatically in Fig. 6. Other investigators have reported similar distributions (2, 3). Gonadotrophs were found in acini populated predominantly by other cell types. Gonadotrophs were either located peripherally with one edge abutting on the stromal wall of the acinus or centrally with blunt cytoplasmic processes extending towards the stromal wall. Vascular spaces were present adjacent to the portion of the acinus containing the entire gonadotropin cell or its blunt processes. In the postero-medial pars distalis, the gonadotrophs were sometimes the only cell type found in the acinus.

The finding that both FSH and LH are present in the same cell raises the question of how their release is controlled and suggests the possibility that a single substance may release both gonadotropins. Recent studies on porcine FSH and LH releasing factors (23) seem to favor the view that one single releasing factor is responsible for release of both FSH and LH.

Comparison of Results with Immunostaining and Histologic Staining Methods

A number of histologic stains were applied to sections serial to those immunostained with gonadotropin antisera in an attempt to determine the histochemical and tinctorial affinities of the gonadotrophs. From these studies

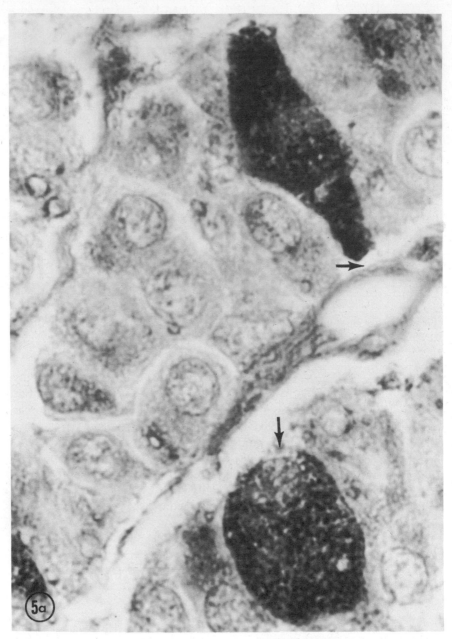

FIG. 5. Two serial sections of the same area of a human hypophysis. (a) Immunostained with antiserum to human FSH. (b) Immunostained with the antiserum to porcine LH. Note that the same cells are immunostained in both sections. Vertical arrow indicates cell occurring in the peripheral portion of an acinus. The other prominently immunostained cell has a blunt cytoplasmic process extending toward a perivascular space and is indicated by a horizontal arrow (X 1300).

18

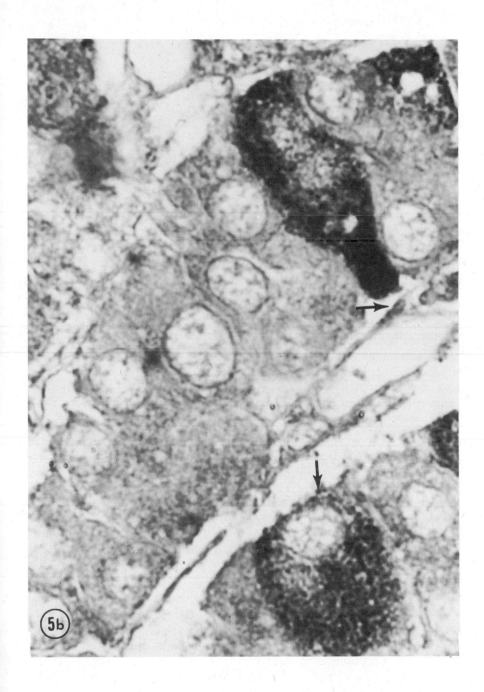

FIG. 5. (continued)

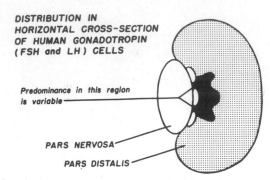

DISTRIBUTION IN HORIZONTAL CROSS-SECTION OF HUMAN GONADOTROPIN (FSH and LH) CELLS

Predominance in this region is variable

PARS NERVOSA

PARS DISTALIS

FIG. 6. Distribution in horizontal cross-section of human gonadotropin (FSH and LH) cells.

five major factors emerged which are considered important in identifying gonadotropin cells stained with various procedures. First, the gonadotrophs often contain two different populations of granules. It should be noted parenthetically that the term granule is used loosely to designate all cytoplasmic inclusions discernible at the light microscopic level. Such inclusions may be aggregates of the actual secretory granules, or may be cell organelles, such as lipofuscins, other than secretory granules. Second, the relative percentage of the two granules in a given cell can vary over a wide range. Third, histochemical properties of one of the granules can vary widely. Fourth, the granules of gonadotrophs appear to be extremely susceptible to the effects of autolysis or the disruptive influences of a histologic procedure. Fifth, with the periodic acid Schiff (PAS) stain some gonadotrophs may be difficult to distinguish from ACTH cells.

In regard to the first of these considerations, certain staining observations indicate the presence of two populations of cytoplasmic granules in gonadotrophs. The two types of granules were best demonstrated with an alcian blue at pH 2.5-periodic acid-silver (AB-PA-silver) procedure. This was performed identically to Mowry's alcian blue-periodic acid Schiff (AB-PAS) technique (24), modified as previously described (19), except that after periodic acid oxidation the sections were exposed to the silver and subsequent solutions employed by Rambourg (25), instead of to Schiff's reagent. With this procedure, the cells were clearly seen to contain coarse granules stained black with silver, and flocculent or ill-defined granules stained turquoise with alcian blue. The black coloring was never observed without a prior periodic acid oxidation, indicating that the silver deposition was due to oxidative induction of aldehydic reducing groups. The turquoise granules also stained intensely with alcian blue at pH 0.2. This staining did not require prior oxidation as, for example, by performic acid (26), to introduce basophilia and thus depended on intrinsic sulfate groups. As would be expected from their reactivity with PA-silver, the black granules often stained an intense red with PAS. Large PAS-positive vesicles, such as those found in human TSH cells and presumed to be lipofuscins, were never seen in gonadotrophs identified in serial sections with immunostaining.

Intensity of immunoreactivity with either the LH or the FSH antiserum appeared to correlate with the intensity of PA-silver or PAS reactivity, and therefore no evidence was obtained that the two granule types correspond to the two different hormones. Exceptions to the usual correlation of intensity of immunostaining and PAS staining were observed in the immunostaining of the hypophysis of a castrated woman. In this gland most of the immunostained cells were completely chromophobic. Possibly stainable granules represent a storage form of hormone, which might not exist in quantity in hypersecreting cells. In such a secretory state, the cytoplasm might be filled with ergastoplasm which could be the site of most of the immunostaining seen in the chromophobic, hypersecreting cells.

The coarse granules have been interpreted as lysosomes because of their acid phosphatase activity (27). From Smith and Farquhar's studies of prolactin secreting cells in the rat hypophysis (28), the suggestion might be made that the coarse granules are a type of lysosome or lysosomal derivative such as a lipofuscin involved in the degradation of excess hormone. However as pointed out above, the most intense immunostaining in the hypophyses of endocrinologically unremarkable patients was usually observed in cells containing the most coarse granules. This finding seems inconsistent with the idea that the coarse granules are involved in hormone degradation, since most of the hormonal antigenic sites appeared to be in the coarse granules.

As concerns the second factor related to the histologic staining properties of the gonadotropin cells, the gonadotrophs of most glands appeared to contain varying amounts of coarse granules evenly dispersed in the cell cytoplasm. Concomitantly present turquoise granules were usually found distributed among the coarse PAS or PA-silver positive granules, but the former were not always demonstrable. Cells colored only turquoise with AB-PAS, and containing little or no PAS-positive granules have been seen in only 10% of the hypophyses studied thus far. No information in the clinical history explained the striking presence of turquoise cells seen in these glands. Cells which stained turquoise predominantly were usually smaller than gonadotropin cells containing prominent PAS-positive granules. When PAS-positive coarse granules were present in small amounts in a turquoise cell, they were usually clustered in one region of the cell. Another type of gonadotroph contained turquoise granules in one-half of the cytoplasm and PAS-positive granules in the other half.

As regards the third histologic staining factor, the variability of the histochemical properties of one granule type, the coarse granules appeared to react inconsistently with the alcian blue in the Mowry/AB-PAS stain, and stained a range of colors from blue-purple to red. The basis for this is not known. However, regardless of their reactivity with alcian blue, coarse granules stained with high iron diamine (29), aldehyde fucsin (29), and 0.1% alcian blue in 0.2M $MgCl_2$. All of the latter three stains selectively bind the sulfate groups (30).

Apparently none of the histochemically demonstrable basophilia of the gonadotropin cell granules was due to the presence of sialic acid, since sialidase digestion has no effect on the basophilia.

The fourth histologic factor to be considered is the apparent susceptibility of the gonadotropin cells to autolysis or disruption by a given stain. The average number of granules in the cells after histologic staining appeared to be inversely proportional to both: 1) the postmortem interval before the hypophysis was fixed; and 2) the harshness of the staining method employed. Thus characteristically in glands obtained more than 4-6 hr postmortem, few granules were demonstrable in the gonadotropin cells, and those few present were invariably only the coarse type. On the other hand, in surgical specimens,[5] stainable granules were nearly always present in gonadotropin cells. In addition, the concomitant presence of coarse PAS-positive and flocculent turquoise granules was most consistently demonstrable in surgical specimens. Other pituitary cell types do not seem to have such a marked propensity for autolysis. It is tempting to speculate that the granules' delicacy might be due to the proteolytic enzymes associated with the gonadotropins in vivo. Proteolytic enzymes have been found associated in vitro with gonadotropin or isolated gonadotropin granules from several species (31,32). Since the other cell types may also contain proteolytic enzymes but do not undergo such marked autolysis, proteolytic activity would not seem to be a sufficient factor by itself. A more likely explanation might be that the gonadotropin granules are by nature more susceptible to physical or chemical damage than are the granules containing other hormones. This possibility is strongly supported by the findings of Hymer and McShan (33), who observed that gonadotropin granules isolated in vitro from the rat hypophysis exhibited more fragility than other granule types.

As regards the disruptive effect of the histologic staining procedure, the permanganate oxidation (27, 34) used in some stains seemed to be especially destructive and, as a rule, only apparent coarse granules, and sometimes only a few of these, remained in the cell after permanganate oxidation. Performic acid did not disrupt the granules as severely but tended to blur morphologic detail.

The susceptibility of the cytoplasmic granules to destruction is probably the basis for several investigators' findings that many immunoreactive gonadotropin cells in normal glands are essentially chromophobic (8, 27 35). Such findings were also made in the present study, in which a cell whose cytoplasm was filled with granules in the immunostaining procedure was often observed to contain only a few granules in the serial section stained with AB-PAS. This procedure, however, seemed the least disruptive of cytoplasmic structure.

The fifth aspect of the histologic observations concerns the difficulty in distinguishing gonadotrophs from that portion of the ACTH cell population that stained red with the AB-PAS method. However, the ACTH cells generally can be

[5]Surgical specimens of human hypophyses were kindly provided by Drs. Jules Hardy, Richard M. Bergland, and Bronson S. Ray.

distinguished because they contain smaller granules. Moreover, an AB-PA-silver stain on the adjacent serial section allowed ready differentiation since ACTH cells were never filled with coarse black granules as were the gonadotropin cells. ACTH cells, stained red with AB-PAS, can also be distinguished from red gonadotrophs by a performic acid (26) or permanganate (27) alcian blue at pH 0.2-PAS procedure, probably because the latter contain cystine or cysteine which is oxidized to cysteic acid. Thus the gonadotrophs which would stain red with AB-PAS became blue-purple after performic acid oxidation and almost turquoise after permanganate oxidation when subsequently stained with the alcian blue at pH 0.2-PAS procedure. Lacking appreciable cystine, the ACTH cells still stain red with the techniques employing oxidation before alcian blue. Parenthetically it may be suggested that the explanation for the blue-purple coloration of gonadotrophs after performic oxidation and turquoise staining after permanganate staining is probably related to the fact that performic acid does not destroy vicinal hydroxyls (36) whereas permanganate oxidizes them to carboxyls. Thus after performic acid oxidation, the coarse granules in gonadotropin cells stain blue-purple as a result of the combined red staining of vicinal hydroxyls and the blue staining of cysteic acid groups. After permanganate treatment, which destroys vicinal hydroxyls, the coarse granules of gonadotrophs have little or no PAS staining, and color almost turquoise, the color of alcian blue alone. This blue staining, attributable to oxidatively engendered cysteic acid groups, may actually represent staining of the gonadotropin hormones, which are relatively rich in cystine (37). Little difference in results was noted when either aldehyde thionine (34) or alcian blue was used after permanganate oxidation. The only change was in basic coloration, the former yielding blue-black staining, and the latter resulting in turquoise staining. Romeis' resorcin fuchsin-azan stain (38, 39) provides a third way of distinguishing between the gonadotropin and ACTH cells indistinguishable with an AB-PAS stain because the coarse granules in gonadotropin cells also stain with aniline blue. Gonadotrophs stain blue whereas ACTH cells stain purplish-brown with the latter staining procedure (29).

The results of histologic staining support in two ways the immunohistologic evidence that FSH and LH are both contained in a single cell population. First, cells reacting with gonadotropin antisera appeared to represent a single chromophilic cell population. Second, all chromophilic cells except for those classifiable as either ACTH cells (19), TSH cells (8), or GH cells (18), reacted with the gonadotropic antisera.

REFERENCES

1. Midgley, A. R., Exp Cell Res 32:606, 1964.
2. Robyn, C., Y. Bossaert, P. Hubinot, J. Pasteels, and M. Herlant, C R Acad Sci 259:1226, 1964.
3. Mosca, L., and G. Chiappino, Lancet 2:1016, 1964.
4. Koffler, D., and M. Fogel, Proc Soc Exp Biol Med 115:1080, 1964.
5. Kracht, J., U. Hachmeister, H. J. Breustedt, and H. D. Zimmermann, Mat Med Nordmark 19:224, 1967.
6. Brozman, M., Rev Czech Med 16:1, 1970.
7. Bain, J., and C. Ezrin, J Clin Endocrinol 30:181, 1970.
8. Phifer, R. F., and S. S. Spicer, read by title at 53rd Annual Meeting of The Endocrine Society, San Francisco, California, June 24-26, 1971.
9. Marshall, J. M., J Exp Med 94:21, 1951.
10. Phifer, R. F., A. R. Midgley, and S. S. Spicer, submitted to J. Clin Endocrinol.
11. Pierce, J. G., T. H. Liao, R. B. Carlsen, and T. Reimo, J Biol Chem 246:866, 1971.
12. Papkoff, H., M. R. Sairam, and C. H. Li, J Amer Chem Soc 93:1531, 1971.
13. Saxena, B. B., and P. Rathnam, J Biol Chem 246:3549, 1971.
14. Rathnam, P. and B. B. Saxena, J Biol Chem 246:7087, 1971.
15. Bahl, O. P., in C. H. Li (Ed.), Protein and Polypeptide Hormones, Academic, New York, in press 1971.
16. Mason, T. E., R. F. Phifer, S. S. Spicer, R. A. Swallow, and R. B. Dreskin, J Histochem Cytochem 17:563, 1969.
17. Midgley, A. R., and L. E. Reichert, in M. Margoulies (Ed.), Protein and Polypeptide Hormones, Excerpta Medica Foundation, Amsterdam, 1968, p 117.
18. Beck, J. S., and A. R. Currie, Vitamins and Hormones 25:89, 1967.
19. Phifer, R. F., S. S. Spicer, and D. N. Orth, J Clin Endocrinol 31:347, 1970.
20. Goluboff, L., and C. Ezrin, J Clin Endocrinol 29:1533, 1969.
21. Nayak, R., read by title at 53rd Annual Meeting of The Endocrine Society, San Francisco, California, June 24-26, 1971 (abstract).
22. Albert, A., E. Rosemberg, G. T. Ross, C. A. Paulsen, and R. J. Ryan, J Clin Endocrinol 28:1214, 1968.
23. Schally, A. V., A. Arimura, Y. G. Baba, R. M. G. Nair, H. Matsuo, T. W. Redding, L. Debeljuk, and W. F. White, Biochem Biophys Res Commun 43:393, 1971.
24. McManus, J. F. A., and R. W. Mowry, Staining Methods, Hoeber, New York, 1960, pp. 63 and 136.
25. Rambourg, A., J. Histochem Cytochem 15:409, 1967.
26. Adams, C. W. M., and K. V. Swettenham, J Pathol Bact 75:95, 1958.
27. Herlant, M., and J. L. Pasteels, Meth Achievm Exp Pathol 3:250, 1967.
28. Farquhar, M. G., in J. T. Dingle, and H. B. Fell (Eds.), Lysosomes in Biology and Pathology, Vol. 2, Wiley, New York, 1969, p. 462.
29. Phifer, R. F., Texas Rep Biol Med 26:438, 1968 (abstract).
30. Spicer, S. S., R. G. Horn, and T. J. Leppi, in B. M. Wagner, (Ed.), The Connective Tissue, Williams and Wilkins, Baltimore, 1967, p. 251.
31. Perdue, J. F., and W. H. McShan, J Cell Biol 15:159, 1962.

32. Reichert, L. E., and A. F. Parlow, Endocrinology 74:809, 1964.

33. Hymer, W. C., and W. H. McShan, J Cell Biol 17:67, 1963.

34. Ezrin, C., and S. Murray, in J. Benoit, and C. Da Lage (Eds.), Cytologie De L'adenohypophyse, Editions D Du C. N. R. S., Paris, 1963, p. 183.

35. Midgley, A. R., J Histochem Cytochem 14:159, 1966.

36. Lillie, R. D., Stain Technol 31:151, 1956.

37. Reichert, L. E., R. H. Kathan, and R. J. Ryan, Endocrinology 82:109, 1968.

38. Romeis, B., Mikroskopische Technik, 15 ed., Leibniz Verlag, München, 1948, p. 363.

39. Romeis, B., in W. v. Möllendorff, (Ed.), Handbuch der mikroskopischen Anatomie des Menschen, Vol 6, Julius Springer, Berlin, 1940, Part 3, p. 99.

ACKNOWLEDGMENT

The authors are grateful to the National Pituitary Agency for generous gifts of antisera to human TSH and HCG and to Dr. N. S. Halmi for his critical reading of the manuscript.

The research was supported by NIH grants AM-10956, AM-11028, and HD-05318.

3. Purification, Amino Acid Composition and N-Terminus of the Luteinizing Hormone Releasing Factor (LRF) of Ovine Origin with Recent Studies on its Biological Activity

Max S. Amoss, Roger Burgus, Richard Blackwell, Wylie Vale, and Roger Guillemin

Following the successful isolation and characterization of the thyrotropin releasing factor (TRF) present in the extract from about 300,000 sheep hypothalamic fragments (1, 2), aliquots taken from the entire effluent of the large (15 cm X 2.5 m) Sephadex G-25 filtration stage were assayed for LRF activity, using a highly specific assay for LRF based on measurements of plasma LH in assay rats by a solid-phase radioimmunoassay (3, 4). Plasma LH is measured before and 10 minutes after injection of the LRF fraction, the level of the +10-min sample being adjusted by covariance. This study revealed that LRF activity was fairly well localized (approximately 0.5 V_0, Fig. 1), but that it overlapped the zone containing TRF. LRF activity was thus followed by the bioassay in the side fractions from the (previously performed) stages that had led to the isolation of TRF (1-3). It was found that LRF and TRF activities completely separated at the level of the first partition chromatography (3). This

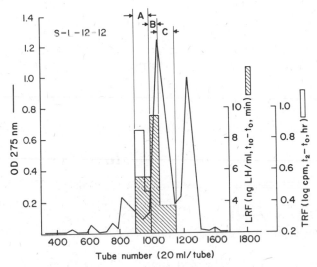

FIG. 1. Gel filtration chromatography of fraction 2, stage 3 (see Table I) on Sephadex G-25 in 0.5M acetic acid. Column dimensions: 15 cm × 2.5 m.

LRF fraction was subsequently used for pilot studies from which, after four more steps of purification (5), 992 μg of an LRF preparation were obtained which moved as a single component (ninhydrin negative, Pauly positive) in four TLC systems (2) as well as thin layer electrophoresis. This preparation of LRF was active at > 25 ng/dose in the bioassay system as above; it contained > 20% amino acids by weight.

In view of the negative reaction with ninhydrin, aliquots of this purified LRF preparation were incubated with the pyrrolidonyl-carboxylyl-peptidase purified by Fellows and Mudge from B. subtilis, which we had used previously to confirm the existence of a pyroGlu N-terminal in TRF (2). In all experiments, biological activity was destroyed. These results were considered compatible with the hypothesis (5) that ovine LRF activity is associated with a polypeptidic structure in which the N terminus is pyrrolidonyl-carboxylyl (PCA), as in the case of TRF (PCA-His-Pro-NH$_2$). This hypothesis was confirmed by partial acid hydrolysis followed by dansylation and finally by mass spectrometry on an aliquot of LRF which revealed peaks at m/e = 84 and 129, characteristic of PCA amides. The mass spectra were obtained on an MS 9 instrument equipped with a chemical ionization probe (courtesy of Dr. H. Fales, NIH, Bethesda, Maryland).

The presence of a Tyr residue in the preparation of highly purified LRF suggested the possibility of attaching a radioactive ^{125}I label on the peptide to be used as a convenient marker. A modification of the method of Greenwood et al. (6) was employed which yielded a specific activity of 1.28 mCi/μg of LRF peptide. The iodinated peptide was separated from unreacted iodine and other reagents by chromatography on a 2 mm × 24 cm column of Sephadex G-10 in 0.5M acetic acid. The addition of the iodine reduced the biological activity to approximately 50% of untreated LRF and to 60% of LRF subjected to the iodination reagents minus the iodine. However, ^{125}I LRF exhibited the same Rf as native LRF (γ counts, Pauly color) in the TLC systems and in TLE utilized previously (5).

Purification of the LRF from the bulk of the LRF-active fraction (fractions B + C in Fig. 1) from the original 300,000 sheep hypothalami was then undertaken, according to the sequence outlined in Table I. An aliquot of 0.2 μg

TABLE I. Sequence of purification of ovine LRF

Stage	Weight	LRF (u/mg)[a]
1. Lyophilized ovine hypothalami	25 kg	
2. Alcohol-chloroform extract	294 g	
3. Ultrafiltration (Diaflo membranes, UM-05)	71 g	1.5
4. Sephadex G-25 in 0.5M acetic acid	51.18 g	1.6
5. Ion exchange chromatography on CMC	61.1 mg	250
6. Column electrophoresis	11.92 mg	600
7. Partition chromatography 11 : 5 : 3, 0.1% HOAc-n-BuOH-pyridine	2.028 mg	3600
8. Partition chromatrography 4 : 1 : 5, n-BuOH-HOAc-H_2O	ca. 200 μg	not ascertained

[a]One LRF U defined as the biological activity of 1 mg of the material designated fraction B on Fig. 1.

of ^{125}I-labeled LRF obtained as above was added to the bulk of the LRF concentrate prior to stage 5. At stages 1 through 7 of the purification sequence described below, the peak of LRF activity was found to coincide with a peak of radioactivity (^{125}I-LRF). At the last step (stage 8), a definite shift was observed, so that the peak of ^{125}I-LRF (localized by γ counts) preceded the peak of biological activity (unlabeled LRF) by as much as 0.25 V_0 (Fig. 2). The stages of the purification sequence for LRF (i.e., not previously used for TRF) are described as follows. Stage 5: Ion exchange chromatography on carboxymethyl cellulose (Whatmann CM32), 10 × 16 cm column, equilibrated with 0.01M ammonium acetate, pH 4.5; step gradients in molarity and pH, first to 75mM, pH 6.5 then to 250 mM, pH 7.0, were utilized; the last step exchanges both LRF and Arg-8-vasopressin present in the starting material. Stage 6: High-voltage column electrophoresis on Sephadex G-25 (LKB Model 3540), in 0.05M pyridine acetate, pH 5.0, 5 hr, 100 mA, 1000 V. Stage 7: Partition chromatography with the system 0.1% acetic acid-n-BuOH-pyridine (11 : 5 : 3) on a 4 mm × 60 cm column of Sephadex G-25 as matrix; this step achieved total separation of LRF from Arg-8-vasopressin. Stage 8: Partition chromatography in the system n-BuOH-acetic acid-H$_2$O (4 : 1 : 5) on a 6 mm × 60 cm column of Sephadex G-25 (Fig. 2).

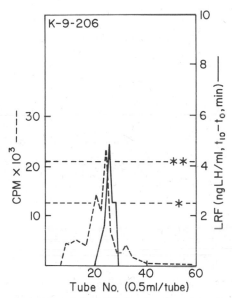

FIG. 2. Partition chromatography of the LRF fraction from stage 7 on Sephadex G-25 in the system (n-butanol-acetic acid-water, 4 : 1 : 5). Column dimensions: 6 mm × 60 cm. LRF activity determined on 25 ng doses/rat.

Hydrolysis (6N HCl) of a 31.5-μg aliquot of the material in tube 25 yielded the following amino acid composition (normalized to Leu): Lys, 0.03; His, 1.06; Arg, 1.24; Asp, 0.17; Ser, 0.85; Glu, 1.20; Pro, 0.78; Gly, 2.02; Ala, 0.02; Leu, 1.00; Tyr, 1.09. These amino acids accounted for 56% of the weight of the aliquot and for 94% of the total peptide present, the over-all yield in the LRF peak being about 200 μg. It is thus reasonable to propose that the preparation of LRF obtained here has the composition His, 1; Arg, 1; Ser, 1; Glu, 1; Pro, 1; Gly, 2; Leu, 1; Tyr, 1; and represents highly purified LRF peptide, the additional material, nonpeptidic in nature, likely being constituted by water-soluble substances eluted from the last columns' matrices.

Nikitovitch-Winer et al. (7) had reported that a purified preparation of ovine LRF was ninhydrin negative; our results are in agreement with their early observation. Recently, Currie et al. (8), using a PCA peptidase from P. fluorescens and crude preparations of bovine LRF, have concluded that bovine LRF is associated with a peptide moiety with an N-terminal PCA, confirming our earlier observations with ovine LRF (5). It is of considerable interest that, working independently and with a different purification sequence, Schally and collaborators (9) have recently obtained for porcine LRF, the same amino acid composition reported here for ovine LRF.

TABLE II. Highly purified LRF on LH and FSH release *in vitro*

Dose of LRF (ng/ml)	Hormone determined	Potency ratio[a] pituitary donors		
		Immature female (30 days)	Immature males (30 days)	Mature males 150 g
0.5	LH	1.77	0.95[b]	1.81
	FSH	1.21[b]	1.12[b]	1.13[b]
2.0	LH	4.22	8.95	2.12
	FSH	2.83	5.28	1.23[b]
10.0	LH	51.47	44.55	53.23
	FSH	7.57	20.40	13.90

[a]Obtained in classical four-point bioassays.

[b]Not significantly different from a potency of 1.0; all other potency ratios, statistically different from 1, at 95 or 99% significance by factorial analysis.

Besides the results obtained in vivo in the assays reported here, the biological activity of LRF was also studied in vitro. In several experiments, hemipituitaries from rats of different age and sex were incubated for 1 hr with increasing doses (0.5-10 ng/ml) of LRF (material from tube 25, see Fig. 2). Four point bioassays of both LH and FSH released in the incubation fluids, as determined by specific murine radioimmunoassays, indicated that LRF elicits concomitant release of LH and FSH (Table II); it is obvious that the functions relating amounts of FSH and LH released to the doses of LRF are of different slopes and different intercepts. These results, obtained with a highly purified preparation of LRF, are at variance with previous claims (10, 11) that preparations of LRF free of FSH releasing activity had been obtained in the very early stages of purification of LRF. That highly purified LRF stimulates concomitantly the secretion of LH and FSH as seen here, does not exclude the possible existence of a specific FRF distinct from LRF, both releasing factors perhaps sharing the activity to release LH and FSH though with different ratios of specific activity. It is also possible that the molecule of LRF could account for all the LH and FSH releasing activities seen in hypothalamic extracts, in which case it could be and probably should be described as the hypothalamic gonadotropin releasing factor.

ACKNOWLEDGMENT

Research supported by AID (contract No. AID/csd 2785), NIH (AM 08290; AM 14894), Ford Foundation and Rockefeller Foundation. We gratefully acknowledge the devoted collaboration of M. Butcher, D. Cedergren, A. Erenea, R. Givens, E. Raines, R. Smith, K. Wendler, and P. Wilson.

REFERENCES

1. Burgus, R., T. F. Dunn, D. Desiderio, and R. Guillemin, C R Acad Sci (Paris) 269:1870, 1969.
2. Burgus, R., T. F. Dunn, D. Desiderio, D. N. Ward, W. Vale, and R. Guillemin, Nature 226:321, 1970.
3. Burgus, R., and R. Guillemin, in J. Meites, (Ed), Hypophysiotropic Hormones of the Hypothalamus, 1 Vol., Williams & Wilkins, Baltimore, 1970, p. 227.
4. Amoss, M.S., and R. Guillemin, Fed Proc 28:381, 1969.
5. Amoss, M., R. Burgus, D. N. Ward, R. E. Fellows, and R. Guillemin, Progr 52nd Meet Endocrine Soc, St. Louis, Missouri, June 1970, p. 61.
6. Greenwood, F. C., W. M. Hunter, and J. S. Glover, Biochem J 89:114, 1963.
7. Nikitovitch-Winer, M. B., A. H. Pribble, and A. D. Winder, Am J Physiol 208:1286, 1965.
8. Currie, B. L., H. Sivertsson, C. Bogentoft, J. K. Chang, K. Folkers, C. V. Bowers, and R. F. Doolittle, Biochem Biophys Res Commun 42:1180, 1971.
9. Schally, A. V., A. Arimura, Y. Baba, R. M. G. Nair, H. Matsuo, T. W. Redding, L. Debeljuk, and W. F. White, in Program 53rd Meet Endocrine Soc, San Francisco, California, June 1971.
10. Dhariwal, A. P. S., S. Watanabe, J. Antunes-Rodrigues, and S. M. McCann, Neuro-endocrinology 2:294, 1967.
11. Schally, A. V., A. Arimura, C. Y. Bowers, A. Kastin, S. Sawano, and T. W. Redding, Rec Prog Horm Res 24:497, 1968.

4.   Recent Progress in the Physiological and Clinical Studies with LH- and FSH-Releasing Hormone

Akira Arimura, Abba J. Kastin, and Andrew V. Schally

The recurrent reproductive periods of mature female mammals, including human beings, are governed by the rhythmic secretion of hormones by the pituitary and ovaries. This rhythm is directed by the central nervous system, particularly by the hypothalamus and related structures of the brain. Involvement of the central nervous system in the male reproductive processes appears to be less obvious than in the female. However, in the male too, control of the reproductive processes can also be analyzed in terms of a "neuroendocrine reflex" (1). Each pituitary gonadotropin, LH and FSH, appears to be identical in the male and female. It is evident that the stimulus which releases LH and FSH both in males and females is mediated by a neurohumoral mechanism involving the hypothalamic LH releasing hormone (LH-RH) and FSH releasing hormone (FSH-RH). These hormones are manufactured by the nerve cells in the hypothalamus, released into the primary plexus of the hypophysial portal vessels and then transported to the pituitary gonadotrophs where they stimulate secretion of LH and FSH. Intensive effort has been made by several investigators, including our group, to purify and isolate LH-RH and FSH-RH from hypothalamic tissue of domestic animals and elucidate their chemical structure. Clarification of the molecular structure of these hormones will lead to synthesis on a large scale which should open the way to vast practical application of these hormones in the clinical field.

ASSAY, PURIFICATION, AND ISOLATION OF LH-RH AND FSH-RH

In order to purify and isolate LH-RH and FSH-RH from crude extracts of hypothalamic tissue, it was necessary to establish reliable and specific assay methods for these hormones. Both in vivo and in vitro methods can be used for detection of the activities of LH-RH and FSH-RH. For LH-RH, we employ an in vivo system originally described by Ramirez and McCann (2) using ovariectomized rats pretreated with progesterone and estrogen. Samples are injected intravenously after anesthesia of the animal and blood is collected 20 min later. In the early phase of our studies, LH levels in plasma from assay rats were determined by bioassay using the ovarian ascorbic acid depletion method of Parlow (3). Later the bioassay was replaced by a specific radioimmunoassay (RIA) for LH using ovine LH and antiovine LH system (OO-Rat-LH-RIA) described by Niswender et al. (4). This RIA system has been found very satisfactory in specificity, accuracy, and sensitivity. Our LH-RH preparation has been found not to interfere with this radioimmunoassay, in other words, the presence of LH-RH in the reaction tube does not inhibit the binding of LH and the antiserum. Using this in vivo assay method for LH-RH followed by RIA, a straight log-dose response regression line was constructed for our LH-RH reference standard, AVS 77-3 #320-339, in the range from 5 to 20 ng; the index of precision was 0.153. It is possible to determine the potency of LH-RH activity in any unknown sample with good accuracy by using factorial determination.

Although iv injection of FSH-RH preparations increased serum FSH levels in ovariectomized, progesterone-estrogen pretreated rats as compared with the preinjection levels, the magnitude of rise of serum FSH was not as great as LH. Furthermore, levels of serum FSH in these assay animals vary considerably from rat to rat. Therefore, for FSH-RH an in vitro assay system described by Mittler and Meites (5) has been adapted for use in our laboratories. This method is based on stimulation of FSH release in vitro from pituitaries of normal intact male rats. The amount of FSH released into the incubation media is determined by the bioassay of Steelman-Pohley (6) with slight modifications (7) or radioimmunoassay (8). A straight log-dose response regression line has been constructed for a highly purified porcine FSH-RH preparation.

The isolation of LH-RH and FSH-RH was accomplished essentially in 11 steps (9):

1. Pulverization of lyophilized porcine hypothalamic tissue on dry ice and defatting with acetone and petroleum ether.

2. Extraction of the defatted powder with 2N acetic acid and lyophilization of the extracts.

3. Concentration of the lyophilized extracts by reextraction with glacial acetic acid and lyophilization of the supernatant.

4. Gel filtration on a preparative column (15.5 × 180 cm) of Sephadex G-25 in 1M acetic acid.

5. Extraction of the LH-RH/FSH-RH active fractions with phenol followed by recovery.

6. Chromatography on carboxymethylcellulose (CMC), using ammonium acetate buffers.

7. Rechromatography on CMC.

8. Free-flow electrophoresis in pyridine acetate buffer at pH 6.3.

9. Countercurrent distribution (CCD) in a system of 0.1% acetic acid-1-butanol-pyridine (11 : 5 : 3 v/v).

10. Partition chromatography in a system consisting of 1-butanol-acetic acid-water-benzene (4 : 1 : 5 : 0.33).

11. Partition chromatography in a system consisting of 1-butanol-ethanol-water-acetic acid-pyridine-benzene (25 : 7 : 30 : 2 : 1 : 10).

After lyophilization, essentially homogenous material was obtained which contained both LH-RH and FSH-RH activity. The amino acid composition, determined after hydrolysis with 6N HCl (22 hr, 110 C), was: His, 1; Arg, 1; Ser, 1; Glu, 1; Pro, 1; Gly, 2; Leu, 1; and Tyr, 1. In addition, one Trp residue was detected by alkaline hydrolysis and by the method of Matsubara and Sasaki (10).

The view that the polypeptide moiety, which consists of 10 amino acids, is essential for biological activity of LH-RH and FSH-RH was supported by experiments with proteolytic enzymes (11). Both LH-RH and FSH-RH activities were simultaneously abolished by incubation with endopeptidases (chymotrypsin, papain, subtilisin, thermolysin) but not by exopeptidases (leucine aminopeptidase, aminopeptidase M, carboxypeptidase A and B). Lack of inactivation by Edman procedure and failure to detect any N-terminal amino acid by the Dansyl method indicated a blocked N terminus. Inactivation by pyrrolidone carboxylyl peptidase (G-200 preparation, supplied by Dr. R. Doolittle) suggested that the N terminus might be occupied by pyroglutamic acid. This was supported by mass spectral fragmentation patterns of free LH-RH. Inactivation with N-bromosuccinimide and diazotized sulfanilic acid suggested that tyrosine and/or histidine are necessary for both biological activities.

Partition chromatography in 10 different solvent systems did not separate FSH-RH activity from LH-RH. The material isolated as described above stimulated the release of both LH and FSH in vivo as well as in vitro. Although the material should be designated as LH-RH/FSH-RH, we will call this LH-RH to avoid any awkwardness in this paper. The complete amino acid sequence of porcine LH-RH has been determined by the use of a microscale of the combined Edman-Dansyl procedure coupled with the selective tritiation method for C-terminal analysis. On the basis of these results, we have proposed the following decapeptide sequence for LH-RH: (pyro)Glu-His-Trp-Ser-Tyr-Gly-Leu-Arg-Pro-Gly-NH$_2$(12 13). This decapeptide was shynthesized by Merrifield's solid-phase method and found active in vivo and in vitro in releasing both LH and FSH (14, 15). Table I shows that does as small as 0.5 ng natural porcine LH-RH/ml

TABLE I. Stimulation of LH and FSH release in vitro from male rat pituitaries by "pure" LH-RH[a]

Beaker no.	Sample added	Dose (ng/ml)	LH[b] (ng/ml/6 hr)	FSH[c] (ng/ml/6 hr)
1	control	—	238	8,000
2	LH-RH	.5	363	9,625
3	LH-RH	1.5	460	12,450
4	LH-RH	4.5	628	16,200
5	LH-RH	13.5	978	24,000

[a]AVS-36-68 #6-13.

[b]Expressed as NIH-LH-S 14, determined by radioimmunoassay.

[c]Expressed as NIAMD-Rat-FSH-RP-1, determined by radioimmunoassay; 10 pituitary halves from normal male rats incubated in 10 ml Krebs-Ringer-bicarbonate solution for 6 hr.

augmented the release of both LH and FSH in vitro as ascertained by bioassay and radioimmunoassay of media. The larger dose stimulated the greater release of both LH and FSH. Table II shows the results of simultaneous determination of serum LH and FSH 10 and 45 min after intracarotid injection of the same material into castrated male rats pretreated with testosterone propionate. The LH levels 10 min after injection were higher than those 45 min after injection. Since considerable variation was found in the preinjection levels of serum FSH among individual animals, FSH-RH activity was assessed by the increment of serum FSH as compared to preinjection levels.

Serum FSH significantly increased 45 min after injection of 25 ng of LH-RH as compared with preinjection levels, but not 10 min after injection. This may be at least partly due to the longer halflife of FSH than that of LH (16) in rats. The maximal percent increase of serum FSH after 25 ng of LH-RH (increase/preinjection levels $\times$ 100) was 26%, which was considerably smaller than the maximal increase of LH. The greater response of LH than FSH in terms of percent increase was observed in most of the in vivo experiments including studies in human beings. This is particularly interesting, since the percent increase of LH and FSH release in vitro induced by the same preparation of LH-RH was similar (Table I).

TABLE II. Serum LH and FSH levels after intracarotid injection of "pure" LH-RH[a] in castrated TP-treated male rats

Sample	Dose (ng)	LH[b] (ng/ml)			FSH[c] (ng/ml)		
		0 min	10 min	45 min	0 min	10 min	45 min
Saline	–	ND[d]	ND	ND	2231 ± 123 (6)[e]	1980 ± 181 (3)	2254 ± 117 (6)
LH-RH	1	ND	12 ± 4.5 (3)	5 ± 1.3 (3)	2937 ± 592 (3)	2883 ± 681 (3)	3671 ± 850 (3)
LH-RH	5	ND	42 ± 4.0 (3)	14 ± 1.7 (3)	2615 ± 240 (3)	2651 ± 153 (3)	2998 ± 234 (3)
LH-RH	25	ND	66 ± 5.9 (6)	28 ± 2.6 (6)	2340 ± 198 (6)	2870 ± 170 (3)	3162 ± 186 (6)

[a] AVS-36-68 #6-13.

[b] Expressed as NIH-LH-S 14.

[c] Expressed as NIAMD-Rat-FSH-RP-1, determined by radioimmunoassay.

[d] Not detectable.

[e] Numbers in the parentheses indicate the number of rats in the group.

Note: When mean serum FSH levels after injection of LH-RH were compared with corresponding mean preinjection levels, only the level 45 min after injection of 25 ng LH-RH was significantly higher than the corresponding preinjection level.

RESPONSE TO LH-RH IN NORMAL ANIMALS

Although castrated animals, regardless of sex, are very sensitive to LH-RH, normal intact animals are relatively insensitive to exogenously administered LH-RH. This trend has been observed in rats and sheep (17). Intracarotid (IC) injection of 1 μg of purified porcine LH-RH preparation (AVS 77-3 #320-339) through a carotid loop into the conscious intact ram and anestrous ewe raised serum LH 2 to 5 ng/ml in terms of NIH-LH-S 14. Maximal responses in the ewe and the ram were obtained with 3 μg LH-RH, a dose which increased serum LH levels 6 to 18 ng/ml at 2.5 to 10 min after IC injections. Higher levels of LH could not be obtained by increasing the dose of LH-RH. On the other hand, in the castrated male sheep (wether), a 20 ng/ml elevation of serum LH was obtained with 1 μg LH-RH and by increasing the dose of LH-RH to 27 μg, serum LH levels as high as 160 ng/ml could be obtained. A typical elevation of serum LH induced by 9.0 μg of purified LH-RH as measured by radioimmunoassay in the ewe, ram, and the wether is shown in Fig. 1.

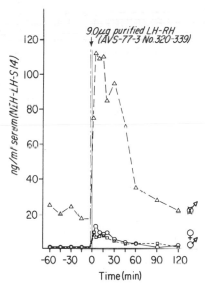

FIG. 1. Typical elevation in serum LH induced by LH-RH as measured by radioimmuno-assay in the sheep (17). Reproduced by permission from The American Society of Animal Science.

INFLUENCE OF GONADAL STEROIDS ON THE PITUITARY RESPONSE TO LH-RH IN NORMAL ANIMALS

In normal cycling female rats, serum LH levels rise in the afternoon of proestrus. The magnitude of the rise of LH reaches as high as 50 to 100 ng/ml in terms of

NIH-LH-S 14. This degree of elevation of serum LH has never been produced in normal rats, even by a comparably large dose of LH-RH. Therefore, we thought that another factor might be interacting with LH-RH or increasing the responsiveness of the pituitary to LH-RH.

At first, we considered the influence of estrogen on the pituitary. A direct influence of estrogen on the pituitary responsiveness, in addition to its hypothalamic action, was first proposed by Döcke and Dörner (18). Recently, Miyake and his associates (19) accumulated evidence in rats for the possibility that a gradual increase of estrogen secretion starting in the morning of proestrus is a necessary trigger for the preovulatory surge of LH which occurs in the afternoon; they emphasized the mediation of the hypothalamus in this. We have recently investigated the effect of pretreatment with estrogen on LH-RH-induced release of LH in intact diestrous rats (20). As shown in Table III, 10 or 20 μg estradiol benzoate in all were injected into 5-day cycling female rats on day 1 (diestrus). On day 2 (diestrus), 0.1 μg of LH-RH (AVS 77-3 #320-339) was injected into the carotid artery. Serum LH levels before and 20 min after the injection were determined by radioimmunoassay. In oil-pretreated control rats, LH-RH injection induced only a slight rise of serum LH. In the estrogen-pretreated rats, the same dose of LH-RH induced a much greater rise in serum LH levels. Estrogen by itself did not affect the level of serum LH.

Substantial reports (21) indicate that progestins suppress LH release mainly by acting on the hypothalamus or some other area of the central nervous system. On the other hand, several investigators reported that the major blocking effect of progestins is on the pituitary. Hilliard et al. (22) reported that ovulation induced by intrapituitary infusion of purified LH-RH in rabbits was blocked by a single injection of norethindrone 15 to 24 hr before the infusion. Spies et al. (23) reported that a single SC injection of progesterone or chlormadinone blocked ovulation induced by intrapituitary infusion of median eminence extracts in rabbits. We also examined the effect of a single injection of progesterone on LH release following intracarotid injection or intrapituitary infusion of small doses of purified porcine LH-RH (24). The results of this study are summarized in Tables IV and V. Control serum LH concentrations were very low both in oil-injected control and progesterone-treated rats. Intracarotid injection of 10 and 50 ng LH-RH into the untreated rats raised serum concentrations by 1.5 and 3.6 ng/ml, respectively. A similar trend was observed in the experiments in which LH-RH was infused into the pituitary. Factorial analysis of variance indicated that progesterone significantly suppressed LH release induced by LH-RH. The magnitude of suppression was approximately 50%. These results may indicate a direct effect of the steroid on the pituitary.

It was suggested that progesterone's suppressive effect on LH-RH-induced LH release took place in a competitive manner (22). Hilliard, Schally, and Sawyer (22) reported that in estrous rabbits, ovulation induced by an intrapituitary infusion of a small dose of LH-RH was prevented by pretreatment of the animals

TABLE III. Serum LH levels before and 20 min after intracarotid injection of 0.1 µg of LH-RH or saline in diestrous rats pretreated with oil or estrogen[a]

Material	Serum LH level (ng/ml)[b]					
	Oil pretreated			Estrogen pretreated		
	Before	After	Δ	Before	After	Δ
					(10 µg of estradiol bz.)	
Saline	1.4 ± 0.89	2.4 ± 1.40	1.0 ± 0.57 (3)	0.3 ± 0.28	0.4 ± 0.29	0.1 ± 0.05 (4)
LH-RH	0.3 ± 0.30	2.5 ± 0.91	2.2 ± 0.70 (5)	0.5 ± 0.22	13.1 ± 2.88[d]	12.6 ± 2.76 (8)
					(20 µg of estradiol bz.)	
Saline	2.6 ± 0.52	2.7 ± 0.16	0.1 ± 0.43 (5)	2.7 ± 1.02	3.1 ± 0.40	0.5 ± 0.75 (4)
LH-RH	2.4 ± 0.32	5.5 ± 0.61[c]	3.1 ± 0.51 (9)	2.0 ± 0.09	10.5 ± 1.56[d]	8.6 ± 1.50 (7)

[a]Number of rats in each group is given in parenthesis, 2×2 factorial analyses of 4 mean values indicate a significant interaction in both experiments.

[b]Expressed in terms of NIH-LH-S 14.

[c]$p < 0.02$.

[d]$p < 0.01$; significant levels in student's "t" test as compared with preinjection level.

From Arimura and Schally (20).

TABLE IV. Serum LH levels (ng/ml) before and 15 min after intracarotid injection of LH-RH into oil- or progesterone-treated rats

Material injected IC	Oil-treated			Progesterone-treated		
	Before LH-RH	After LH-RH	Δ	Before LH-RH	After LH-RH	Δ
Saline	0.2 ± 0.19^b	0.1 ± 0.07	-0.1 ± 0.21	0	0.1 ± 0.05	0.1 ± 0.05
10 ng LH-RH	0.4 ± 0.24	1.9 ± 0.44	1.5 ± 0.29	0	0.5 ± 0.30	0.5 ± 0.30
50 ng LH-RH	0.9 ± 0.54	4.5 ± 1.15	3.6 ± 0.75	0	1.6 ± 0.06	1.6 ± 0.06

Duncan's new multiple range test for

10 ng LH-RH/oil vs. Saline/oil	0.05
50 ng LH-RH/oil vs. Saline/oil	0.01
10 ng LH-RH/prog vs. Saline/prog	NS
50 ng LH-RH/prog vs. Saline/prog	0.05
10 ng LH-RH/prog vs. 10 ng LH-RH/oil	NS
50 ng LH-RH/prog vs. 50 ng LH-RH/oil	0.01

[a] Mean serum LH concentrations, ng/ml ± SE, expressed as NIH-LH-S 14; 4 rats used/group; 2 × 3 analysis of variance indicates a significant (p 0.025) interaction between the effect of progesterone and that of LH-RH on serum LH levels.

[b] Difference in serum LH levels before and after injection.

From Arimura and Schally (24).

TABLE V. Effect of intrapituitary infusion of saline or LH-RH on serum LH levels in cycling rats treated with oil or progesterone

Materials	Oil-treated	Progesterone-treated
Saline	$0.1 \pm 0.06 \ (15)$[a]	$0 \ (5)$
2 ng LH-RH	$7.6 \pm 1.70 \ (8)$	$3.8 \pm 0.47 \ (8)$
10 ng LH-RH	$12.5 \pm 1.68 \ (8)$	$6.1 \pm 0.85 \ (9)$

2 × 3 analysis of variance shows the significant interaction between the effects of progesterone and LH-RH, indicating that the difference between simple effects of LH-RH in oil- and progesterone-pretreated rats is significant.

Duncan's new multiple range test:

Saline/oil	vs. 2 ng LH-RH/oil	0.01
Saline/prog	vs. 2 ng LH-RH/prog	0.05
2 ng LH-RH/prog	vs. 2 ng LH-RH/oil	0.05
10 ng LH-RH/prog	vs. 10 ng LH-RH/oil	0.01

[a]Mean serum LH concentrations, ng/ml $\pm$ SE, expressed by NIH-LH-S 14. Numbers in parentheses indicate number of rats used.

From Arimura and Schally (24).

with 2 mg progesterone but ovulation following a large dose of LH-RH was not affected by progesterone. They stated that the ability of LH-RH to overcome progesterone blockade is directly related to the dose of LH-RH administered. In

TABLE VI. Effects of the pretreatment with estradiol benzoate and/or progesterone on LH-RH-induced release of LH (ng/ml) in diestrous female rats[a]

Pretreatment	LH (ng/ml)[b]	
	Injection of saline	Injection of LH-RH
Oil	$0.9 \pm 0.2 \ (12)$[c]	$15.2 \pm 2.4 \ (14)$
Estradiol + progesterone	$0.03 + 0.1 \ (7)$	$5.9 \pm 1.2 \ (8)$[d]
Estradiol	$1.1 \pm 0.5 \ (7)$	$34.9 \pm 9.5 \ (9)$[d]
Progesterone	$1.5 \pm 0.5 \ (8)$	$16.6 \pm 2.2 \ (7)$

[a]Dose of estradiol benzoate: 20 μg; dose of progesterone: 5 mg.

[b]Expressed as NIH-LH-S 14.

[c]Number of animals in parentheses.

[d]Significantly different from oil pretreated LH-RH injected group.

Note: Steroids were injected 48 hr before the injection of saline or 1 μg LH-RH (AVS 77-3 #320-339). Blood was collected before and 15 min after injection of LH-RH from the jugular vein under urethane anesthesia.

our recent experiments (25), normal diestrous rats were pretreated with 5 mg progesterone. Elevation of serum LH induced by a large dose (1 μg) of LH-RH (AVS 77-3 #320-339) was not suppressed by the pretreatment with progesterone. On the other hand, pretreatment with 20 μg estradiol benzoate augmented LH release induced by LH-RH, although the resting level remained at the same level after estrogen administration. It is interesting that combined administration of 20 μg estrogen and 5 mg progesterone significantly suppressed the response to 1 μg LH-RH (Table VI).

STUDIES IN HUMAN SUBJECTS

The possible clinical application of porcine LH-RH and lack of species specificity for the human being were suggested by our recent studies (26, 27). Igarashi et al. (28) and Root et al. (29) also reported limited experiments in which administration of large amounts of comparatively crude hypothalamic preparation of bovine or ovine origin caused the elevation of plasma FSH (28) and LH (29). Our clinical studies were performed in collaboration with Dr. C. Gual and Dr. A. R. Midgley, Jr.

In the weeks prior to the administration of LH-RH, many of the subjects received an intravenous injection of vasopressin as a control solution, a dose approximately equivalent to the vasopressin contained in the administered LH-RH. Blood samples were withdrawn from an indwelling iv catheter immediately before injection of the vasopressin or LH-RH at various times afterwards. Serum LH and FSH were determined by specific radioimmunoassay (30, 31) and expressed in terms of mIU of 2nd IRP-HMG/ml serum.

Resting serum LH and FSH levels varied considerably from one subject to another. In this review, an absolute increment of the concentration of serum LH and FSH (mIU/ml) will be utilized to express the magnitude of response. Because the biological dose response regression line is generally constructed as a sigmoid curve, at low doses several-fold increases of LH or FSH secretion might not necessarily stimulate gonadal function to a significant extent. Therefore, we thought that the absolute increment of serum LH and FSH levels after injection of LH-RH may be suitable index of the physiological response.

In the initial studies (26), 1.5 mg of a porcine LH-RH preparation containing 0.35 U of pressor activity was injected. The healthy subjects tested in this study included 2 untreated men, 2 untreated women, 2 men who received 1.5 mg of ethinyl estradiol for each of the 3 days, and 2 normal women who received the oral contraceptive Lyndiol (Mestranol + Lynestrenol, Organon, Inc.) for 2 weeks prior to the tests. Administration of 1.5 mg LH-RH caused a significant increase in both serum LH and FSH levels when compared with the values obtained after injection of a control solution of vasopressin. The results are shown in Table VII.

In one of the untreated women, administration of LH-RH resulted in an absolute increase in serum LH of 73 mIU/ml and serum FSH of 68.8 mIU/ml. She was on day 15 of her menstrual cycle and the resting LH and FSH levels

TABLE VII. Maximal increment in serum LH and FSH levels (Δ mIU/ml) after administration of HL-RH[a] in human subjects

Subjects		LH LH-RH	FSH LH-RH
Untreated men	1	11.4	2.0
	2	15.5	6.2
Untreated women	1	73.0	68.8
	2	7.4	2.2
Men treated with estrogen	1	14.5	4.3
	2	41.4	35.0
Women treated with oral contraceptive	1	3.3	1.4
	2	2.2	0.1

[a]Purified porcine LH-RH, a single dose of 1.5 mg LH-RH was given IV in all subjects.

were elevated (34.7 mIU/ml and 42.8 mIU/ml respectively). As was the case in our experiments with sheep (32), the pituitary responsiveness to LH-RH appeared to be highest when the preovulatory surge of LH occurs. Thus women near the midcycle of their menstrual period might show the greater response to exogenous LH-RH. In other stages of the cycle, the response to LH-RH in women appeared to be of the same magnitude as the response in untreated men.

In one of the men pretreated with estrogen, administration of LH-RH resulted in an increment of serum LH and FSH levels of 41.4 mIU/ml and 35 mIU/ml, respectively. Similar findings were obtained in the second study (27). It is possible that estrogen pretreatment augmented pituitary responsiveness to LH-RH in human beings in the same way as was seen in the experiments with rats (20) and sheep (33).

On the other hand, the magnitude of response to LH-RH appeared to be the smallest in women treated with oral contraceptives, drugs which are a mixture of progestagen and estrogen. It is interesting to recall the experiments in intact female rats in which response to LH-RH was suppressed by pretreatment with progesterone and estradiol benzoate (25).

In the second series of experiments, the observations were extended in additional selected human subjects using a more potent preparation of porcine LH-RH (AVS 77-3 #320-339). The subjects tested included 2 untreated women, 2 untreated postmenopausal women, 2 postmenopausal women treated with Lyndiol and 2 women with secondary amenorrhea pretreated with Pergonal for 8 days so that a rise in estrogen excretion was reflected in the cytology of the vaginal smears, two normal men who received 1.5 mg of ethynyl estradiol for each of 3 days, and 2 normal untreated men. Most of these subjects received an intravenous injection of 0.1 IU of vasopressin as a control solution 2 weeks prior to the administration of LH-RH. The dose of LH-RH was 0.7 mg for all subjects except the 2 women with secondary amenorrhea and the 2 normal women in day 9 of their menstrual cycle. These subjects received a single dose of 1.4 mg of LH-RH in an attempt to induce ovulation.

TABLE VIII. Maximal increment of serum LH and FSH levels (Δ mIU/ml) after administration of LH-RH[a] in human subjects

Group		LH	FSH
1			
untreated men	1	16.8	8.6
	2	23.6	9.3
untreated women on day 9	1	28.4	14.4
	2	19.7	12.0
2			
postmenopausal women treated with	1	15.8	8.2
Lyndiol	2	18.2	9.9
women with secondary amenorrhea	1	10.9	1.8
	2	9.3	3.1
3			
men treated with estrogen[b]	1	38.6	22.2
	2	10.5	3.7
4			
postmenopausal women, untreated	1	28.2	36.2
	2	41.6	87.0

[a]Highly purified porcine LH-RH (AVS 7703 #320-339). A single dose of 0.7 mg of LH-RH was given iv in all subjects except for 2 untreated women and 2 women with secondary amenorrhea who received 1.4 mg LH-RH.

[b]LH-RH was injected SC in these subjects.

The results of this study are shown in Table VIII. LH-RH induced an over-all mean maximum increase in serum LH of 460% as compared with a mean maximum increase of 10% after injection of the vasopressin control solution. LH-RH also increased serum FSH levels by 92% as compared with 10% mean increase after vasopressin. There was considerable variation among the subjects regarding the time at which the maximum increase in serum LH and FSH occurred following administration of LH-RH. In each case, however, there was a delay of at least 16 min before the maximum effect was observed. A typical pattern of serum LH and FSH levels after IV injection of LH-RH is shown in Fig. 2.

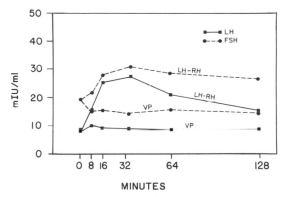

FIG. 2. Serum LH and FSH levels (mIU/ml) after administration of porcine LH-RH and lysine vasopressin (VP) to a normal woman on day 9 of her menstrual cycle.

The results can be summarized in several separate groups of subjects. The first group was composed of subjects with "normal" resting levels of serum LH. This group consisted of 2 untreated men and 2 untreated women on day 9 of their menstrual cycle. The magnitude of the rise of serum LH after injection of LH-RH appeared to be the same between men and women. On the other hand, a greater rise of serum FSH was observed in women, although preinjection levels of serum FSH in women were higher than those in men (Table VIII).

The second group consisted of subjects with suppressed resting levels of serum LH. Postmenopausal women treated with Lyndiol illustrate this group. Resting serum LH levels in these women were lower than those in unsuppressed postmenopausal women. The magnitude of the response to LH-RH in these suppressed postmenopausal women was considerably smaller than those in unsuppressed postmenopausal women (Table VIII).

Two women with secondary amenorrhea pretreated with Pergonal might be included in this group because their resting serum LH levels were lower than those of untreated women on day 9 of their menstrual cycle. The magnitude of the rise of both LH and FSH after LH-RH in these 2 women was the smallest of all of the subjects tested (Table VIII).

The third group consisted of 2 men pretreated with estradiol benzoate in whom the LH-RH was administered subcutaneously. In subject 1, resting levels of serum LH were not different from those of the untreated man. There was observed, however, a considerably greater response to LH-RH as compared to that which was observed in the other subject not receiving estrogen. In the other subject, both the resting levels of serum LH and the response to LH-RH appeared to be slightly suppressed by pretreatment with estrogen. These findings may suggest a complex effect of estrogen on pituitary responsiveness to LH-RH. The readers might recall aforementioned animal experiments with large doses of LH-RH, in which estrogen augmented the response to LH-RH, and a combined pretreatment of estrogen and progesterone suppressed it, even if progesterone alone was not sufficient to suppress the response (25). Although the mechanism by which estrogens augment or suppress pituitary responsiveness to LH-RH in human beings is unknown, it is possible that circulating endogenous steroids interact with administered estrogen in modulating the pituitary response to LH-RH.

The fourth group consisted of 2 untreated postmenopausal women with elevated resting levels of serum LH and FSH. The magnitude of the response to LH-RH, particularly the rise of FSH, was the largest of all of the subjects.

Another interesting finding in this study is that the FSH/LH ratio after injection of LH-RH was larger than 1 in only unsuppressed menopausal women, whereas in other subjects it was smaller than 1. At present, LH-RH and FSH-RH are inseparable. One releasing hormone probably controls both LH and FSH secretion, but other factors appear to govern the preferential response of the pituitary to LH-RH.

The single dose of LH-RH employed in this study, however, did not produce ovulation in the women with secondary amenorrhea or normal women on day 9 of their menstrual cycle. These amenorrheic subjects previously had shown that they were able to ovulate after suitable treatment with Pergonal and HCG. It seemed probable that a more prolonged stimulation by repeated injections or continuous infusion of LH-RH would be required to induce ovulation.

In order to further study this problem, a 34-year-old woman who had irregular menses since menarche was selected. For several previous years she had secondary amenorrhea and sterility. In the control period, Pergonal was injected IM on each of three days and basal body temperature, cervical mucus, vaginal cytology, and urinary pregnanediol, pregnanetriol, and total estrogens followed at various times for a month. At the end of this time, vaginal bleeding was induced with chlormadinone (4 mg orally for 2 days); Pergonal was then administered in the same schedule as before. Ten days later, the infusion of LH-RH was started. LH-RH, 600 μg, was infused for 24 hr, supplemented with rapid iv injection of 300 μg of LH-RH at 8 and 24 hr. Serum LH levels remained elevated (100 mIU/ml) during most of the infusion of LH-RH. The rapid injection of LH-RH resulted in a further increase in serum LH levels which lasted between 2 and 4 hr. The patient then returned home. The estrogenic effect of Pergonal upon cervical mucus disappeared five days after the infusion of LH-RH. By this time, basal body temperature had risen and urinary pregnanediol values had increased to 1.56 mg/24 hr. Pregnanediol levels continued to increase; one month later the immunological pregnancy test was positive. Pregnancy has been subsequently confirmed. The total dose of LH-RH, although much greater than the minimum required to release LH, was still less than the single injection given to other women in an attempt to induce ovulation (34).

These clinical data indicate the effectiveness of the highly purified LH-RH preparation of porcine origin in human beings. Synthetic LH-RH, which will be available soon, should greatly facilitate development of clinical uses of this substance.

ACKNOWLEDGMENT

These studies were supported in part by grants from Research Service VACO, NIH grants AM-09094, AM-07467, and the Population Council, New York, New York.

REFERENCES

1. Davidson, J. M., in L. Martini and W. F. Ganong (Eds.), Neuroendocrinology, Academic, New York, 1966, p. 565.
2. Ramirez, V. D., and S. M. McCann, Endocrinology 73:193, 1963.
3. Parlow, A. F., in A. Albert (Ed.), Human Pituitary Gonadotropins, Charles C Thomas, Springfield, Ill., 1961, p. 300.
4. Niswender, G. D., A. R. Midgley, Jr., S. E. Monroe, and L. E. Reichert, Jr., Proc Soc Exp Biol Med 128:807, 1968.
5. Mittler, J. C., and J. Meites, Endocrinology 78:500, 1966.
6. Steelman, S. L., and F. Pohley, Endocrinology 53:604, 1953.
7. Kuroshima, A., Y. Ishida, C. Y. Bowers, and A. V. Schally, Endocrinology 76:614, 1965.
8. Parlow, A. F., A. T. Daane, and A. V. Schally, Abstracts Endocrine society, 51st Meeting, New York, New York, 1969, p. 83.
9. Schally, A. V., A. Arimura, Y. Baba, R. M. G. Nair, H. Matsuo, T. W. Redding, L. Debeljuk, and W. F. White, Biochem Biophys Res Commun 43:393, 1971.
10. Matsubara, H., and R. Sasaki, Biochem Biophys Res Commun 35:175, 1969.
11. Schally, A. V., Y. Baba, A. Arimura, and T. W. Redding, Biochem Biophys Res Commun 42:50, 1971.
12. Matsuo, H., Y. Baba, R. M. G. Nair, A. Arimura, and A. V. Schally, Biochem Biophys Res Commun 43:1334, 1971.
13. Baba, Y., H. Matsuo, and A. V. Schally, Biochem Biophys Res Commun in press, 1971.
14. Arimura, A., H. Matsuo, Y. Baba, L. Debeljuk, J. Sandow, and A. V. Schally, Endocrinology, submitted, 1971.
15. Schally, A. V., A. Arimura, A. J. Kastin, H. Matsuo, Y. Baba, T. W. Redding, R. M. G. Nair, L. Debeljuk, and W. F. White, Science, submitted, 1971.
16. Bogdanove, E. M., and V. L. Gay, in E. Rosemberg (Ed.), Gonadotropins 1968, Geron-X, Inc., Los Altos, Calif., 1968, p. 131.
17. Reeves, J. J., A. Arimura, and A. V. Schally, J Anim Sci 31:933, 1970.
18. Döcke, F., and G. Dörner, J Endocrinol 33:491, 1965.
19. Miyake, T., Endocrinol, Japan Suppl 1:83, 1969.

20. Arimura, A., and A. V. Schally, Proc Soc Exp Biol Med 136:290, 1971.
21. Flerkó, B., in L. Martini and W. F. Ganong (Eds.) Neuroendocrinology, Academic, New York, 1966, p. 613.
22. Hilliard, J., A. V. Schally, and C. H. Sawyer, Endocrinology 188:730, 1971.
23. Spies, H. G., K. R. Stevens, J. Hilliard, and C. H. Sawyer, Endocrinology 84:297, 1969.
24. Arimura, A., and A. V. Schally, Endocrinology 87:653, 1970.
25. Debeljuk, L., A. Arimura, and A. V. Schally, in preparation.
26. Kastin, A. J., A. V. Schally, C. Gual, A. R. Midgley, Jr., C. Y. Bowers, and A. Diaz-Infante, J Clin Endocrinol 29:1046, 1969.
27. Kastin, A. J., A. V. Schally, C. Gual., A. R. Midgley, Jr., C. Y. Bowers, and F. Gomez-Perez, Amer J Obst Gyn 108:177, 1970.
28. Igarashi, M., N. Yokota, Y. Ehara, R. Mayuzumi, T. Hirano, S. Matsumoto, and M. Yamasaki, Amer J Obst Gyn 100:867, 1968.
29. Root, A. V., G. P. Smith, A. P. S. Dhariwal, and S. M. McCann, Nature 221:570, 1969.
30. Midgley, A. R., Jr., Endocrinology 79:10, 1966.
31. Midgley, A. R., Jr., J Clin Endocrinol 27:295, 1967.
32. Reeves, J. J., A. Arimura, and A. V. Schally, J Anim Sci 32:123, 1971.
33. Reeves, J. J., A. Arimura, and A. V. Schally, J Anim Sci, accepted, 1971.
34. Kastin, A. J., A. Zarate, A. V. Schally, A. R. Midgley, Jr., and E. S. Canales, submitted to N Eng J Med.

5. The Role of Monoamines in the Control of Gonadotropin and Prolactin Secretion

Samuel M. McCann,[1] P.S. Kalra,[2] S.P. Kalra,[2] A.O. Donoso, W. Bishop, H.P.G. Schneider, C.P. Fawcett, and L. Krulich

Early evidence for participation of catecholamines in the regulation of gonadotropin secretion was obtained by Sawyer and co-workers who demonstrated that dibenamine would block ovulation (1). More recent work has shown that drugs such as reserpine which deplete monoamines can also block ovulation (2) and lead to the development of pseudopregnancy in animals (3). Reserpine can also induce lactational changes in man (4). If the depletion of monoamines is prevented by the administration of monoamine oxidase inhibitors such as pargyline or of precursors of catecholamines, the effects of reserpine are reversed which indicates that they are due to the depletion of amines (5, 6).

Additional evidence supporting a role for catecholamines in the regulation of gonadotropin secretion has been provided by the demonstration of fluctuations in monoamine oxidase levels in states where gonadotropin secretion is altered (7, 8) and by the demonstration of changes in the hypothalamic content and turnover of catecholamines in states of altered gonadotropin release (9-11).

The anatomical substrate for adrenergic control of gonadotropin secretion has been localized by the use of fluorescence microscopy to demonstrate catecholaminergic and serotoninergic nerve endings in the hypothalamus (12). In particular, there appears to be a dopaminergic pathway with neurons whose cell

[1] Supported by NIH grant #AM10073, by a Ford Foundation grant and by a grant from The Texas Population Crisis Foundation.

[2] Postdoctoral fellow of the Ford Foundation.

49

bodies lie in the arcuate nucleus and whose axons project to the median eminence. Norepinephrine-containing terminals are also located in this region and in the suprachiasmatic region as well. Alterations in the content and turnover of catecholamines in the catecholaminergic neurons in the arcuate-median eminence region have been reported in the situations associated with altered gonadotropin and prolactin release (12, 13). In the meantime it has become clear that the final common pathway linking the hypothalamus to the pituitary is bridged by a family of neurohormones known as releasing and inhibiting factors (hormones) which are secreted into the hypophyseal portal capillaries in the median eminence and pass down the portal veins to alter release of each and every pituitary hormone (14, 15).

We became interested in reexamining the role of monoamines in the regulation of gonadotropin secretion and set out initially to determine if monamines might actually be releasing factors, if they might potentiate the action of releasing and inhibiting factors at the pituitary level or, finally, if they might act as synaptic transmitters to alter release of the releasing factors from the hypothalamus. Several approaches were used in these studies. The first approach was to examine the effects of monoamines on the release of hormones from pituitaries incubated in vitro and on the releasing factors from ventral hypothalamic fragments incubated in vitro. Then, the effects of these agents in vivo after intraventricular administration were examined, and lastly, the effects of drugs which selectively modify catecholamine and indoleamine synthesis in the hypothalamus were examined to determine the effects of deficiency or excess of monoamines on gonadotropin and prolactin release. Hormones were measured in early in vitro studies by bioassay but in most of the studies radioimmunoassay was used.

EFFECTS OF MONOAMINES ON RELEASE OF HORMONES FROM PITUITARIES INCUBATED IN VITRO

Serotonin, an indoleamine, had no effect on the release of FSH (16) or LH (17) from pituitaries incubated in vitro. Relatively large doses of norepinephrine and epinephrine were capable of stimulating the release of FSH and LH (16, 17). Dopamine had no effect on the release of FSH and LH from pituitaries incubated in vitro but at high does it inactivated both gonadotropins (16, 17). Relatively low doses of dopamine were capable of inhibiting prolactin release from the gland (18). The inhibitory effect of dopamine on prolactin release in vitro is in agreement with other studies (19, 20).

EFFECT OF MONOAMINES ON RELEASE OF RELEASING AND INHIBITING FACTORS FROM VENTRAL HYPOTHALAMIC FRAGMENTS INCUBATED IN VITRO

The coincubation with pituitaries of ventral hypothalamic fragments which included the median eminence and arcuate nucleus plus adjacent hypothalamic tissue produced a slight increase in the release of FSH and LH and a slight decrease in the release of prolactin from the glands, presumably because of the release of gonadotropin releasing factors and prolactin inhibiting factor (PIF) from the fragments (17, 18, 21). When dopamine was added to the incubation medium, it produced a stimualtion of LH and FSH release from the glands and the response was dose-related up to a dose of 2.5 μg of dopamine/ml of medium (Fig. 1). Above this dose the increase in release was less (17, 21). The increase of

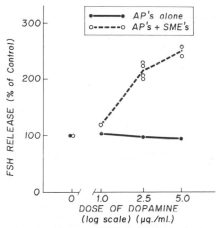

FIG. 1. Effect of dopamine on release of FSH from pituitaries incubated alone or together with stalk-median eminence fragments (21). Each point represents a separate assay. Reproduced by permission from J. B. Lippincott Company.

gonadotropin release provoked by dopamine in the coincubation system appeared to be due to a release of gonadotropin releasing factors from the hypothalamic fragments since dopamine failed to alter the response of the incubated pituitaries to releasing factors. Thus no potentiating action of dopamine on the action of releasing factors was demonstrated. Dopamine also provoked a release of prolactin inhibiting factor (PIF) from the hypothalamic fragments incubated in vitro; however, because of the fact that dopamine also inhibited prolactin release by a direct action on the pituitary, it was necessary to use a blocking drug, haloperidol, to block the action of dopamine at the pituitary level in order to demonstrate the release of PIF from hypothalamic fragments incubated alone in vitro (18). Haloperidol did not block the response of the pituitaries to the PIF which was released.

    In an attempt to define the receptor involved in dopamine-induced release of hypothalamic factors, several adrenergic blocking agents were added to the incubation medium, and it was found that the α-adrenergic blocking drugs, phentolamine and phenoxybenzamine, could block the effect of dopamine on FSH releasing factor (FRF) and/or LH releasing factor (LRF) discharge.

Haloperidol, presumably a blocker of both alpha and dopamine receptors (22), blocked the release of both FRF and LRF; the β blocker, pronethalol, did not interfere with the releasing action of dopamine (17, 21).

EFFECT OF MONOAMINES INJECTED INTO THIRD VENTRICLE ON GONADOTROPIN AND PROLACTIN RELEASE

To determine whether the action of dopamine could be demonstrated in vivo, cannulae were implanted chronically in the third ventricle of rats and monoamines were injected in microliter volumes into the third ventricle. Dopamine was capable of elevating LH as determined by radioimmunoassay in normal male rats, in female rats in late diestrus and proestrus, and in ovariectomized females in which the release of LH had been inhibited by the administration of gonadal steroids (23). No response could be demonstrated in ovariectomized animals in the absence of steroid blockade. The response to dopamine was rapid and quite large in the case of proestrous rats and steroid-blocked, ovariectomized animals.

Norepinephrine was much less effective in elevating plasma LH than dopamine. On the other hand, 5-hydroxytryptamine produced a dramatic inhibition of LH release in the untreated, ovariectomized females (23). There was no clear-cut effect of 5-hydroxytryptamine in rats at various stages of the estrous cycle; however, Kamberi et al. (24) have demonstrated a slight decrease in normal males following the third ventricular injection of the indoleamine. The systemic injection of dopamine had no effect on plasma LH which indicates that the site of action of dopamine in vivo as in vitro is on the hypothalamic-pituitary unit (25).

In order to determine if dopamine was acting to release LRF in vivo as in vitro, the amine was injected into the third ventricle of hypophysectomized rats and the peripheral circulating LRF levels in these animals were assayed in ovariectomized, estrogen- progesterone-blocked rats (25, 26). The hypophysectomized animals had low but detectable levels of circulating LRF which were dramatically elevated within 10 min of the intraventricular injection of dopamine. Kamberi et al. (27) have also demonstrated that intraventricular dopamine can elevate LRF levels in hypophyseal portal blood of anesthetized male rats and that its perfusion into a portal vessel had no effect on LH release in confirmation of the early work indicating that dopamine did not influence LH release from pituitaries incubated in vitro (17).

Dopamine is also capable of elevating FSH levels following its intraventricular injection in anesthetized male rats and this is accompanied by an increase in FRF in portal blood (28). Dopamine again was ineffective when perfused into a portal vessel indicating that it had no effect on the release of FSH from the pituitary itself (28).

The intraventricular injection of dopamine has been found to be capable of lowering the elevated levels of plasma prolactin present in lactating female rats which were suckling their pups (18). Similarily, dopamine lowered prolactin levels in normal male rats and this was accompanied by an increase in PIF levels in hypophyseal portal blood (29). Infusion of dopamine into a hypophyseal portal vessel failed to alter prolactin release (29). This observation is in opposition to the finding that dopamine will reduce prolactin release from pituitaries incubated in vitro (18-20).

Experiments in male rats with different doses of intraventrically administered catecholamines have revealed that dopamine is much more potent than norepinephrine and that epinephrine is the least potent in elevating levels of FSH and LH and in depressing levels of prolactin (24, 28 29), in agreement with the earlier in vitro studies (17,21). On the other hand, Rubinstein and Sawyer (30) found epinephrine to be the most potent drug in inducing ovulation in proestrus rats following its intraventricular administration. Obviously, there is a discrepancy here which has not yet been resolved, but all studies are in agreement that catecholamines can augment gonadotropin and inhibit prolactin release.

EFFECT OF ESTROGEN ON RESPONSE TO DOPAMINE IN VITRO AND IN VIVO

To determine if estrogen might exert some of its feedback actions by blocking the dopaminergic release of LRF, estrogen was added to coincubates of hypothalami and pituitaries in vitro to ascertain if it would alter the response to dopamine (31). Estradiol was found to block the release of LRF provoked by dopamine in vitro. In animals bearing chronic third ventricular cannulae, administration of estradiol into the third ventricle two hours prior to treatment

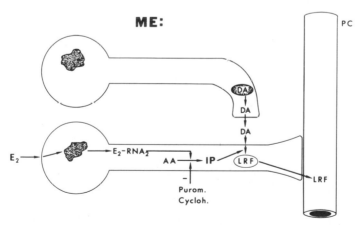

FIG. 2. Schematic representation of a possible cellular mode of action of estradiol (E_2) to reduce LH release by affecting median eminence (ME). Key to symbols: DA = dopamine; E_2-RNA_2 = RNA induced by E_2; AA = amino acids; IP = inhibiting protein or peptide; PC = portal capillary; Purom. = puromycin; Cycloh. = cycloheximide.

with dopamine blocked the increase in LRF observed in saline-injected controls treated with dopamine (25). Since inhibitors of protein synthesis, puromycin and cycloheximide, reversed the estrogen blockage of dopamine action in vitro (31), it was postulated that estrogen was taken up by LRF-secreting neurons and transported to the nucleus where it induced RNA synthesis responsible for the formation of an inhibitory peptide or protein which blocked the action of dopamine in releasing LRF (Fig. 2). This would be analogous to the mechanism of action of estrogen in other target tissues.

EFFECTS OF DRUGS THAT MODIFY BRAIN MONOAMINE CONCENTRATIONS ON PLASMA GONADOTROPIN AND PROLACTIN LEVELS IN THE RAT

DL-α-methyl-tyrosine methyl ester (α-MT) which blocks catecholamine synthesis by inhibiting tyrosine hydroxylase, thereby lowering levels of hypothalamic catecholamines (32) (Fig. 3), produced a dramatic rise in plasma prolactin within

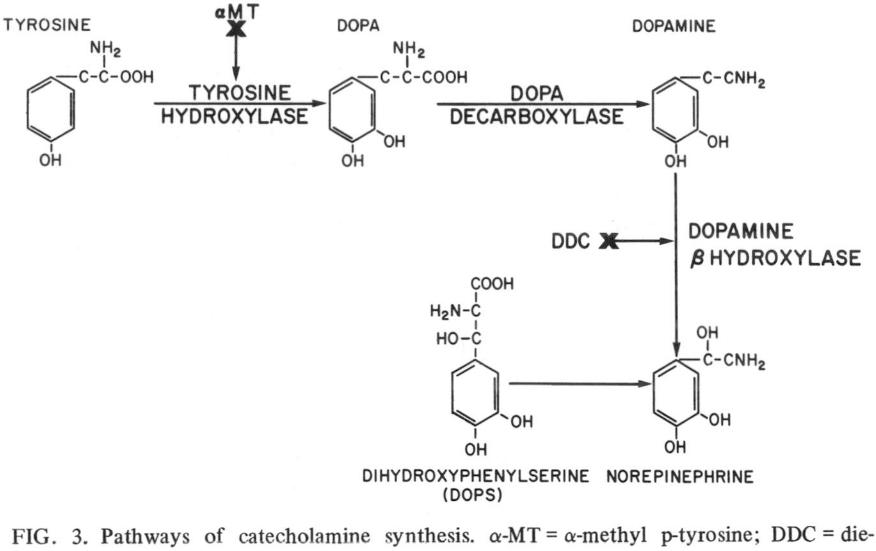

FIG. 3. Pathways of catecholamine synthesis. α-MT = α-methyl p-tyrosine; DDC = diethyldithiocarbamate.

30 min of its injection in castrated rats of either sex (Fig. 4). Treatment with α-MT for four days resulted in continued high levels of plasma prolactin and resulted in an elevation of pituitary prolactin concentration and content. These results indicate that chronic depletion of central catecholamines stimulates not only increased release but also increased synthesis of prolactin.

In order to determine which catecholamine was involved in prolactin release, selective blockade of norepinephrine biosynthesis was accomplished with

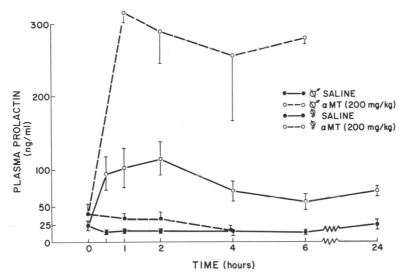

FIG. 4. Effect of α-MT on plasma prolactin (36). Vertical bars = SEM. Reproduced by permission from J. P. Lippincott Company.

diethyldithiocarbamate (DDC), an agent which blocks the conversion of dopamine to norepinephrine by inhibiting dopamine-β-oxidase (33) (Fig. 3). Selective blockade of norepinephrine biosynthesis with DDC failed to alter prolactin levels. Similarly, blockade of serotonin biosynthesis with parachloro-phenylalanine (PCPA) (34) failed to modify plasma levels of prolactin, whether it was administered alone or concomitantly with α-MT. These results indicate that serotonin plays little if any role in the regulation of prolactin release.

When L-dihydroxyphenylalanine (L-DOPA) was administered to elevate brain catecholamines (35), it lowered plasma prolactin. This lowering still occurred if conversion of dopamine to norepinephrine was blocked by prior administration of DDC. Even in animals with elevated plasma prolactin as a result of depletion of catecholamines by α-MT treatment, L-DOPA administration to bypass the block and normalize catecholamine biosynthesis produced a dramatic lowering of plasma prolactin (Fig. 5), which, again, was not prevented by administration of DDC.

In other animals treated with α-MT, dihydroxyphenylserine (DOPS) which normalizes only norepinephrine synthesis leaving a deficit in dopamine (Fig. 3) resulted in a further elevation in prolactin levels (Fig. 5). Treatment of animals with DOPS alone to elevate norepinephrine levels selectively also elevated prolactin.

When monoamine oxidase was inhibited by pargyline to elevate levels of both catecholamines and serotonin by inhibiting their breakdown, there was a lowering of plasma prolactin.

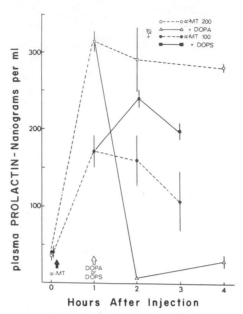

FIG. 5. Effect of ip injection of α-MT (100 or 200 mg/kg) at 0 time on plasma prolactin (36). One hr after α-MT, a catecholamine precursor, DOPA or DOPS, was given ip to reverse the effect of α-MT. Reproduced by permission from J. B. Lippincott Company.

In every case, an expected alteration in brain dopamine was associated with a converse change in prolactin providing strong support for the thesis that dopamine is an inhibitory transmitter which suppresses prolactin release (Table I) (36). The suppression may be mediated by a stimulation of PIF release from the PIF secretory neurons in the hypothalamus. On the other hand, since elevated levels of norepinephrine were found to increase prolactin, it appears possible that norepinephrine may stimulate release of prolactin releasing factor (PRF); however, alternate explanations of these latter findings are possible.

In contrast to the dramatic results observed with prolactin, alterations in levels of central monoamines had little effect on the release of gonadotropins. In the case of FSH, none of the treatments mentioned above produced a significant alteration in the hormone, whereas in the case of LH, lowered levels of norepinephrine produced by administration of DDC were associated with a lowering of plasma levels (36). It is possible that the drugs at the doses used did not produce sufficient changes in central stores of catecholamines to bring out an alteration in the levels of FSH and LH.

Since there was considerable evidence from the early literature to indicate that adrenergic blocking agents could block ovulation (37), it appeared likely that an adrenergic link was involved in the ovulatory surge of gonadotropins and

TABLE I.

Drug	Expected effect on MA activity[a]			Effect on plasma prolactin
	DA	NE	5-HT	
α-MT	−	−	0	+
p-CPA	0	0	−	0
p-CPA + α-MT	−	−	−	+
pargyline	0	+	+	−
α-MT + DOPA	0	0	0	0
DDC	0	−	0	0
DDC + DOPA	+	−	0	−
DDC + DOPS	0	,0	0	0
DOPA	+	+	0	−
DOPS	0	+	0	+

[a] − = decrease,
+ = increase,
0 = no change,
−,0 = decrease followed by return towards normal.

in the stimulatory effect of estrogen and progesterone on gonadotropin release. Progesterone has been shown to evoke a dramatic discharge of FSH and LH in ovariectomized rats which have been pretreated with estrogen (38, 39).

We took this model to study the effect of alterations in central catecholamines on the progesterone-induced stimulation of gonadotropin release. It was first found that the peaks of plasma LH and FSH induced 6 hr after the injection of progesterone were completely abolished by prior treatment with phenoxybenzamine and haloperidol, while the β-adrenergic receptor blocker, propranolol, had no effect (39). These results indicated the involvement of an α-adrenergic receptor mechanism and catecholamines in the transmission of the progesterone stimulus.

Further experiments were performed to identify the catecholamine involved in transmission of this stimulus by using drugs which modify brain catecholamine levels (40). The expected elevations of plasma LH and FSH from progesterone were effectively blocked by administration of α-MT to block synthesis of catecholamines. DDC which blocks the conversion of dopamine to norepinephrine, and 1-phenyl-3-(2-thiazolyl)-2-thiourea (U-14,624, Upjohn) which also blocks conversion of dopamine to norepinephrine, were both effective in blocking the progesterone-induced stimulation of gonadotropin release. Selective resynthesis of norepinephrine by injection of DOPS (Fig. 3) to animals in which norepinephrine synthesis had been blocked either with DDC, or U-14,624 reversed the blockade, whereas treatment with DOPA in these animals to elevate only dopamine failed to reverse the block. These results suggest the involvement of norepinephrine in the transmission of stimulatory effects of progesterone on the release of LH and FSH by an α-adrenergic receptor mechanism.

From the results of all of these experiments, it appears quite clear that adrenergic pathways are involved in the control of gonadotropin and prolactin release. In the case of prolactin, it appears that a dopaminergic inhibitory pathway is involved. It is most reasonable to speculate that this pathway involves the dopaminergic neurons which have cell bodies in the arcuate nucleus and axons which project to the median eminence. Presumably these neurons synapse with the PIF secreting neurons, and, when the pathway is active, a release of PIF occurs which inhibits prolactin discharge. A possible effect of dopamine at the pituitary level cannot be ruled out at this stage in view of the inhibitory effects of dopamine on release of prolactin from pituitaries incubated in vitro.

The situation in the case of the gonadotropins is more complicated. Since it is clear that dopamine can stimulate the release of FRF and LRF both in vitro and in vivo, it is tempting to postulate a dopaminergic transmission to stimulate the discharge of the gonadotropin releasing factors. This may be localized to the same part of the hypothalamus as the dopaminergic inhibitory pathway for prolactin. It would involve the arcuate nucleus-median eminence dopaminergic tract, and activity in these fibers would stimulate the release of both FRF and LRF. This pathway may be involved in the so-called tonic discharge of gonadotropins and in the negative feedback action of gonadal steroids. Evidence is presented here that estrogen can block the response of the LRF neurons to dopamine. These presumed pathways are shown schematically in Fig. 6.

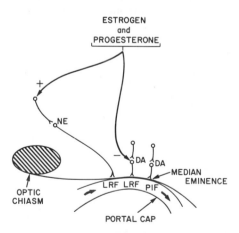

FIG. 6. Schematic representation of possible adrenergic synapses in the hypothalamus affecting discharge of LRF and PIF, and the effect of estrogen and progesterone at these sites.

The stimulatory effects of gonadal steroids which are thought to bring about ovulation in the normal animal are presumably mediated more rostally in the suprachiasmatic region and preoptic area. This conclusion is based upon the fact that lesions in the suprachiasmatic region prevent ovulation (41) and block the progesterone-induced elevation of gonadotropins (42), whereas implantation of estrogen in this area can advance puberty in the rat (43). Moreover, knife cuts which separate the preoptic region from the remainder of the hypothalamus also block ovulation (44). The studies carried out with progesterone-induced gonadotropin release support the hypothesis that an adrenergic synapse is also involved in mediating the stimulatory effect of progesterone on gonadotropin release. In this case it would appear that the transmitter is norepinephrine rather than dopamine on the basis of the pharmacological studies reported here. We would postulate that a similar mechanism may mediate the stimulatory effects of estrogen and that the ovulatory release of gonadotropin is under the control of a noradrenergic synapse (Fig. 6).

REFERENCES

1. Sawyer, C. H., J. E. Markee, and W. H. Hollinshead, Endocrinology 1:395, 1947.
2. Barraclough, C. A., and C. H. Sawyer, Endocrinology 57:32, 1955.
3. Barraclough, C. A., and C. H. Sawyer, Endocrincology 65:563, 1959.
4. Rabinowitz, P., and I. S. Friedman, J Clin Endocrinol 21:1489, 1961.
5. Coppola, J. A., R. G. Leonardi, W. Lippman, J. W. Perrine, and I. Ringler, Endocrinology 77:485, 1965.
6. Mayerson, B. J., and C. H. Sawyer, Endocrinology 83:170, 1968.
7. Kobayashi, T., T. Kobayashi, J. Kato, and H. Minaguchi, Endocrinol Japan 11:283, 1964.
8. Zolovich, A., J. R. Pearse, K. W. Boehlke, and B. E. Eleftheriou, Science 154:649, 1966.
9. Donoso, A. O., and M. B. De Gutierrez Moyano, Proc Soc Exp Biol Med 135:633, 1970.
10. Donoso, A. O., M. B. De Gutierrez Moyano, and R. Santolaya, Neuroendocrinology 4:12, 1969.
11. Coppola, J.A., Neuroendocrinology 5:75, 1969.
12. Fuxe, K., and T. Hökfelt, in W. F. Ganong and L. Martini (Eds.), Frontiers in Neuroendocrinology, Oxford, New York, 1969, p. 47.
13. Lichtensteiger, W., Progr Histo Chem Cytochem 1:185, 1970.
14. McCann, S. M., and J. C. Porter, Physiol Rev 49:240, 1969.
15. Meites, J. (Ed.), Hypophysiotropic Hormones of the Hypothalamus, Assay and Chemistry, Williams and Wilkins, Baltimore, 1970.
16. Kamberi, I. A., and S. M. McCann, Endocrinology 85:815, 1969.
17. Schneider, H. P. G., and S. M. McCann, Endocrinology 85:121, 1969.
18. Kuhn, E., L. Krulich, M. Quijada, P. Illner, P. S. Kalra, and S. M. McCann, Program of the 52nd Meeting of the Endocrine Society, St. Louis, Missouri, 1970, p. 126.
19. Macleod, R. M., Endocrinolgoy 85:916, 1969.

20. Birge, C. A., L. S. Jacobs, C. T. Hammeo, and W. H. Daughaday, Endocrinology 86:120, 1970.

21. Kamberi, I. A., H. P. G. Schneider, and S. M. McCann, Endocrinology 86:278, 1970.

22. Anden, N. E., A. Carlsson, and J. Haggendal, Ann Rev Pharmacol 9:119, 1969.

23. Schneider, H. P. G., and S. M. McCann, Endocrinology 86:1127, 1970.

24. Kamberi, I. A., R. S. Mical, and J. C. Porter, Endocrinology 87:1, 1970.

25. Schneider, H. P. G., and S. M. McCann, Endocrinology 87:249, 1970.

26. Schneider, H. P. G., and S. M. McCann, J Endocrinol 46:401, 1970.

27. Kamberi, I. A., R. S. Mical, and J. C. Porter, Science 166:388, 1969.

28. Kamberi, I. A., R. S. Mical, and J. C. Porter, Endocrinology 88:1003, 1971.

29. Kamberi, I. A., R. S. Mical, and J. C. Porter, Endocrinology 88:1012, 1971.

30. Rubinstein, L., and C. H. Sawyer, Endocrinology 86:988, 1970.

31. Schneider, H. P. G., and S. M. McCann, Endocrinology 87:330, 1970.

32. Spector, S., A. Sjoerdsma, and S. Udenfriend, J Pharmacol Exp Ther 147:86, 1965.

33. Carlsson, A., K. Fuxe, T. Hökfelt, and M. Lindqvist, J Pharmacol 18:60, 1966.

34. Koc, B. K., and A. Weissman, J Pharmacol Exp Ther 154:499, 1966.

35. Corrodi, H., and L. C. F. Hanson, Psychopharmacologia 10:116, 1966.

36. Donoso, A. O., W. Bishop, C. P. Fawcett, L. Krulich, and S. M. McCann, Endocrinology, 89:774, 1971.

37. Everett, J. W., Physiol Rev 44:373, 1964.

38. Caligaris, L., J. J. Astrada, and S. Taleisnik, Acta Endocrinol 59:177, 1968.

39. Kalra, P. S., L. Krulich, M. Quijada, S. P. Kalra, and C. P. Fawcett, Program of the 52nd Meeting of the Endocrine Society, St. Louis, Missouri, 1970, p. 126.

40. Kalra, P. S., Program of the 53rd Meeting of the Endocrine Society, San Francisco, California, 1971, p. 78.

41. McCann, S. M., A. P. S. Dhariwal, and J. C. Porter, Ann Rev Physiol 30:589, 1968.

42. Bishop, W., P. S. Kalra, and S. M. McCann, unpublished observation, 1970.

43. Smith, E. R., and J. M. Davidson, Endocrinology 82:100, 1968.

44. Halasz, B., and R. A. Gorski, Endocrinology 80:608, 1967.

DISCUSSION

B. LUNENFELD. Dr. Phifer has shown that the "gonadotropin producing cells" in the pituitary react both with anti-FSH and anti-LH. I would like to ask Dr. Phifer whether his anti-FSH cross-reacted with either subunit of LH and whether his anti-LH reacted with the α or β subunit of FSH. Since during biosynthesis of the gonadotropins, subunits might be present in the cells, I wonder whether you have established that such cross-reactions do not occur?

R. F. PHIFER. As a matter of fact we did. Dr. Saxena was kind enough to send us some of his α and β subunits of human FSH and LH. We did not obtain as big a differential as we did with the whole hormone preparations in each case, but in the case of LH, β subunit virtually abolished all immunostaining of the LH antiserum, while the same amount of α subunit of LH did not. The same was true for FSH antiserum and FSH subunits. We were not able to obtain big differentials with the subunits of the opposite gonadotropin. Thus, whereas a certain amount of β subunit of LH virtually abolished all immunostaining obtained with LH antiserum, eight times more of α or β subunits of FSH, although not completely abolishing immunostaining, still markedly decreased it. The same was relatively true for FSH antiserum and increasing amounts of LH subunits. The point is that each antiserum appeared to react predominantly with its antigen's β chain, as might be expected from antisera specific for each gonadotropin.

M. S. AMOSS. Dr. Phifer, several years ago Dr. Paul Nakane working on a similar system with Dr. Midgley, visited our laboratory. In some of his preliminary work he reported that the central core of the pituitary had cells in which granules containing both FSH and LH were present. If I remember correctly, he mentioned that as one looks at cells closer to the periphery, they seem to preferentially contain LH. Were you aware of the study or has any more been done?

R. F. PHIFER. I do not think he has done any more. A great deal of caution has to be taken in dealing with the gland's periphery, especially in terms of fixative penetration. We have stained 20 to 30 human pituitaries and noted no differential distribution except in cases where the glands were not well fixed. When we did not allow the fixative to go in long enough, there was intense immunostaining for both FSH and LH peripherally, whereas the center of the gland was not fixed and did not immunostain.

A. R. MIDGLEY. The antisera that Dr. Nakane used in his study have since been examined in the same type of system that Dr. Phifer just described, in other words, determining whether the antisera would bind electrophoretically isolated, labeled LH and FSH of rat origin. These studies have indicated the presence of some cross-reaction with those particular antisera. Therefore, I cannot be certain that Dr. Nakane independently localized the two hormones. Steroids can influence the ratio of LH to FSH in the pituitary gland and thus it would not be surprising to find, under appropriate conditions, some cells which have predominantly FSH and others which have predominantly LH. The point being made is that both hormones can be found within the same cell. I think this conclusion is going to hold up. Recent studies in our laboratory using well-characterized antisera indicate that rat LH and FSH can each be found in the same cell.

L. MARTINI. I want to make a comment on Dr. McCann's paper. I think we should not disregard acetylcholine as a possible trigger for the release of LH-RF and FSH-RF. Using an in vitro system similar to the one which Dr. McCann proposed a few years ago, we have recently found that the addition of acetylcholine to the incubation media containing hypothalamic fragments and anterior pituitary tissue brings about a tremendous secretion of both LH and FSH; this pehnomenon can be abolished by the addition of atropine to the system. It is interesting that acetylcholine does not do anything when added to incubation media containing only anterior pituitary tissue. This implies that acetylcholine releases the gonadotropin releasing factors from the hypothalamic fragments, which in turn induce the secretion of LH and FSH from the anterior pituitary tissue. The presence of the hypothalamus is therefore necessary for the secretion of anterior pituitary hormones. The work on LH was performed in my laboratory by Dr. F. Fiorindo and that on FSH by Dr. I. Simonovic.

M. S. AMOSS.   I guess I have to ask the obvious question, Dr. Arimura. You mentioned a synthetic molecule that would release LH. We would like to know a little more about this molecule, especially its amino acid sequence.

A. ARIMURA. The chemistry of LH-RH in detail will be presented in San Francisco during the Endocrine Society meeting. However, Dr. Matsuo, who has been engaged in the amino acid sequence and synthesis of this material, may like to comment.

H. MATSUO. The data on synthetic LH-RH which Dr. Arimura presented today is the first evidence that the structure of LH-RH is correct. I think this is the first synthetic peptide which shows real LH-RH activity.

M. S. AMOSS. Dr. Matsuo, I have two comments. One to ask you if you can tell us whether the peptides that Dr. Arimura showed on the slide do in fact represent native LRF. Is that true?

H. MATSUO. Yes, it is.

M. S. AMOSS. Might I draw the conclusion then that you are injecting this material in doses of 2.5 to 10 μg. We know, from the use of TRF as a model, that the nanogram range constitutes an active dose. I would have to conclude at least on the basis of the present information that this could not in fact be native LRF.

H. MATSUO. Dr. Amoss is asking why we have to use such a large dose like 10 μg for inducing ovulation? The dosage which Dr. Arimura used in his experiment was expressed as dry weight but no actual content of LH-RH. We purified the synthetic peptide by countercurrent distribution and electrophoresis. The purified LH-RF which Dr. Arimura used in the present study was chromatographically and electrophoretically homogeneous and identical with natural LH-RH. This sample, however, still had some contamination with cellulose and nonpeptide material.

F. C. GREENWOOD. Question to Dr. McCann: Can you tell me what happens to the prolactin in the model system of estrogen-progesterone LH release?

S. M. MCCANN. You touched on a sensitive point there because we have not really got that well worked out yet and, therefore, I did not want to talk about it. This is an ovariectomized animal injected with a single priming dose of 5 μg of estradiol benzoate and progesterone two days later. In that animal the prolactin level is already elevated as a response to the initial estrogen injection. We are not really prepared to say yet, exactly what happens to prolactin when we use the various agents that alter central levels of catecholamines.

E. KNOBIL. Progesterone seems to reduce the sensitivity of the pituitary to any given dose of LRH. I would like to ask Dr. Arimura why he uses an estrogen-progesterone primed rat as the test animal to measure the biological activity on his LH-RH preparations.

A. ARIMURA. The suppression by progesterone on LH release by LH-RH could be related to dose as suggested by Sawyer's group. Therefore, if the LH-RH exceeds a certain limit, progesterone's suppressive effect cannot be observed. In our previous studies using ovariectomized, estrogen-progesterone treated animals, we reported that progesterone did not suppress LH release induced by LH-RH. This animal preparation is, however, supersensitive to LH-RH so that the dose of LH-RH used in that experiment may already have exceeded the threshold dose of LH-RH. Similar results were observed in normal animals using a large dose of LH-RH. As I have shown here in normal rats, progesterone even in a very large dose of 5 mg did not block the LH-RH-induced LH release, but the combined administration of progesterone and estrogen could block the LH release.

6. On the Mechanism of Action of the Hypothalamic Gonadotropin Releasing Factors

Marian Jutisz, Bernard Kerdelhue, Annette Berault, and M. Paloma de la Llosa

The regulation of the gonadotropic function of the anterior pituitary gland is controlled by two hypothalamic principles, LH releasing factor (LRF) and FSH releasing factor (FRF). Highly purified preparations of the two releasing factors (RFs) from different species have been obtained (1-3). Recently, Schally et al. (4) reported the isolation from porcine hypothalamic extracts of a polypeptide which has both LRF and FRF activity. In these authors' opinion, this peptide represents the hypothalamic hormone which controls the secretion of both LH and FSH from the pituitary.

In this laboratory, partially purified preparations of LRF (5) and FRF (6) from ovine material have been obtained. It appeared, on the basis of in vitro assays, that each one of these preparations contained both activities but in a given preparation one of the activities was always predominant. Only isolation of both activities in homogeneous state will answer the question of their unity or duality. For the time being, we will admit the existence of two chemically different entities, one carrying LRF and another FRF activity.

Most of the work on the mechanism of action of RFs was done using in vitro procedures in which halves of rat pituitary glands were incubated in a Krebs-Ringer-bicarbonate-glucose buffer (KRB) saturated with $93\% O_2/7\% CO_2$. The development in our laboratory of radioimmunoassays (RIA) for rat LH (7) has provided a sensitive and precise technique for assaying these gonadotropins in plasma, in incubation media, and in tissues. In our standard in vitro method, four hemipituitaries/flask were incubated as described elsewhere (8). Ten μl of media were withdrawn at 30- to 60-min periods during the incubation and were stored frozen until assayed. Results are expressed in terms of a highly purified rat LH laboratory reference preparation (S15 B, mean potency: 0.95 X NIH-LH-S1).

For the assay of adenyl cyclase three types of experiments were performed. In experiment 1, homogenates of the anterior pituitaries of male rats (3 mg) were incubated in a Tris buffer for 15 min at 37C, according to Chase and Aurbach (9). Different substances tested were added into incubation media and cyclic adenosine 3',5'-monophosphate (cAMP) generated during the incubation was assayed according to Krishna and Birnbaumer (10). In experiment 2, whole male rat pituitary glands were incubated for 30 min in a Tris buffer as previously, either in the presence of LRF or NaF. In experiment 3, male rat hemipituitaries were incubated during a 4-hr period in a KRB medium in the presence of LRF or in a high [K$^+$] KRB. At the end of the incubation, tissues were ground and aliquots corresponding to about 1 mg of tissue were incubated in the presence of ^{32}P-ATP for the assay of adenyl cyclase as indicated above.

For the incorporation studies, pituitary halves of ovariectomized rats treated with estradiol benzoate and progesterone (EBP rats) were incubated for 1 hr either in a KRB medium without or with LRF (0.4 μg/mg tissue). After this period of time, the media were replaced by new media containing the same substances plus 2.5 μCi/ml of ^{3}H-L-leucine (at 35 Ci/mM) and incubation proceeded for a further 1.5 hr. In some cases, after this second period, the media were again replaced as above and incubations took place for another 1.5-hr period. In another experiment, pituitaries of ovariectomized rats were incubated as above for 1-hr + 1.5-hr + 1.5-hr periods. At the end of the incubation, pituitaries were ground, extracted and total LH was assayed in these extracts using RIA. Then aliquots of the extracts corresponding to a constant amount of LH were withdrawn. LH was precipitated using the double antibody technique as in RIA and the radioactivity of the tritiated LH was counted in a liquid scintillation spectrometer.

CELLULAR MECHANISM OF ACTION OF LRF AND FRF

The mechanism of action of hypothalamic releasing factors has been studied in several laboratories during the past few years. Well documented reviews have recently been published on this subject (11-14). As time and space are limited, we shall only discuss the two main problems developed in our research: first, the possibility of cyclic AMP being an intermediate of the releasing action of RFs, and second, some evidence against a direct participation of RFs in the mechanism by which FSH and LH are synthesized.

Cyclic AMP as Intermediate of the Releasing Action of RFs

The following arguments are in favor of the participation of cAMP in the mechanism of action of RFs.

1. Cyclic AMP, like FRF and LRF, is able to release FSH and LH <u>in vitro</u> from rat pituitaries, giving rise to a similar log dose-response curve. On the other hand, theophylline, by inhibiting the destruction of cAMP by phosphodiesterase, significantly potentiates the response of pituitary tissue to both FRF and LRF (8, 15).

2. NaF which activates adenyl cyclase (16), also stimulates the release of LH. Fig. 1 shows the results of an experiment in which one pair of four

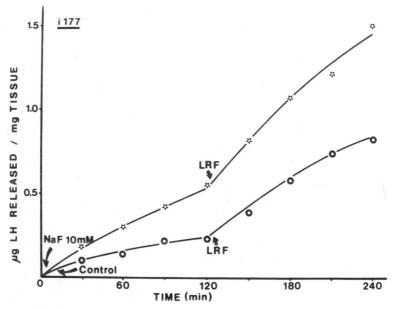

FIG. 1. Kinetics of the <u>in vitro</u> response to NaF and LRF of pituitaries of EBP rats. One group of hemipituitaries was incubated in a 10mM NaF-KRB medium and another in normal KRB. After a 2-hr period, LRF (4 μg/ml) was added to each flask and incubation continued for a further 2 hr.

hemipituitaries of EBP rats was incubated, one group in KRB in which 10mM of NaCl were replaced by 10mM of NaF, and another in normal KRB. After a 2-hr period, LRF (4 μg/ml) was added to each flask and incubation continued for a further 2 hr. It is evident from this experiment, that NaF alone stimulates the release of LH and that it potentiates the action of LRF.

3. LRF activates <u>in vitro</u> adenyl cyclase of pituitary tissue. Adenyl cyclase was assayed in pituitaries of male rats incubated in 3 different manners:

1) pituitary homogenates incubated for 15 min in a Tris buffer (9); 2) whole pituitaries incubated for 30 min in the same way, and 3) hemipituitaries incubated for 4 hr in a KRB buffer. It can be concluded from the results shown in Table I that: 1) adenyl cyclase of homogenates is not activated during 15 min incubation with LRF nor with 59mM [K$^+$] but is activated with 10mM NaF and crude hypothalamic extract; 2) adenyl cyclase of whole pituitaries is activated during 15 min incubation either with LRF or with NaF; and 3) adenyl cyclase of hemipituitaries incubated for 4 hr is activated by LRF but is not activated by 59mM [K$^+$] KRB.

TABLE I. Effect of various treatments on adenylcyclase activity in male rat anterior pituitaries incubated in different conditions

Experiment	Conditions of incubation	Treatment	Adenyl cyclase activity cpm^{32}P-cyclic AMP prod/mg tissue[a]
1	Homogenate, 15 min, 37C Tris buffer pH 7.4 (cf. 9)	Control	87 ± 27
		LRF, 0.3 µg/mg	75 ± 20
		LRF, 1.7 µg/mg	72 ± 6
		59 mM K$^+$	76 ± 7
		10 mM NaF	392 ± 46
		Control	41 ± 9
		Crude hypothal extract, 37 µg/mg	120 ± 49
		Idem, 185 µg/mg	243 ± 68
2	Whole pituitaries, 30 min, 37C, Tris buffer pH 7.4 (cf. 9)[b]	Control	183 ± 67
		LRF, 0.4 µg/mg	260 ± 43
		10 mM NaF	9527 ± 3436
		Control	320 ± 23
		LRF, 1.2 µg/mg	607 ± 175
3	Hemipituitaries, 4 hr, 37C, KRB medium	Control	533 ± 159
		LRF, 0.18 µg/mg	652 ± 157
		LRF, 0.36 µg/mg	733 ± 359
		LRF, 1.80 µg/mg	1310 ± 108
		Control	487 ± 127
		59 mM K$^+$ - KRB	478 ± 216

[a]The results are the average ± SEM of triplicate determinations.

[b]In experiment 2 the results are given as cpm/pituitary.

RFs and In Vitro Synthesis of Gonadotropins.

The results previously reported from our laboratory (cf. 17) showed that: 1) the total amounts (tissues + medium) of FSH significantly increase during 2-hr and 4-hr incubations of hemipituitaries of EBP rats in the presence of FRF; 2) FSH also increases after incubation of pituitaries in normal KRB containing cAMP (0.3mM) or after incubation in 59mM [K⁺] KRB; and 3) LH does not increase after incubation of pituitaries in a high [K⁺] medium. These results led us to the conclusion that synthesis of FSH is not under direct control of FRF but that synthesis of LH may be a complex phenomenon.

We now report some new data on the incorporation of ^{3}H-leucine into LH synthesized during incubation of the pituitaries of ovariectomized rats and EBP rats. The results recorded in Table II show that: 1) there is a very discreet, if any, increase of total LH after 1.5- and 3-hr incubations of pituitaries of ovariectomized rats and EBP rats; and 2) LRF has either a very discreet or no action on the incorporation of ^{3}H-leucine into LH isolated from both types of pituitaries.

It now seems well established that RFs exert their primary effects on the release of gonadotropins from the pituitary gland. As this effect on the release is not abolished by inhibitors of either protein or RNA synthesis, it is postulated that the mechanism of release does not involve de novo synthesis of any protein or nucleic acid. Many results are in favor of an action of RFs on a membrane receptor which activates adenyl cyclase. Cyclic AMP is therefore a mediator of the action of LRF and FRF. Zor et al. (18, 19) have already shown that a crude hypothalamic extract stimulates adenyl cyclase activity in vitro either in homogenates of rat anterior pituitary glands or in whole pituitaries. Our results (Table I) confirm this data. They show furthermore that purified LRF does not activate adenyl cyclase in homogenates of pituitaries but only in whole pituitaries or hemipituitaries. It is not easy to explain why LRF does not stimulate formation of cyclic AMP in pituitary homogenates; maybe in the conditions used, the hormonal receptor was in some way disconnected from the site of activation of adenyl cyclase as was already shown in the case of the adenyl cyclase system in plasma membranes isolated from rat liver (20). The fact that fluoride ion activated adenyl cyclase in homogenates and LRF did not, suggests that they act at separate sites.

How cyclic AMP promotes release of gonadotropins is still unknown. Two recent theories can be considered in particular: cyclic AMP may stimulate specific protein kinases (21) and thus act on phosphorylation of microtubules; this step is considered as an initial event in vesicle secretion (22). The relationship between secretory vesicles, microtubules, and the plasma membrane must ultimately be determined. Rasmussen and Tenenhouse (23) consider cyclic AMP and Ca^{2+} as key elements in most of the releasing processes induced by hormones. They postulate that cyclic AMP acts either by altering the permeability of the membrane to Ca^{2+} or by affecting the binding of Ca^{2+} to

TABLE II.   Incorporation of ^{3}H-leucine into LH during incubation of rat pituitaries[3]

Experiment	Treatment	Total LH[b]		Labeled LH	
		μg/mg tissue	% Control	Ci/30.000 g LH	% Control
Pituitaries of EBP rats incubated for 1.5 hr					
1.	Control	7.73		37.3	
	LRF (0.4 μg/mg)	8.24	106	26.8	72
2.	Control	4.89		2.0	
	LRF (0.4 μg/mg)	4.88	100	2.6	130
Pituitaries of EBP rats incubated for 3 hr (media replaced after 1.5 hr)					
1.	Control	8.13		40.0	
	LRF (0.4 μg/mg)	8.31	102	80.0	200
2.	Control	4.16		9.5	
	LRF (0.4 μg/mg)	4.44	106	10.1	106
Pituitaries of ovariectomized rats incubated for 3 hr (media replaced after 1.5 hr)					
1.	Control	6.00		26.3	
	LRF (0.4 μg/mg)	6.40	106	33.4	127
2.	Control	4.60		6 1	
	LRF (0.4 μg/mg)	4.98	108	6.7	110

[a]Total LII was assayed (tissues + supernatant) using RIA, then LH was isolated from aliquots of tissue extracts using double antibody technique and radioactivity of labeled LH was counted.

[b]In terms of NIH-LH-S1.

membranes (11). This hypothesis is mainly based on the theory advanced by Douglas and Rubin (24) which postulated that the role of a stimulus for secretion is to modify the permeability of the plasma membrane to Ca^{2+} and Na^+. It is the increase of Ca^{2+} in the cell which promotes the secretory process. Indeed, it was shown that the presence of Ca^{2+} in the external medium is necessary for in vitro LH (25) and FSH (26) release. As to the exact role of Ca^{2+} in the release process, several hypotheses can be formulated (11, 12). Ca^{2+} intervenes in many intracellular enzymatic processes and it is probable that Ca^{2+} or Ca^{2+} and cyclic

AMP either activate protein kinases (22) or provoke conformational modifications in membrane proteins participating in the release mechanism.

An additional finding supports the hypothesis of a central role of Ca^{2+} in the release process, in other words, the fact that a high $[K^+]$ in the external medium can function as a nonspecific stimulus for release of either LH (25) or FSH (27). This effect of high $[K^+]$ is also inhibited when incubation is performed in Ca^{2+}-free medium containing EDTA (25, 26). Therefore this process requires Ca^{2+}, as does the release stimulated by an RF. One could have postulated that elevated $[K^+]$ activates the adenyl cyclase system, but it was shown that this is not true in the case of the pituitary tissue (19, see also Table I). The effect of high $[K^+]$ can best be attributed to an action on the increase in intracellular $[Ca^{2+}]$, as a high $[K^+]$ medium has been shown to markedly enhance the uptake of $^{45}Ca^{2+}$ by the posterior pituitary gland (28).

Do releasing factors have a direct action on the synthesis of gonadotropins? The results previously obtained in our laboratory (13, 14) showed that the total amount of FSH increased significantly over that of controls when pituitaries of EBP rats, or male rats, were incubated either with FRF, or with cAMP (025mM) or in a high $[K^+]$ medium. The synthesis of FSH did not occur in Ca^{2+}-free media (26, 17). These results led us to the conclusion that FRF has no direct action on the synthesis of FSH, as the synthesis is also enhanced by incubation with cyclic AMP or in a high $[K^+]$ medium.

The situation with LH was slightly different. Samli and Geschwind (29) reported that in a 4-hr incubation, crude hypothalamic extract had no effect on the incorporation of either ^{14}C-leucine or ^{14}C-glucosamine into LH. The absence of Ca^{2+} did not inhibit, nor did high $[K^+]$ stimulate, the incorporation of ^{14}C-leucine into LH. Using in our work a biological assay method of LH (17), we did not find any significant difference between the total amount of LH in the controls and in the pituitaries incubated either with LRF or in a high $[K^+]$ medium. In agreement with the data obtained in the two laboratories, our recent results, recorded in Table II, show that although there is some de novo synthesis of LH in pituitary tissues of both ovariectomized and EBP rats, LRF has either a very discret or no action on incorporation of ^{3}H-leucine into LH.

Thus although no difference was observed in the mechanisms by which the two gonadotropins are released, serious differences seem to exist between processes inducing synthesis of FSH and LH. Further research is still necessary to find out whether these differences are apparent or real.

REFERENCES

1. Schally, A. V., A. Arimura, C. Y. Bowers, A. J. Kastin, S. Sawano, and T. W., Redding, Rec Progr Hormone Res 24:497, 1968.
2. Burgus, R., and R. Guillemin, Ann Rev Biochem 39:499, 1970.
3. Jutisz, M., in E. Rosemberg and C. A. Paulsen (Eds.), The Human Testis, Plenum, New York, 1970, p. 207.

4. Schally, A. V., A. Arimura, Y. Baba, R. M. G. Nair, H. Matsuo, T. W. Redding, L. Debeljuk, and W. F. White, Biochem Biophys Res Commun 43:393, 1971.

5. Jutisz, M., A. Berault, M.-A. Novella, and G. Ribot, Acta Endocrinol (Kubh) 55:481, 1967.

6. Jutisz, M., and M. P. de la Llosa, Endocrinology 81:1193, 1967.

7. Kerdelhue, B., A. Berault, C. Courte, and M. Jutisz, CR Acad Sci Ser D 269:2413, 1969.

8. Jutisz, M., B. Kerdelhue, and A. Berault, in E. Rosemberg and C. A. Paulsen (Eds.), The Human Testis, Plenum, New York, 1970, p. 221.

9. Chase, L. R., and G. D. Aurbach, Science 159:545, 1968.

10. Krishna, G., and L. Birnbaumer, Anal Biochem 35:393, 1970.

11. Geschwind, I. I., in J. Meites, (Ed.), Hypophysiotropic Hormones of the Hypothalamus: Assay and Chemistry, Williams & Wilkins, Baltimore, 1970, p. 298.

12. Geschwind, I. I., in E. Rosemberg and C. A. Paulsen (Eds.), The Human Testis, Plenum, New York, 1970, p. 171.

13. Jutisz, M., M. P. de la Llosa, A. Berault, and B. Kerdelhue in L. Martini, M. Motta, and F. Fraschini (Eds.), The Hypothalamus, Academic, New York, 1970, p. 293.

14. Jutisz, M., J Neuro-Visceral Relations, Suppl X:22, 1971.

15. Jutisz, M., and M. P. de la Llosa, C R Acad Sci Ser D 268:1636, 1969.

16. Sutherland, E. W., T. W. Rall, and T. Menon, J Biol Chem 237:1220, 1962.

17. Jutisz, M., M. P. de la Llosa, A. Berault, and B. Kerdelhue, Proceedings of the Colloque de Neuroendocrinologie of the C.N.R.S. No. 927, Paris, 1970, p. 287.

18. Zor, U., T. Kaneko, H. P. G. Schneider, S. M. McCann, I. P. Lowe, G. Bloom, B. Borland, and J. B. Field, Proc Nat Acad Sci USA 63:918, 1969.

19. Zor, U., T. Kaneko, H. P. G. Schneider, S. M. McCann, and J. B. Field, J Biol Chem 245:2883, 1970.

20. Birnbaumer, L., S. L. Pohl, and M. Rodbell, J Biol Chem 246:1857, 1971.

21. Walsh, D. A., J. P. Perkins, and E. G. Krebs, J Biol Chem 243:3763, 1968.

22. Goodman, D. B. P., H. Rasmussen, F. Dibella, and C. E. Guthrow, Jr., Proc Nat Acad Sci USA 67:652, 1970.

23. Rasmussen, H., and A. Tenenhouse, Proc Nat Acad Sci USA 59:1364, 1968.

24. Douglas, W. W., and R. P. Rubin, J Physiol (London) 167:288, 1963.

25. Samli, M. H. and I. I. Geschwind, Endocrinology 82:225, 1968.

26. Jutisz, M., and M. P. de la Llosa, Endocrinology 86:761, 1970.

27. Jutisz, M., and M. P. de la Llosa, Bull Soc Chim Biol 50:2521, 1968.

28. Douglas, W. W., and A. P. Poisner, J Physiol (London) 172:19, 1964.

29. Samli, M. H. and I. I. Geschwind, Endocrinology 81:835, 1967.

7. Role of Estrogen in the Positive and Negative Feedback Control of LH Secretion During the Menstrual Cycle of the Rhesus Monkey

E. Knobil, D. J. Dierschke[1], T. Yamaji[2], F. J. Karsch[2], J. Hotchkiss, and R. F. Weick[2]

The time course of circulating luteinizing hormone (LH) during the menstrual cycle of the rhesus monkey (1), like that of man, is characterized by low, relatively constant levels interrupted, once every 28 days on the average, by abrupt elevations in the concentration of the hormone lasting two to three days (Fig. 1). By analogy to the schema postulated for the rat (2), these circulating levels of LH in primates may be thought of as resultants of tonic secretion and intermittant, or cyclic, discharges of the hormone, the latter eventuating in ovulation some 24 to 36 hours later.

NEGATIVE FEEDBACK CONTROL OF TONIC LH SECRETION.

It has been recognized for several decades that LH secretion in primates is under negative feedback control by the gonadal hormones, but the dynamics and other details of this control system have become apparent only recently with the

[1] Special Fellow of the National Institute of Child Health and Human Development (1 FO3 HD 19799).

[2] Fellow of the Ford Foundation.

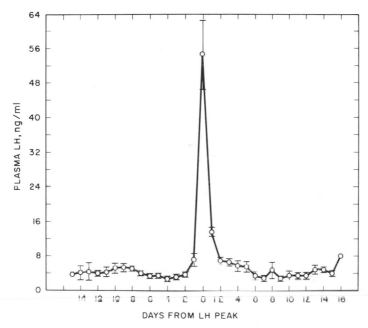

FIG. 1. Time course of plasma LH concentrations during the menstrual cycle of the rhesus monkey (1). These data from 9 normal cycles are normalized to the day of the LH peak. Reproduced by permission of J. B. Lippincott Company.

advent of radioimmunoassay and kindred techniques for the measurement of the gonadotropins and gonadal steroids in peripheral plasma.

Interruption of the negative feedback loop by gonadectomy results, within 2 days, in a significant increase in plasma LH concentration. Circulating levels of this hormone continue to rise until they reach a plateau at approximately 10 times the initial basal concentrations in about 20 days after the operation (3). The functioning of this negative feedback system is considerably delayed in sexually immature animals, even in immediately premenarchial females in which estrogens are clearly measurable at the time of ovariectomy (4).

In chronically ovariectomized female monkeys, the elevated plasma LH concentrations are not the result of continuous high rates of LH secretion as initially supposed. Rather, they represent the intergration of pulsatile discharges of LH from the pituitary with a mean frequency of one LH burst/hr, hence the appelation "circhoral" (5). This striking phenomenon, which we have not been able to observe in intact animals as yet, is illustrated in Fig. 2.

The administration of estradiol-17β by single, intravenous injection resulting in brief elevations of circulating estrogen (Fig. 3), interrupts the pulsatile discharges of LH with a consequent decline in mean plasma LH concentrations (6). It is noteworthy that the pulsatile discharges are inhibited long after the

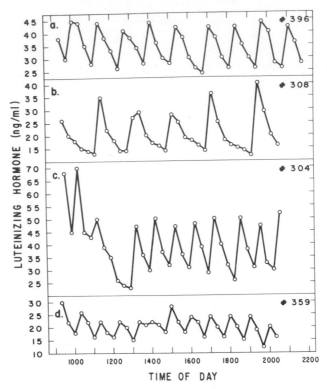

FIG. 2. Circhoral patterns of plasma LH concentrations in 4 ovariectomized rhesus monkeys (5). Reproduced by permission of J. B. Lippincott Company.

circulating levels of estrogen have returned to unmeasurable levels. Furthermore, the duration of inhibition appears to be directly related to the magnitude of the estrogen pulse (6). This sustained response to a brief exposure of the system to estrogen is probably indicative of an initial steroid-receptor interaction (7) which entrains subsequent intracellular events leading to an inhibition of gonadotropin secretion.

That more physiologic increments in plasma estrogen concentrations have the same effect is shown in Fig. 4. In these studies (6), circulating estrogens were increased from nondetectable levels to those characteristic of the early follicular phase of the cycle (8), or less, where they were maintained by constant infusion. In most of these experiments, the resumption of pulsatile LH secretion, even after prolonged periods of quiescence, was remarkably abrupt. Notably, however, these reinitiated oscillations were usually of lower frequency and of larger magnitude than those during the control period. When similarly low plasma estrogen concentrations (~50 pg/ml) were maintained chronically over a period of several months by subcutaneously implanted Silastic capsules

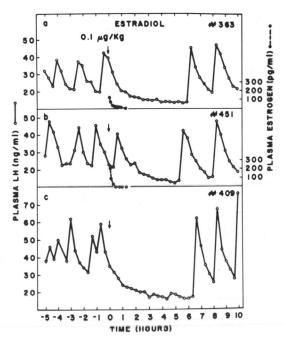

FIG. 3. Effects of single intravenous injections of estradiol-17β (arrows) on circulating LH patterns in ovariectomized rhesus monkeys.

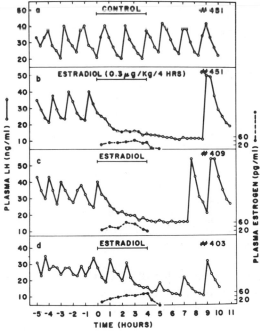

FIG.4. Effects of estradiol-17β infusions (horizontal lines) on circulating LH patterns in ovariectomized rhesus monkeys.

containing estradiol-17β, a procedure which permits the control of circulating estrogen levels in ovariectomized monkeys as precisely as constant infusion pumps, the resulting LH concentrations were maintained, over these same periods, at concentrations characteristic of the follicular phase of the cycle (9).

The acute closure of the negative feedback loop by estrogen injection as described above is mimicked, in every detail, by single doses also injected intravenously, of chlorpromazine, haloperidol, and of the α-adrenergic blocking agents phenoxybenzamine or phentolamine (6). Fig. 5 illustrates the striking similarity between the action of estradiol and phenoxybenzamine in their inhibitory effects on pulsatile LH secretion. The β-blocker propanolol on the other hand, even in extremely high doses, was totally ineffective in this regard (6). Similarly, deep sodium pentobarbital anesthesia, which effectively inhibits growth hormone secretion in the rhesus monkey (10) failed to interfere with the oscillatory discharge of LH in ovariectomized animals (6).

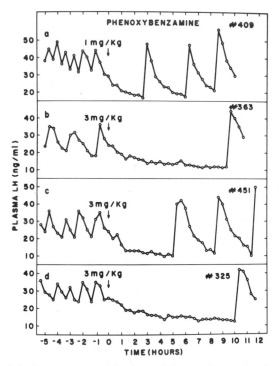

FIG. 5. Effects of single, intravenous injections of phenoxybenzamine (arrows) on plasma LH concentrations in ovariectomized rhesus monkeys.

It should also be mentioned in this regard that the infusion of ovine and human LH as well as of HCG into ovariectomized monkeys, with resultant "physiological" or "supraphysiologic" circulating levels of these gonadotropins, did not inhibit the circhoral discharges of endogeneous LH (unpublished observations). Since these substances have full biological activity in the rhesus monkey in terms of their gonadotropic effects (cf 11), it may be concluded that the circhoral pattern of LH secretion cannot, in all probability, be explained in terms of the operation of a simple, short-loop negative feedback mechanism. In light of the foregoing, a more likely view is that the circhoral pulses of LH are the consequence of signals from the CNS relayed by LRH.

Lastly, and somewhat surprisingly, the acute administration of progesterone alone to ovariectomized monkeys, resulting in plasma concentrations of this steroid a thousandfold greater than those normally observed during the luteal phase of the cycle, was without significant effect on the open-loop pattern of LH secretion (Fig. 6). Similarly, chronic progesterone administration failed to depress the elevated circulating LH levels in such animals (unpublished).

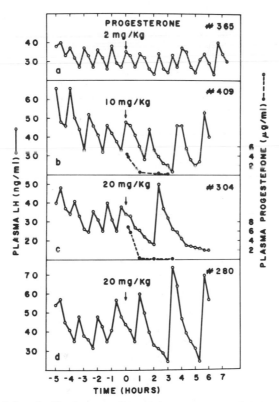

FIG. 6. The relative ineffectiveness of acute progesterone administration (single IV injection at arrows) on LH secretion in ovariectomized monkeys. Note the magnitude of the resulting progesterone concentrations. Luteal phase progesterone levels in the monkey average 4 ng/ml.

The foregoing observations permit the conclusion that tonic LH secretion, as reflected in the circulating levels of this hormone during the follicular phase of the cycle, can be accounted for by the negative feedback action of estrogen alone and that, as in the rat (12), this negative feedback loop probably involves a dopaminergic and/or an α-adrenergic component.

POSITIVE FEEDBACK CONTROL OF THE PREOVULATORY LH SURGE

Although progesterone administration can, under certain experimental circumstances, trigger an acute release of LH in experimental animals and man (12-14) it is unlikely that it does so in a physiologic context. The reason for this assertion is that the initiation of the preovulatory LH discharge in man (15, 16), the rhesus monkey (1, 17), and the rat (27), has not been found to be preceded by an increment in plasma progesterone concentration. Furthermore, the nature of the LH surge evoked by progesterone differs markedly from that observed during the normal menstrual cycle. In contrast to the foregoing, however, circulating estrogen levels, clearly and consistently, rise several days before the initiation of the LH surge in the rhesus monkey (8) and in man (16). The temporal relationship between these two hormones during the menstrual cycle of the rhesus monkey is illustrated in Fig. 7. A nearly identical relationship between estrogen and LH secretion has been described in the abbreviated ovarian

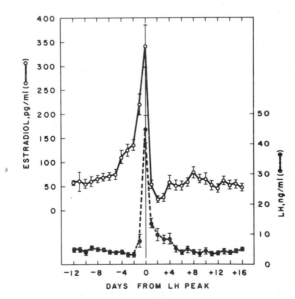

FIG. 7. Composite of mean daily serum estradiol and LH concentrations of 10 normal rhesus monkey menstrual cycles normalized to the day of the LH peak (8). Reproduced by permission of J. B. Lippincott Company.

cycle of the rat (18) in which it has been convincingly demonstrated that the neutralization of this increment in circulating estrogen by the administration of antisera to estradiol, but not to progesterone, effectively inhibits ovulation (19).

The inference that this increase in circulating estrogens may be the primary stimulus for the preovulatory LH discharge has been strengthened by the observation in sheep (20) and rats (21) that estrogen administration leads to an acute release of LH.

Our initial attempts to elicit an LH surge in the rhesus monkey by estrogen administration were consistently unsuccessful. In these early experiments estradiol-17β was given intramuscularly in oil or subcutaneously in the form of crystalline suspensions beginning on the second or third day of the menstrual cycle. In response to these treatments, plasma estradiol concentrations, as monitored by radioimmunoassay (8), rose to very high levels (in excess of 2000 pg/ml) but these were not sustained for longer than 12 hr (22). When the absorption of the estradiol was delayed, however, and the increment in circulating estrogen sustained for longer than 12 hr (by the multiple subcutaneous injection, in oil, of estradiol benzoate, rather than the free alcohol) premature LH surges essentially identical, qualitatively and quantitatively, to those occurring spontaneously were uniformly elicited (Fig. 8a). This regimen of estrogen administration resulted in circulating estrogen patterns (22) which mimicked those normally observed prior to the onset of the spontaneous LH surge in normal menstrual cycles. As shown in Fig. 8b, single injections of estradiol benzoate were similarly effective and have since been utilized as a convenient test system for the continued study of the positive feedback action of estrogen on LH secretion.

In the foregoing experiments the increment in estrogen levels above the control values of approximately 75 pg/ml, resulted in an initial decline in plasma LH concentration, attributable to the negative feedback action of the steroid, followed by an abrupt rise 36 to 60 hr after the initiation of multiple estrogen injections or 24 to 48 hr after the single injection. In the latter circumstance, circulating estrogen levels, in most instances, were beginning to fall at the time when the LH surge was initiated (22). This biphasic time course in LH concentrations (a decline in LH levels preceding the surge) is also observed during the normal monkey menstrual cycle (1).

Similarly, the administration of a single dose of estradiol benzoate to ovariectomized females evokes an LH surge but this is preceded by a more dramatic decrease in LH concentrations from their elevated control values (Fig. 12a).

Our studies to date (22) have failed to reveal a clear dose-response relationship between the estradiol benzoate administered and the magnitude or duration of the LH surge. They suggest, rather, that the discharge of LH in response to the increment in circulating estrogen is an "all or none" phenomenon if this increment is sustained for 12 hr or longer. The effective increment in plasma estrogen concentrations, if maintained for this period, need

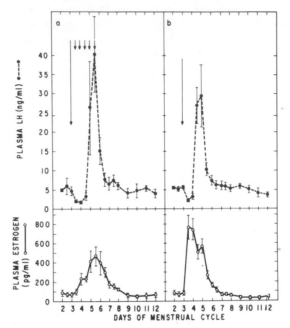

FIG. 8. Mean plasma concentrations of LH and estrogen in 4 intact rhesus monkeys treated with estradiol benzoate, in oil, in 6 divided doses (7 μg/kg) given at 12 hr intervals beginning on day 3 of the cycle (a) and in 7 intact females (b) given a single subcutaneous injection of 42 μg/kg of this steroid, in oil, on the 3rd day of the cycle (22). Reproduced by permission of J. B. Lippincott Company.

not be large since an increase in 60 pg/ml has been shown to evoke an LH surge (22). It would appear, therefore, that the sensor component of the positive feedback system responds not to a threshold concentration in circulating estrogen as such but to an incremental pattern in estrogen levels. This positive feedback action of estrogen on LH secretion is not demonstrable in sexually immature females (4). Our findings to date suggest that this control system becomes operative only some time after the advent of menarche and could explain the anovulatory cycles associated with this period of sexual development.

In contrast to the striking inhibition of tonic LH secretion by α-adrenergic blocking agents and by drugs with antidopaminergic activity we have not succeeded at the time of this writing to block the LH surge, whether spontaneous or induced, with these agents. Acute or chronic administration of β-adrenergic blocking drugs have also been ineffective in this regard. Progesterone, on the other hand, which was shown to be essentially inert in the negative feedback regulation of tonic LH secretion completely inhibits the estrogen-induced LH surge (4). This is demonstrable when exogenous progesterone is administered at the same time as the test dose of estradiol benzoate on day 3 of the menstrual cycle and, in most instances when progesterone is injected 12 hr later (Fig. 9). Similarly, and in a more physiological setting, an LH surge cannot be induced by estradiol benzoate administration during the luteal phase of the

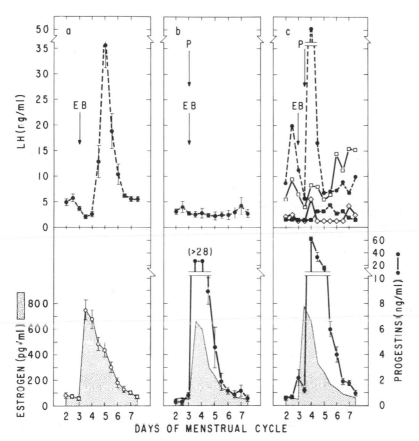

FIG. 9. Effects of estradiol benzoate alone (a); with progesterone, 5 mg/kg (b); and with progesterone given 12 hr later (c), on plasma LH concentrations in intact monkeys. Panels (a) and (b) represent composites of 8 and 14 monkeys, respectively, while panel (c) shows the plasma LH levels of individual animals.

cycle (Fig. 10a) when plasma progesterone concentrations are normally elevated (4). Since, once an LH surge is evoked, the system is refractory to subsequent estrogen stimulation for approximately 3 days (unpublished observations), the results of this experiment could be interpreted in terms of such a refractory period consequent to the spontaneous LH discharge which occurred a few days before. That such is not the case was shown by the removal of the newly formed corpus luteum and repeating the experiment at approximately the same day of the cycle. As illustrated in Fig. 10b, estradiol benzoate administration was again fully effective in inducing an LH surge when plasma progesterone had declined to undetectable levels.

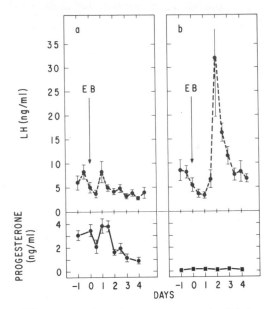

FIG. 10. Plasma LH concentrations in response to estradiol benzoate administration (arrows) during the early luteal phase of the menstrual cycle. The data are normalized to the time of EB injection. (a) Corpora lutea in situ (8 animals); (b) corpora lutea excised (5 animals). The lower panels show circulating levels of endogenous progesterone.

It may be concluded at this juncture that, in the rhesus monkey, the negative and positive feedback actions of estrogen on LH secretion appear to involve different pathways. Viewed in this light, the tonic secretion of LH and the surge, or cyclic, secretion of this gonadotropin seem to be controlled by different mechanisms, one containing an adrenergic component which senses low, relatively constant, levels of estrogen, while the other responds to sustained increments in the plasma concentration of this hormone. Clearly, these two control systems must be coexistent since the LH surge is normally superimposed on the tonic secretory pattern once every 28 days on the average, and can be induced experimentally during the follicular phase of the cycle when LH secretion is normally suppressed by the estrogen circulating at that time.

That the negative and positive feedback controls of LH secretion by estrogen are mediated by the operation of two concurrent mechanisms was demonstrated in ovariectomized monkeys bearing chronically implanted Silastic capsules containing estradiol-17β (9). In these experiments, as described earlier, constant levels of circulating estrogen were achieved which approximated those ($\sim$50 pg/ml) normally observed during the early follicular phase of the menstrual cycle. These, in turn, maintained the low plasma LH concentrations characteristic of this portion of the cycle (negative feedback action). When such animals were given our standard test dose of estradiol, with a consequent increment in circulating estrogen which was superimposed on the levels resulting from the estradiol released from the implant, an essentially normal LH surge (positive feedback action) could be induced at will. Figure 11 illustrates one of these experiments. In this instance the negative feedback effect of the implanted estrogen was interrupted by an LH surge occasioned by the initial pulse in plasma estrogen concentration attributable to a surface contamination of the Silastic capsule by the steroid. When this was avoided, by prior incubation of the estradiol-containing capsules in an appropriate medium, LH concentrations fell uninterruptedly from castrated to basal levels where they remained unless and until a subcutaneous injection of estradiol benzoate was given.

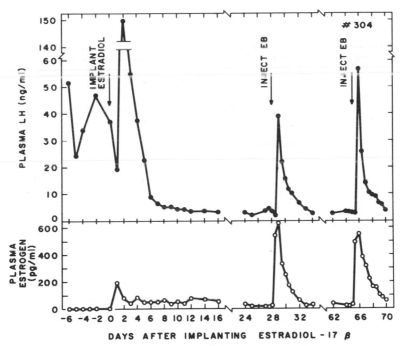

FIG. 11. Effects of single injections of estradiol benzoate (last 2 arrows) on plasma LH concentration in an ovariectomized monkey bearing an implant of estradiol-17β (see text for details).

The results of this study are consonant with the view that the basic pattern of LH secretion throughout the menstrual cycle (tonic secretion interrupted by an LH surge) can be accounted for entirely by the changes in ovarian estrogen secretion known to occur during the cycle. That the sizable increments in plasma estrogen levels usually observed in man, and occasionally in the rhesus monkey, during the luteal phase of the cycle do not elicit clear LH surges is readily explained by the presence of progesterone.

This conclusion implies that the "clock" or "zeitgeber" which determines the timing of ovulation in primates is not resident in the brain, as appears to be the case in the rat, but in the ovary which is reposited in a less lofty anatomic locale.

Whether the increment in estrogen secretion by the preovulatory follicle which evokes the LH surge acts at the level of the CNS or the pituitary, or both, remains to be determined in primates. In any event, a CNS component in the positive feedback action of estrogen on LH secretion need not be postulated at present since estrogen has been demonstrated to have a direct effect on LH release at the level of the pituitary (23, 28) and that it increases the sensitivity of the gland to LRH (24) in the rat. Similarly, progesterone appears to block LH release at the level of the pituitary in this species (25). One may postulate, therefore, that in the rhesus monkey an increment in circulating estrogen may increase the sensitivity of the gonadotrophs to constant levels of LRH with a resultant release of LH. Clearly, however, additional information may modify this view.

The foregoing speculations inevitably lead to a consideration of the male pattern of LH secretion which, classically, is held to be of the tonic type and controlled in a manner analogous to that of tonic LH secretion in the female. It would be reasonable to suppose that, if the fundamental difference between the tonic and cyclic patterns of LH secretion in primates is in the pattern of circulating estrogen, the administration of estradiol benzoate to males should also result in a discharge of LH from the pituitary gland. When such experiments were conducted in intact male rhesus monkeys, however, the results were unequivocally negative (22). The responses of castrated males to the injection of estrogen, on the other hand, did not differ qualitatively from those of castrated females (Fig. 12). As in the ovariectomized female, the initial response of the orchidectomized male to the increment in circulating estrogen levels, was a decline in plasma LH concentrations followed by an abrupt increase. The resulting maximal LH concentrations in the males, however, did not exceed control values (22). Since in the gonadectomized males, as in the gonadec-tomized females, the increase in LH concentrations occurred in the presence of elevated estrogen levels, it may be argued that the estrogen stimulated LH secretion in both instances but did so to a lesser degree in the male. It has been shown in more recent studies that when the dose of estradiol benzoate given to castrated males was increased, the resultant pattern in LH secretion was similar to that observed in the females illustrated in Fig. 12. If one assumes that the responses of gonadectomized males and females to the positive feedback action of estrogen are qualitatively the same, differing but quantitatively, then the decline in plasma LH concentrations below control levels, in both sexes, approximately 3 days after the injection of the steroid may be accounted for by a sustained negative feedback action of the estrogen which has been temporarily overridden by its stimulatory effect (22). The inability of estrogen to demonstrably elicit LH secretion in the intact male may be due to the presence of testosterone which has recently been shown to block LH release in response to estrogen stimulation in the rat (26), much as progesterone does in the female monkey.

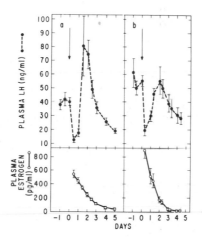

FIG. 12. Mean plasma LH and estrogen concentrations in 8 ovariectomized (a); and 4 orchidectomized (b), rhesus monkeys given estradiol benzoate in oil (subcutaneously) at the time indicated by the arrows (22). Reproduced by permission of J. B. Lippincott Company.

While much of the foregoing is admittedly speculative, the continued investigation of the questions raised will, hopefully, lead us to a much-needed better understanding of the manner in which reproductive phenomena are regulated in primates.

ACKNOWLEDGMENT

This work was supported by grants H003969 and RR00298 from the NIH and by a grant from the Ford Foundation.

REFERENCES

1. Monroe, S. E., L. E. Atkinson, and E. Knobil, Endocrinology 87:453, 1970.
2. Schwartz, N. B., Rec Progr Hormone Res 25:1, 1969.
3. Atkinson, L. E., A. N. Bhattacharya, S. E. Monroe, D. J. Dierschke, and E. Knobil, Endocrinology 87:847, 1970.
4. Yamaji, T., D. J. Dierschke, F. J. Karsch, R. F. Weick, J. Hotchkiss, and E. Knobil, Program of the 53rd Meeting of The Endocrine Society, San Francisco, 1971, p. A-78 (abstract).

5. Dierschke, D. J., A. N. Bhattacharya, L. E. Atkinson, and E. Knobil, Endocrinology 87:850, 1970.

6. Dierschke, D. J., T. Yamaji, A. N. Bhattacharya, L. E. Atkinson, and E. Knobil, Program of the 52nd Meeting of The Endocrine Society, St. Louis, Missouri, 1970, p. 60 (abstract).

7. McGuire, J. L., and R. D. Lisk, Proc Nat Acad Sci USA 61:497, 1968.

8. Hotchkiss, J., L. E. Atkinson, and E. Knobil, Endocrinology 89:177, 1971.

9. Karsch, F. J., D. J. Dierschke, T. Yamaji, J. Hotchkiss, R. F. Weick, and E. Knobil, Fed Proc 30:254, 1971 (abstract).

10. Knobil, E., and V. Meyer, Ann NY Acad Sci 148:459, 1968.

11. Knobil, E., and J. B. Josimovich, Endocrinology 69:139, 1961.

12. McCann, S. M., this symposium, p. 49.

13. Odell, W. D., and R. S. Swerdloff, Proc Nat Acad Sci USA 61:529, 1968.

14. Leyendecker, G., S. Wardlaw, and W. Nocke, this symposium, p. 720.

15. Neill, J. O., E. D. B. Johansson, J. K. Datta, and E. Knobil, J Clin Endocrinol 27:1167, 1967.

16. Vande Wiele, R. L., J. Bogumil, I. Dyrenfurth, M. Ferin, R. Jewelewicz, M. Warren, T. Rizkallah, and G. Mikhail, Rec Progr Hormone Res 26:63, 1970.

17. Kirton, K. T., G. D. Niswender, A. R. Midgley, Jr., R. B. Jaffe, and A. D. Forbes, J Clin Endocrinol 30:105, 1970.

18. Brown-Grant, K., D. Exley, and F. Naftolin, J Endocrinol 48:295, 1970.

19. Ferin, M., A. Tempone, P. E. Zimmering, and R. L. Vande Wiele, Endocrinology 85:1070, 1969.

20. Goding, J. R., K. J. Catt, J. M. Brown, C. C. Kaltenbach, I. A. Cumming, and B. J. Mole, Endocrinology 85:133, 1969.

21. Caligaris, L., J. J. Astrada, and S. Taleisnik, Endocrinology 88:810, 1971.

22. Yamaji, T., D. J. Dierschke, J. Hotchkiss, A. N. Bhattacharya, A. H. Surve, and E. Knobil, Endocrinology 89:1034, 1971.

23. Piacsek, B. E., and J. Meites, Endocrinology 79:432, 1966.

24. Arimura, A., and A. V. Schally, Proc Soc Exp Biol Med 136:290, 1971.

25. Arimura, A., and A. V. Schally, Endocrinology 87:653, 1970.

26. Klawon, D. L., S. Sorrentino, Jr., and D. S. Schalch, Endocrinology 88:1131, 1971.

27. Barraclough, C. A., R. Collu, R. Massa, and L. Martini, Endocrinology 88:1437, 1971.

28. Schneider, H. P. G., and S. M. McCann, Endocrinology 87:330, 1970.

8.   Active Immunization
with Estradiol-17 β
Bovine Serum
Albumin in Monkeys

F. Susan Cowchock, Michelle Ferin, Inge Dyrenfurth, Peter Carmel, Earl Zimmerman, A. Brinson, and Raymond Vande Wiele

Steroids can be made antigenic when covalently coupled to proteins (1). In previous studies, we have shown that antisera to estradiol-17β, produced in ewes, are capable of inhibiting the uterine weight increase evoked by estradiol in immature rats (2). When these antibodies are given to cycling rats, the ovulatory LH surge is suppressed (3).

In the course of our studies on steroid-sensitive feedback areas for LH in the central nervous system, the need for an intact primate who was anovulatory became apparent. For this reason, regularly cycling rhesus monkeys were actively immunized to estradiol-17β-BSA.[1] This report concerns the production in these monkeys of antibodies to estradiol and their effect on spontaneous cyclic ovulation.

MATERIALS AND METHODS

Immunization

Six female rhesus monkeys (Maccaca mulata) with regular menstrual cycles for at least 3 months preceding the experiment were used. The animals were housed in an air-conditioned room. The sole light source was controlled in a 12-hr

[1] E_2 = estradiol-17β, anti-E_2 = antiserum to estradiol, and BSA = bovine serum albumin.

day/12-hr night pattern. Four of these animals were injected with estradiol-17β-succinyl-BSA as the antigen. The E_2 conjugate, in a dose of 1.5 or 3 mg, was dissolved in 0.5 ml of saline and suspended in an equal volume of complete Freund's adjuvant. This dose was injected into 4 different subcutaneous sites, near to axillary and inguinal lymph nodes. The usual immunization schedule consisted of 4 weekly injections followed by monthly boosters. The 2 animals (No. 60 and 194) treated with 1.5 mg of the E_2 conjugate received a preliminary series of 6 weekly injections, first with the antigen in Freund's, then 5 injections of the antigen in saline. Since no antibodies were produced, Freund's adjuvant was added and the regular schedule was resumed. The monkeys were checked daily for menstrual bleeding by vaginal swabs. In addition, stained vaginal smears were prepared and blood samples drawn 3 times a week.

Antiestradiol titers

The monkey sera were tested for antibodies by using the principle of the radioimmunoassay for estradiol (4). In this assay, estradiol antibodies are adsorbed onto the walls of plastic tubes in proportion to the amount present in the serum sample. A constant amount of labeled estradiol (approximately 4000 cpm of 2,4,6,7-^{3}H-estradiol in buffer is added. The amount of radioactive steroid bound to the walls of the tube, after an equilibration period of 2 hr at room temperature, can be used as a relative measurement of the amount of antibodies present in the antiserum. This binding capacity, expressed as percent, will be referred to as the "titer" of the antiserum. These antibody titers were measured at serum dilutions of 1:10 to 1:50,000. Examples of dilution curves are shown in Figs. 6 and 7. A maximum occurred constantly at a dilution of 1:100. Therefore, this particular dilution was selected to determine the "titer" of antibodies throughout immunization.

Immunodiffusion discs

Immunodiffusion was performed in a commercially prepared gel disc with a dye indicator (Miles Laboratory, Kankakee, Ill.). The discs were developed at 5 C for at least one week. Undiluted serum samples were used and the presence of a precipitate with the E_2 conjugate or BSA was noted.

Progesterone and "progestin" levels

A modification of the competitive protein-binding method originated by Neill et al. (5) was used to measure serum progesterone. The TLC plates were developed in a system of 80% chloroform and 20% ethylacetate. Exposure of the equilibrated samples to the florisil was timed precisely. Later, thin layer chromatography was omitted from the procedure for routine assays. This abbreviated method measures the serum "progestins" which include progesterone and its 20-reduced and 17-hydroxylated forms (6).

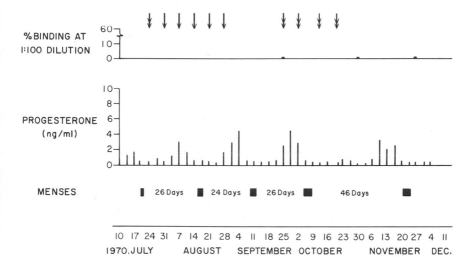

FIG. 1. Control animal injected with saline only (↓) or saline suspended in Freund's complete adjuvant (⇂).

RESULTS

Immunization

In the 2 control monkeys who received only saline and Freund's adjuvant (Fig. 1) no anti-E_2 titer was found. The results from the 2 monkeys (No. 60 and 194) who received an immunizing dose of 1.5 mg of the E_2 conjugate are shown in Figs. 2, 3. Three weeks after the first series of injections of the conjugate mixed with saline, the antibody titers were below 10%. They reached maxima of 33 and 43% within 10 days after the fourth and last weekly injection. The titers declined thereafter at a similar rate in both animals and reached a nadir in the week of the first booster injection. Approximately 10 days after each booster injection, an increase in anti-E_2 titers occurred, followed by a rapid decline. One exception was observed: a rise in titer failed to occur after the second booster injection in monkey 194 (Fig. 3). In Fig. 2 only the percent of estrogen bound to the antibody at a dilution of 1:100 is plotted. Fig. 6 shows full dilution curves for a selected number of sera from monkey 60 during the early period of immunization. While no antibodies were demonstrable on Sept. 25, sera obtained from Oct. 6 to 30 show a clear maximum in the assay at a dilution of 1:100. Fig. 7 shows the dilution curves obtained from samples collected at later period of immunization when high levels of anti-E_2 binding (40 to 58%) were present. E_2 binding was maximal at a dilution of 1:100 as in the earlier samples (Fig. 6) but the most recent serum (April 7) which had the greatest binding at 1:100 (57%) also showed some residual binding (24%) at dilutions as high as 1:50,000.

90

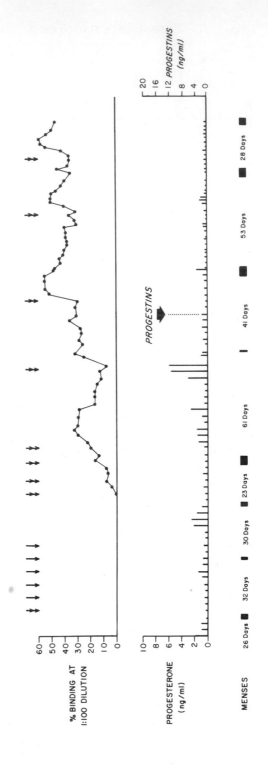

FIG. 2. Monkey 60 injected with 1.5 mg E$_2$ conjugate in saline only ($\downarrow$), or suspended in Freund's adjuvant ($\Uparrow$).

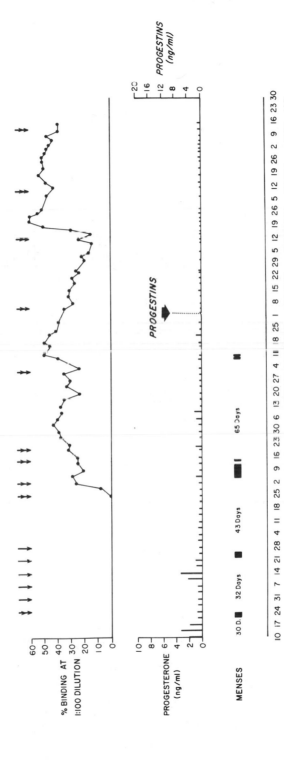

FIG. 3. Monkey 194 injected with 1.5 mg E$_2$ conjugate in saline only ($\downarrow$), or suspended in Freund's adjuvant ($\Updownarrow$).

91

Two other monkeys (No. 443 and 461) received a larger dose of the E_2 conjugate (3.0 mg) mixed with Freund's adjuvant (Figs. 4, 5). Monkey 443

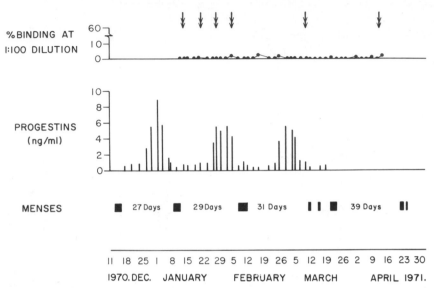

FIG. 4. Monkey 461 injected with 3 mg E_2 conjugate suspended in Freund's adjuvant ($\downarrow$). No increase in serum binding of estradiol is seen.

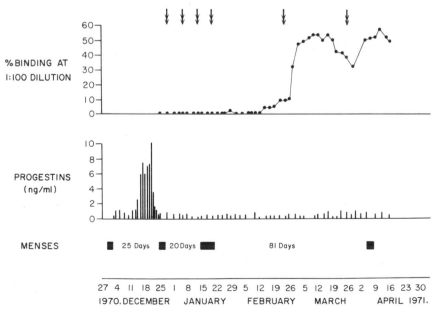

FIG. 5. Monkey 443 injected with 3 mg E_2 conjugate suspended in Freund's adjuvant ($\downarrow$).

developed a very slight increase in anti-E_2 (5%) about 4 weeks after the last weekly injection. The first booster was given one month later and the anti-E_2 titers rose very rapidly to levels of over 50%. These levels remained high for a period of 2 weeks, in contrast to those in monkeys injected with 1.5 mg of the antigen, in which they declined rapidly. The titers then fell to 32% but were restored by the second booster. Monkey 461 had not produced any antibodies

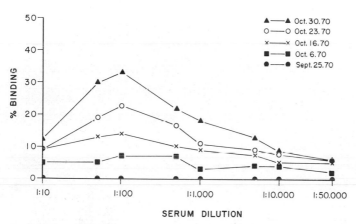

FIG. 6. Binding of estradiol by serum samples (monkey 60) at increasing serum dilutions, early in the course of immunization.

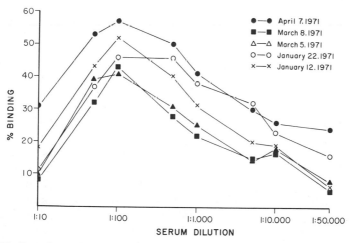

FIG. 7. Binding of estradiol at increasing serum dilutions with samples chosen from periods of highest binding late in immunization (monkey 60).

at the time of the second booster under the same immunization schedule.

Immunodiffusion discs which demonstrate the precipitated complex between antisera from these monkeys and the E_2-BSA conjugate or BSA alone are shown in Plates 1 and 2 respectively. Sera from the 2 animals who have been immunized for 5 months or more can be seen to form an antigen-antibody line against BSA in the center well while sera from monkeys immunized for only 1 to 3 months form a precipitate only with the E_2 conjugate.

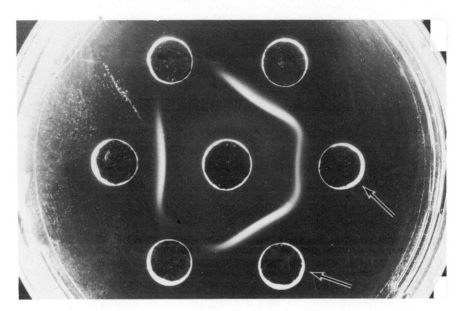

PLATE 1. Immunodiffusion disc with E_2 conjugate in the center well. Sera from two monkeys immunized for at least 5 months are indicated by arrows. The other precipitate lines are from monkeys in an earlier stage of immunization.

Effects of immunization on the menstrual cycles

The two control animals who received only saline with Freund's adjuvant had regular menstrual cycles as did the other animals before immunization occurred. The average length of these 34 cycles was 28.2 days with a range from 24 to 34 days. Two cycles were longer and lasted 46 and 60 days. In 21 of these cycles, the progesterone or progestin levels were determined. Progesterone or progestin levels greater than 2 ng/ml were considered indicative of ovulation. By this criterion, all these control cycles, even the 46-day cycle, were ovulatory.

All three animals who produced antibodies to estradiol became anovulatory. Vaginal bleeding became irregular and the interval period was prolonged as much as 81 days. At no time did progesterone or progestin reach ovulatory levels. Monkeys 194 and 443 became anovulatory before the first booster (Figs. 3 and 5). In monkey 60 an ovulation occurred during the initial immunization period

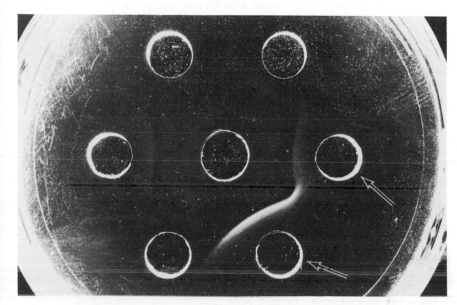

PLATE 2. Immunodiffusion disc with BSA in the center well. Sera from two monkeys immunized for 5 months are indicated by arrows.

(Fig. 3). During administration of E$_2$ conjugate in saline the cycles remained ovulatory.

The vaginal smears did not become hypoestrogenic after significant amounts of antibodies were found. On the contrary, an increase in the number of cornified cells together with a decrease in parabasal cells was often evident as soon as serum estradiol binding reached maximum levels. No abnormally high cornification was seen during the administration of the E$_2$ conjugate at the beginning of the immunization.

DISCUSSION

Female rhesus monkeys immunized with an estradiol-protein conjugate suspended with Freund's adjuvant produced antibodies within one month. The menstrual cycles in these immunized animals became irregular and no serum progesterone or progestin levels indicative of an ovulatory surge of LH were seen. The vaginal smears lost significant cyclic variations and cornified cells were always present. The inherent estrogenic activity of the estradiol-protein conjugate (1) was not responsible for these effects. Indeed, during immunization the animals retained cyclic variations in the serum progestin and progesterone levels and vaginal smears until antibody titers started to rise.

The presence of vaginal cornification in these animals immunized to estrogens is puzzling. In immature rats treated with E_2 and anti-E_2, even large amounts of anti-E_2 did not completely abolish the uterine weight increase induced by the estrogens (2). These persistent cornified cells seen after immunization are reminiscent of the constant vaginal estrus syndrome in rats. This syndrome was attributed to the constant secretion of estrogens as a consequence of an abnormal gonadotropin secretion (7). It is interesting to note that serum LH levels measured by radioimmunoassay in one monkey were slightly but consistently higher after immunization.

The antibodies produced in the first months of immunization appeared to be homogeneous. The sera formed a single line with the estradiol-BSA conjugate in immunodiffusion discs. No precipitate was seen with BSA alone until the fifth month of immunization. Previous studies have shown that, in ewes, this same antigen induced antibodies which are specific for estrogens when tested in vitro and in vivo. In radioimmunoassay, they do not significantly cross-react with any other class of steroids (4, 8). In spontaneously cycling rats, antiserum to estrogen, but not antisera to progesterone or testosterone, inhibited the LH surge and ovulation (3). This last evidence and the specificity of these antibodies imply that the absence of ovulatory LH surges in these immunized monkeys is due to the inactivation of the serum estrogens which control the LH surge.

Such immunized monkeys are ideal for the intimate study of the LH feedback mechanism. Previous studies have shown that diethylstilbestrol, a synthetic estrogen which is not inhibited by anti-E_2 (2), can restore the LH surge in rats in which ovulation was blocked by anti-E_2 (3). It can also induce LH release in actively immunized ovariectomized ewes (9). In our monkeys such experiments can be performed as frequently as pituitary LH reserve will permit without regard to spontaneous LH release. We plan to study both the location in the central nervous system of this feedback mechanism and the role played by steroids other than estrogens and nonsteroid substances such as catecholamines.

ACKNOWLEDGMENT

Supported by NIH grant 1-P01-HD0507702. The immunization of monkeys 60 and 194 was started at Rockefeller University. We would like to thank Dr. L. K. Gulton for a generous gift towards the expenses for the primate colony.

REFERENCES

1. Lieberman, S., B. Erlanger, S. Beiser, and J. Agate, Rec Prog Hormone Res 15:165, 1959.
2. Ferin, M., P. E. Zimmering, S. Lieberman, and R. Vande Wiele, Endocrinology 83:565, 1968.
3. Ferin, M., A. Tempone, P. E. Zimmering, and R. Vande Wiele, Endocrinology 85:1070, 1969.
4. Abraham, G. E., J Clin Endocrinol 29:866, 1969.
5. Neill, J., E. Johansson, J. Datta, and E. Knobil, J Clin Endocrinol 27:1167, 1967.

6. Johansson, E., Acta Endocrinol 61:592, 1969.

7. Barraclough, C. A., in L. Martini and W. Ganong (Eds.), Neuroendocrinology, Academic, New York, 1967.

8. Mikhail, G., H. W. Chung, M. Ferin, and R. Vande Wiele, in F. Peron and B. Caldwell (Eds.), Immunologic Methods in Steroids Determination, Appleton-Century-Crofts, New York, 1970, p. 113.

9. Caldwell, B. V., R. Scaramuzzi, S. Tillson, and I. Thorneycroft, in F. Peron and B. Caldwell (Eds.), Immunologic Methods in Steroids Determination, Appleton-Century-Crofts, New York, 1970, p. 183.

DISCUSSION

S. M. McCANN. I thought that in discussing these papers we would begin with Dr. Jutisz's paper since that one is more or less unrelated to the last two papers presented by Dr. Knobil and Dr. Cowchock. Are there any questions on Dr. Jutisz's paper? If not, then I would like to ask him a question. It's rather interesting that there are a number of stimuli which will increase gonadotropin release. One of them is a releasing factor, then you can also stimulate with cyclic AMP or with high potassium. Now, it may well be that the normal mechanism of action is cyclic AMP. When potassium is added, there is no change in the adenylcyclase or cyclic AMP level, if I have read your data correctly. I would like you to explain the secretory response to the potassium since we seem to have a difference in the mechanism of action.

M. JUTISZ. Well, I have no explanation. I think that potassium has a different mechanism of action than LH and FSH releasing factors. Potassium acts in a different way on the cell membrane. Maybe it acts on the membrane potential or on the increase in intracellular Ca^{2+} as it has been shown by Douglas and Poisner. We know that high potassium is a nonspecific stimulus. It releases all pituitary hormones.

J. GOLDZIEHER. In reference to that particular question, Howard Rasmussen's article in the May 1961 issue of the American Journal of Medicine has a discussion of intracellular calcium-induced flux of sodium across intracellular membranes. Possibly that would apply equally well to the situation in these cells as it does in the systems that he was discussing.

M. JUTISZ. I agree completely with what you are saying.

D. T. ARMSTRONG. Have you explored effects of steroids, administered in vivo or added to the incubation medium in vitro, either on LH release from the pituitary in response to cyclic AMP, or on pituitary adenyl cyclase activity in response to LRF?

M. JUTISZ. I think that Dr. McCann has done work on this problem. Maybe he can answer this question.

S. M. McCANN. As far as I know, nothing has been done on the effects of steroids on the responsiveness, let's say, to cyclic AMP or any agent of that kind. Releasing factors have been added to see whether estrogen can block at the pituitary level. It does not appear to have a very strong blocking action at the pituitary level in acute in vitro experiments.

A. R. MIDGLEY. Dr. Knobil, I want to congratulate you on what has to be an elegant presentation concerning the mode of regulation of luteinizing hormone in the primate. I noted that you have been unable to demonstrate oscillation of luteinizing hormone in the intact animal. As a result of studies done in collaboration with Dr. Jaffe involving sampling at hourly intervals, it has become very clear that the same type of pattern occurs in women throughout the menstrual cycle. The periodicity appears to be less frequent than that which you have observed in the castrated monkey with bursts of LH occurring at 2 to 3 hr intervals. The same phenomenon can be observed throughout the duration of the major LH peak which occurs at midcycle. The latter lasts for some 24 to 48 hr in the human, and it is characterized by a series of little surges that work their way up and then work their way back down. In the luteal phase of the cycle, it is clear that the oscillations of LH are much greater in amplitude than they are during the follicular phase. The opposite appears to be true for FSH. This suggests that progesterone might act to enhance the amount of LH released with each burst. I was interested to note that your slides also indicated that progesterone might act to give LH surges of greater magnitude. Studies done in collaboration with Scott Monroe and Robert Jaffe have indicated that administration of estradiol benzoate to women during the follicular phase of the cycle can induce release of LH, giving, in some cases, peaks similar to those observed at midcycle. These estradiol-induced peaks have not been followed by ovulation as assessed by serum progesterone levels and basal body temperature recordings. Instead, LH levels tend to remain at or above normal follicular phase levels followed, after a period approximating two weeks, by another major LH peak which usually results in ovulation.

E. KNOBIL. I am fascinated by your observation that these pulsatile patterns of LH secretion can also be demonstrated in intact human females. We have looked for this, as you know, but have not been able to see it in the intact monkey. Neither have we seen oscillations during the LH surge in rhesus monkeys, but we only sampled once every three hours, and observed a rather smooth rise and fall of circulating LH. It may be that our assay is not sensitive enough, that our sampling frequency was inappropriate or that the monkey differs from the human in this regard.

A. R. MIDGLEY. It is important to note, I think, that the one really major difference between the human and the monkey is in the duration of the LH surge at midcycle. It is very brief in the monkey, is it not?

E. KNOBIL. No, it is two to three days.

A. R. MIDGLEY. That is not what we found earlier.

E. KNOBIL. In our monkeys it is anyway. As far as the effect of progesterone is concerned, we have done a large number of experiments and have selected for illustration those in which progesterone seemed to do something. The magnitude of the pulsatile discharge is directly related to the frequency. Therefore, the slower the frequency of the pulses, the larger the discharge. The oscillation frequency does vary considerably from animal to animal, although the mean happens to be about one an hour with a relatively reasonable standard deviation.

Because of the tremendous doses given in these acute experiments, as well as the inability of chronic progesterone administration, by itself, to reduce mean plasma LH level as measured once a day over a period of several weeks, we are led to the conclusion that if it has any negative feedback action at all, it is very small indeed and would not be expected to be demonstrable at physiologic concentrations.

G. LEYENDECKER. We have conducted practically the same experiments in the human female and we can show also that estradiol benzoate can exert a positive feedback with a latency of one to two days. I want to ask Dr. Knobil whether he ever found in the rhesus monkey the biphasic LH peak that was described in the human being by Thomas and Ferin?

E. KNOBIL. As I mentioned a moment ago, we have monitored the spontaneous LH surge during the normal menstrual cycle of several monkeys at 3-hr intervals, just to answer the question that you have raised. Within the limitations of this experimental design, we have not seen double peaks. Regarding the importance of progesterone in the normal preovulatory discharge of LH, all I can say at the moment is that we can induce normally appearing LH surges, essentially at will, by estradiol benzoate injection in ovariectomized females in whom LH is reduced to low, follicular phase levels by chronically implanted silastic capsule containing estradiol-17β. These animals have no circulating progesterone detectable by our assay system.

R. S. SWERDLOFF. Dr. Knobil, I was hoping you might have some information on estrogen-induction of FSH peaks in the monkey. I am particularly interested in that while Drs. Jacobs, Odell, and myself were able in the castrate female rat to induce LH peaks with ethinyl estradiol administration, we were not able to induce FSH peaks. That was also true of our studies on estrogen-treated intact humans. In contrast, when we added progesterone to estrogen-treated castrated women we were able to induce both LH and FSH peaks. In the experiments with castrate rats, when 20α-hydroxyprogesterone was added to doses of estrogen which alone failed to induce LH peaks, both LH and FSH peaks were seen.

E. KNOBIL. We shared your hope but, unfortunately, we have not so far been able to measure FSH reliably in the rhesus monkey.

S. REICHLIN. Dr. Seyler, Dr. Malacara, and myself have been interested in the positive feedback action of estrogen on LH release, and the problem obviously is whether or not the activated phase of estogen effects is due to a stimulation of LRF release at midcycle or a sensitization of the pituitary to a tonic level of LH releasing factor secretion or both. In work which Dr. Seyler and Dr. Malacara reported in Atlantic City at the American Federation for Clinical Research last month, they used an assay for LRF which is sensitive enough to detect the circulating hormone in the blood of normal women. They found a significant correlation between the rise at midcycle of LH and the rise at midcycle of LH releasing factor. Also, in men treated with large doses of estrogen, there appears in the blood relatively large amounts of luteinizing hormone releasing factor activity. The conclusion from these studies has been that estrogen induces the release of LH releasing factor at midcycle. I wonder if either you or Dr. Knobil would comment on the possible effect of estrogen in sensitizing the pituitary. In other circumstances this may occur, but in the chronic high dose estrogen-treated man, one sees high LRF-like activity in the blood and very low LH levels, which could only be brought about by an inhibition of the pituitary in association with the stimulation of the hypothalamus.

S. M. McCANN. Well, I am very excited about Dr. Reichlin's results which I heard him present, and I certainly think it does favor the idea that LRF is involved in the preovulatory gonadotropin surge. I think there is a tremendous amount of evidence in favor of that. There is a good possibility that there may be some effects at the pituitary level. The weakness so far in the pituitary-level story is usually that we do not know whether this is really working at physiological levels that occur, let's say, during the cycle.

J. WEISZ. I would like to refer to some data which I think are quite relevant. They relate to the very rapid fall in LH observed in the castrate monkey following estradiol, and to the difficulty of distinguishing where the site of action of the estradiol might be. Is it the hypothalamus, the pituitary, or both? This question can only be considered by looking at experiments as artificial as those involving implantation of steroids or in vitro systems. We have chosen to use the latter. We have adapted the superfusion system of the Tails, developed for studies of the adrenal, to study the dynamics of gonadotropin secretion by the pituitaries.

In this system of incubation, the medium flows over the pituitaries at a fixed rate. It is possible to add to the medium for fixed periods of time hypothalamic extract, steroids, or anything else one may wish to investigate. The superfusate is collected in a refrigerated fraction collector and analyzed for its content of trophic hormones. The work to which I refer was carried out by three of our associates, Drs. A. Dowd, N. Chaudhuri, and A. Barofsky.

The superfusion system turned out to be very pretty. The pituitaries responded in a reproducible manner over many hours in terms of, for instance, LH output following stimulation for a brief period; for example, 10 to 15 min, with a given dose of stalk median eminence extract. The coefficient of variation of the response in terms of ng of LH released by any given pool of pituitaries to a given dose of hypothalamic extract is remarkably small, 2 to 7%, depending on the duration of the stimulus pulse. In this system we find that after the pituitaries have been exposed for 60 min to a level of estradiol of the order of 3×10^{-9}M, the amount of LH they put out in response to a given dose of hypothalamic extract is significantly reduced. Under these conditions the estradiol can clearly reduce the responsiveness of the pituitary. The inhibiting effect persists for at least up to 30 min after the withdrawal of the estradiol. The effect that Dr. Knobil observed may have been due also to an immediate inhibiting effect of estradiol on the pituitaries of the monkeys in vivo. It is intriguing to try and speculate on what mechanisms might be involved in so rapid an effect.

H. NANKIN. Dr. Philip Troen and I have been interested in characterizing the pattern of circulating LH in normal individuals. I would like to expand a little on Dr. Midgley's comment. We have noted that the level of LH can vary by as much as two- to three-fold from day to day or within a single day in normal men. We attempted to devise a study to characterize the pattern of circulating LH. The first thing we did was to take four normal men and sample blood every 15 min from 6 am to 6 pm and we found a repetitive pattern of LH peaks throughout the day. There were 21 LH peaks during the total of 48 hr of sampling. When we took the highest value for each man and made a comparison to his lowest value we got ratios of 2.1 to 2.9 in the 4. Obviously, you cannot do 12 hr studies routinely, so we then decided to devise a protocol for clinical use and by doing shorter multiple-sampling studies of 2.5 hr with blood drawings at 10-min intervals we find that in normal men and during the follicular and luteal phases in normal women, LH peaks occur. We think that the presence or absence of a peak, and the absolute LH concentration of the peak and lowest trough value, and the ratio of the highest peak value to the lowest trough concentration may be important in detecting individuals with mild hypogonadotropism or mild hypogonadism. We are presently widening the use of these shorter multiple-sampling studies.

C. LLOYD. Could I ask Dr. Cowchock about the final point she brought up; that is the possibility of using the antibody to examine the LH releasing area. Do you have any data suggesting any differences in sensitivity of the uterus and of the LH releasing areas to the estrogen you are giving in the presence of the antibody? In other words, you have shown that diethylstilbestrol will override the antibody to estradiol. Do you have any data that would let you know whether the sensitivity of the pelvic structures and the sensitivity of the brain structures are the same to the estrogen?

F. S. COWCHOCK. No, we have not yet studied the effects of immunization or the change in sensitivity after immunization to diethylstilbestrol as far as pelvic structures are concerned, except for the note I made about vaginal smears. Perhaps I did not make it clear that our work has been on hypothalamic injections of estrogen. We have studied castrates and immunized animals. It might be of interest to Dr. Knobil that we have also looked for bursts of LH in our immunized animals. Indeed, they do have a periodic rhythm, but the amplitude is much lower, the fluctuations are of lesser value than in the castrate animals.

G. LEYENDECKER. I would like to ask Dr. Knobil how he would explain that the positive feedback to estradiol is an all-or-none reaction and then saying that it is probably due to the fact that the pituitary gland is made more sensitive for LRH by estradiol. If you keep the concentration of estradiol in blood high for a couple of days, over a threshhold dose, let's say of about 100 pg/ml, then you only get one short peak of LH. If it is true that sensitization of the pituitary gland to LRH would be the reason, then you would expect a longer duration of that peak.

E. KNOBIL. This is a good question, and I really don't have an answer to it. Whether the apparent all-or-none response to estrogen which, by the way, remains to be established, is consonant with the hypothesis that the site of the positive feedback action of this steroid is at the level of the pituitary is an interesting point. With reference to Dr. Weisz's comment, we specifically attempted to look for a dose of estrogen which would be high enough to block LH release. We never succeeded in finding such a dose; we quit at 500 μg/kg, which led to circulating levels of estrogen in excess of several thousand pg/ml, and felt that there was not too much point in going beyond that. Your observations are interesting and may be related to the initial negative feedback effect of administered estrogen which we always see prior to the initiation of the LH surge.

I. ROTHCHILD. The data presented by Dr. Knobil and by Dr. Cowchock has certainly answered several questions that many of us have puzzled over, particularly how the brain can be sensitive to both the inhibitory and the stimulatory effects of estrogen on gonadotropin secretion and yet know when to react to one and not to the other. There is still one question, however, which seems to be unanswered. Although estrogen, under the conditions you described, will induce an LH peak, how is it that we can inhibit ovulation by the continuous administration of estrogen, starting early in the cycle? Is there an LH peak that follows the first treatment, but without induction of ovulation, and then the maintenance of a system in which further LH peaks cannot occur?

E. KNOBIL. Dr. Rothchild, Dr. Midgley actually answered your question earlier, and we found exactly the same thing. What we find in many of the animals in which a premature LH surge is elicited by the injection of estrogen on day 3 of the cycle is that this LH surge is not followed by a spontaneous LH surge before the onset of the next menstruation and ovulation does not occur. In the remainder of the cycle one does observe a spontaneous LH surge later, but this is delayed by some 15 to 20 days and is followed by ovulation and a normal luteal phase of 14 to 15 days in duration. This is in response to a single injection of estrogen early in the cycle and I would assume that, if one administers estrogen continuously, the chances of preventing ovulation would be great indeed. The most likely reason that the induced surge did not induce ovulation in any of the animals that we have looked at so far is that the follicles just are not ripe enough to respond to the LH surge early in the follicular phase of the cycle.

J. W. GOLDZIEHER. In reply to both Dr. Leyendecker and the last comment, I might mention that Dr. V. Stevens and our group published (Am J Obst Gyn 102:95, 1968) some clinical studies showing that 10 μg of ethynyl estradiol per day starting on cycle day 1 produces a large and sustained increase in urinary gonadotropin. If you start with 50 μg or higher, you go immediately to a low level. At least from the clinical point of view, there is no question of the biphasic action of estrogen.

Isolation, Chemistry, and Structure of Gonadotropins

9.　Human FSH:

Purification, Properties, and Some Structure-Function Relationships

Leo E. Reichert, Jr.

The need for homogeneous preparations of human gonadotropins to allow precise definition of endocrine function, to permit investigation of structure-function relationships, and for development of immunoassay procedures for their measurement have proven powerful stimuli to studies on the purification of these hormones as well as their chemical, biologic, and immunologic characterization. Recent exciting advances in our understanding of the subunit structure of bovine TSH and LH (1, 2), ovine LH (3, 5), HCG (6, 7) and HLH (8) have stimulated the imagination of scientists from a number of disciplines and will undoubtedly have important consequences for future studies on the mechanism of action of these hormones. Much less is known about FSH. The quantities of purified hormone available from the most accessible source, ovine pituitaries, is discouragingly miniscule (9). Bovine pituitary FSH has been particularly resistant to attempts at purification, possibly because of certain apparently unique pharmacologic properties (10), and the cost of the required large quantities of porcine and equine pituitaries is rather formidable. The availability of human FSH is also limited for obvious reasons. Nevertheless, the National Institute of Arthritis and Metabolic Diseases (NIAMD) through the National Pituitary Agency, has succeeded in making available reasonable amounts of gonadotropin-enriched human pituitary fractions for further separation and purification and the resulting materials have already been applied to a variety of important problems in human reproductive physiology. In this report we wish to consider specifically human FSH (HFSH) and describe recent advances in its purification and characterization as well as in our understanding of certain aspects of its structure-function relationships.

REFERENCE PREPARATIONS FOR MEASUREMENT OF HFSH

HFSH may be validly bioassayed in terms of ovine FSH when using the Steelman-Pohley assay (11, 12). This permits use of the readily available NIH-FSH-S (ovine) series of well-characterized preparations for this purpose. Activity is usually expressed in terms of NIH-FSH-S1, the first member of the series, one unit being the activity present in 1 mg of the NIH-FSH-S1. Activity may also be expressed in terms of IU using a reference preparation distributed by the World Health Organization International Laboratory for Biological Standards (Mill Hill, London) and designated the 2nd International Reference Preparation of Human Menopausal Gonadotropin (2nd IRP-HMG). It has been shown that one NIH-FSH-S1 U of FSH activity is approximately equivalent to 25 IU (2nd IRP-HMG). Recently, the NIAMD has made available a human pituitary gonadotropin fraction carefully characterized in terms of IU (2nd IRP-HMG), designated LER-907. This latter material has been widely used for the bioassay and radioimmunoassay of human pituitary and plasma FSH. For a discussion of this and other pertinent aspects relating to bioassay and radioimmunoassay of human pituitary and/or urinary gonadotropins and appropriate reference preparations, the reader is referred to Refs. 13 and 14 in the bibliography.

BIOLOGICAL ASSAY FOR HFSH

The Steelman-Pohley bioassay (11) depends on the ability of FSH to stimulate an increase in the ovarian weight of intact, immature rats which have been simultaneously treated with an augmenting dose of HCG. We routinely employ 40 IU of HCG for this purpose. It is recommended that the claimed potency of commercially available HCG be checked for accuracy prior to routine use, as preparations from several sources have occasionally been found to be considerably less active than anticipated. As originally proposed for measurement of porcine FSH (11), this assay called for three subcutaneous injections of FSH and HCG per day for each of three days with autopsy on the morning of the fourth day. It has been shown, however, that two injections/day are adequate when assaying human or ovine FSH (12). Adequate log dose-response relationships are obtained with 90 and 180 μg-equivalents of NIH-FSH-S1, or with 3 and 6 IU 2nd IRP-HMG. For meaningful quantitative measurements it is essential that accepted bioassay design be employed with resulting data processed by standard statistical methods for parallel line bioassays (15).

It is interesting to recall here the observation by Parlow (16) that administration of an entire assay dose of FSH in a single injection followed by continued twice daily injections of HCG over the usual three day period,

TABLE I. Effects of variations in injection schedule on the response to HFSH

Preparation	Schedule	Ovarian wt (mg)	Mean
A. 0.9% Saline	+ 40 IU HCG given 6X 0.5 ml inj. twice a day for 3 days. Autopsy morning of day 4.	46, 54, 43, 48	48
B. HFSH	180 μg HFSH + 40 IU HCG prepared as single solution (0.9% saline) given 6 x 0.5 ml inj. twice a day for 3 days. Autopsy morning of day 4.	179, 110, 174, 127	148
C. HFSH	180 μg HFSH given 0.5 ml (0.9% saline) morning of day 1. HCG given as under A.	165, 155, 96, 166	146

resulted in good ovarian weight gain in the rat. Parlow did not specify what species FSH was used in his study. However, we have confirmed this observation in a preliminary study with HFSH (Table I). Thus it appears that the ovarian weight gain which we are measuring is triggered by an initial pulse of FSH which then requires a maintenance does of HCG for final expression.

BIOLOGICAL ACTIVITY OF VARIOUS PREPARATIONS OF HUMAN FSH

Several laboratories have reported purification of HFSH to a high degree of biological activity. The most potent preparations have been reported by Roos (17), between 12,000 and 14,000 IU/mg, and by Peckham and Parlow (18), 304 NIH-FSH-S1 units/mg or about 7600 IU/mg. Preparations having a lesser degree of activity, about 5000 IU (19) and 2500 IU/mg, have been obtained in other laboratories (20-22) and, interestingly, these appear to have chemical and physical properties quite similar to the more active fractions (22, 23). Further, they appear to be of immunochemical-grade purity (12). A variety of interesting studies have also been reported by Butt and co-workers (23-25) using preparations of even lower specific activity, about 1000 IU/mg, but also showing evidence of a high order of chemical purity. A variety of speculations can be put forth to explain these differences in potency among highly purified preparations (24, 26) but their true basis remains uncertain.

PREPARATION OF IMMUNOCHEMICAL- AND CLINCIAL-GRADE HFSH FRACTIONS FOR THE NATIONAL PITUITARY AGENCY-NATIONAL INSTITUTE OF ARTHRITIS AND METABOLIC DISEASE HORMONE DISTRIBUTION PROGRAM

For some years our laboratory has worked in collaboration with the above agencies in a program to make available small amounts of chemically or biologically pure human gonadotropin preparations for use in clinical studies or for radioimmunoassay (12). Gonadotropin-rich fractions are generally derived from acetone-stored and -dried glands by differential extraction with ammonium sulfate (27) or with ammonium acetate-ethanol (28). A major separation of FSH and LH activities is then achieved by ion exchange chromatography on DEAE-cellulose (29), the LH being unadsorbed under the conditions of the experiment, and the FSH being absorbed, but selectively eluted between 0.05 and 0.1N NaCl. The specific FSH activity at this point is about 500 IU/mg and LH contamination is approximately 100 IU/mg.

The FSH can be brought to immunochemical-grade purity by gel filtration through Sephadex G-100. Highly purified FSH emerges as the major component with a V_e/V_o ratio of about 1.65 (21). Fractions LER-869-2 and LER-1366, distributed by the NIAMD for use in its HFSH radioimmunoassay kits, were prepared in this fashion. The specific activity of the final product usually lies between 2000 and 4000 IU/mg, with an LH contamination of about 50 IU/mg.

For clinical studies, it is desirable that HFSH be as devoid as practicable of contamination with LH. It is possible to significantly lower the LH activity in HFSH fraction by its selective inactivation with α-chymotrypsin (30). The initial lot of clinical-grade HFSH distributed by the NIAMD program, LER-862, (FSH activity = 750 IU/mg) had its LH activity decreased from an initial level of 150 IU/mg to 7 IU/mg by this procedure. Two possible disadvantages of this approach should be recognized. First, the final product contains a slight amount of chymotrypsin (about 10 μg enzyme/mg of hormone preparation). Clinical experiences with this preparation, however, have thus far revealed no untoward effects as a result of the presence of the chymotrypsin. Second, the chymotrypsin-hydrolyzed LH fragments also remain present, and these have been shown to retain some of their immunologic activity (31, 32). This may be a complicating factor where radioimmunoassay studies on serum HLH levels are being done as part of the study.

Several laboratories have reported that incubation of ovine gonadotropins with urea results in a selective inactivation of the LH component, leaving the FSH activity only slightly diminished. Saxena and Rathnam (33) reported retention of HFSH activity following dialysis against 8M urea for from 24 to 72 hr at 4 C. We have observed a marked decrement in FSH biologic activity after incubation with 8M urea for 24 hr at room temperature (32). The studies of Butt et al. (34) with HFSH and those of Hermier et al. (35) with ovine FSH, however, indicate that the urea inactivation processes are complex and are probably dependent on pH, concentration, temperature, and time. It is obvious that great care must be taken if this technique is to be applied to the selective inactivation of HLH in the presence of FSH.

CHEMICAL AND PHYSICAL PROPERTIES OF HFSH

The complete amino-acid and carbohydrate analysis of highly purified HFSH from several laboratories have been compared by Butt (23) and, in general, good agreement was noted. Perhaps the only major discrepancy detected was the relatively high value for cysteine reported by Roos (17) for his very active HFSH preparation. A representative amino acid and carbohydrate analysis for HFSH is given in Table II. The best estimate of the molecular weight of HFSH is probably

TABLE II. Amino acid and carbohydrate composition of HFSH[a]

A. Amino acid composition

Amino Acid	μM/mg		
		Tyrosine	0.084
		Phenylalanine	0.207
Aspartic acid	0.467	Lysine	0.308
Threonine	0.405	Histidine	0.160
Serine	0.402	Arginine	0.196
Glutamic Acid	0.563		
Proline	0.341	B. Carbohydrate Composition	
Glycine	0.406		
Alanine	0.368	Carbohydrate	Dry wt (%)
Valine	0.368	Sialic acid	5.2
½ Cystine	0.140	Hexose (as mannose)	11.6
Methionine	0.055	Hexosamine	9.1
Isoleucine	0.170	Protein (Lowry-BSA)	78.0
Leucine	0.350	Total	103.9

[a]Data taken from Ref. 21.

that reported by Ryan et al. (22) of 35,000 ± 1000. There is some uncertainty concerning the sedimentation coefficient (S) of HFSH when examined at near neutral pH's. Values ranging from 1.67 S (36) to 4.63 S (37) have been reported. However, values for the most highly purified HFSH vary between 2.04 S (33) and 2.9 S (17, 22). Human FSH appears to have a Stokes radius of from 32 to 35Å (22, 31). We have recently completed an extensive series of studies designed to determine the isoelectric point (pI) of pituitary FSH from human and other sources, by the method of electrofocusing (38). HFSH fractions with biologic activity were detected between pH 3.36 and 5.55. This wide range of activity is probably due to a variable content of sialic acid among molecules in the HFSH preparation. In parallel studies with HLH, such apparent heterogeneity was resolved following digestion of the hormone with neuraminidase (38). Values of 3.0 (39), 4.25 (33) and 5.6 pI (37) have also been reported for HFSH.

SIALIC ACID REQUIREMENTS FOR BIOLOGICAL ACTIVITY OF HFSH

Amir et al. (23) have reported a complete loss of HFSH activity following incubation with neuraminidase. However, these workers did not specify what type of bioassay was used, nor did they provide details of their sialic acid or bioassay analysis. Mori (40) using a highly purified HFSH fraction prepared by us, also reported "0% residual activity" compared to control values, following neuraminidase digestion for 30 min. He did not indicate what amount of hormone had been tested in the exclusion assay; it is therefore difficult to assess below what level activity could actually by excluded. Morell et al. (41) working with the immunochemical grade HFSH preparation LER-869-2, described it as becoming "biologically inert" following neuraminidase incubation. Again, details of the bioassay were not provided.

In preliminary experiments with HFSH, we have observed a marked decrease, but not an absolute abolishment, of biologic activity, as measured in the Steelman-Pohley bioassay following treatment with neuraminidase (11). Interpretation of results of desialylation experiments are somewhat difficult. With neuraminidase in the enzyme digest, and in view of the sensitivity of HCG to this enzyme, separate site injections of the treated FSH preparation and HCG are, of course, required. Also, the problem of interpreting the degree of desialylation is complicated by an apparently nonspecific color development which occurs when using the standard Warren method (42) to compare the amount of sialic acid released by sulfuric acid (presumably all the sialic acid on the molecule) with that released after enzymic digestion. When such comparisons are made, an incorrect impression may be made that all sialic acid has been released when, in fact, it has not. The experiments summarized in Table III illustrate this point (compare A-1 and A-2). A second analysis for total sialic acid content by acid hydrolysis, carried out on the enzyme-treated preparation itself, is necessary to permit an accurate assessment of degree of desialylation.

As can be seen, an HFSH preparation which has had approximately 95% of its original sialic acid content removed by two consecutive digestions with neuraminidase still retained biological activity when tested at a sufficiently high dose level. This residual activity could be due to the small number of molecules apparently not desialylated. On the other hand, current concepts of glycoprotein metabolism suggest that terminal sialic acid residues are necessary for persistence of the molecule in the circulation (41). It has also been shown that desialylated HLH (43) and HCG (44) retain some biologic activity. By analogy, therefore, it might not be too surprising to find desialylated HFSH capable of eliciting an in vivo biologic response.

Regardless of whether further studies reveal the presence or absence of traces

TABLE III. Biological activity of desialylated HFSH

A Sialic acid (SA) analysis (41)

Preparation	Dose tested (mg)	OD 549 mμ	μM SA	μg SA	% SA (by wt)	% SA released
1 Precursor HFSH (825 IU/mg) SA released by sulfuric acid digestion	1	1.145	0.085	26.6	2.6	
2 SA released from HFSH by first neuraminidase digestion (conditions as in (42))	1	1.388	0.104	32.4	3.2	122
3 SA released from HFSH by a second neuraminidase digestion	1	0.103	0.007	2.38	0.24	8.9
4 SA released from A3 by sulfuric acid digestion, after it had been dialyzed and lyophilized	1	0.059	0.004	1.36	0.14	5.1

B Biologic activity of HFSH after two neuraminidase digestions

Preparation	Dose (μg)	Ovarian weights[a] (mg)	Mean
Saline		82, 62, 64, 58	66
Precursor HFSH	4.5	154, 143, 99, 191	147
Desialylated HFSH, A-3	1000.0	160, 156, 110, 151, 148, 91	136

[a]Bioassay (12) with augmenting dose of HCG = 40 IU. Separate injection sites for hormone and HCG.

of in vivo biologic activity in "desialylated" HFSH preparations, it is clear that, at least as measured by classical bioassay methods, sialic acid is vital for full expression of biologic activity. It seemed of interest, therefore, to explore whether an intact sialic acid moiety was required for such activity. The development of methods for generation of eight or seven carbon analogs of sialic acid on glycoproteins rendered such a study feasible, and they were undertaken in collaboration with Drs. M. Suttajit and R. J. Winzler (45). The general approach was to subject the HFSH to periodate oxidation, followed by borohydride reduction to yield sialic acid analogs shortened by one or two carbons. Oxidations were carried out at molar ratios of periodate to sialic acid content of HFSH ranging from 1.0 to 3.5. The results summarized in Table IV, indicate that an intact 3-carbon polyhydroxy side chain in sialic acid is not required for HFSH activity.

TABLE IV. Effect of modification of sialic acid on the biological activity of HFSH[a]

IO_4^-/sialic acid	Relative potency (IU/mg)[b]	% initial activity	Sialic acid content (μM/mg)		
			Intact	8-C	7-C
Control	1107.5		0.10	0	0
1.0	715.0	65	0.05	0.02	0
2.5	677.5	61	0.01	0.04	0.02
3.5	532.5	48	Trace	0.02	0.05

[a]Data taken from (44).

[b]Results expressed in terms of IU (2nd IRP-HMG), using the Steelman-Pohley assay (11, 12).

We have not mentioned the relationship of sialic acid to immunologic activity of HFSH. There appears to be general agreement, however, that desialylation does not cause a decrease in immunologic activity of HFSH and, in preliminary experiments carried out in collaboration with Drs. J. T. Vaitukaitis and G. T. Ross, it appears that similar results are obtained when the sialic acid is modified to the 8- or 7-carbon analogs by careful oxidation and reduction, as discussed above.

The Subunit Nature of HFSH

The subunit composition of ovine, bovine, HLH, bovine TSH, and HCG has been well established, and will be discussed in detail elsewhere during this symposium. A preliminary report has appeared dealing with the isolation of subunits of ovine

FSH (46). The material utilized for the subunit separation had a specific activity of 37 NIH-FSH-S1 U/mg. Recently, however, Sherwood et al. (9) have described preparation of an ovine FSH fraction having a biologic activity of 133 NIH-FSH-S1 U/mg, and our laboratory has had the opportunity to confirm this potency estimate. Thus the interpretation of the experiments described in Ref. 46 are as yet somewhat uncertain, although the difficulties encountered in the bioassay of highly purified ovine FSH preparations may be similar to those discussed earlier in relation to HFSH.

Gray (47) has described gel filtration studies with HFSH which suggest that it can exist in a monomeric form of about 17,000, but is capable of forming dimers and tetramers in milieu of decreasing ionic strength. In addition, he found peaks corresponding to all three molecular weight forms to be "active in the ovarian augmentation assay." In studies carried out in collaboration with Dr. A. Reese Midgley (31) we treated highly purified HFSH with 8M urea at room temperature for 24 hr. Before urea treatment the human FSH behaved as a single component on gel filtration through G-100 emerging with a K_{av} of 0.24 and a Stokes radius of 34.6Å. After urea treatment, an additional component was generated, emerging with a K_{av} of 0.41 and a Stokes radius of 22.3Å. These results could be interpreted as reflecting generation of a HFSH subunit component, or a mixture of dissimilar subunits. Interestingly, the 34.6Å component noted after urea treatment showed only 12% of the biologic and 7% of immunologic activity of the precursor hormone which had identical gel filtration characteristics. The 22.3Å component showed 4 and 14% of the immunologic activity of the precursor hormone.

Ryan et al. (22) have studied the physical properties of human FSH following treatment with guanidine hydrochloride. The molecular weight of the precursor HFSH fraction was 35,000 while a 16,000 molecular weight component was formed after incubation with the dissociating agent. The Stokes radius for the intact hormone was 32.2Å, while that for the dissociated form, considered to represent the HFSH subunits, was 23.2Å. These results were in excellent agreement with our earlier studies (31). An interesting observation was that dissociation appeared to be incomplete and also irreversible (22). This is apparently not the situation encountered when propionic acid is used as the dissociating agent (vide infra).

Treatment of HFSH with 1M propionic acid (10 mg/ml, room temperature, 16 hr) resulted in a greater than 99% decrease in FSH activity (Table V). After removal of the propionic acid by lyophilization and subsequent incubation (2 mg/ml, 0.01M phosphate buffer, pH 7.0, 16 hr, 40 C) activity was restored to a level 27-fold higher than present prior to incubation. By analogy with similar results reported with bovine LH and TSH (48) and ovine FSH (46), our data were interpreted as reflecting a dissociation of HFSH into subunits in the first instance, followed by their recombination. Addition of bovine LHα subunit (2, 48) to the HFSH subunit mixture prior to incubation did not affect the recovery of FSH biologic activity. Addition of bovine LH β subunit (2, 48), however,

TABLE V. Biological activity of HFSH before and after treatment with propionic acid and following incubation with and without bovine LH subunits[a]

Description	No. of assays	R.P. (IU/mg)[b]	% original activity
A Activity of HFSH prior to propionic acid incubation	3	812.5	—
B Activity after incubation of (A) with propionic acid, followed by lyophilization	1	< 8.0	< 1.0
C Activity of (B) after incubation[c]	4	217.5	27
D Activity of (B) after incubation with bovine-LH α	3	297.5	37
E Activity of (B) after incubation with bovine LH β	2	70.0	9

[a]Data taken from (48).

[b]Results expressed in terms of IU (2nd IRP-HMG), using Steelman-Pohley bioassay (11, 12).

[c]For details see text.

resulted in a significant decrease in biologic activity (Table V) (49). These results can be explained on the basis of a subunit structure for HFSH. Let us assume that HFSH is composed of subunits of the α (common) and β (hormone specific) types, and that the activity of any associated α-β dimer is determined by the nature of the hormone specific β subunit, which is the generally accepted notion (2, 46, 48). Let us also assume that a sufficient relatedness exists between HFSH α and bovine LH α to allow each to compete for binding sites on HFSH β or bovine LH β. Then bovine LH α would not be expected to affect the FSH activity of the reassociating HFSH subunits, since either HFSH α or bovine LH α could combine with HFSH β to give a dimer having FSH activity. Bovine LH β, however, could be expected to compete with HFSH β for combining sites on HFSH α, which would be limiting. The expected results with regard to FSH activity clearly have been shown to occur (compare C, D, and E in Table V). We recognize that if no similarity existed between bovine LH α and human FSH α, the results obtained in D would still be expected. However, the results obtained upon addition of bovine LH β (see E), would seem inconsistent with the alternate interpretation.

Further, we have observed similar results in parallel studies using subunits of human chorionic gonadotropin kindly supplied by Dr. Robert E. Canfield. In these experiments, propionic acid dissociated subunits from highly purified HFSH (4200 IU/mg) were first separated from undissociated and aggregated components by gel filtration through Sephadex G-100 prior to the biologic studies. Incubation of the human FSH subunit fraction in the presence of HCG β subunit resulted in a marked decrease in recovery of FSH biologic activity compared to that obtained in the absence of any HCG subunit or in the presence of HCG α subunit. In addition, when the HCG β subunit was added there was a concomitant increase in the LH potency of the mixture, presumably reflecting association of the HCG β subunit with FSH α subunit to give a hybrid molecule with the biologic characteristics of intact HCG. This increase in LH activity was not seen when the HCG α subunit was added.

These biologic studies, in addition to supporting the subunit concept for HFSH, also indicate a close relationship exists in the structures of human, bovine, and HCG α subunits.

Our results do not rule out the possibility that HFSH consists of two identical subunits, similar to bovine LH α and HCG α, and capable of recombining to give high biologic activity. However, this would imply that the α subunits isolated from LH, TSH, and HCG are also capable of associating to form molecules with FSH activity, and there has been, as yet, no indication that this can occur.

ACKNOWLEDGMENT

The study was supported by USPHS grant AM-3598, and is publication #1010 from the Division of Basic Health Sciences, Emory University.

It is a pleasure to acknowledge the able technical assistance of Mrs. Rosemary Ramsey, Mrs. Maria Wertz, Miss Donna Howell, and Mr. William Fugate in various phases of this work.

REFERENCES

1. Pierce, J. G., T. H. Liao, R. B. Carlsen, and T. Reimo, J Biol Chem 246:866, 1971.
2. Reichert, L. E., Jr., M. A. Rasco, D. N. Ward, G. D. Niswender, and A. R. Midgley, Jr., J Biol Chem 244:5110, 1969.
3. Papkoff, H., M. R. Sairam, and C. H. Li, J Amer Chem Soc 93:1531, 1971.
4. Liu, W. K., H. S. Nahm, C. M. Sweeney, H. N. Baker, W. L. Lamkin, and D. N. Ward, Res Comm Chem Pathol Pharmacol 2:168, 1971.
5. Liu, W. K., C. M. Sweeney, H. S. Nahm, G. N. Holcomb, and D. N. Ward, Res Comm Chem Pathol Pharmacol 1:463, 1970.
6. Morgan, F. J., and R. E. Canfield, Endocrinology 88:1045, 1971.
7. Swaminathan, N., and O. P. Bahl, Biochem Biophys Res Commun 40:422, 1970.
8. Reichert, L. E., Jr., A. R. Midgley, Jr., G. D. Niswender, and D. N. Ward, Endocrinology 87:534, 1970.
9. Sherwood, O. D., H. J. Grimek, and W. H. McShan, J Biol Chem 245:2328, 1971.
10. Reichert, L. E., Jr., Endocrinology 81:1180, 1967.
11. Steelman, S. L., and F. M. Pohley, Endocrinology 53:604, 1953.

12. Parlow, A. F., and L. E. Reichert, Jr., Endocrinology 73:740, 1963.

13. Albert, A., E. Rosemberg, G. T. Ross, C. A. Paulsen, and R. J. Ryan, J Clin Endocrinol 28:1214, 1968.

14. Albert, A., J Clin Endocrinol 28:1683, 1968.

15. Bliss, C. I., The Statistics of Bioassay, Academic, New York, 1952.

16. Parlow, A. F., in E. Rosemberg (Ed.), Gonadotropins 1968, Geron-X, Inc., Los Altos, 1968, p. 450.

17. Roos, P., Human Follicle Stimulating Hormone, Almqvist and Wiksells AB, Uppsala, 1967.

18. Peckham, W.D., and A. F. Parlow, Endocrinology 84:953, 1969.

19. Saxena, B.B., and P. Rathnam, J Biol Chem 242:3769, 1967.

20. Reichert, L. E., Jr., and A. F. Parlow, Proc Soc Exp Biol Med 115:286, 1964.

21. Reichert, L. E., Jr., R. Kathan, and R. J. Ryan, Endocrinology 82:109, 1968.

22. Ryan, R. J., N. S. Jiang, and S. Hanlon, Biochemistry 10:1321, 1971.

23. Butt, W. R., in E. Diczfalusy (Ed.), Karolinska Symposium on Research Methods in Reproductive Endocrinology, 1st Symposium, Stockholm, 1969, p. 13.

24. Amir, S. M., S. A. Barker, W. R. Butt, and A. C. Crooke, Nature (London) 209:1092, 1966.

25. Butt, W., in G. E. Lamming and E. C. Amorose (Eds.), Reproduction in the Female Mammal, Butterworths, London, 1967, p. 113.

26. Ryan, R. J., N. S. Jiang, and S. Hanlon, Rec Prog Hormone Res 26:105, 1970.

27. Parlow, A. F., A. E. Wilhelmi, and L. E. Reichert, Jr., Endocrinology 77:1126, 1965.

28. Hartree, A. S., Biochem J 100:754, 1966.

29. Reichert, L. E., Jr., and A. F. Parlow, Endocrinology 74:236, 1964.

30. Reichert, L. E., Jr., J Clin Endocrinol 27:1065, 1967.

31. Reichert, L. E., Jr., and A. R. Midgley, Jr., in E. Rosemberg (Ed.), Gonadotropins 1968, Geron-X, Inc., Los Altos, 1968, p. 26.

32. Reichert, L. E., Jr., in Colloques Internationaux Du Centre National De La Recherche Scientifique No. 177, Paris, 1969, p. 315.

33. Saxena, B. B., and P. Rathnam, in E. Rosemberg (Ed.), Gonadotropins 1968, Geron-X, Inc., Los Altos, 1968, p. 3.

34. Butt, W. R., A. C. Crooke, and A. Wolfe, in G. E. Wolstenholme and J. Knight (Eds.), Gonadotropins: Physicochemical and Immunologic Properties, Ciba Foundation Study Group #22, Churchill, Ltd., London, 1965, p. 85

35. Hermier, C., P. de la Llosa, and M. Jutisz, Endocrinology 87:1364, 1970.

36. Li, C. H., P. G. Squire, and U. Gröschel, Arch Biochem 86:110, 1960.

37. Papkoff,H.,L. J. Mahlmann, and C. H. Li, Biochemistry 6:3976, 1967.

38. Reichert, L. E., Jr., Endocrinology 88:1029, 1971.

39. Bettendorf, G., M. Brickwoldt, P. J. Czygan, A. Fock, and T. Kunsaaka, in E. Rosemberg (Ed.), Gonadotropins 1968, Geron-X, Los Altos, 1968, p. 13.

40. Mori, K. F., Endocrinology 85:330, 1969.

41. Morell, A. G., G. Gregoriadis, I. H. Scheinberg, J. Hickman, and G. Ashwell, J Biol Chem 246:1461, 1971.

42. Warren, L., J Biol Chem 234:1911, 1959.

43. Braunstein, G. D., L. E. Reichert, Jr., E. V. Van Hall, J. L. Vaitukaitis, and G. T. Ross, Biochem Biophys Res Commun 42:962, 1971.

44. Van Hall, E. V., J. L. Vaitukaitis, G. T. Ross, J. W. Hickman, and G. Ashwell, Endocrinology 88:456, 1971.
45. Suttajit, M., L. E. Reichert, Jr., and R. J. Winzler, J Biol Chem, in press, 1971.
46. Papkoff, H., and M. Ekblad, Biochem Biophys Res Commun 40:619, 1970.
47. Gray, C. J., Nature 216:1112, 1967.
48. Liao, T. H., and J. G. Pierce, J Biol Chem 245:3275, 1970.
49. Reichert, L. E., Jr., Endocrinology, 89:925, 1971.

10. Subunits of FSH from Human Pituitary Glands[1]

P. Rathnam and B. B. Saxena[2]

Since 1964, several investigators have attempted to isolate FSH in a high state of purity (1, 2). The specific activities of FSH have ranged from 45 to 555 NIH–FSH–SI U/mg (3, 4). Species specificity and low yield of highly purified FSH and LH from a scarce source like human pituitaries necessitated the development of procedures to isolate hormones of the anterior pituitary from the same batch of glands. Collection and provision made by the National Pituitary Agency in the United States have permitted significant advances in this endeavor. A procedure developed in our laboratory for the preparation of anterior pituitary hormones is summarized in Fig. 1.

ISOLATION AND PROPERTIES OF FSH

Human pituitary glands were extracted to obtain a glycoprotein fraction containing predominantly FSH, LH, and TSH. This fraction was further purified by ascending chromatography on Sephadex G-100 (5) and ion exchange chromatography on CM-Sephadex C-50. As shown in Fig. 2, fractionation on CM-Sephadex C-50 resulted in a significantly purer FSH fraction than that obtained from CM-cellulose resin columns (6). The FSH was isolated by zone electrophoresis on cellulose and polyacrylamide gel (5).

The physicochemical characterization of human pituitary FSH has been

[1]This study was supported by grants AM-11187 and T1-AM-5350 from the National Institutes of Health, and by grant M71.26 from the Population Council, Rockefeller University, New York.

[2]Career Scientist Awardee, Health Research Council, City of New York Contract I-621.

partly described earlier (6). A continuous absorption spectrum of a 0.01% solution of FSH measured between 200 and 340 mμ is shown in Fig. 3. An absorption maximum at 278 mμ was obtained. The effect of various chemical and enzymatic treatments on the biological activity of FSH is shown in Table I.

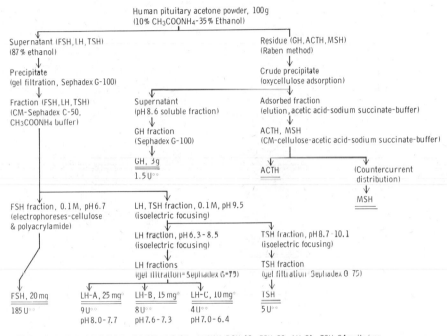

Sialic acid content - LH-A 0.5%; -B 1.3%; -C 1.8%   NIH-BGH-10; -FSH-S3; -LH-S1; -TSH-S4 units / mg

FIG. 1.   Isolation of the hormones of the anterior pituitary gland.

The biological activity was found to be stable to dialysis in water and 8M urea, to pH changes from 5.5 to 9.5, and at temperatures between 25 to 37 C. The loss of activity caused by the removal of sialic acid and neutral sugars suggests that an essential role is played by the carbohydrate moiety in the biological activity of FSH. Chemical cleavage with cyanogen bromide also caused a loss of activity indicating that one or more methionine residues may constitute a part of the active core of the hormone. Biological activity was not lost by the reduction of disulfide groups with mercaptoethanol followed by alkylation with iodoaceta-mide indicating that some of these bonds may not be essential for the biological activity of FSH. However, the oxidation by performic acid destroyed the biological activity of FSH. Enzymatic digestion of FSH with DFP-treated carboxypeptidase-A, pepsin, trypsin, chymotrypsin, trypsin + chymotrypsin, papain, and pronase did not destroy the biological activity of FSH. In 1969, we described the isolation and preliminary characterization of a biologically active glycopeptide from FSH by papain digestion (7). In addition to the earlier suggestion of the existence of FSH in more than one of its polymeric forms (5), circular dichroism studies revealed a high random coil and a low α-helical configuration of the FSH molecule. Hence a systematic study on the physical behavior of FSH in the analytical ultracentrifuge was undertaken.

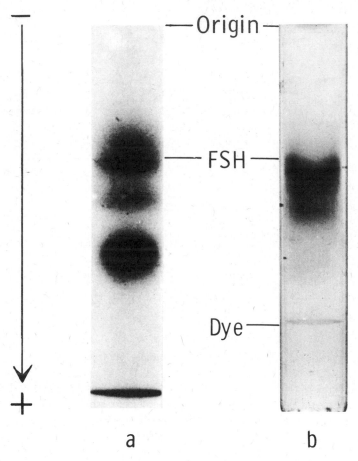

a   b

FIG. 2. Comparison of disc electrophoretic patterns of FSH fraction from (a) CM cellulose column (6); and (b) CM-Sephadex C-50 column (5).

As shown in Fig. 4, the sedimentation rate of FSH is concentration dependent. When extrapolated to zero protein concentration, values of 1.98S and 2.89S were obtained which fit into a monomer-dimer model (8). In 8M urea however, FSH showed a reduction in the sedimentation rate to 0.61 S (Table II).

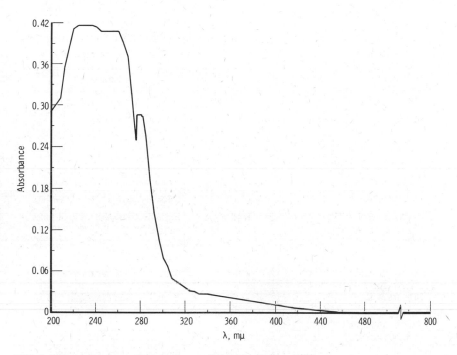

FIG. 3. Ultraviolet absorption spectrum of human pituitary FSH.

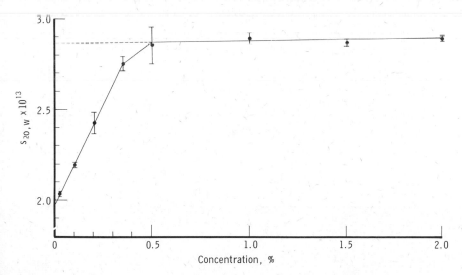

FIG. 4. The variation of the sedimentation rate of human pituitary FSH with concentration.

TABLE I. The effect of various treatments on the biological activity of human pituitary FSH.

Treatment	Biological activity	Remarks
Dialysis against H_2O, 72 hours at 4	Retained	
Dialysis against 8M urea in H_2O, 72 hours at 4	Retained	Effect on hydrogen bonds
0 to 50 , 24 hours	Retained	
Removal of sialic acid	Lost	
Cyanogen bromide	Lost	Cleavage at methionine residues
Performic acid	Lost	Oxidative cleavage of disulfide bonds
Mercaptoethanol, 0.1M, 24 hours followed by iodoacetamide, 0.1M, 24 hours	Retained	Reductive cleavage of disulfide bonds and alkylation of sulfhydryl groups
DFP	Retained	
Carboxypeptidase A enzyme: substrate 1:50; pH 8.0; 20 hours at 37	Retained	Cleavage of C-terminal residues
Pepsin enzyme: substrate 1:20 and 1:50; pH 5; 24 hours at 37	Retained	
Trypsin enzyme; substrate 1:20; pH 8.0; 24 hours at 37 and 50	Retained	Cleavage at lysine and arginine residues
Chymotrypsin enzyme: substrate 1:20; pH 8.0; 24 hours at 37 and 50	Retained	Cleavage at aromatic residues
Trypsin + chymotrypsin enzyme: substrate 1:20; pH 8.0; 24 hours at 50	Retained	
Papain enzyme: substrate 1:20; pH 6.0; 24 hours at 50	Retained	
Pronase enzyme: substrate 1:50; pH 8.0; 40 hours at 37	Retained	
Renin enzyme: substrate 1:50; pH 7.0; 24 hours at 37	Lost	Cleavage at leu-leu residues

TABLE II. Physical properties of human pituitary FSH

Protein concentration (%)	Sedimentation rate
	($S_{20,w}$ in S/sec)
2.0	2.89 ± .01[a]
1.5	2.86 ± .02
1.0	2.89 ± .03
0.5	2.86 ± .10
0.35	2.75 ± .04
0.20	2.43 ± .06
0.10	2.20 ± .01
0.025	2.04 ± .01
Extrapolated to 0.000	1.98
	2.89
In 8M urea[b]	0.61 ± .10
Diffusion coefficient ($D_{20,w}$)[b]	7.504×10^{-7} cm^2/sec
Frictional coefficient	7.898×10^{-8}
Partial specific volume ($\bar{v}$)	0.72
Molecular weight[b]	32,600
Stokes radius	
FSH (22.6 mg)	31.3Å
FSH labeled with ^{131}I (2 μg)	23.7Å

[a]SD.

[b]At 0.5% concentration.

ISOLATION AND PROPERTIES OF THE SUBUNITS OF FSH

The retention of biological activity (Table I), and the markedly lower $S_{20,w}$ of FSH in 8M urea suggested the dissociation of FSH into moieties of smaller molecular weights. Evidence on the subunit nature of HCG (9, 10), and ovine LH (11) also suggested the possibility of the dissociation of FSH into subunits. Hence 20 mg of FSH was treated with 8M urea in 0.04M Tris-phosphate buffer of pH 7.5 at 40 C for two hr and the urea digest was fractionated on a column of DEAE-Sephadex A-50. As shown in Fig. 5, two major protein fractions designated as α and β subunits were eluted.

The α and β subunits of FSH were purified by gel filtration on a 2 x 100 cm column of Sephadex G-100 (Fig. 6). The α subunit eluted with a V_e/V_o of 1.77 as a single peak and the β subunit eluted with a V_e/V_o of 2.13. An additional peak with V_e/V_o of 1.80 was also eluted with the β subunit. This peak had a higher mobility in disc electrophoresis than the α subunit, and may represent undissociated or reassociated FSH, or a polymerized subunit as suggested for ovine FSH (12). The V_e/V_o values of the α and β subunits suggested slight dissimilarity in their molecular weights.

As shown in Fig. 7a, the disc electrophoresis of FSH at pH 8.6 showed a single band. The patterns of the α and β subunits of FSH revealed two basic and three acidic bands, respectively (Figs. 7c and d). The presence of more than one band in the α and β subunits may be due to the electrophoretic microheterogeneity similar to that encountered in the subunits of glycoprotein hormones such as HCG (9), bovine LH (13), and bovine TSH (14).

The yield and biological activity (15, 16) of the subunits of FSH are summarized in Table III. From 20 mg FSH, 4 mg of the α subunit were obtained. The yield of the β subunit prior to and following gel filtration was 11 and 5 mg respectively. The α and β subunits of FSH were incubated (1 : 1 w/w) in 0.2M phosphate buffer of pH 6.8, for 16 hr at 37 C (17). The bioassays of the incubated subunits, prior to gel filtration on Sephadex G-100, revealed 50 U/mg

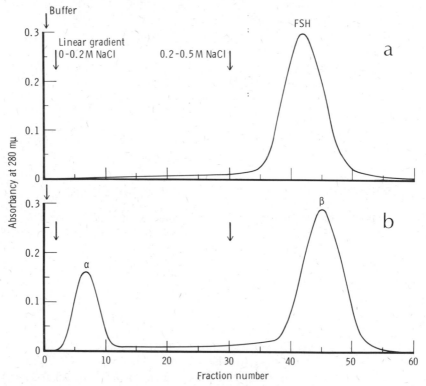

FIG. 5. Ion exchange chromatography on a 1.5 × 50 cm column of DEAE-Sephadex A-50 of (a) 20 mg FSH; (b) 20 mg of urea-treated FSH. Flow rate: 6 ml/hr.

representing approximately a sixfold augmentation over the predicted FSH activity, suggesting the reassociation of the subunits. Incomplete reassociation due to the absence of optimal ratio of subunits and conditions of incubation used in these studies as well as those with the subunits of HCG (9, 10), ovine LH (11, 18), bovine LH and TSH (17, 19), and human LH (20, 21) may account for not achieving activities closer to that of the native molecule. It may be of interest that the biological activity of FSH in 8M urea (Table I) was greater than that of the α and β subunits. This may be due to the recombination of the naturally occuring ratio of α and β subunits in the aliquot of urea-treated FSH used in the assay, as compared to 1 : 1 (w/w) ratio of the subunits used in the present reassociation studies.

Liao and Pierce (19), and Papkoff and Ekblad (12) have suggested a homology of the α subunits of ovine LH and TSH, and of ovine LH and FSH, respectively. Reichert et al. (20) presented evidence that following recombination of C-II subunits of bovine LH with the C-I subunit of human LH, some biological activity could be reconstituted. Similar homology with respect to human gonadotropins was examined by incubation of the α subunits of FSH, LH, and HCG with the β subunits of each of these hormones, using conditions described above. The results of specific bioassays of FSH (15), LH (16), and the incubated products are shown in Table IV. The α and β subunits of FSH and

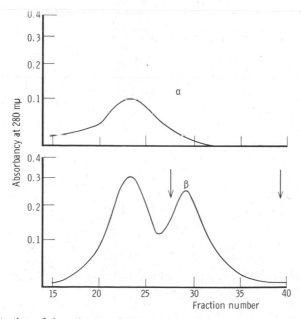

FIG. 6. Gel filtration of the subunits of FSH on a 2 × 100 cm column of Sephadex G-100. Flow rate of 6-10 ml/hr. Buffer: 0.05M phosphate containing 0.05M NaCl.

HCG could be substituted for the α subunit of LH to generate 4.6 and 6.9 NIH–LH–S1 U/mg, representing augmentation. Further, the α subunit of FSH substituted for the α subunit of HCG to generate almost entire activity of the native HCG molecule. In the incubation experiments, the β subunits prior to gel filtration were used; however, the augmentation of the biological activity over the predicted additive or average values support the reassociation of the α and β subunits. These observations confirm the hormone specificity of the β subunits and suggest a homology of the α subunit of FSH, LH, and HCG.

In Table V, analyses of 24-hr hydrolysates of the α and β subunits of FSH are compared with those of the subunits of LH (22) and of HCG (9). The α subunits are nonidentical with the β subunits for example in Met, Tyr, and His content. The α subunits of FSH, LH, and HCG exhibit certain common characteristics, for example, a high content of glutamic acid, and a Lys/Arg ratio of >1.0. The Lys/Arg ratio of the β subunits of LH and HCG are reciprocal to that of the β subunit of FSH.

These results confirm the homology of the α subunits of FSH, LH, and HCG, and the hormone specificity of the β subunits.

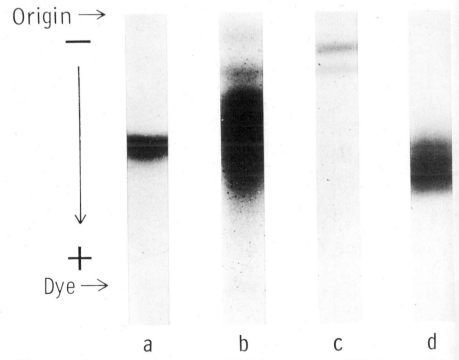

FIG. 7. Disc electrophoretic pattern at pH 8.6 of (a) human pituitary FSH; (b) urea-treated FSH; (c) α subunit of FSH; and (d) β subunit of FSH.

TABLE III. Yield and biological activity of the subunits of FSH

Fraction	Yield (mg)	FSH Specific $U^{a,b}$/mg	FSH Total U^a	Recovery (%)
FSH	20	185.0 ± 10.0	3700	100.0
α subunit	4	3.3 ± 1.2	13	0.4
β subunit[d]	11	12.0 ± 1.4	132	3.6
$\alpha + \beta$ subunits[c] (1:1 w/w)		50.0 ± 3.8		

[a] 1 unit is equivalent to 1 mg NIH-FSH-S3 = 1.1 mg NIH-FSH-S1 = 1.43 mg LER-907 = 29.15 IU of 2nd IRP-HMG.

[b] Mean ± SD.

[c] Yield, total activity, and recovery were not calculated as the optimal ratio in which the α and β subunits recombine is not determined (see text).

[d] Yield of β subunit following gel filtration was 5.1 mg.

TABLE IV. Homology of α subunits of FSH, LH, and HCG

Fraction	Specific activity $(U/mg)^a$ FSH	Specific activity $(U/mg)^a$ LH[b]
FSH α + LH β	n.d.[c]	4.6(3.0– 8.3)
FSH α + HCG β	n.d.	18.0(9.6–48.4)
LH α + FSH β	22.6 ± 5.0	1.2(0.8– 1.9)
LH α + HCG β	n.d.	7.9(1.1–14.0)
HCG α + LH β	n.d.	6.9(3.6–22.6)
HCG α + FSH β	53.4 ± 9.2	0.8(0.4– 1.6)

[a] NIH-FSH-S3 U ± SE or in NIH-LH-S1 U (95% confidence limits).

[b] 1 unit NIH-LH-S1 = 588 IU 2nd IRP-HMG; 1 unit NIH-LH-S1 = 513 U HCG-2nd International Standard.

[c] Not detectable.

129

TABLE V. Amino acid analyses[a] of the subunits of FSH, LH, and HCG

Amino acid residue	FSH		LH		HCG (9)	
	α	β	α	β	α	β
			g/100 g protein			
Lysine	5.6	6.5	5.3	3.9	7.8	3.5
Histidine	3.2	1.6	3.3	3.8	3.9	1.1
Arginine	4.0	3.0	5.3	8.0	4.2	10.7
Aspartic acid	8.7	8.7	8.1	6.8	7.3	9.7
Threonine	6.3	7.0	7.2	5.6	8.0	6.6
Serine	5.1	4.2	5.4	5.3	7.2	7.8
Glutamic acid	11.4	11.2	10.3	8.3	12.7	8.9
Proline	7.4	10.3	8.2	14.7	6.9	13.8
Glycine	3.4	2.2	2.7	2.8	2.5	3.3
Alanine	4.8	4.6	3.6	4.1	3.3	3.9
Valine	5.9	5.8	7.6	7.9	7.0	6.6
Cysteine	5.1	12.0	8.2	5.8	9.4	7.4
Methionine	6.4	1.3	2.2	2.1	3.0	0.4
Isoleucine	3.6	4.1	4.9	5.2	0.9	2.9
Leucine	4.8	5.1	5.0	6.4	4.0	8.4
Tyrosine	1.7	4.3	6.0	3.3	5.9	3.0
Phenylalanine	5.4	4.0	5.3	4.3	5.8	2.2

[a]24-hr hydrolysates.

ACKNOWLEDGMENT

We are grateful to Dr. R. E. Canfield of Columbia University, New York for kindly supplying us with the subunits of HCG; to the National Pituitary Agency, Baltimore, Md. for supplying us with human pituitary glands; to the Endocrine Study Section of the National Institutes of Health, Bethesda, Md., for supplying NIH—FSH—S3.

REFERENCES

1. Geschwind, I. I., Gen Comp Endocrinol Supple 2:180, 1969.
2. Geschwind, I. I., in H. H. Cole, (Ed.), Gonadotropins, Freeman, San Francisco, 1964.
3. Butt, W. R., Acta Endocrinol (Kbh) 63(Suppl 142):13, 1969.
4. Hellema, M. J. C., J Endocrinol 49:393, 1971.
5. Saxena, B. B., and P. Rathnam, in E. Rosemberg (Ed.), Gonadotropins 1968, Geron-X, Inc., Los Altos, 1968, p. 3.

6. Saxena, B. B., and P. Rathnam, J Biol Chem 242:3769, 1967.

7. Rathnam, P., and B. B. Saxena, in Proceedings of Workshop on the Chemistry of Gonadotropins (1969), Birmingham, England, Livingston, Edinburgh, 1971, p. 107.

8. Schachman, H. K., Ultracentrifugation in Biochemistry, Academic, New York, 1959, p. 242.

9. Swaminathan, N., and O. P. Bahl, Biochim Biophys Res Commun 40:422, 1970.

10. Morgan, F. J., and R. E. Canfield, Endocrinology 88:1045, 1971.

11. de la Llosa, P., C. Courte, and M. Jutisz, Biochim Biophys Res Commun 26:411, 1967.

12. Papkoff, H., and Ekblad, M., Biochim Biophys Res Commun 41:614, 1970.

13. Liao, T. H., G. Hennen, S. M. Howard, B. Shome, and J. G. Pierce, J Biol Chem 244:6458, 1969.

14. Hennen, G., G. Maghun-Rogister, and G. Mamoir, FEBS Lett 9:20, 1970.

15. Steelman, S. L., and F. M. Pohley, Endocrinology 53:604, 1953.

16. Parlow, A. F. in A. Albert (Ed.), Human Pituitary Gonadotropins, Charles C. Thomas, Springfield, Ill, 1961, p. 300.

17. Reichert, L. E., Jr., M. A. Rasco, D. N. Ward, G. D. Niswender, and A. R. Midgley, J Biol Chem 244:5110, 1969.

18. Papkoff, H., and T. S. A. Samy, Fed Proc 27:371, 1968.

19. Liao, T. H., and J. G. Pierce, J Biol Chem 245:3275, 1970.

20. Reichert, L. E., Jr., A. R. Midgley, Jr., G. D. Niswender, and D. N. Ward, Endocrinology 87:534, 1970.

21. Reichert, L. E., Jr., and A. R. Midgley, Jr., in E. Rosemberg (Ed.), Gonadotropins 1968, Geron-X, Inc., Los Altos, 1968, p. 25.

22. Saxena, B. B., and P. Rathnam, Fed Proc 30:473, 1971.

11. Comparative Studies of Ovine, Bovine, and Human LH

Darrell N. Ward, Leo E. Reichert, Jr., Wan-Kyng Liu, Hyun S. Nahm, and William M. Lamkin

In this presentation we shall attempt to show two things: 1) that the peptides from the specific degradation of ovine and bovine luteinizing hormones are identical in behavior and composition, thus presumably indicating an identical amino acid sequence; and 2) that human luteinizing hormone, by the behavior and properties of its subunits, differs considerably from the reported properties of ovine, bovine, porcine, and murine luteinizing hormone (LH) subunits.

The number of chromatograms, degradation procedures, and amino acid analyses required to detail our results for item 1) are prohibitive for this presentation. Instead what we shall attempt to do is summarize the peptide isolations involved by reference to the amino acid sequences we have proposed for ovine LHα (1) and the ovine LHβ (2). These sequences are presented in Figs. 1 and 2. In the case of the ovine LHβ sequence we were led to reexamine the sequencing of two of the peptides of our original sequence proposal for two reasons; first, the bovine peptides appeared to be different in terms of composition and second, these particular peptides showed a disagreement with the recent sequence proposal of Papkoff, Sairam, and Li (3). As a result of our reinvestigation we have inserted an additional threonine residue at position 28 in agreement with the proposal of Papkoff et al. (3). We have also inserted a half-cystine residue at positions 34 and 89, which is not in agreement with that of Papkoff et al. (3). The revised sequence of LHβ in Fig. 2 in all has 20 amino acids located differently from the sequence proposed by Papkoff et al. (3). The LHα sequence in Fig. 1 has two amino acids inverted from that proposed by Papkoff et al. (3).

[R]$^+$ - Gln - Gly - CysAE - Pro   Gln - CysAE - Lys - Leu - Lys - Glu - Asn - Lys - Tyr - Phe - Ser - Lys - Pro
         10   15   20   25

Asp - Ala - Pro - Ile - Tyr - Gln - CysAE - Met - Gly - CysAE - CysAE - Phe - Ser - Arg - Ala - Tyr - Pro - Thr -
                      30   35   40

Pro - Ala - Arg - Ser - Lys - Lys - Thr - Met - Leu - Val - Pro - Lys - Asn (CHO$_{S\alpha}$) - Ile - Thr - Ser - Glu -
     45   50   55   60

Ala - Thr - CysAE - CysAE - Val - Ala - Lys - Ala - Phe - Thr - Lys - Ala - Thr - Val - Met - Gly - Asn - Val -
                         65   70

Arg - Val   Glu - Asn (CHO$_{S\beta}$) - His - Thr - Glu - CysAE   His - CysAE - Ser - Thr - CysAE - Tyr - Tyr - His
         80   85   90

Lys - Ser - OH †[R] = H - Phe - Pro - Asn - Gly - Gln - Phe - Thr - Met -
                                                   1   5

FIG. 1. Amino acid sequence of the S-aminoethylated ovine luteinizing hormone S-subunit
(LH-α).

In addition to 20 amino acid placement differences in LHβ there are three additional differences between the two laboratories which should be mentioned. First, we find an acyl group on the NH$_2$-terminus of LHβ (4), although recent evidence indicates this acyl group is very labile or present on only a portion of the molecules. Further research is required on this point.

The second difference relates to the COOH-terminus of the LH β. We found a COOH-terminal aspartic acid (4), while Samy, Papkoff, and Li reported initially a -Cys-Ile-Leu-OH sequence, but recently revised this to an -Asp-Ile- Leu·OH (3). As first noted by Dr. Rasco studying bovine LH β in our laboratory (6), there is apparently a proteolytic removal of Ile-Leu in positions 119 and 120 of the LH β. We have now found this reaction to be almost quantitative for ovine pituitary glands in the isolation procedure we employ (7), but by heat denaturation of proteases similar to the step applied by Papkoff et al. (8), we can avoid this reaction at least partially. Bovine pituitaries appear to have somewhat less of this particular protease activity (6). Thus the difference we long held between our studies and those of C. H. Li's laboratory was an operational difference. What we were seeing as COOH-terminal was residue 118 in the sequence for LH β, and we agree that residues 119 and 120 must now be included. We should also mention at this point that the preparations obtained by Dr. Reichert, one of the co-authors, showed a COOH-terminal leucine (9). Recent work has shown in one of his preparations (LER-1373) an 11 amino acid peptide is obtained as the COOH-terminal peptide after tryptic digestion. Therefore, one may isolate an LH β which terminates with the leucine residue at position 116, too. Thus unless one specifically examines it, a COOH-terminal leucine may indicate a 116 amino acid subunit, 120 amino acid subunit, or combinations of both. One may also conclude that the presence of absence of these last four amino acids does not greatly affect the biological activity.

Acyl – Ser – Arg – Gly – Pro – Leu – Arg – Pro – Leu – CysCM – Gln – Pro – Ile – Asn(CHO) – Ala – Thr – Leu – Ala – Ala –
5   10   15

Glu – Lys – Glu – Ala – CysCM – Pro – Val – CysCM – Ile – Thr – Phe – Thr – Thr – Ser – Ile – CysCM – Ala – Gly – Tyr – CysCM –
20   25   30   35

Pro – Ser – Met – Lys – Arg – Val – Leu – Pro – Val – Ile – Leu – Pro – Pro – Met – Pro – Gln – Arg – Val – CysCM –
40   45   50   55

Thr – Tyr – His – Glu – Leu – Arg – Phe – Ala – Ser – Val – Arg – Leu – Pro – Gly – CysCM – Pro – Pro – Gly – Val – Asp –
60   65   70   75

Pro – Met – Val – Ser – Phe – Pro – Val – Ala – Leu – Ser – CysCM – His – CysCM – Gly – Pro – CysCM – Arg – Leu – Ser –
80   85   90   95

Ser – Thr – Asp – CysCM – Gly – Pro – Gly – Arg – Thr – Glu – Pro – Leu – Ala – CysCM – Asp – His – Pro – Pro – Leu – Pro –
100   105   110   115

Asp – Ile – Leu – OH
120

FIG. 2. Amino acid sequence of S-carboxymethylated A-subunit of ovine LH (LH-β).

The third difference we should mention may just be an apparent one. We found an NH_2-terminal heterogeneity on the LHα subunit. We find this on both bovine and ovine LHα. Liao et al. found a similar NH_2-terminal heterogenity on bovine TSHα (10) as apparently did Bates and Condliffe (11). This heterogeneity was not mentioned in the report of Papkoff et al. (3), who showed simply an NH_2-terminal phenylalanine, although their earlier reports had indicated only NH_2-terminal proline detected as the PTH derivative (5). In this same report they mention, however, "DNS-proline could not be identified with certainty because of the multiplicity of spots on the chromatogram" (5).

The designation of amide residues (glutamine or asparagine) in Figs. 1 and 2 has been based on best available evidence as judged by chromatography or electrophoresis, although in several instances this has been confirmed by direct analysis as the methyl thiohydantoin derivative obtained from the Edman degradation of the appropriate peptide.

In Fig. 3 is presented the scheme for the degradative approach applied initially to ovine LHα (1) and subsequently to bovine LHα. The peptides obtained in both instances appear identical. The sequence determination for several of those derived from bovine LHα have been completed and in all instances have been identical to those established for ovine LHα. These observations are in complete accord with those of Pierce et al. (12) who find the

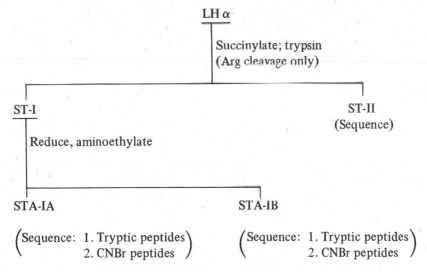

FIG. 3. LH α degradation scheme for sequence determination.

tryptic peptides from bovine LHα to be identical with those of bovine TSHα. Our laboratory, in turn, found the ovine LHα amino acid sequence (1) to be identical to the bovine TSHα amino acid sequence reported by Liao et al. (10). By the location in Table I we have attempted to summarize the overlap peptides obtained using the scheme shown in Fig. 3 applied to both ovine and bovine LHα. The numbers given are the inclusive numbers for the amino acid residues in Fig. 1.

TABLE I. Ovine and bovine LH α peptides for sequencing, arranged by degradation source and assigned overlaps[a]

Peptide:	STA-IB-CNBr	STA-IB-T	ST-II	STA-IA-CNBr	STA-IA-T
	1-8	1-14			
		15-32			
	9-33	33-35			
		36			
	34-39	37-39			
			40-46		
				47-51	47-63
					64
					65-69
				52-75	70-77
					78-79
					80-86
					87-88
					89-91
					89-92
			76-96		92-96

[a]Numbers refer to Fig. 1; peptides designated as in Fig. 3.

In Fig. 4 we summarize the scheme employed for the determination of the amino acid sequence of ovine LHβ (2), which has also been applied to bovine LHβ. Again in Table II we attempt to summarize the overlap peptides in terms of the inclusive residue numbers from Fig. 2. As noted earlier the apparent differences in bovine and ovine LHβ eventually led to a revision of our ovine sequence. Our studies to date will allow us to state that the amino acid sequence of ovine and bovine LH is identical to within a 98% certainty.

At this point we briefly call attention to the sequence interrelationships between TSH and LH, which has been so nicely established largely as a result of the work of Dr. Pierce and collaborators at UCLA (12, 13). As noted earlier the LHα and TSHα homology is identical or nearly so. We do not know how the carbohydrate sequences compare as yet nor whether the disulfide bonds close the same. Since the subunit of TSH or LH may be used interchangeably to combine with TSHβ or LHβ, presumably the disulfide bond closures must be identical in the α subunit from either source, but this is as yet unproven.

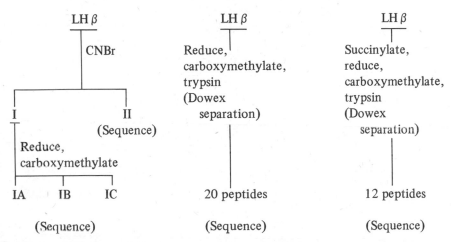

FIG. 4.   LH β degradation scheme for sequence determination.

As Dr. Pierce pointed out in the Laurentian Hormone Conference last fall (14) the areas of homology between TSHβ and LHβ very likely represent areas involved in the binding of the β to α subunit. For reference a bar is placed above the areas of identity or near identity in the case of the one long run. In the understanding of protein subunit interactions, this system has unique features which allow a theoretical delimitation not found in other protein subunit recombination systems.

The converse to the above may also be stated, namely, the areas of difference between LHβ and TSHβ must relate to the nature of any specific receptor site in their respective target organ. If we pursue this reasoning further one might expect the α subunit to perform a common function in either target organ.

Since evidence is accumulating that the subunit relationships of the LH-TSH system are also shared by HCG (15-17) and FSH (18-20), it is attractive to speculate that the knowledge of sequence for these hormones can be more readily applied to detailed studies on their mechanism of action than has proved possible for the other protein hormone sequences. We yet need some ingenious investigators to make our prediction true.

We would next turn to some studies on human LH(HLH) which are far too early for sequence comparisons as with the bovine and ovine LH. In Fig. 5 is shown a typical countercurrent distribution pattern obtained with the Papkoff-Samy system (21) applied to ovine, bovine, porcine, or murine LH. All of these species show the same pattern: a very low partition coefficient for the α subunit, and a very high coefficient for the β subunit. When we tried to apply this

TABLE II. Ovine and bovine LH β peptides for sequencing, arranged by degradation source and assigned overlaps[a]

Peptide:	CNBr-IA	Succinyl-SCM-T	CNBr-II	CNBr-IC	CNBr-IB	SCM-T
						1-2
		1-2				3-6
	1-41	3-43	42-53			7-20
						3-20
						21-42
						43
		44-56		54-80		44-56
		57-64				57-64
		65-69				65-69
		70-80				70-80
		70-87			81-120	70-87
		81-95				81-87
		88-95				81-95
		96-105				88-95
		106-120				96-105
						106-120

[a]Numbers refer to Fig. 2; peptides designated as in Fig. 4.

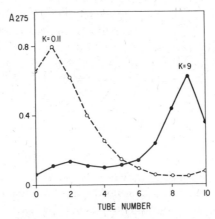

FIG. 5. Countercurrent distribution pattern for 10 mg rat LH, n = 10, solvent system of Papkoff and Samy (21) with the modifications of Reichert et al. (22). Similar distribution patterns are obtained with ovine, bovine, and porcine LH. Dotted line = A_{275} of lower phase; solid line, upper phase.

countercurrent distribution system to human LH a rather different result was obtained. One of our first patterns is shown in Fig. 6. Our initial impression was that the dissociation of subunits was too difficult. Subsequently Dr. Reichert obtained evidence this was not the case. We would now interpret this pattern as simply indicating failure to achieve a true partition equilibrium. We routinely

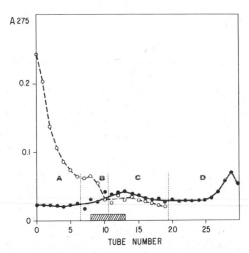

FIG. 6. Early attempt to apply the countercurrent distribution system described in Fig. 5 to 20 mg of HLH, n = 30. The fraction D represents an upper phase withdrawal beginning at transfer number 20. Cross-hatched area designates an interphase precipitate (denaturation?). Dotted line = A_{275}, lower phase; solid line, upper phase.

apply the modifications to the Papkoff-Samy procedure which we found necessary for reproducible separations of the subunits (22). However, in all of our subsequent attempts to use countercurrent distribution with HLH we have employed the following additional devices: first, the time of mixing each tube was increased threefold (90 sec on a Vortex mixer, 0.5 to 1.0 ml/phase); second, the sample was equilibrated overnight with 6M guanidine hydrochloride prior to starting the distribution (the sample was diluted 1 : 4 with lower phase—the guanidine remains in the first tube). In one experiment the distribution was conducted at 37 C, but with no apparent advantage. Under these conditions the pattern shown in Fig. 7 was obtained.

The countercurrent distribution pattern (Fig. 7) suggested that a separation of subunits of HLH had been achieved. This was substantiated by recombination studies (23) and hybridization with human LHα and bovine LHβ (24) using biological activity as an endpoint. There is one serious drawback to the Papkoff-Samy procedure for subunit separation for HLH which concerns the removal of the high salt content employed in the solvent (21). This was particularly difficult since our separations generally involved 0.4 to 20 mg of

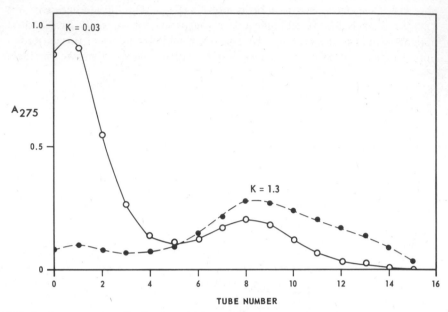

FIG. 7. Countercurrent distribution of 17 mg of HLH, pretreated for 16 hr in 6M guanidine hydrochloride, then submitted to countercurrent distribution (n = 15) as in Fig. 5, but with increased mixing at each transfer. Solid line, A_{275} lower phase; dotted line, upper phase.

human LH. The major difficulty concerns the recovery of the HLHβ, which was influenced by adsorption on glassware, dialysis membranes, or ultrafiltration membranes. Using a variety of techniques we have often recovered only a few percent of this subunit, but seldom as much as 50% of the theoretical quantity. As a result, both our biological and chemical studies of subunits have suffered. A more efficient procedure is clearly indicated, and studies are in progress which we hope will provide this. In the interim, we present our best analyses of the preparations so far in Table III. We do not regard these as definitive composition studies for several reasons; namely, at the level of material analyzed we anticipate losses of the sulfur-containing amino acids during hydrolysis; analyses are on 24-hr hydrolysates only and no corrections for decomposition or difficult hydrolyses have been made; and the complete removal of salt during the isolation has not been insured, thus the data are presented only as μmoles per 100 μmoles analyzed, a presentation which suffers distortion from losses in analysis, and so on. Nevertheless, the data are sufficient to indicate that HLHβ is quite different from ovine LHβ, both in its physical properties (i.e., the lower partition coefficient) and its composition. Less can be said concerning HLHα since the partition coefficient observed implies virtually complete exclusion from the upper phase (as is true of the other LH α subunits examined in this system), thus the system is not constituted to detect differences in this instance.

TABLE III. Amino acid composition of the subunits of HLH[a]

Amino acid	LH α	LH β	Amino acid	LH α	LH β
Lysine	6.6	2.6	Alanine	5.4	4.9
Histidine	3.9	2.6	Half-cystine	7.0[b]	7.7[b]
Arginine	4.0	7.7	Valine	7.9	10.2
Aspartic acid	6.9	6.7	Methionine	2.6[b]	1.8[b]
Threonine	8.1	6.2	Isoleucine	2.6	3.9
Serine	8.5	5.1	Leucine	5.7	7.8
Glutamic acid	9.8	7.3	Tyrosine	3.7	3.4
Proline	6.6	14.4	Phenylalanine	3.6	2.0
Glycine	6.9	6.3			

[a]Values are nm amino acid/100 nm analyzed; 24-hr hydrolyses only.

[b]Under the conditions of hydrolysis the sulfur-containing amino acids will give low values.

Also the composition studies do not suggest large differences, thus we can at least be led to expect more minor differences in the HLHα compared to ovine LHα, and so on, than one anticipates for the HLHβ compared to ovine LHβ, and so on. We hope to say more concerning these chemical comparisons by the time the next International Symposium on Gonadotropins convenes.

Finally, since it has been reported HLH has more sialic acid than ovine or bovine LH (25-27), we wished to determine whether removal of sialic acid by neuraminidase would materially alter the distribution pattern. For this experiment 480 μg of asialo HLH, preparation LER 1486-2b$_1$ of the study by Braunstein et al. (26), were iodinated with ^{125}I according to the procedure of Sonoda and Schlamowitz (28) with conditions designed to add no more than one iodine per molecule. Excess iodine-iodide was removed on a Sephadex G-100 column, 1.2 × 100 cm, and the labeled HLH recovered at $V_e/V_o = 1.6$ to 1.7. Under these conditions no "damaged" LH was observed at the void volume. Upon submitting the labeled asialo HLH to 6M guanidine hydrochloride overnight, and subjecting this material to the countercurrent distribution procedure described above the pattern obtained in Fig. 8 as measured by ^{125}I labeling was obtained. Two things are evident. First, the removal of 94% of the sialic acid (26) failed to alter the distribution pattern of HLH. Second, from the relative area under the curve, the labeling of the two subunits was very nearly equal. This also demonstrates how one may test a variety of separation conditions with very little expenditure of material, a point already made by Ryan (29) and Reichert (22) in their studies on LH and long utilized by all the radioimmunoassayists in the audience.

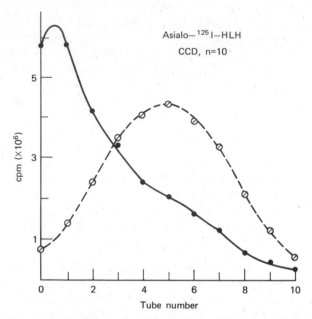

FIG. 8. Countercurrent distribution (n = 10) of 480 μg of iodinated asialo HLH (see text), using the conditions described for Fig. 7, but with iodine counting in upper and lower phase aliquots to measure the distribution; solid line, counts for 100 μl aliquot lower phase; dotted line upper phase; total vol/phase, 500 μl.

ACKNOWLEDGMENT

This research was supported in part by research grants from The USPHS, NIH: AM-3598 (LER) and AM-9801; from The Robert A. Welch Foundation G-147; and contract 69-2221 from the Center for Population Research. We are indebted to Dr. Shunro Sonoda for iodinating the asialo HLH used in this study.

REFERENCES

1. Liu, W-K., H. S. Nahm, C. M. Sweeney, H. N. Baker, W. M. Lamkin, and D. N. Ward, Res Commun Chem Pathol Pharmacol 2:168, 1971.

2. Liu, W-K., C. M. Sweeney, H. S. Nahm, G. N. Holcomb, and D. N. Ward, Res Commun Chem Pathol Pharmacol 1:463, 1970.

3. Papkoff, H., M. R. Sairam, and C. H. Li, J Amer Chem Soc 93:1531, 1971.

4. Liu, W-K., C. M. Sweeney, and D. N. Ward, Res Commun Chem Pathol Pharmacol 1:214, 1970.

5. Samy, T. S. A., H. Papkoff, and C. H. Li, Arch Biochem Biophys 130:674, 1969.

6. Rasco, M. A., Ph.D. Dissertation, The University of Texas Graduate School of Biomedical Sciences, Houston, Texas, January 1970.

7. Ward, D. N., M. A. Mayne, N. Ray, D. E. Balke, J. Coffey, and M. Showalter, Gen Comp Endocrinol 8:44, 1967.

8. Papkoff, H., D. Gospodarawicz, A. Candiotti, and C. H. Li, Arch Biochem Biophys 111:431, 1965.

9. Reichert, L. E., Jr., Endocrinology 78:186, 1966.

10. Liao, T-H., and J. G. Pierce, J Biol Chem 246:850, 1971.

11. Bates, R. W., and P. G. Condliffe, Recent Prog Hormone Res 16:309, 1960.

12. Pierce, J. G., T-H. Liao, R. B. Carlsen, and T. Reimo, J Biol Chem 246:866, 1971.

13. Liao, T-H., and J. G. Pierce, J Biol Chem 245:3275, 1970.

14. Pierce, J. G., T-H. Liao, S. M. Howard, B. Shome, and J. S. Cornell, Recent Prog Hormone Res, in press, 1970.

15. Swaminathan, N., and O. P. Bahl, Biochem Biophys Res Commun 40:422, 1970.

16. Bell, J. J., R. E. Canfield, and J. J. Schiarra, Endocrinology 84:298, 1969.

17. Reichert, L. E., Jr., unpublished results.

18. Papkoff, H., and M. Ekblad, Biochem Biophys Res Commun 40:614, 1970.

19. Reichert, L. E., Jr., this symposium.

20. Rathnam, P., and B. B. Saxena, J Biol Chem 246:3549, 1971.

21. Papkoff, H., and T. S. A. Samy, Biochim Biophys Acta 147:175, 1967.

22. Reichert, L. E., Jr., M. A. Rasco, D. N. Ward, G. D. Niswender, and A. R. Midgley, Jr., J Biol Chem 244:5110, 1969.

23. Reichert, L. E., Jr., D. N. Ward, G. D. Niswender, and A. R. Midgley, Jr., In W. Butt, and A. Crooke (Eds.), Gonadotrophins and Ovarian Development, E. & S. Livingston, Edinburgh, 1971, p. 149.

24. Reichert, L. E., Jr., A. R. Midgley, Jr., G. D. Niswender, and D. N. Ward, Endocrinology 87:534, 1970.

25. Kathan, R. H., L. E. Reichert, Jr., and R. J. Ryan, Endocrinology 81:45, 1967.

26. Braunstein, G. D., L. E. Reichert, Jr., F. V. Van Hall, J. L. Vaitukaitis, and G. T. Ross, Biochem Biophys Res Commun 42:962, 1971.

27. Gröschel, U., and C. H. Li, Biochim Biophys Acta 37:375, 1960.

28. Sonoda, S., and M. Schlamowitz, Immunochemistry 7:885, 1970.

29. Ryan, R. J., Biochemistry 8:495, 1969.

12. The Chemistry of Ovine Interstitial Cell Stimulating Hormone

M. R. Sairam, Harold Papkoff, and Choh Hao Li

The pioneering work of Smith and Engle (1) established the presence of gonadotropic factor(s) in the anterior pituitary gland. Fevold et al. (2) in 1931 showed that two factors present in the anterior pituitary were necessary for maintenance of normal reproductive cycles in the female. After obtaining a partial separation of the two factors they were designated follicle stimulating hormone (FSH) and luteinizing hormone [LH, interstitial cell stimulating hormone (ICSH)]. Li, Simpson, and Evans (3) first reported the isolation of ICSH from sheep pituitary glands, and Shedlovsky et al. (4) from porcine glands. The interest in the study of the detailed chemistry of ICSH was rekindled by the development of two new procedures for the isolation of the ovine hormone (5-7). These studies have shown that ovine ICSH is a homogeneous protein with a molecular weight of 30,000, containing carbohydrate. Following the demonstration that under acidic conditions ovine ICSH behaves as a monomer of molecular weight 16,000 (8) and the suggestion that ovine ICSH may consist of 2 nonidentical subunits (9), Papkoff and Samy (10) realized the separation of the two subunits of ovine ICSH molecule by means of countercurrent distribution. The two dissimilar subunits were designated CI—material having a low K value and found in the lower aqueous phase, and CII—the material concentrated in the upper phase and having a high K value. Recently the ovine ICSH subunits, CI and CII have been redesignated ICSH α and ICSH β, respectively. After the initial observation of Papkoff and Samy (10) on the separation of ovine ICSH subunits a number of reports have appeared on the separation of subunits of ICSH from different species such as bovine (11-13), porcine (14), and human (15, 16).

In this paper some of the recent investigations conducted in our laboratory on the chemical aspects of ovine ICSH are reviewed.

ISOLATION OF OVINE ICSH AND ITS SUBUNITS

Ovine ICSH was isolated according to procedures previously described (5, 6, 17). Biological activity of the ICSH as determined by the ovarian ascorbic acid depletion (OAAD) method (18) was shown to be 2.5 times the potency of NIH-S1 preparation. Immunochemical characterization of the hormone and its subunits have also been described (19).

The separation (10) of the two subunits of the hormone achieved by the countercurrent distribution procedure is illustrated in Fig. 1. The organic phase

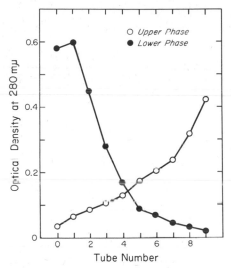

FIG. 1. Countercurrent distribution of 50 mg of ovine ICSH. Solvent system: 40% ammonium sulphate (w/v)-0.2% dichloroacetic acid-n-propanol-ethyl alcohol (60:60:27:33); 5 ml of each phase; the lower phases of tube 0 to 3 represent the ICSH α fraction and upper phases of tubes 6 to 9 represent the ICSH β fraction.

contains exclusively the β subunit while the aqueous phase consists of the α subunit contaminated with undissociated ICSH. A clear separation of the α subunit from the undissociated ICSH is achieved by gel filtration on Sephadex G-100, in 0.05M ammonium bicarbonate (Fig. 2).

PHYSICOCHEMICAL PROPERTIES OF THE HORMONE AND ITS SUBUNITS

Some of the physicochemical properties of the hormone and its subunits are tabulated in Table I. The molecular weight of the hormone as determined by the

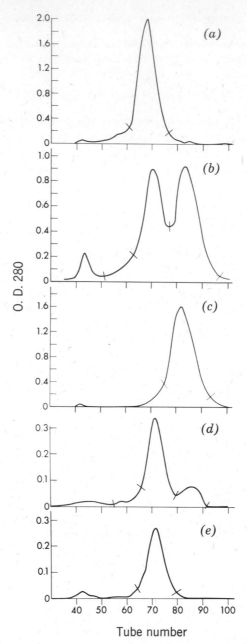

FIG. 2. Gel filtration pattern of native ovine ICSH, α fraction and reassociated ICSH. Sephadex G-100, 3.4 × 78 cm. equillibrated with 0.05 M ammonium bicarbonate containing 0.02% sodium azide, room temperature, 4.8 ml/fraction 30 to 35 ml/hr. (a) Elution pattern of native ICSH. (b) Elution pattern of CCD lower phase material. F 63 to 76, undissociated ICSH; F 77 to 96, α fraction. (c) Rerun of F 77 to 96 from B. (d) Elution pattern of reassociated ICSH molecule. 25 mg each of the α and β subunits were dissolved in 2.5 ml 0.1M phosphate buffer pH 6.0, and incubated at room temperature for 24 hr. The mixture was directly chromatographed. F 67 to 79 represents reassociated molecule. (e) Rerun of F 67 to 79 from D.

ultracentrifugation technique is dependent upon pH; at pH 6.8, an S_{20} value of 2.47 S corresponding to a molecular weight of 28,000 to 30,000 is obtained, while at acidic pH the hormone behaves as a monomer with an S^{20} value of 1.64 S and an average molecular weight of 16,300. Ovine ICSH is a neutral protein with an isoelectric point at pH 7.1 to 7.3. The α subunit has an amino terminal phenylalanine and carboxyl terminal serine, while the β subunit begins with an amino terminal serine and terminates in leucine.

TABLE I. Some physicochemical properties of ovine ICSH and subunits

Property	ICSH	α	β
Molecular weight	30,000	13,700[a]	14,600[a]
S_{20} pH 6.8	2.74		
pH 1.3	1.64		
Isoelectric point	7.3		
Partition coefficient in CCD (K)		low K	high K
Carbohydrates, %	15	18	11
Terminal amino acids			
N-	Phe Ser	Phe	Ser
C-	Ser Leu	Ser	Leu
Tyrosine, %	4.5	6.6	2.5
Tryptophan	Absent	Absent	Absent

[a]Calculated from structure (21).

The amino acid composition of the performic acid oxidized ICSH and its subunits as listed in Table II reveals some striking features. There is a somewhat reciprocal relationship in the content of the basic amino acid lysine and arginine in the two subunits, while the histidine content is identical. Both subunits have a large number of half-cystines. The content of hydrophobic amino acids in the β subunit is unusually high, comprising nearly 43% of the total number in contrast to 28% in the α subunit. The α subunit has twice the number of aromatic residues in the β. The methionine content of the two subunits also differ.

Analysis of the carbohydrate moiety of the two subunits (Table III) shows that the α subunit has nearly twice (18%) that of the β (11%).

TABLE II. Amino acid composition of performic acid oxidized ICSH and subunits[a]

Amino acid	ICSH		α subunit		β subunit		Reassociated[b]	
	Experimental	Theoretical	Experimental	Theoretical	Experimental	Theoretical	Experimental	Theoretical
Lysine	12.9	12	9.8	10	3.4	2	13.4	
Histidine	6.0	6	3.0	3	3.0	3	6.0	
Arginine	11.4	11	2.9	3	8.0	8	10.0	
Cysteic acid	20.4	22	9.3	10	11.0	12		
Aspartic acid	10.5	11	5.8	6	5.0	5	11.3	
Methionine sulfone	6.7	7	3.8	4	2.7	3		
Threonine	15.0	16	8.6	9	6.6	7	16.0	
Serine	13.1	14	5.8	6	7.0	8	13.4	
Glutamic acid	14.1	14	8.1	8	6.9	6	14.5	
Proline	26.9	28	7.0	7	24.1	21	28.5	
Glycine	10.7	11	4.1	4	7.0	7	11.0	
Alanine	14.2	15	6.6	7	8.3	8	15.3	
Half-cystine							21.1	22
Valine	11.4	13	5.2	5	7.0	8	10.7	
Methionine							5.8	7
Isoleucine	6.0	7	1.9	2	3.7	5	6.2	
Leucine	12.9	14	2.3	2	10.3	12	13.6	
Tyrosine	5.6	7	3.5	5	1.8	2	5.2	
Phenylalanine	7.0	8	4.2	5	3.0	3	6.9	

[a]Hydrolyzed for 22 hr at 110 C, values expressed as molar ratios; Thr and Ser values are uncorrected.

[b]Has not been oxidized.

TABLE III. Carbohydrate composition of ovine ICSH and
subunits

Preparation	Hexose	Hexosamine	Fucose
ICSH[a]	12.0	10.7	2.9
α subunit[b]	7.7	5.9	1.3
β subunit[b]	4.0	4.0	1.0

[a]Residues/30,000.

[b]Residues/15,000.

IMMUNOLOGICAL AND BIOLOGICAL PROPERTIES

Ovine ICSH is an excellent antigen and a rabbit antiserum to the native hormone is capable of neutralizing the biological activity of ICSHs from different species (20) indicating structural similarity of the antigenic determinants in the molecule. Of the two subunits of ovine ICSH, it appears that the β subunit is more strongly antigenic than the α and thus a major contributor to the antigenicity of the whole ICSH molecule (19). A summary of the cross-reactions obtained with antisera to the hormone and subunits is given in Table IV. It is interesting to note that the biological activity of the native ICSH could be neutralized only by an antiserum to ICSH and the β subunit, but not by an antiserum to the α subunit.

The subunits α and β of ICSH are by themselves virtually inactive in the OAAD test. Incubation of the two subunits under proper conditions (see Table V for details) leads to regeneration of biological activity. The reassociated molecule is indistinguishable from the native in its behavior on Sephadex G-100 (Fig. 2e), amino acid analysis (Table II) and immunological behavior (19).

PRIMARY STRUCTURE OF THE α AND β SUBUNITS (21-23)

The general approach to the elucidation of the primary structure of the subunits is indicated in Table VI. The determination of sequence of 40 residues at the C-terminus of the β subunit is herein described in some detail as an example. This fragment was isolated by gel filtration on Sephadex G-50 in 20% formic acid as one of the four reaction products of the CNBr treated, reduced, and carbamidomethylated β subunit. The amino acid composition of these 4 fragments along with the theoretical values computed from the final structure of the subunit is given in Table VII. The detailed sequence analysis of the C-terminal 40 amino acid fragments is summarized in Table VIII. Tryptic digestion of a fraction containing this fragment yielded three peptides, CB4-T1, CB4-T2, and CB4-T3, the sum of whose amino acids corresponded nicely to the

TABLE IV. Immunological cross-reactivity of ICSH and subunits[a]

Antigen	A/S ICSH			A/S ICSH β		
	Equivalence Region (μg)	Precipitate[b] (μg)	Cross Reaction (%)	Equivalence Region (μg)	Precipitate (μg)	Cross Reaction (%)
ICSH	25-30	330	100	5	220	78
β subunit	20	230	70	5	280	100
α subunit		60	18		50	18

[a]Taken from (19).
[b]Precipitate at or near the equivalence region.

150

TABLE V. Biological activity of subunits and the reassociated molecule

Preparation	Specific activity	95% limits	λ
ICSH	2.06	1.02-4.2	0.24
α subunit	0.014	0.011-0.018	0.090
β subunit	0.032	0.027-0.038	0.062
Reassociated ICSH[a]	1.2	0.7-2.29	0.25

[a]Was prepared by incubating equal amounts of the subunits at 10 mg/ml concentration in 0.1 M phosphate buffer pH 7.0 for 24 hr. The mixture was directly diluted with saline for assay.

TABLE VI. General approach to the analysis of sequence

1. CNBr treatment and performic acid oxidation; reduction and alkylation followed by CNBr treatment.

2. Maleylation and trypsin digestion of oxidized materials.

3. Chymotrypsin digestion.

4. Subtilisin degradation of complicated peptides.

5. Leucine aminopeptidase and carboxypeptidase kinetic studies.

6. Edman-dansyl-subtractive procedure.

total composition of the RA-CB-4 fraction. The three tryptic peptides were digested further with subtilisin to obtain smaller fragments suitable for sequence analysis. The peptides CB-T1 and CB-T3 containing three cysteic acid residues and four proline residues, respectively, were the most difficult ones dealt with in this portion of the β subunit. Because of the presence of these unusually large numbers of cysteic acid and proline residues, the peptides were resistant to the action of chymotrypsin and pepsin. Only subtilisin digestion yielded fragments suitable for complete structural elucidation. Since the peptide CB4-T1 begins with valine which is also the amino terminal of the RA-CB-4 fragment this should obviously be the N-terminal peptide, and the peptide CB4-T3 having the C-terminal sequence -Ile-Leu, identical with the RA-CB-4 fraction as well as the oxidized β subunit itself, must be C-terminal peptide of RA-CB-4 and hence of the β subunit. From this information the ordering of the three tryptic peptides in this CNBr fragment would be CB4-T1 $\longrightarrow$ CB4-T2 $\longrightarrow$ CB4-T3.

In a manner analogous to the sequencing of the RA-CB4 fraction, the entire amino acid sequence of the two α and β subunits of ovine ICSH have thus been recently determined (21) as shown in Figs. 3 and 4.

TABLE VII. Amino acid composition of the CNBr fragments of reduced and carbamidomethylated β subunit[a]

Amino acid	CB-1		CB-2		CB-3		CB-4	
	Actual values	Theoretical	Actual values	Theoretical	Actual values	Theoretical	Actual values	Theoretical
Lys	1.0	1	1.1	1	1.0	1	0.3	2
His	0.3		0.1			1	1.7	2
Arg	2.0	2	1.0	1	2.5	3	2.0	5
SCMC	4.0	5			1.4	2	4.1	3
Asp	1.0	1	0.14		0.9	1	2.5	3
Thr	2.6	4	0.10		0.8	1	1.9	2
Ser	2.5	3	0.14		0.6	1	3.0	4
Glu	2.6	3			2.1	2	1.4	1
Pro	8.4	5	6.6	4	7.8	5	7.6	7
Gly	1.9	2	0.28		2.0	2	2.8	3
Ala	3.9	5	0.20		1.4	1	2.2	2
Val	1.2	1	1.6	2	2.6	3	2.3	2
Ile	2.1	3	0.7	1			0.5	1
Leu	3.0	3	2.0	2	2.2	2	4.4	5
Tyr	0.6	1			0.8	1	0.1	
Phe	0.9	1	0.12		1.0	1	1.0	1
Homoserine	Present	1	Present	1	Present	1		
Carbohydrate	Present							
NH₂ terminal	Ser		Lys		Pro		Val	
Total No. of residues	41		12		27		40	

[a]The values obtained after 22-hr hydrolysis are expressed in terms of molar ratios. Thr, Ser, and SCMC values have not been corrected for hydrolytic destruction. Homoserine where present is assumed to be equivalent to 1 residue.

TABLE VIII. Amino acid sequence of the C-terminal cyanogen bromide fragment of ICSH β subunit

RA-CB-4	Val-Ser-Phe-Pro-(Val, Ala, Leu,Ser,Cys,[a] His,Gly,Pro,Cys,[a] Cys,[a] Arg,
	$\rightarrow$ $\rightarrow$ $\rightarrow$ $\rightarrow$
CB-4-T1[b]	Val-Ser-Phe-Pro- Val(Ala, Leu,Ser,Cys,[c] His,Gly,Pro,Cys[c])Cys[c]-Arg
	$\rightarrow$ $\rightarrow$ $\rightarrow$ $\rightarrow$ $\rightarrow$ $\leftarrow$ $\leftarrow$
CB-4-T1S1[d]	Val(Ser,Phe,Pro, Val)Ala- Leu
	$\leftarrow$ $\leftarrow$
CB-4-T1S2	Ser-Cys[c]-His-Gly-Pro-Cys[c]-Cys[c]-Arg
	$\rightarrow$ $\rightarrow$ $\rightarrow$ $\rightarrow$ $\rightarrow$ $\rightarrow$ $\leftarrow$ $\leftarrow$

Sequence	Val-Ser-Phe-Pro- Val-Ala- Leu-Ser-Cys -His-Gly-Pro-Cys -Cys -Arg
	81 85 90 95

RA-CB-4 (cont.)	Leu,Ser,Ser,Thr,Asx,Cys,[a] Gly,Pro,Gly,Arg,Thr,Glx,Pro,Leu,Ala,Cys[a]
CB-4-T2[b]	Leu-Ser-Ser-Thr-Asp-Cys[c]-Gly(Pro,Gly)Arg
	$--\rightarrow$ $--\rightarrow$ $--\rightarrow$ $--\rightarrow$ $--\rightarrow$ $--\rightarrow$ $--\rightarrow$
	$\rightarrow$ $\rightarrow$ $\rightarrow$ $\rightarrow$ $\rightarrow$ $\rightarrow$ $\rightarrow$
CB-4-T2S1[d]	Leu(Ser,Ser,Thr)
	Asp-Cys[c]-Gly-Pro-Gly-Arg
	$\rightarrow$ $\rightarrow$ $\rightarrow$ $\rightarrow$ $\rightarrow$ $\leftarrow$
CB-4-T3[b]	Thr-Glu-Pro-Leu-Ala(Cys[c]
	$--\rightarrow$ $\rightarrow$ $\rightarrow$ $\rightarrow$ $\rightarrow$
CB-4-T3S1	Thr-Glu-Pro-Leu[e]
	$\rightarrow$ $\rightarrow$
CB-4-T3S2	Ala-Cys[c]
	$\rightarrow$ $\rightarrow$

Sequence	Leu-Ser-Ser-Thr-Asp-Cys -Gly-Pro-Gly-Arg-Thr-Glu-Pro-Leu-Ala- Cys
	96 100 105 110

RA-CB-4 (cont.)	Asx,His,Pro,Pro,Leu,Pro,Asx)Ile-Leu
	$\leftarrow$ $\leftarrow$
CB-4-T3 (cont.)	Asx,His,Pro,Pro,Leu,Pro,Asx)Ile-Leu
	$\leftarrow$ $\leftarrow$
CB-4-T3S2 (cont.)	Asp-His-Pro-Pro-Leu-Pro-Asp-Ile-Leu
	$\rightarrow$ $\rightarrow$ $\rightarrow$ $\rightarrow$ $\rightarrow$ $\rightarrow$ $\leftarrow$ $\leftarrow$

Sequence	Asp-His-Pro-Pro-Leu-Pro-Asp-Ile-Leu
	115 120

Note: $--\rightarrow$ Leucine aminopeptidase digestion; $\longrightarrow$ Indicates sequence by Edman-Dansyl method; $\longrightarrow$ Sequence determination by Edman-Dansyl-subtractive method; $\longleftarrow$ Carboxypeptidase A digestion; $\longleftarrow$ Carboxypeptidase A and B digestion; $\longleftarrow$ Carboxypeptidases A and B and hydrazinolysis.

[a] Present as S-carbamidomethylcysteine in this fragment.

[b] Tryptic peptide isolated from mixture of CNBr fragments of the β subunit.

[c] Present as cysteic acid in this peptide.

[d] Obtained from a subtilisin digest.

[e] Determined by hydrazinolysis.

H-Phe-Pro-Asp-Gly-Glx-Phe-Thr-Met-Glx-Gly-Cys-Pro-Glx-Cys-[Lys]-Leu-
                                      10

[Lys]-Glu-Asn-[Lys]-Tyr-Phe-Ser-[Lys]-Pro-Asx-Ala-Pro-Ile-Tyr-Gln-Cys-
          20   30

Met-Gly-Cys-Cys-Phe-Ser-[Arg]-Ala-Tyr-Pro-Thr-Pro-Ala-[Arg]-Ser-[Lys]-
                              40

                                   CHO
[Lys]-Thr-Met-Leu-Val-Pro-[Lys]-Asn-Ile-Thr-Ser-Glu-Ala-Thr-Cys-Cys-
    50   60

Val-Ala-[Lys]-Ala-Phe-Thr-[Lys]-Ala-Thr-Val-Met-Gly-Asn-Val-[Arg]-Val-
                70   80

CHO
Glx-Asn-His-Thr-Glx-Cys-His-Ser-Cys-Thr-Cys-Tyr-Tyr-His-[Lys]-Ser-OH
                                      90

FIG. 3. Amino acid sequence of ICSH α subunit.

                                             CHO
H-Ser-[Arg]-Gly-Pro-Leu-[Arg]-Pro-Leu-Cys-Glu-Pro-Ile-Asn-Ala-Thr-Leu-Ala-Ala-Glu-[Lys]-
                               10   20

Glu-Ala-Cys-Pro-Val-Cys-Ile-Thr-Phe-Thr-Thr-Ser-Ile-Gly-Ala-Tyr-Cys-Cys-Pro-Ser-
                              30   40

Met-[Lys-Arg]-Val-Leu-Pro-Val-Pro-Pro-Leu-Ile-Pro-Met-Pro-Gln-[Arg]-Val-Cys-Thr-Tyr-
                              50   60

His-Gln-Leu-[Arg]-Phe-Ala-Ser-Val-[Arg]-Leu-Pro-Gly-Pro-Cys-Pro-Val-Asp-Pro-Gly-Met-
                              70   80

Val-Ser-Phe-Pro-Val-Ala-Leu-Ser-Cys-His-Gly-Pro-Cys-Cys-[Arg]-Leu-Ser-Ser-Thr-Asp-
                              90   100

Cys-Gly-Pro-Gly-[Arg]-Thr-Glu-Pro-Leu-Ala-Cys-Asp-His-Pro-Pro-Leu-Pro-Asp-Ile-Leu-OH
                   110   120

FIG. 4. Amino acid sequence of ICSH β subunit.

DISCUSSION.

Nearly three decades after the first isolation of ovine ICSH, the primary structure of the hormone has been worked out. The ICSH molecule consists of two dissimilar subunits bound by noncovalent linkages and contains a total of 216 amino acid residues. One of the subunits, α begins with an amino terminal phenylalanine and terminates with a serine, whereas the β subunit has serine at the amino terminus and leucine at the carboxyl terminal end. The α subunit has 96 amino acids and nearly twice as much carbohydrate as the β subunit which has 120 amino acid residues. The two carbohydrate moieties in the α subunit are linked at different places to asparagine residues at positions 56 and 82, while in the β subunit the single carbohydrate moiety is linked to asparagine at position 13. A perusal of the amino acid sequence around the point of attachment of the carbohydrate reveals a general pattern Asn-X-Thr, where X is another amino acid

$$\text{CHO}$$

residue. This general sequence has also been found in the subunits of another pituitary glycoprotein hormone, TSH (24, 25). Eylar (26) theorizes that this may be a signal for the enzyme to attach the carbohydrate moiety to the asparagine in the biosynthesis of the glycoprotein.

The primary structures of the α and β subunits have certain remarkable features. Both have a large number of half-cystine residues: 10 and 12, respectively; in each there are areas in which they occur in succession or in clusters, for example $\alpha_{45,46}$, $_{63,64}$, $_{86,91}$, and $\beta_{74,76}$, $_{47,48}$ and $_{93,94}$. The three histidine residues of the α subunit are all found near the C-terminus, and so are two of the five tyrosine residues in the molecule. The distribution of the large number of hydrophobic residues in the β subunit is very unusual; they occur in clusters in regions 70-79, 44-54 and 114-120.

Recently Liu et al. (27) have also proposed the amino sequence for the A chain (equivalent to β) of ovine ICSH. A comparison of this structure with our proposal reveals certain differences. A total of five residues are lacking in their proposal, two half-cystines, and one each of threonine, leucine, and isoleucine located at positions 38, 94, 28, 119, and 120, respectively, in our formulation.[1]

The subunits, particularly α, exhibit microheterogeneity. The heterogeneity in the α subunit occurs at the amino terminus: tryptic peptides beginning with Phe_1, Asp_3 and Gly_4, were isolated from digests of the oxidized material. Further by the dansyl chloride technique, these same amino acids were detected as N-terminus in the oxidized α subunit. The same degree of heterogeneity has been found in the case of bovine TSH α and bovine ICSH α subunits too (24). Although no heterogeneity has been detected in our preparations of the β subunit, Liu et al. (27) indicate that their structure for the A chain terminates in Asp, which is the third residue from the C-terminus of our β structure. This would indicate that in their preparations the dipeptide -Ile-Leu is missing from the original molecule. Interestingly, TSH β also has heterogeneity at the

[1] D. N. Ward (private communication) has now confirmed the presence of the additional threonine and two half cystines found in our structure of ICSH β subunit. Ward and co-workers (32) have also recently postulated the amino acid sequence of the ovine ICSH α subunit.

C-terminus (25). Thus, the overall picture emerges that in the two chains of both ICSH and TSH, the heterogeneity seems to be located at the amino terminus of the α subunit and at the carboxyl terminus of the β subunit. The pituitary gland is notoriously active in peptidases (28). These enzymes might be responsible for cleavage of certain residues at the termini. It should be pointed out that particular care should be taken to eliminate such proteolytic activity during the purification procedures employed (17). In addition to the heterogeneity of the peptide portion, there may also be heterogeneity in the carbohydrate moiety.

A comparison of the structures of the two subunits of ovine ICSH with bovine TSH indicate striking similarities. In fact, the amino acid sequences of the two α subunits are nearly identical. The β subunit structure also reveals identity or close similarity in a sufficiently large number of regions; Fig. 5 sketches the similarities in the two β subunit structures. It can also be seen that there is excellent similarity in the spacing of the half-cystine residues in the two sequences.

```
                                                     18
H-Ser-Arg-Gly-Pro-Leu-Arg-Pro-Leu-Cys-Glu-Pro-Ile-Asn-Ala-Thr-Leu-Ala-Ala-
                  H-Phe-Cys-Ile-Pro-Thr-Glu-Tyr-Met-Met-His-Val-Glu-
                                                     12

                                                          37
    Glu-Lys-Glu-Ala-Cys-Pro-Val-Cys-Ile-Thr-Phe-Thr-Thr-Ser-Ile-Gly-Ala-Tyr-Cys-
    Arg-Lys-Glu-Cys-Ala-Tyr-Cys-Leu-Thr-Ile-Asn-Thr-Thr-Val-Cys-Ala-Gly-Tyr-Cys-
                                                               31

                                                          55
    Cys-Pro-Ser-Met-Lys-Arg-Val-Leu-Pro-Val-Pro-Pro-Leu-Ile-Pro-Met-Pro-Gln-
    Met-Thr-Arg-Asx-Val-Asx-Gly-Lys-Leu-Phe-Leu-Pro-Lys-Tyr-Ala-Leu-Ser-Gln-
                                                               49

                                                          74
    Arg-Val-Cys-Thr-Tyr-His-Gln-Leu-Arg-Phe-Ala-Ser-Val-Arg-Leu-Pro-Gly-Pro-Cys-
    Asp-Val-Cys-Thr-Tyr-Arg-Asp-Phe-Met-Tyr-Lys-Thr-Ala-Gln-Ile-Pro-Gly-Cys-Pro-
                                                               68

                                                     92
    Pro-Val-Asp-Pro-Gly-Met-Val-Ser-Phe-Pro-Val-Ala-Leu-Ser-Cys-His-Gly-Pro-
    Arg-His-Val-Thr-Pro-Tyr-Phe-Ser-Tyr-Pro-Val-Ala-Ile-Ser-Cys-Lys-Cys-Gly-
                                                     86

                                                          110
    Cys-Cys-Arg-Leu-Ser-Ser-Thr-Asp-Cys-Gly-Pro-Gly-Arg-Thr-Glu-Pro-Leu-Ala-
    Lys-Cys-Asx-Thr-Asx-Tyr-Ser-Asx-Cys-Ile-His-Glu-Ala-Ile-Lys-Thr-Asn-Tyr-
                                                               104

                    120
Cys-Asp-His-Pro-Pro-Leu-Pro-Asp-Ile-Leu-OH
Cys-Thr-Lys-Pro-Gln-Lys-Ser-Tyr-Met-OH
                    113
```

————   *Bovine TSH-β structure of Pierce and co-workers, 1970.

FIG. 5. Comparison of the amino acid sequences of ICSH β and TSH β (taken from 31). Areas of identity are enclosed in the box.

The separation of the subunits in two other glycoprotein hormones [ovine FSH (29) and HCG (30)] also show that the two subunits are nonidentical.[2] The

[2] The only glycoprotein hormone for which a subunit nature has not been demonstrated is pregnant mare serum gonadotropin (PMSG).

availability of these subunits have made possible the preparation of hybrids (15, 29, 31), and study of their biological and immunological properties. The general concept which emerges from these studies is that each of these glycoprotein hormones is composed of two chemically dissimilar subunits, one of which can be termed a "common or carrier" subunit, and another "the hormone specific" subunit. Thus, the α subunit would be the common subunit and the β subunit the hormone specific. The biological center (ICSH, FSH, TSH activity) is contained in the β subunit and it is expressed only when suitably combined with the α subunit.

Finally, it may be pointed out that the elucidation of the primary structures of ovine ICSH, bovine TSH, and the realization of the subunit nature of other glycoprotein hormones (FSH, HCG) have opened new avenues for important investigations on the biosynthesis, mode of action, validity of immunoassay, and structure-function relationships of these glycoprotein hormones.

ACKNOWLEDGMENT

We take the opportunity to thank Dr. T. S. Anantha Samy for his participation in the earlier phases of this study. In addition, we thank Mr. Daniel Gordon, Mr. J. D. Nelson, and Mrs. Susanna Liles for their expert technical assistance. This work was supported in part by grants from the National Institute of Arthritis and Metabolic Diseases (AM-6097), National Institutes of Health and the Geffen Foundation. One of us (H.P.) is a Career Development Awardee of the National Institute of General Medicine Sciences, National Institutes of Health.

REFERENCES

1. Smith, P. E., and E. T. Engle, Amer J Anat 40:159, 1927.
2. Fevold, H. L., F. L. Hisaw, and S. L. Leonard, Amer J Physiol 97:291, 1931.
3. Li, C. H., M. E. Simpson, and H. M. Evans, Endocrinology 27:803, 1940.
4. Shedlovsky, T., A. Rothen, R. O. Greep, H. B. Van Dyke, and B. F. Chow, Science 92:178, 1940.
5. Squire, P. G., and C. H. Li, Science 127:32, 1958.
6. Squire, P. G., and C. H. Li, J. Biol Chem 230:524, 1959.
7. Ward, D. N., R. F. McGregor, A. C. Griffin, Biochim Biophys Acta 32:305, 1959.
8. Li, C. H. and B. Starman, Nature 202:291, 1964.
9. Ward, D. N., M. Fujino, and W. M. Lamkin, Fed Proc 25:348, 1966.
10. Papkoff, H. and T. S. A. Samy, Biochim Biophys Acta 147:175, 1967.
11. Papkoff, H. and J. Gan, Arch Biochem Biophys 136:522, 1970.
12. Reichert, L. E., M. A. Rasco, D. N. Ward, G. D. Niswender, and A. R. Midgley, J Biol Chem 244:5110, 1969.

13. Liao, T. H., and J. G. Pierce, J Biol Chem 245:3275, 1970.

14. Hennen, G., Z. Prusik, and G. M. Rogister, Eur J Biochem 18:376, 1971.

15. Reichert, L. E., A. R. Midgley, G. D. Niswender, and D. N. Ward, Endocrinology 87:534, 1970.

16. Saxena, B. B., and P. Rathnam, Fed Proc 30:1553, 1971.

17. Papkoff, H., D. Gospodarowicz, A. Candiotti, and C. H. Li, Arch Biochem Biophys 111:431, 1965.

18. Parlow, A. F., in A. Albert (Ed), Human Pituitary Gonadotropins, Charles C Thomas, Springfield, Ill., 1961, p. 300.

19. Papkoff, H., J. S. Wallckermann, M. Martin, and C. H. Li, Arch Biochem Biophys, in press, 1971.

20. Moudgal, N. R., and C. H. Li, Arch Biochem Biophys 95:93, 1961.

21. Papkoff, H., M. R. Sairam, C. H. Li, J Amer Chem Soc 93:1531, 1971.

22. Sairam, M. R., H. Papkoff, and C. H. Li, in preparation.

23. Sairam, M. R., T. S. A. Samy, H. Papkoff, and C. H. Li, in preparation.

24. Pierce, J. G., T. H. Liao, R. B. Carlson, and T. Reimo, J Biol Chem 246:866, 1971.

25. Liao, T. H., and J. G. Pierce, J Biol Chem 246:850, 1971.

26. Eylar, E. H., J Theoret Biol 10:89, 1965.

27. Liu, W.-K., C. M. Sweeney, H. S. Nahm, G. N. Holcomb, and D. N. Ward, Res Commun Chem Pathol Pharmacol 1:463, 1970.

28. McDonald, J. K., T. J. Reilly, B. B. Zeitman, and S. Ellis, J Biol Chem 241:1494, 1966.

29. Papkoff, H., and M. Ekblad, Biochem Biophys Res Commun 40:614, 1970.

30. Swaminathan, N., and O. P. Bahl, Biochem Biophys Res Commun 40:422, 1970.

31. Pierce, J. G., T. H. Liao, S. M. Howard, and B. Shome, Rec Prog Hormone Res, in press, 1971.

32. Liu, W. K., H. S. Nahm, C. M. Sweeney, H. N. Baker, W. M. Lamkin, and D. N. Ward, Res Commun Chem Pathol Pharmacol 2:168, 1971.

13.   Isolation of Human FSH and Human LH Controlled by Isoelectric Focusing

D. Graesslin, H. Chr. Weise, and G. Bettendorf

Several investigators have purified FSH and LH from human pituitaries to a high degree (1-5). The most potent preparations described biological activities of 12,000 to 14,000 IU FSH/mg (3), and 5200 IU/mg for LH (4). The protein concentration was calculated by UV absorption (3) or based on the Lowry technique (4).

This report describes the isolation of a highly purified FSH and a homogeneous LH preparation from human pituitaries. The isoelectric focusing in polyacrylamide gel was employed as a sensitive criterion for purity.

MATERIALS AND METHODS

Crude gonadotropin (E_3) was extracted from human pituitaries as described earlier (6). All procedures were performed at 4 C. About 80 to 100 mg of E_3 were obtained from 100 pituitaries. Biological activities varied between 100 and 200 IU/mg FSH and 100 and 600 IU/mg LH. All potency estimations are based on dry weight.

Ion exchange chromatography of crude gonadotropin on QAE-Sephadex A-50 was performed as reported earlier (7).

Bioassay

FSH activity was measured by the augmentation test of Steelman and Pohley (8), and LH by the OAAD test according to Karg (9) and Parlow (10).

159

Gel Filtration on Sephadex

To study the homogeneity, a small quantity of the purified LH fraction was chromatographed on a 0.9 × 85 cm column of Sephadex G-100 with distilled water as the elution solvent.

Column Isoelectric Focusing

Preparative isoelectric focusing was carried out in a 110-ml capacity column. An Ampholine concentration of 1% covering a pH range from 3 to 10 and a density gradient with sucrose was used (ultrapure quality, Serva, Heidelberg). The voltage was 300V for 108 hr. Refocusing was performed in the more selective pH range of 3 to 6 at 500V for 84 hr. Precipitation of proteins was never observed. The column was eluted using a peristaltic pump (Perpex, LKB). Fractions of 2.5 ml were collected and monitored for transmittance at 278 mμ. The pH gradient was measured in each tube with a glass micro electrode at 4 C. Sucrose and carrier ampholytes were removed from protein by dialysis with stirring in a dialysis bag "20/32" (Visking, Unicarbide, New York) for 3 days.

Gel Isoelectric Focusing

Isoelectric focusing in polyacrylamide gel is an analytical technique which results in extremely sharp banding of proteins. It was performed essentially according to Awdeh et al. (11). A slab of large pore gel was used as stabilizing medium. The carrier ampholyte, Ampholine, with a concentration of 2% (w/v), covered a pH range of 3 to 10. The polyacrylamide concentration was 5%, the comonomer relation was 1 : 35, no TEMED was used. Riboflavin served as catalyst. Protein samples between 20 and 800 μg, dissolved in 20 μl of distilled water were soaked in filter paper discs of 1 cm^2 which were put on a gel slab of 12 × 18 cm and 1 mm thickness. As many as six samples can be analyzed simultaneously. It is important to apply proteins with acid isoelectric points near the cathode and vice versa.

The slab was developed for 5 hr at a constant voltage of 330V. The amperage decreases from 32 to 2 mA during the run. Subsequently the pH gradient was determined by punching a line of about 25 gel disc with a cork borer and transferred into 0.5 ml of redistilled water for determination of pH.

The gel slab was immediately stained in a 0.1% solution of Coomassie brilliant blue R250 (Serva, Heidelberg, Germany) in water:ethanol:acetic acid, (55 : 40 : 5) with gentle shaking. The background became colorless within 2 or 3 hr.

Disc Electrophoresis

The polyacrylamide gel electrophoresis was carried out by the Davis technique (12) in 7.5% acrylamide, with "running" pH 8.9, in Tris-glycine buffer, 3 mA/tube, and stained with amido black.

Carbohydrate Analysis

Sialic acid was tested by the thiobarbituric acid method (13), the neutral sugars were determined by the orcinol method (14).

RESULTS

The results of a typical isoelectric focusing (IEF) experiment are shown in Fig. 1. Crude gonadotropin, 30 mg, (E_3MN_{70}) with a specific biological activity of 190 IU FSH and 580 IU LH had been applied to a column covering the pH range 3 to 10. Fractions were pooled as indicated. Fifty-six percent of the total LH activity and 52% of the total FSH activity were recovered. The recovery of protein was 72%.

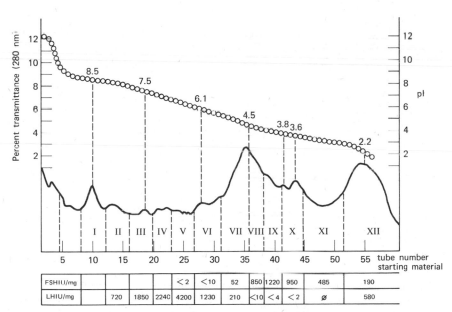

	I	II	III	IV	V	VI	VII	VIII	IX	X	XI	XII	starting material
FSHIU/mg					<2	<10	52	850	1220	950	485	190	
LHIU/mg		720	1850	2240	4200	1230	210	<10	<4	<2	ø	580	

FIG. 1. Column isoelectric focusing of crude gonadotropin E_3MN_{70}, pH 3 to 10. Solid line: transmittance at 278 mµ; dotted line: pH.

The protein fractions in the pH range 8.35 to 5.40 (F II to F VI), containing LH activity were separately pooled, dialyzed, and lyophilized. Protein yields varied between 0.9 and 2.1 mg. The highest LH activity was found in fraction V (pH 6.25 and 6.95). The biological activity was found to be 4200 IU/mg containing less than 2 IU/mg FSH. The specific activities of fractions F II, F III, and F IV, varied between 700 IU and 2250 IU.

Isoelectric focusing fractions ranging in pH between 4.5 and 3.0 contained little if any LH activity, however, high FSH potencies were found, as summarized in Fig. 1. On the basis of their gel isoelectric focusing patterns (Fig. 2), these partially purified FSH fractions of three preparative IEF runs were

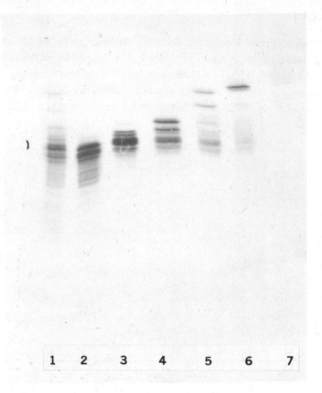

FIG. 2. Gel isoelectric focusing patterns of FSH fractions obtained from first column IEF. Staining with Coomassie brilliant blue. The anode is at the top. (1) Starting material, (2 to 6), fractions F VII-F XI.

pooled and subjected to a second run. Results obtained in the narrower range of pH 3 to 6 are illustrated in Fig. 3. Although further chemical purification was achieved, no increase of biological potency was noted. The highest FSH activity was found in fraction VI (pH 4.25 and 4.65) with 1120 IU/mg and less than 4 IU/mg LH.

Disc electrophoresis of the most active LH fraction of the first IEF (F V) showed a single band (Fig. 4). The homogeneity of this LH preparation could also be demonstrated by isoelectric focusing in polyacrylamide gel, revealing a sharp single zone with only faint traces of contaminants (Fig. 5). The isoelectric point measured in the gel slab was found to be 6.9. In contrast, the isoelectric focusing pattern of the starting material revealed a heterogeneous spectrum of at

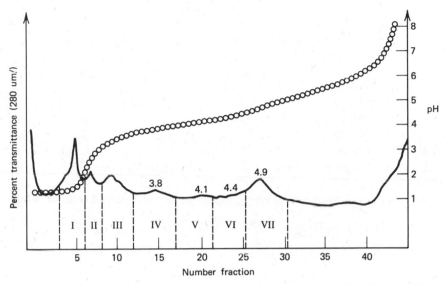

FIG. 3. Second column isoelectric focusing of pooled FSII fractions F VII-F XI, pH 3-6.

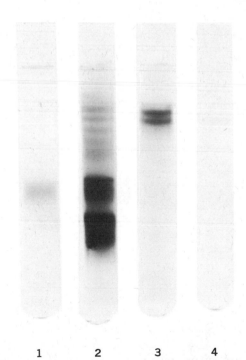

1 2 3 4

FIG. 4. Disc electrophoresis at pH 8.9 (7.5% polyacrylamide, 3 mA/tube) of human pituitary preparations. Staining with amido black. The anode is at the bottom. (1) FSH preparation from second IEF, F VI. (2) Starting material E_3MN_{70}. (3) LH fraction from QAE-Sephadex ion exchange chromatography. (4) LH preparation from first IEF, F V.

least 20 bands (Fig. 5). The components ranged in isoionic points from 3.5 to 8.4. Major contaminants of normal serum proteins could be identified as albumin, prealbumin, and acid α_1-glycoprotein at pI 4.9, 4.7, and 3.5, respectively. On disc electrophoresis only 10 bands could be separated, when crude gonadotropin was applied (Fig. 4).

A complex protein pattern, however, occurred when the FSH-containing fractions of the first preparative IEF run, ranging in pH from 4.5 to 3.0, were subjected to analytical IEF, as illustrated in Fig. 2. The pooled, refocused FSH-containing fractions resulted in a high-purity FSH when controlled by gel IEF. Two distinguishable bands appeared in the limited pI range 4.5 to 4.7 (Fig. 5). On column IEF the pH of this FSH fraction ranged from 4.3 to 4.7 Disc electrophoresis, however, revealed the presence of a single zone (Fig. 4), which

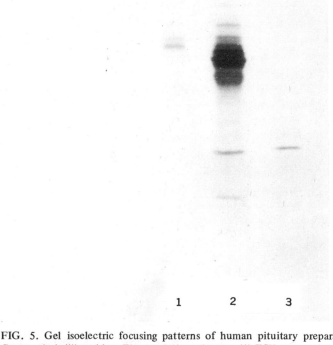

FIG. 5. Gel isoelectric focusing patterns of human pituitary preparations. Staining with Coomassie brilliant blue. The anode is at the top. (1) FSH preparation of second IEF, F VI. (2) Starting material. (3) LH preparation of first IEF, F V.

migrates slower than albumin. In addition to disc electrophoresis and gel isoelectric focusing, the highly potent LH (F V) was run on Sephadex G-100 and emerged as a single symmetrical peak. The isolated LH preparation contained 0.6% sialic acid and 5.8% neutral sugars.

DISCUSSION

Crude gonadotropin (E_3), extracted from human pituitaries by a modified procedure of Koenig and King (6, 15), contained relatively high biological activities of FSH and LH. The protein pattern of E_3 (Fig. 5) after analytical isoelectric focusing in flat gel offered a good chance for separation of LH fractions from the major contaminants of plasma proteins and FSH. Hence by this technique, applied in preparative scale, a homogeneous LH fraction could be isolated. Only partial separation of FSH from albumin and prealbumin was achieved, due to their closely related isoelectric points.

Refocusing of pooled FSH fractions in a narrower pH range resulted in an FSH of a higher degree of purity. Despite the increased purity, the biological activity did not increase. This may be due to losses of activity during dialysis and lyophilization. Similar results were reported by Amir and co-workers (16).

The isoelectric point of LH was found to be 6.9. This value agrees fairly well with those obtained by Rathnam and Saxena (4). Squire and co-workers (17), however, reported a pI of 5.4. The low amount of sialic acid found in our LH preparation accounts for one residue/molecule LH. Since sialic acid is important for the isoelectric point of a glycoprotein, this low value may explain the neutral pI.

The percentage of total hexoses in LH reported here, as well as the sialic acid content, are in good agreement with the findings of Papkoff and Li (18), whereas Rathnam and Saxena (4) have calculated a higher content of neutral sugars.

It should be noted that the resolving power of gel isoelectric focusing is superior to that of disc electrophoresis. Nevertheless, both separation techniques complement each other to become, when used together, a valuable tool in analytical protein chemistry because of their different separation principles, loading, and molecular size.

ACKNOWLEDGMENT

This work was supported by a grant from Deutsche Forschungsgemeinschaft (SFB 34).

REFERENCES

1. Parlow, A. F., P. G. Condliffe, L. E. Reichert, Jr. and A. E. Wilhelmi, Endocrinology 76:27, 1965.
2. Hartree, A. S., Biochem J 100:754, 1966.
3. Roos, P., Human Follicle–Stimulating Hormone, Almqvist a. Wiksells AB, Uppsala, 1967.
4. Rathnam, P., and B. B. Saxena, J Biol Chem 245:3725, 1970.
5. Peckham, W. D., and A. F. Albert, Endocrinology 84:953, 1969.
6. Bettendorf, G., M. Breckwoldt, P.-J. Czygan, A. Fock, and T. Kumasaka, in E. Rosemberg, (Ed.), Gonadotropins 1968, Geron-X, Inc., Los Altos, 1968, p. 13.
7. Graesslin, D., Y. Yaoi, and G. Bettendorf, Hormone Metab Res 2:51, 1970.
8. Steelman, S. L., and F. M. Pohley, Endocrinology 53:604, 1953.
9. Karg, H., Klin Wschr 35:643, 1957.
10. Parlow, A. F., in A. Albert, (Ed.), Human Pituitary Gonadotropins 1961, Charles C Thomas, Springfield, Ill., 1961, p. 300.
11. Awdeh, Z. L., A. R. Williamson, and B. A. Askonas, Nature (London) 219:480, 1968.
12. Davis, B. J., Ann NY Acad Sci 121:404, 1964.
13. Warren, L., J Biol Chem 234:1971, 1959.
14. Winzler, R. J., Methods Biochem Anal 2:279, 1955.
15. Koenig, V. L. and E. King, Arch Biochem 26:219, 1950.
16. Amir, S. M., S. A. Barker, W. R. Butt, and A. C. Crooke, Nature (London) 209:1092, 1966.
17. Squire, P. G., C. H. Li, and R. N. Andersen, Biochemistry 1:412, 1962.
18. Papkoff, H. and C. H. Li, in W. R. Butt, A. C. Crooke, and M. Ryle (Eds.), Gonadotrophins and Ovarian Development, E. & S. Livingstone, Edinburgh, 1971, p. 138.

14. Purification and Properties of Human Pituitary LH and its Subunits

Aida Nureddin, Anne Stockell Hartree, and Paley Johnson

Studies of the physicochemical and biological properties of human pituitary luteinizing hormone (HLH) and of subunits derived from it are in progress in our laboratories in Cambridge. We report here an improved method for preparation of highly purified LH and studies of its sedimentation behavior as determined by ultracentrifugation in a synthetic boundary cell. We also report on procedures for isolating subunits of urea-dissociated human LH and their recombination with restoration of biological activity. The subunits have been further characterized by amino acid analysis and polyacrylamide gel electrophoresis. Some of these findings will shortly be published elsewhere (1).

EXPERIMENTAL

Preparation of HLH

HLH, fraction DEAE-I, (potency approximately 3.5 mg NIH-LH-Sl/mg) was prepared from acetone-dried human pituitaries and was further purified by ion exchange chromatography on Amberlite IRC-50. This preparation, designated IRC-2, has a potency of approximately 5 mg NIH-LH-Sl/mg (2). Subsequently a more convenient procedure was devised for final purification of fraction DEAE-I in which the hormone (200 mg) was dissolved in 0.08M sodium acetate buffer at pH 5 and applied to a column (1 X 46 cm) of CM-cellulose (Whatman microgranular CM-32) at 4 C previously equilibrated with the same buffer. After elution of a small amount of material absorbing at 280 nm, a linear gradient from 0.14M to 0.16M sodium acetate buffer at pH 5 was applied to the column.

The protein solution eluted under these conditions (CM-LH) was dialyzed at 4 C against distilled water and freeze-dried. The average yield was 43% by weight of the starting material (fraction DEAE-I). The biological activity of preparation CM-LH as determined by Dr. V. C. Stevens by the ovarian ascorbic acid depletion method was 6.4 mg NIH-LH-Sl/mg with 95% fiducial limits of 5.2 to 7.6 mg NIH-LH-Sl/mg. Another batch of CM-LH was assayed by Dr. D. B. Crighton by the same method. The potency in this case was 5 mg NIH-LH-Sl6/mg with 95% fiducial limits of 3.3 to 7.5 mg NIH-LH-Sl6/mg.

Sedimentation in The Ultracentrifuge

These studies were performed in the Beckman Spinco Model E ultracentrifuge at 59,780 rpm using a synthetic boundary cell at accurately measured temperatures near 20 C. Phosphate buffer at pH 6 was used with NaCl added to the required ionic strength (I), usually 0.1. Schlieren patterns were photographed at appropriate intervals, usually 8 min. Migration of the peak on each plate (measured using a microcomparator) was determined as a function of time. The sedimentation coefficients were corrected to the viscosity and density of water at 20 C.

Polyacrylamide Gel Electrophoresis

This was performed by the method of Davis (3) using Tris-glycine buffer, pH 8.3, in the reservoirs. The gels were 7% polyacrylamide and samples (approximately 50 μg each) were applied in 40% sucrose solution. Electrophoresis was carried out at 1 mA/tube for 15 min to allow the sample to enter the gel and then at 2.5 mA/tube for 2¼ hr. The gels were stained for 1 hr in a solution of 1% amido black in 7% acetic acid, and were destained by immersion overnight in 7% acetic acid with stirring.

RESULTS AND DISCUSSION

Studies of CM-LH

Polyacrylamide gel electrophoresis of this purified preparation of HLH compared to the precursor (fraction DEAE-I) is illustrated in Fig. 1. At least five distinct electrophoretic components are present in the precursor fraction but only three remain in the purified CM-LH preparation. These are assumed to be the three active species isolated by Peckham and Parlow (4). Sedimentation velocity behavior of CM-LH at pH 6, I = 0.1, was examined as a function of protein concentration (Fig. 2). The reduced sedimentation coefficients ($S_{20,w}$) were found to increase with increasing protein concentration up to 0.4 g/100 ml. At higher concentrations an approximately constant value of 3.4 S were observed. At I = 0.2, a similar but not identical curve of $S_{20,w}$ versus protein concentration was obtained. It seems clear that the protein molecule is involved in some type of association-dissociation equilibrium whose details require further investigation.

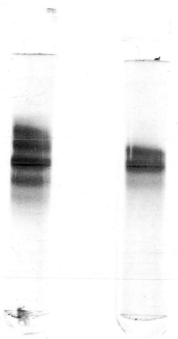

FIG. 1. Polyacrylamide gel electrophoresis of HLH at pH 8.3. Left tube: preparation DEAE-I; right tube: preparation CM-LH.

Preparation of Subunits

HLH has previously been shown to dissociate into subunits on treatment with acid. The pH at which the hormone is 50% dissociated is approximately pH 1.9, and complete dissociation is obtained in the neighborhood of pH 1 (5). In order to prepare subunits without using extremes of pH which might irreversibly damage the protein, urea has been used to dissociate the hormone. Preparation IRC-2 (103 mg) was incubated overnight at 4 C in 5 ml freshly prepared 8M urea (Analar). After removal of urea by gel filtration at 4 C on Sephadex G-100, equilibrated with 0.08M sodium acetate buffer at pH 5, the preparation was chromatographed at 4 C on a column of CM cellulose (Whatman microgranular CM-32) previously equilibrated with the same buffer. An unadsorbed fraction (A) was eluted immediately and was followed by smaller amounts of material (fraction B) eluted with the starting buffer. A third fraction (C) was eluted by increasing the buffer concentration to 0.15M sodium acetate. The gel-filtration patterns of the fractions on Sephadex G-100 suggested that fraction A was a subunit while fraction C was a mixture of subunit and reassociated LH. Protein was precipitated from fraction A with 80% ethanol and the precipitate washed with ethanol and ether and dried in vacuo to yield 19.2 mg (subunit A).

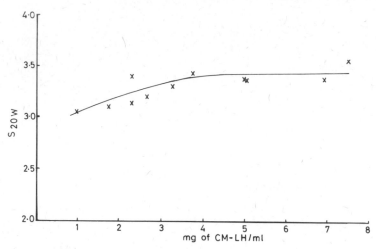

FIG. 2. Sedimentation coefficient ($S_{20,w}$) of HLH at different protein concentrations. Determinations were made in phosphate buffer at pH 6 containing sodium chloride at ionic strength of 0.1 at controlled temperatures near 20 C.

In another experiment human LH (207 mg of preparation DEAE-I) was dissociated by incubation overnight at 4 C in 10 ml freshly prepared 8M urea (Analar). After removal of urea by dialysis against 0.01M ammonium acetate at pH 5 the material was freeze-dried. It was then submitted to countercurrent distribution in the system described by Papkoff and Samy (6), composed of 40% ammonium sulphate-0.2% dichloroacetic acid-1-propanol-ethanol in proportions of 60 : 60 : 27 : 33 by volume. The procedure was carried out at room temperature and equal volumes (20 ml) of each phase were used for each transfer. After sixteen transfers, three fractions (I, II, and III) were separated and each was concentrated by rotary evaporation, dialyzed against 2mM phosphate buffer at pH 7, and submitted to gel filtration on Sephadex G-100. From the elution patterns obtained, it was assumed that fraction I was native or reassociated LH, fraction II was a mixture of subunit and reassociated LH, and fraction III was a subunit. The latter fraction was concentrated, dialyzed against distilled water, and freeze-dried to yield 18.2 mg (subunit III). Amino acid analyses of subunit A and of subunit III confirmed that the composition of each was very different, the contents of arginine, proline, glycine, half-cystine, valine, isoleucine, and leucine being significantly higher in subunit III. The average content of each amino acid in the subunits was approximately equal to the composition of the native hormone (1).

A more efficient procedure was subsequently used for isolation of subunits. A preparation of CM-LH (50 mg) was treated with 2.5 ml 8M urea for 24 hr at 4 C and the solution applied to a column of CM cellulose (46 × 1 cm) equilibrated with 0.08M sodium acetate buffer, pH 5.0 at 4 C. Subunit A was eluted with the starting buffer and the remaining subunit plus reassociated LH were eluted together with a linear gradient from 0.14M to 0.16M sodium acetate buffer at pH 5. This latter fraction was dialyzed against distilled water, concentrated by rotary evaporation, and submitted to gel filtration at room temperature on a column of Sephadex G-75 (135 × 2.5 cm) in 0.1M sodium phosphate buffer at pH 7. Two separate peaks containing material absorbing at 280 nm were eluted. The first peak, eluted near the void volume of the column, was assumed to be native or reassociated LH and the second peak was assumed to be a subunit

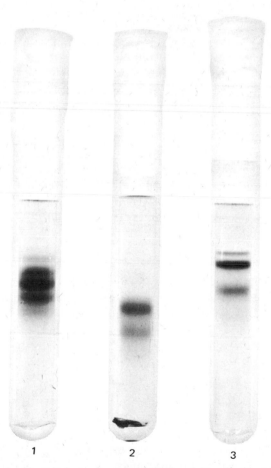

FIG. 3. Polyacrylamide gel electrophoresis of HLH and its subunits at pH 8.3. Tube 1: preparation CM-LH; tube 2: subunit A; and tube 3: subunit Seph-B.

(subunit Seph-B). Each fraction was dialyzed against distilled water and freeze-dried. The weight yields were as follows: subunit A, 8.8 mg; reassociated LH, 8.1 mg; and subunit Seph-B, 6.2 mg. The polyacrylamide gel electrophoretic pattern of each subunit compared with native LH (CM-LH) is illustrated in Fig. 3. In addition to the three components of native LH, this preparation of CM-LH has faint bands with mobilities corresponding to the bands seen in the subunits. This suggests the presence of very small amounts of dissociated material in CM-LH, which may arise on storage of the preparation. Subunit A contains two components both of greater mobility than the components of native LH. Subunit Seph-B contains three electrophoretic components, two of which are of lesser mobility than native LH, the other being similar to LH in this sytem.

Recombination of Subunits

This was accomplished by mixing equal weights (8.3 mg) of subunit A and of subunit III dissolved in 0.5 mg of 0.1M sodium phosphate buffer at pH 7. The mixture was left at 4 C for 65 hr and was then submitted to gel filtration on Sephadex G-100. The elution pattern showed a peak in the position expected for native LH with a shoulder eluted in the position expected for subunits. The protein from the main peak was recovered by precipitation with ethanol in a yield of 8 mg. Bioassays of each subunit and of the reassociated subunits were performed by Dr. E. T. Bell and Dr. D. W. Christie using the ovarian ascorbic acid depletion method (7). The activities were as follows: subunit A, 0.53 mg NIH-LH-Sl2/mg; subunit III, 0.13 mg NIH-LH-Sl2/mg; and reassociated subunits, 3.73 mg NIH-LH-Sl2/mg (1). It is apparent, therefore, that each of the isolated subunits is of relatively low biological activity, but their recombination results in restoration of the biological activity of the native hormone.

ACKNOWLEDGMENTS

We are indebted to several colleagues for their help in performing bioassays on preparations of LH and its subunits and to Misses M. B. Thomas and D. J. Reed for expert technical assistance. Human pituitary glands and a grant in support of this work were provided by the Medical Research Council of Great Britain, and one of us (A.N.) is the recipient of a postdoctoral fellowship from the Population Council. We also thank Professor F. G. Young, F. R. S., for his interest and encouragement.

REFERENCES

1. Stockell Hartree, A., M. Thomas, M. Braikevitch, E. T. Bell, D. W. Christie, G. V. Spaull, R. Taylor, and J. G. Pierce, J Endocrinol, 51:169, 1971.
2. Stockell Hartree, A., Biochem J 100:754, 1966.
3. Davis, B. J., Ann NY Acad Sci 121:404, 1964.
4. Peckham, W. D., and A. F. Parlow, Endocrinology 85:618, 1969.

5. Braikevitch, M., and A. Stockell Hartree, in W. R. Butt, and A. C. Crooke (Eds.), Gonadotrophins and Ovarian Development, E. & S. Livingstone, Edinburgh, 1971, p. 131.

6. Papkoff, H., and T. S. A. Samy, Biochim Biophys Acta 147:175, 1967.

7. Bell, E. T., J. A. Loraine, S. Mukerji, and P. Visutakul, J Endrocinol 32:1, 1965.

15. Purification and Characterization of Human Postmenopausal Gonadotropins

Paul Roos

The discovery by Ascheim (1) more than 40 years ago of the occurrence of gonad-stimulating activity in urine of postmenopausal women has been followed by numerous papers dealing with different aspects on urinary gonadotropins. A selection of those papers with a demonstrated intention of separating urinary FSH and LH from each other and of purifying one or both of these substances radically reduces the number. If characterization studies are required as well only very few papers remain.

In this paper reference will be made to work on urinary LH by Donini et al. (2, 3), Anderson et al. (4), and Stevens et al. (5), and on urinary FSH by Roos and Gemzell (6), Roos (7), and Donini et al. (3).

URINARY LH

Purification

Donini et al. (2, 3) have described a procedure for the purification of urinary LH. The starting material was prepared as reported earlier by utilizing kaolin-acetone precipitation (8), extraction with 70% ethanol containing 10% ammonium acetate, batchwise fractionation on DEAE-cellulose (9), and a chromatographic step on permutit. This starting material with an LH potency of 58.3 IU/mg was subjected to two consecutive batchwise separations on DEAE-cellulose and on CMC-70. Subsequently the crude LH fraction was successively purified by column chromatography on Sephadex G-100, DEAE-

Sephadex, and Sephadex G-200. From 5.46 g of starting material, urinary LH was prepared in a yield of 20.4 mg with a biological potency of 982 IU/mg. FSH activity was undetectable at the dose level assayed. Investigation of the homogeneity of the urinary LH preparation by analytical polyacrylamide gel electrophoresis revealed the presence of at least two bands.

Essentially the same procedure was employed by Anderson et al. (4) to prepare urinary LH which was further fractionated by column chromatography on SE-Sephadex C-50 and by preparative polyacrylamide gel electrophoresis. In spite of utilization of all these methods, the final product lacked homogeneneity in analytical polyacrylamide gel electrophoresis and immunoelectrophoresis. After DEAE cellulose[1] column chromatography, the LH fraction became unstable and during the first five months of storage this fraction (lyophilized form) lost about 70% of its original biological activity reported to be 753 IU/mg. The immunological activity determined by radioimmunoassay did not, however, seem to change appreciably. No biological activity of the final product was reported, the radioimmunologically determined potency was 740 IU/mg. No corresponding lability of urinary LH preparations was mentioned in the papers by Donini et al. (2, 3).

Stevens et al. (5), also starting with crude material (8), reported purification of urinary LH by DEAE cellulose column chromatography and two consecutive runs on Sephadex G-100. From a starting material with a biological LH potency of 90 IU/mg they obtained a preparation with a potency of 740 IU/mg. Simultaneously there was a decrease in FSH potency from 57 to 15 IU/mg. No attempts were made to study the homogeneity of the preparation.

The biological potencies referred to in this section were all determined by the rat ovarian augmentation test for FSH (10) and by the ovarian ascorbic acid depletion test for LH (11). In summary, procedures have been described for purification of urinary LH but no preparation so far has been shown to fulfill any criterion for homogeneity.

URINARY FSH

Purification

Roos and Gemzell (6), and Roos (7) have developed a procedure for the isolation of urinary FSH. The different fractionation steps involved and the yield of the fractions utilized in the progressive fractionation of the hormone are given in Table I. Biological assays were performed by the rat ovarian augmentation test (10) and by the seminal vesicle test in immature intact rats (12). The starting material was an experimental batch prepared from postmenopausal urine by N. V. Organon, Oss, Holland. A total amount of 10 g was available. The FSH and LH potencies of the starting material were 8.6 and 210 IU/mg, respectively. Separation of FSH and LH was achieved by column chromatography on DEAE-

[1] Utilized instead of DEAE-Sephadex (2, 3).

TABLE I. Purification of human urinary FSH according to Roos (7)

Methods of preparation	Yield/g starting material[a] (mg)		Potency[a] (IU/mg)	
Starting material[b]	1000		8.6	(3)
DEAE-cellulose chromatography	43	(3)	120	(5)
Molecular-sieve chromatography (two consecutive runs on Sephadex G-100)	8.6	(2)	380	(5)
Hydroxylapatite chromatography	3.0	(3)	620	(5)
Polyacrylamide gel electrophoresis	0.85	(3)	780	(5)

[a]Mean values with the numbers of observations in parenthesis.

[b]Prepared by N. V. Organon, Oss, Holland (unpublished procedure).

cellulose using stepwise increase in buffer concentration. Under the conditions initially used, FSH was adsorbed but LH passed unretarded through the column. The potency of the final preparation of urinary FSH was 780 IU/mg which is 90 times higher than the potency of the starting material. The limited supply of urinary FSH did not allow the performance of bioassays for LH activity. Reliance was placed upon the more sensitive radioimmunological technique (13). The LH content was estimated to be 15 IU/mg. The FSH preparation has been subjected to physical, chemical, and immunological characterization. Only 7 mg were available for these studies which will be discussed in the following sections.

Recently Donini et al. (3) have described the preparation of a highly purified urinary FSH. The starting material (8) had an FSH potency of 82.8 IU/ing and an LH potency of 58.3 IU/mg. All bioassays were performed by the rat ovarian augmentation test (10) and by the ovarian ascorbic acid depletion test (11). The initial step was a batchwise separation of FSH and LH on DEAE-cellulose utilizing the conditions described by Roos and Gemzell (6). The crude FSH fraction was subjected to column chromatography on DEAE cellulose according to Reichert and Parlow (14), and to Donini et al. (15). Further fractionation was achieved by molecular-sieve chromatography on Sephadex G-100 and finally by preparative polyacrylamide gel electrophoresis. The final yield from 5.46 g of starting material was 104.3 mg. The FSH potency was 1255 IU/mg, a 15-fold increase in potency over that of the starting material. The potency is the highest reported for any urinary FSH preparation. The LH potency of the preparation evaluated by radioimmunological technique (16) was 3.26 IU/mg. The characterization of the preparation will be discussed in the following sections.

Sedimentation Coefficient

The sedimentation velocity of urinary FSH of Roos was studied in a Spinco Model E ultracentrifuge utilizing schlieren optics. Runs were performed at three different protein concentrations in a 0.01M sodium phosphate buffer, pH 7.0, containing 0.1M NaC1. Pictures taken during one of these runs are shown in Fig. 1. Conversion of the calculated values to standard conditions followed by linear

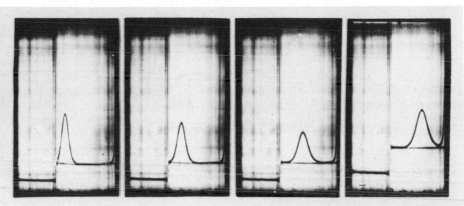

FIG. 1. Sedimentation of urinary FSH in the ultracentrifuge at 59,780 rpm (7). Protein concentration 5.8 mg/ml. Pictures taken 58 min, 90 min, 154 min, and 218 min after the centrifuge was up to speed.

extrapolation to zero protein concentration gave $S_{20,w}^{0} = 2.2$ S. The value utilized for the partial specific volume (v) was $0.69/(g)(cm^3)$ calculated from amino acid and carbohydrate analyses. The results from the three runs are recorded in Table II.

TABLE II. Sedimentation studies of human
urinary FSH according to Roos (7)

Protein concentration (mg/ml)	$(S_{20,w})$
5.8	1.96
4.8	2.00
3.3	2.07
Infinite dilution	2.21

Donini et al. have reported $S_{20,w} = 1.94$ S from a run performed at a protein concentration of 0.6% in a 0.1M phosphate buffer, pH 6.5 for their preparation.

This value is in very good agreement with that obtained by the author at a protein concentration of 0.58% (Table II).

Diffusion Coefficient

Determination of the diffusion coefficient ($D_{20,w}$) by Donini et al. gave a value of $5.98 \times 10^{-7} cm^2/sec^{-1}$. Neither the method used nor any experimental conditions were given.

Molecular Weight

The Roos preparation was subjected to ultracentrifugation utilizing low-speed sedimentation equilibrium technique. The protein concentration at the start was 0.46% and the same solvent was used as in the sedimentation velocity runs. The experimental data were analyzed by plotting the log of the concentration in fringes as function of the square of the radial distance (Fig. 2). From the slope

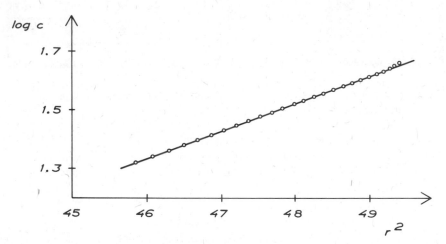

FIG. 2. Analysis of urinary FSH (7) by sedimentation equilibrium centrifugation at 10,587 rpm. Initial protein concentration 4.6 mg/ml.

of the straight line an apparent molecular weight was calculated to be 26,700 ($\bar{v} = 0.69/(g)(cm^3)$). According to the Svedberg equation, in its original form the true molecular weight is proportional to $S^0_{20,w}/D^0_{20,w}$. From the values in Table II, the sedimentation coefficient for urinary FSH is about 9% lower at a protein concentration of 0.46% than at zero concentration. If the concentration dependence of the diffusion coefficient is considered negligible when compared with the dependence of the sedimentation coefficient, the true value for the molecular weight would be 29,400. As a compromise, a value of 28,000 has been chosen to represent the molecular weight of urinary FSH.

Donini et al. have calculated a value of 31,600 for the apparent molecular weight of their urinary FSH. Their calculation was based on the values of $S_{20,w}$

and $D_{20,w}$. The value utilized for $\bar{v}$ was not reported. The difference in molecular weight for the two preparations can not be established as significant since different techniques were used and complete information concerning experimental details are not cited.

Electrophoretic Studies

The electrophoretic homogeneity of Roos' FSH preparation was studied in a Hjerté apparatus for free zone electrophoresis (17). Urinary FSH was recorded as a single symmetrical peak throughout the course of the experiment (Fig. 3). After completion of the run fractions were withdrawn for bioassays. Full evidence was obtained that the FSH activity was associated with the material corresponding to the peak. The mobility of urinary FSH at 0 C in the buffer utilized (0.1M Tris-HCl buffer, pH 8.7) was calculated to be -6.17×10^{-5} $cm^2/(sec)(volt)$. By simultaneously running a sample of pituitary FSH, it was possible to establish that the two forms of FSH differed significantly in mobility. The difference was 6%; urinary FSH had the greater mobility.

Donini et al. subjected their urinary FSH to analytical polyacrylamide gel electrophoresis at pH 8.3. After destaining only one band was observed.

Amino Acid Analysis

Averaged data from analyses according to Spackman et al. (18) of urinary FSH prepared by Roos and by Donini et al. are given in Table III. The integers reported by Roos were obtained by a mathematical treatment of analysis data which provided the most probable number by which the different amino acids are present in the hormone molecule. Consequently a reliable value for the molecular weight of the protein moiety of urinary FSH was obtained. The integers published by Donini et al. were based on the assumption that the molecular weight of the protein moiety of FSH is 21,500. From the data in Table III it is obvious that the amino acid compositions of the two preparations of urinary FSH differ considerably.

Carbohydrate Composition

The carbohydrate content of the two preparations are listed in Table IV. Both preparations were analyzed by a similar technique for total hexose (19) and for N-acetylneuraminic acid (20). For the determination of hexosamine, Roos utilized the amino acid analysis procedure and Donini et al. used the method of Rondle and Morgan (21). The analysis data for the different components are expressed as nearest integer of residues/mole of FSH. The original percent values given by Donini et al. were converted by using the reported value of 31,600 for the molecular weight of FSH. The molecular weights of the carbohydrate moieties of FSH were calculated to be[2] 4500 (Roos) and 9000 (Donini et al.), indicating a pronounced difference in carbohydrate composition. The molecular

---

[2] Hexosamine included an N-acetylglucosamine

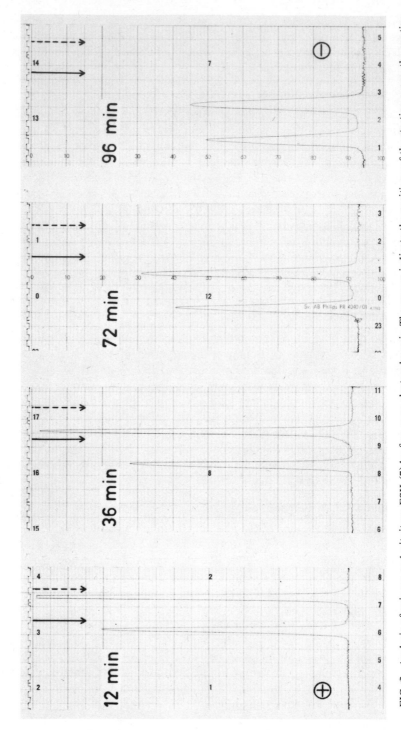

FIG. 3. Analysis of urinary and pituitary FSH (7) by free zone electrophoresis. The arrows indicate the positions of the starting zones, the continuous arrow represents urinary FSH. Current: 3mA; temperature 2.3 C.

180

TABLE III. Amino acid composition of human urinary FSH

Amino acid	Residues/mole	
	FSH according to Roos (7)	FSH according to Donini et al. (3)
Lysine	7	8
Histidine	4	7
Arginine	8	8
Aspartic acid	27	17
Threonine	12	13
Serine	16	13
Glutamic acid	21	23
Proline	19	17
Glycine	25	11
Alanine	12	13
Half-cystine	32	18
Valine	11	9
Methionine	1	3
Isoleucine	5	4
Leucine	11	12
Tyrosine	4	6
Phenylalanine	7	13
Tryptophan	2	2
Total[a]	208	188
Molecular weight of protein moiety	23,600	21,500[b]

[a]Half-cystine included as 16 (Roos) and 9 (Donini et al.) cystine residues.
[b]Value according to Donini et al. (3).

TABLE IV. Carbohydrate components of human urinary FSH

Sugar	Residues/mole	
	FSH according to Roos (7)	FSH according to Donini et al. (3)
Hexose	14	18
N-acetylglucosamine	8	17
N-acetylneuraminic acid	2	9
Molecular weight of carbohydrate moiety	4500	9000

weight for the protein moiety of FSH prepared by Donini et al. would thus be 22,600. It seems justifiable to use this value for the evaluation of the amino acid analysis data instead of an assumed value of 21,500. The higher value would give an increase of about 5% for all the residual numbers cited for the preparation of Donini et al. (Table IV).

Immunological Properties

Pituitary and urinary FSH of Roos were analyzed by Ouchterlony gel diffusion technique against a guinea pig antiserum to a pituitary FSH preparation (Fig. 4). Under the conditions employed, urinary FSH (Fig. 4, well 1) gave a reaction of partial identity with pituitary FSH (Fig. 4, well 2).

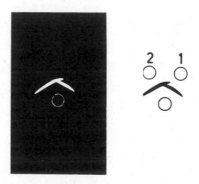

FIG. 4. Analysis of urinary and pituitary FSH (7) by gel diffusion. Center well: antiserum to a pituitary FSH preparation; well 1: urinary FSH; well 2: pituitary FSH.

Immunoelectrophoresis (22) of the urinary FSH preparation of Donini et al. against an unabsorbed rabbit antiserum to a crude urinary gonadotropin preparation gave two precipitation lines, raising doubts about the homogeneity of the urinary FSH preparation.

Concluding Remarks

Two urinary FSH preparations have been compared. Some data for the preparations are listed in Table V. The starting material used by Roos was a urinary concentrate prepared by others according to an unpublished method. The starting material of Donini et al. was about 10 times more potent and prepared by them from unconcentrated collections of urine. The FSH potency reported for the final preparation of Donini et al. was higher than that reported for the preparation according to Roos. The significance in the difference in LH activity seems more uncertain as the potencies were low and different assay techniques were used.

Urinary FSH prepared by Roos was homogeneous when examined by free zone electrophoresis and by ultracentrifugation (both sedimentation velocity

TABLE V. Some parameters determined for urinary FSH preparations

Parameter	Preparation according to ref. 7	Preparation according to ref. 3
Biological FSH potency, IU/mg		
starting material	8.6	82.7
final preparation	780	1255
Radioimmunological LH activity (IU/mg)	15	3.26
Sedimentation coefficient (S)		
0.6 mg FSH/ml	1.9 (6)	1.94
infinite dilution	2.21	
Molecular weight amino acid and carbohydrate		
analyses data	28,100	
ultracentrifugation	28,000	31,600
Residues/mole		
amino acid	208	188
hexose	14	18
N-acetylglucosamine	8	17
N-acetylneuraminic acid	2	9

and sedimentation equilibrium centrifugation). Supporting evidence for the homogeneity of the preparation according to Donini et al. was obtained by analytical polyacrylamide gel electrophoresis and by sedimentation velocity centrifugation. In immunoelectrophoresis, however, there were indications of the presence in the preparation of more than one component.

The values for the sedimentation coefficients were similar and the difference in the molecular weights was not too great. The differences in the amino acid and carbohydrate compositions were, however, considerable.

Taking all the evidence into account, it seems justifiable to conclude that the FSH preparations of Roos and Donini et al. were not of identical composition. Assuming homogeneity for both preparations the discrepancy could possibly be explained by differences in the handling of the urine before its working-up or by differences in the initial chemical procedures utilized. For example a high pH value may have caused splitting of disulfide bonds (in FSH and in other molecules) resulting in the formation of altered molecules by subsequent aggregation. However, the possibility of the occurrence of impurities in either of the two preparations, or in both, should of course not be completely overlooked.

REFERENCES

1. Aschheim, S., Lecture to Berliner gyn. Gesellschaft, December 14, 1928.
2. Donini, P., D. Puzzuoli, I. D'Alessio, G. Bergesi, and S. Donini, in E. Rosemberg (Ed.), Gonadotropins 1968, Geron-X, Inc., Los Altos, 1968, p. 37.
3. Donini, P., D. Puzzuoli, I. D'Alessio, G. Bergesi and S. Donini, in W. R. Butt, A. C. Crooke, and M. Ryle, Gonadotrophins and Ovarian Development, E. & S. Livingstone, Edinburgh, 1971, p. 39.
4. Anderson, D. G., P. Donini, and V. C. Stevens, in W. R. Butt, A. C. Crooke, and M. Ryle, Gonadotrophins and Ovarian Development, E. & S. Livingstone, 1971, p. 22.
5. Stevens, V. C., D. G. Anderson, and J. E. Powell, Ibid.
6. Roos, P., and C. A. Gemzell, Biochim Biophys Acta 93:217, 1964.
7. Roos, P., Acta Endocrinol (Kbh) 59 (Suppl 131):9 1968.
8. Donini, P., D. Puzzuoli, and R. Montezemolo, Acta Endocrinol (Kbh) 45:321, 1964.
9. Albert, A., J. Leiferman, and J. Derner, J Clin Endocrinol 21:1, 1961.
10. Steelman, S. L., and F. M. Pohley, Endocrinology 53:604, 1953.
11. Parlow, A. F., in A. Albert (Ed.), Human Pituitary Gonadotropins, Charles C Thomas, Springfield, Ill., 1961, p. 301.
12. van Hell, H., R. Matthijsen, and G. A. Overbeck, Acta Endocrinol (Kbh) 47:409, 1964.
13. Wide, L., and J. Porath, Biochim Biophys Acta 130:257, 1966.
14. Reichert, L. E., Jr., and A. F. Parlow, J Clin Endocrinol 24:1040, 1964.
15. Donini, P., D. Puzzuoli, I. D'Alessio, B. Lunenfeld, A. Eshkol, and A. F. Parlow, Acta Endocrinol (Kbh) 52:169, 1966.
16. Donini, S., and P. Donini, Acta Endocrinol (Kbh) 63 (Suppl 142):257, 1969.
17. Hjertén, S., Free Zone Electrophoresis, Almqvist a. Wiksells, Uppsala, 1967.
18. Spackman, D. H., W. H. Stein, and S. Moore, Anal Chem 30:1190, 1958.
19. Winzler, R. J., in S. Glick (Ed.), Methods of Biochemical Analysis, Vol II, Interscience, New York, 1955, p. 279.
20. Warren, L., J Biol Chem 234:1971, 1959.
21. Rondle, C. J. M., and W. T. G. Morgan, Biochem J 61:586, 1955.
22. Scheidegger, J. J., Int Arch Allergy 1:103, 1955.

16. Purification and Some Properties of Human Urinary FSH and LH

H. van Hell, A. H. W. M. Schuurs, and F. C. den Hollander

The most potent urinary FSH as prepared by Donini et al. (1) had a biological FSH potency of 1255 IU/mg and contained only 3.2 IU LH/mg by radio-immunoassay. Although this preparation behaved as a homogeneous protein in the ultracentrifuge and in polyacrylamide gel electrophoresis, heterogeneity was found in the immunoelectrophoretic studies. The most potent urinary LH as isolated by Donini et al. (2) had a potency of 982 IU/mg by bioassay ovarian ascorbic acid depletion (OAAD) method, and 1166 IU/mg by radioimmunoassay. In this chapter the preparation of urinary FSH and LH of much higher potency is reported. A preliminary characterization is also presented.

MATERIALS AND METHODS

The starting material was prepared from the urine of healthy postmenopausal women by selective adsorption and desorption using a technical adsorbant and precipitation of the gonadotrophins by ethanol. This material was subjected to fractionation with ethanol (3) followed by treatment with calcium phosphate in order to remove pyrogens. The further purification was performed as shown in the flow sheet in Fig. 1.

Bioassay

The FSH potency was determined by a modification (3) of the augmentation method described by Steelman and Pohley (4). The LH potency was determined with the seminal vesicle test in intact immature rats (3). To all solutions to be

185

Flow sheet of the purification of FSH and LH

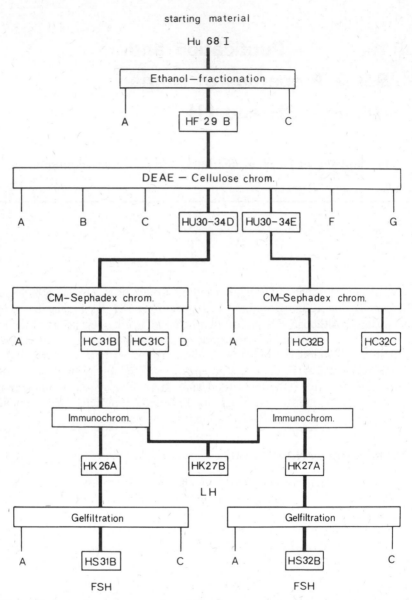

FIG. 1. The heavy lines represent the purification route of the two main FSH preparations and the LH preparation obtained. The small rectangles symbolize the intermediate products. Side fractions not used for further purification are not recorded by their full code but given as capital letters.

tested, both standard and unknown, bovine serum albumin (Cohn Fraction V) was added to make a 0.1% (w/v) solution. FSH and LH potencies were expressed as IU 2nd IRP-HMG.

Radioimmunoassay of FSH

A highly purified urinary FSH preparation with a biological potency of 1160 IU/mg was used for labeling.

Labeled FSH and antisera raised to urinary FSH were extensively purified. The specificity of the radioimmunoassay was tested using gonadotrophin preparations with very different FSH/LH ratios. The immunochemical FSH potencies correlated well with the biological FSH activities irrespective of the LH potencies. The system reacted with HCG but only in high doses (200 IU); similarly, concentrated urine from children or hypophysectomized patients did induce a reaction but only in high doses. All these data indicate that the test system was specific for FSH.

Radioimmunoassay of LH

For the radioimmunoassay of LH, an HCG-anti-HCG system was used. HCG for labeling was prepared by subjecting HCG with a potency of about 9000 IU/mg (6) to successive gel filtration, isoelectric focusing and final gel filtration. Details of both tests will be published later. Starch-gel zone electrophoresis was carried out as described earlier (5, 6), except that a 50 μg sample was introduced directly into the gel. Polyacrylamide gel electrophoresis was carried out as described by Akroyd (7) using approximately 100 μg of protein. Starch gel immunoelectrophoresis was performed as described by Slater (8). Analyses of sialic acid were carried out as described by Goverde et al. (9). An outline of the purification procedure, described below, is given in Fig. 1.

Fractionation with Ethanol

Twenty-five grams of crude HMG was dissolved in 2500 ml, 10% aqueous ammonium acetate solution, with a pH of 7. Absolute ethanol, 3750 ml, was then slowly added and the precipitate which appeared after one night of standing was separated by centrifugation, washed twice with ethanol, and dried (HF 29 A). Ethanol, 3680 ml, and 300 ml glacial acetic acid were added to the clear supernatant. The precipitate which appeared after one night of standing was separated in the usual manner (HF 29 B). A final fraction was obtained by the addition of 3870 ml ethanol (HF 29 C). The whole procedure was carried out at temperatures varying between 0 and 2 C. All liquids added had a temperature of 20 C.

Chromatography with DEAE Cellulose

Preparation HF 29 B was subjected to chromatography with DEAE-cellulose. Details of the procedure are given in Fig. 2. The fractions were pooled according to the elution pattern and the results of the immunoassay of FSH in the fractions. Pooled fractions were concentrated by means of ultrafiltration (Diaflo, UM 10 filter). The protein was isolated from the concentrated fractions by ethanol precipitation (4 vol), and dried.

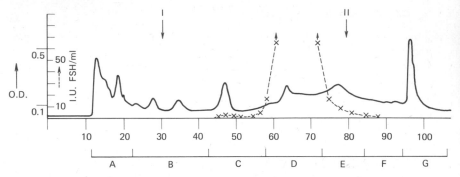

FIG. 2. DEAE-cellulose chromatography of HMG. The column (5.2 × 70 cm) was equilibrated with a 0.05M Tris-(hydroxymethylaminomethane)chloride, pH 7.5. The protein load of the columns was 2.4 mg/ml gel. The elution speed was 8.1 ml/(cm²)/(hr). Buffers: I. Elution with a concave concentration geadient from 0.05 to 0.2M Tris-(hydroxymethyl-aminomethane)chloride pH 7.5; II. Elution with 1.0M Tris-(hydroxymethylaminomethane)-chloride pH 7.5. The change of eluting buffer is indicated by vertical arrows. The optical densities of the fractions at 278 nm and the immunochemical FSH activity/ml of the eluate are recroded along the ordinate by a solid and a broken line respectively. The fractions (60 ml) are recorded along the abscissa. The horizontal bars below the abscissa represent the pooling of the fractions.

Chromatography with CM Sephadex C-25

To fractionate preparation HU 30-34 D and preparation HU 30-34 E, CM-Sephadex chromatography was used essentially as was described previously for HCG (6). Pooled fractions were concentrated by ultrafiltration (Diaflo, UM 10 filter) and the protein isolated by precipitation with ethanol (4 vol), and dried.

Immunochromatography

The LH activity was removed from the fractions HC 31 B and HC 31 C by immunochromatography with an anti-HCG-Sepharose column. Anti-HCG serum was obtained by immunization of rabbits with highly purified HCG (10). The immunoglobulin fraction was precipitated by Na_2SO_4 (180 mg/ml serum) (11). This fraction was coupled to Sepharose 4B (Pharmacia Fine Chemicals, Uppsala, Sweden) using the CNBr-method developed by Axén et al. (12). The ratio between protein and Sepharose during the coupling was 1 : 1 (dry weight).

The LH was adsorbed onto the immunoadsorbent packed in a column from a 5% (w/v) solution of the preparations in a 0.05M sodium citrate buffer pH 5.0. For an optimal separation of FSH and LH, it is essential to use only a slight excess (10 to 30%) of anti-HCG. Too much anti-HCG leads to losses of FSH. After the FSH had been washed from the column with the 0.05M sodium citrate buffer pH 5.0, the LH was eluted with 4M M_gCl_2. The solutions containing the

FSH were diluted with 3 parts of distilled water, the FSH precipitated by the addition of 4 vol of ethanol and isolated in the usual manner (HK 26 A and HK 27 A). The solutions containing the LH from both experiments were pooled, concentrated, and desalted on a UM 10 filter (Diaflo). After lyophylization the last traces of salt were removed by gel filtration with Sephadex G-25. The LH was finally lyophilized and dried (HK 27 B).

Gel Filtration of FSH

The FSH preparations HK 26 A and HK 27 A were subjected to gel filtration with Sephadex G-75 in 0.1M $CaCl_2$ using the recycling technique introduced by Porath and Bennich (13) and as described in the LKB Manual 1-4900 A - E02. The protein was pumped into the column as a 5% solution in 0.1M $CaCl_2$ (0.3 mg protein/ml gel). Elutes of pooled fractions (Figs. 4 and 5) were concentrated and partially desalted on a Diaflo UM 10 filter. Complete desalting was accomplished by gel filtration with Sephadex G-25, after which the purified hormones were recovered from their solutions by lyophilization.

RESULTS

Fractionation with ethanol effects a small increase in the FSH and LH potency of the starting material (Table I) in a quantitative yield (Table IV). Although the fractionation procedure seems to be rather ineffective, it was found essential to obtain good results in the subsequent purification procedure.

TABLE I. Ethanol fractionation of HMG

| Fraction | FSH pot. IU/mg 95% conf. lim. | | LH pot. IU/mg 95% conf. lim. | FSH |
	Bioassay	RIA[a]	RIA	i/b
HF 29 A	4.9(4.0-5.9)	6.0(5.2-7.1)	1.94(1.63-2.31)	1.2
HF 29 B	40(34 - 46)	32.7(30.1-35.6)	21.2(19.0-23.6)	0.82
HF 29 C	2.2	0.76(0.65-0.89)	4.4(3.7-5.3)	3.5

[a]Radioimmunoassay. The i/b ratio for FSH is the quotient of the immunochemical FSH potency and the biological FSH potency.

Chromatography with DEAE-cellulose of fraction HF 29 B (see flowsheet) resulted in a concentration of most of the FSH activity in fraction HU 34 D (Fig. 2, Table II). Some FSH activity was also recovered from fraction HU 34 E. The i/b ratios of these two fractions, however, differ considerably. The bulk of the immunochemical LH activity is eluted from the column a little earlier than the FSH (Table II) indicating that some separation of the two hormones was accomplished.

TABLE II. Results of column chromatographic experiments

Fraction isolated	FSH pot. IU/mg, 95% conf. lim.		LH pot. IU/mg, 95% conf. lim.		FSH i/b
	Bioassay	RIA[a]	Bioassay	RIA	
DEAE Cellulose					
starting material HF 29 B	40(34-46)	32.7(30.1-35.6)		21.2(19.0-23.6)	0.82
HU 34 A	1.4	0.21(0.18-0.24)		4.9(4.3-5.5)	0.15
B	1.5	0.49(0.43-0.55)		35(31-41)	0.32
C	3.3	3.8(3.4-4.3)	23(16-34)	36(32-41)	1.2
D	250(220-300)	120(107-135)	29(20-42)	39(35-45)	0.48
E	10.3(8.7-12.0)	33(30-38)	29(20-42)	4.8(4.2-5.5)	3.2
F	2.9(2.5-3.3)	5.4(4.8-6.1)		4.8(4.2-5.5)	1.9
G	1.9(1.5-2.4)	1.77(1.58-2.00)		3.8(3.3-4.3)	0.93
CM Sephadex					
starting material HU 30-34D	268(238-301)	142(131-154)		66(61-72)	0.53
HC 31 A	3.9(3.3-4.6)	3.6(3.1-4.2)		3.1	0.92
B	1530(1370-1710)	460(430-510)		500(420-600)	0.30
C	1470(1330-1610)	1110(1020-1210)		267(239-297)	0.76
D	190(140-250)	115(98-134)		28(23-22)	0.60
CM Sephadex					
starting material HU 30-34E		35(31-39)		4.6(4.1-5.3)	
HC 32 A		1.1(0.96-1.27)		0.31	
B	260(220-310)	261(230-297)		21.3(18.5-24.6)	1
C	≤160	840(740-960)		53	≥5.2

[a] ... The i/b ratio for FSH is the quotient of the immunochemical biological FSH potency

As the reproducibility of the chromatographic separation with DEAE-cellulose proved to be very good, corresponding fractions carrying FSH activity were pooled. Recovery of biological FSH activity in the pooled fractions D (preparation HU 30-34 D) (Table IV) was very good (86%). The recovery of the immunochemical FSH activity in this preparation, however, was considerably lower (Table IV). Another 15% of the total immunochemical FSH activity brought on the columns was recovered in the pooled fractions E (preparation HU 30-34 E) (Table IV). CM-Sephadex chromatography of preparation HU 30-34 D and HU 30-34 E (Fig. 3; Table II) considerably increased the FSH

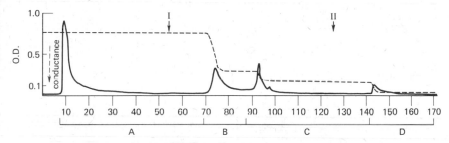

FIG. 3. CM Sephadex C-25 chromatography of HMG. The column (4.8 × 32 cm) was equilibrated with 0.05M ammoniumacetate buffer pH 5.0. The protein load of the columns was 1.7 mg/ml gel. The elution speed was 5 ml/(cm^2/(hr). Buffers: I. 0.3M ammonium-acetate buffer of pH 5.0; II. 0.5M ammoniumacetate buffer of pH 5.0. The change of eluting buffer is indicated by vertical arrows. The optical densities of the fractions at 278 nm and the conductivity of the eluate are recorded along the ordinate by a solid and a broken line respectively. The fractions (30 ml) are recorded along the abscissa. The horizontal bars below the abscissa represent the pooling of the fractions.

potency without effecting a separation between FSH and LH activity (Table II). From the elution pattern shown in Fig. 3, it appears that FSH activity is eluted in two clearly separated peaks by the same buffer. The material recovered from these two peaks proved to have different i/b ratios. The material with the higher ratio was consistently eluted in the second of these two peaks in both experiments.

The isolation of FSH preparations with different i/b ratios after both DEAE-cellulose chromatography and CM-Sephadex chromatography indicates that these preparations have different physicochemical properties. Immuno-chromatography with an anti-HCG Sepharose column was found to effectively remove LH activity from the FSH preparations (Table III). The FSH activity is not affected as is apparent from the specific FSH activities of HK 26 A and HK 27 A (Table III) and the FSH yields of these preparations (Table IV). The LH preparation HK 27 B which was recovered by eluting the immunoadsorbent with 4M MgCl$_2$ had a very high biological LH potency (9400 IU/mg) but still contained some FSH (Table III). On polyacrylamide (Fig. 4) and starch gel electrophoresis this preparation produced no discrete bands; but colored

TABLE III. Immunochromatography and gelfiltration of FSH and LH

Fraction isolated	FSH pot. IU/mg, 95% conf. lim.		LH pot. IU/mg, 95% conf. lim.		FSH i/b[b]	FSH/LH[c]
	Bioassay	IRA[a]	RIA	Bioassay		
Immunochromatography						
starting material						
HC 31 B	1530(1370-1710)	460(430-510)	225(194-256)		0.30	2.1
HK 26 A	1440(1280-1620)	470(430-520)	8.0(7.0-9.1)		0.32	59
starting material						
HC 31 C	1470(1330-1610)	1110(1020-1210)	267(239-297)		0.76	4.3
HK 27 A	1370(1220-1540)	1110(1010-1230)	6.7(5.8-7.6)		0.81	166
HK 27 B		250(210-300)	9100(8200-10100)	9400(7100-12600)		0.03
Gel filtration						
starting material						
HK 26 A	1440(1280-1620)	470(430-520)	8.0(7.0-9.1)		0.32	59
HS 31 A	630(550-730)	179(152-209)	16.5(13.9-19.6)		0.28	11
HS 31 B	4720(4080-5400)	930(790-1090)	15.0(12.6-17.8)		0.20	62
HS 31 C	160	86(73-101)	1.98(1.67-2.36)			43
starting material						
HK 27 A	1370(1220-1540)	1110(1010-1230)	6.7(5.8-7.6)		0.81	166
HS 32 A	460(400-530)	187(159-219)	2.3(1.9-2.7)		0.40	78
HS 32 B	2190(1950-2460)	1680(1540-1830)	9.6(8.6-10.6)		0.77	175
HS 32 C	<183	380(320-440)	0.85(0.72-1.02)		>2.1	450

[a]Radioimmunoassay.

[b]Ratio of immunochemical FSH potency to biological FSH potency.

TABLE IV. Over-all picture of the purification of FSH

Preparation	FSH pot. IU/mg, 95% conf. lim.		LH pot. IU/mg 95% conf. lim. RIA	FSH biol. (%)	Yield	
	bioassay	RIA[a]			FSH RIA (%)	LH RIA (%)
HU 68-I	26.8(24.3-29.7)	23.3(21.1-25.7)	14.9(13.0-17.1)	100	100	100
HF 29 B	40(34-46)	32.7(30.1-35.6)	21.2(19.0-23.6)	108	102	102
HU 30-34 D	268(238-301)	142(131-154)	66(61-72)	86	53	38
HU 30-34 E		35(31-39)	4.6(4.1-5.3)			
HC 31 B	1530(1370-1710)	460(430-510)	225(194-256)	39	14	10
HC 31 C	1470(1330-1610)	1110(1020-1210)	267(239-297)	30	26	10
HC 32 B	260(220-310)	261(230-297)	21.3(18.5-24.6)			
HC 32 C	≤160	840(740-960)	53			
HK 26 A	1440(1280-1620)	470(430-520)	8.0(7.0-9.1)	34	13	0.33
HK 27 A	1370(1220-1540)	1110(1010-1230)	6.7(5.8-7.6)	27	24	0.23
HS 31 B	4720(4080-5400)	930(790-1090)	15.0(12.6-17.8)	26	6.0	0.15
HS 32 B	2190(1950-2460)	1680(1540-1830)	9.5(8.6-10.6)	19	17	0.15

[a]Radioimmunoassay. All yields were calculated as overall yields.

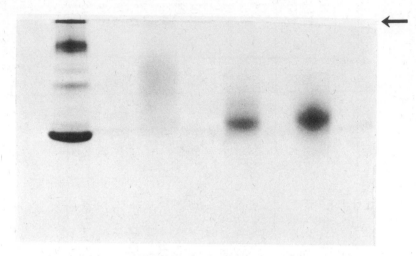

FIG. 4. Polyacrylamide gel electrophoresis of FSH and LH.

Code	Preparation	Biological potenciy, IU/mg
HK 27 B	LH	9400
HS 31 B	FSH	4720
HS 32 B	FSH	2190

The site of application of the sample is indicated by an arrow.

material was detectable from the site of application up to the position of the bovine serum albumin band. Starch gel immunoelectrophoresis showed the presence of a precipitation arc against an antiserum raised against highly purified HCG. HK 27 B produced no line against anti-FSH serum R 50 indicating that no anti-LH was detectable in this serum in the concentration used (Fig. 5).

As a final purification, FSH preparations HK 26 A and HK 27 A were subjected to gel filtration using the recycling technique. The results with HK 26 A are shown in Fig. 6 and Table III. Eluate of the first shoulder appearing in the elution pattern was allowed to run out of the column and collected, eluate of the first real peak was reintroduced into the column (recycled) as indicated in Fig. 6. Eluate of the second real peak was also collected.

After one recycling a pattern of two overlapping peaks appeared as shown in Fig. 6 (the peaks situated between the fractions 30 and 45). No second recycling was attempted. Material with a very high biological FSH potency was isolated (HS 31 B, Table III) from the pooled fractions 29 up to 36 as indicated in Fig. 6. As can be expected from the overlap of the first shoulder with the first real peak, the separation between the fractions HS 31 A and HS 31 B is not complete: HS 31 A still showing considerable FSH activity.

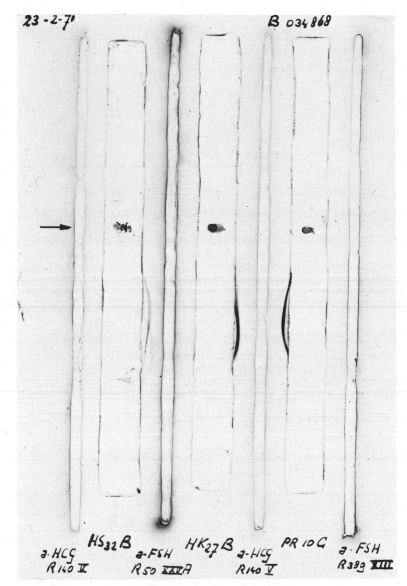

FIG. 5. Starch gel immunoelectrophoresis of FSH, LH, and HCG.

Code	Preparation	Biological potency, IU/mg
HS 32 B	FSH	2190
HK 27 B	LH	9400
PR 10 C	HCG	7300

R 140 V: Antiserum raised to HCG with a potency of at least 14,000 IU/mg. R 50 XXV and R 389 XIII Antisera against FSH preparations with potencies from 150 to 1000 IU/mg containing varying amounts of LH.

The site of application of the sample is indicated by an arrow.

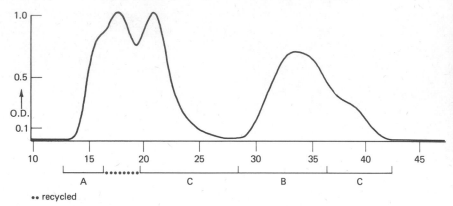

FIG. 6. Gel filtration of FSH preparation HK 26 A on Sephadex G-75 with the recycling technique. The column (1.5 × 142 cm) was equilibrated and eluted with 0.1M calcium chloride. The protein load of the column was 0.55 mg protein/ml gel. The elution speed was 9.5 ml/(cm²)(hr). The optical densities of the fractions at 278 nm are recorded along the ordinate. The fractions (5.7 ml) are recorded along the abscissa. The horizontal bars below the abscissa represent the pooling of the fractions.

Preparation HK 27 A which was recycled three times as indicated in Fig. 7, produced, contrary to expectation, a preparation with a lower biological FSH potency than HS 31 B (Table III). However, the immunochemical FSH potency of HS 32 B is almost twice as high as that of HS 31 B. The side fractions obtained from the latter experiment still contained FSH activity indicating that further fractionation should be possible by continued recycling (Fig. 7). The preparations HS 31 B and HS 32 B showed very different i/b ratios (Table III).

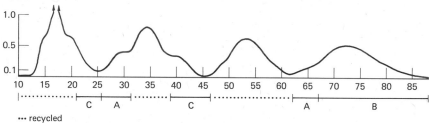

FIG. 7. Gel filtration of FSH preparation HK 27 A on Sephadex G-75 with the recycling technique. The column (1.5 × 142 cm) was equilibrated and eluted with 0.1M calcium chloride. The protein load of the column was 0.43 mg protein/ml gel. The elution speed was 10 ml/(cm²)(hr). The optical densities of the fractions at 278 nm are recorded along the ordinate. The fractions (6.0 ml) are recorded along the abscissae. The horizontal bars below the abscissa represent the pooling of the fractions.

Polyacrylamide (Fig. 4) and starch gel electrophoresis of preparations HS 31 B and HS 32 B showed the presence of a broad band with an electrophoretic mobility slightly less than that of bovine serum albumin for both preparations.

Some tailing was also observed. In starch gel immunoelectrophoresis HS 31 B and HS 32 B both produced at least two lines against anti-FSH sera, indicating heterogeneity. HS 32 B produced no line against an antiserum raised against highly purified HCG (Fig. 5). This is in agreement with the low immunochemical LH content found for this preparation. NANA contents of 6.2 and 6.5%, respectively, were found for preparations HS 31 B and HS 32 B.

An over-all picture of the purification of FSH is shown in Table IV. Using the flowsheet in Fig. 1 as a key for the interpretation of the results in Table IV, the following can be remarked: Concentration of biological FSH activity is effected by ethanol fractionation, chromatography with DEAE-cellulose and CM-Sephadex, and gel filtration. Separation of FSH and LH activity was mainly accomplished by immunochromatography. Considering the number of purification steps the over-all yield of 45% of biological FSH activity recovered in the two final preparations is satisfactory.

The over-all yield of 27% of immunochemical FSH activity for these preparations, however, is considerably lower. This probably means that immunochemical FSH activity is lost in side fractions. Different i/b ratios are consistently found for preparations throughout the whole purification procedure.

DISCUSSION

The properties of the two final FSH preparations obtained (HS 31 B and HS 32 B) can be summarized as follows:

1. The biological potency of preparation HS 31 B is more than twice that of HS 32 B but the immunological potency is only about half that of HS 32 B (Table III). This difference can be conveniently expressed as the quotient of the i/b ratios of these preparations which is about a factor 4.

2. The very low LH contents illustrate the effectiveness of immunochromatography.

3. Analytical thin layer gel filtration on Sephadex G-100 (details not reported here) revealed that HS 31 B behaved as if it had slightly larger molecular dimensions than HS 32 B. Both FSH preparations proved to have smaller molecular dimensions than HCG and bovine serum albumin.

4. Polyacrylamide and starch gel electrophoresis demonstrated that the main band of the two preparations had the same electrophoretic mobility, which was slightly less than that of bovine serum albumin.

5. The NANA contents are 6.2 and 6.5% for HS 31 B and HS 32 B, respectively.

6. Starch gel immunoelectrophoresis revealed the presence of at least two precipitation lines against rabbit anti-HMG for both preparations indicating heterogeneity for both.

Ratios varying from 0.15 i/b to at least 5 were found for other preparations obtained during the purification procedure (Table II and III).

The following explanation for these observations are offered: as the i over b quotient for FSH is considered not to be affected by other (than FSH) urinary proteins present in the preparations, different i/b ratios suggest that FSH as found in menopausal urine consists of a number of different molecular entities.

A comparison of the present FSH preparations with those isolated by some other investigators are summarized as follows:

Investigator	Source	Biol. FSH potency (IU/mg)	Imm. FSH potency (IU/mg)	NANA content (%)
Donini		1,255		
et al. (1, 2)	urine	1,157	1095	8.6
	urine			
	HS 31 B	4,720	930	6.2
van Hell	HS 32 B	2,190	1720	6.5
Roos (14)	pituitary	14,000		7.0
Reichert				
et al. (15)	pituitary	3,798		5.1
Peckham				
et al. (16)	pituitary	8,100		

There seems to be no relationship between the NANA content of these preparations and their biological FSH activity as was shown for HCG. In polyacrylamide gel electrophoresis HS 31 B and HS 32 B show a resemblance to the preparation isolated by Peckham et al. (16).

It may be concluded that the present preparations differ from those isolated by Donini et al. (1, 2), but also from the preparations obtained from pituitary material. For the present preparations degradation of the active material during isolation and purification is not likely because of the mild conditions used during these procedures (pH 4.5 to 7.5, temperatures below 8 C).

Urinary LH (HK 27 B) with a biological potency of 9400 IU/mg and an immunochemical potency of 9100 IU/mg was isolated after immunochromatography of already extensively purified HMG. This high potency is remarkable for a urinary preparation. The most potent urinary LH obtained by Donini (2) had a biological potency of 982 IU/mg and an immunochemical potency of 1166 IU/mg, whereas pituitary LH obtained by Peckham et al. (17) had a biological potency of $6.4 \times$ NIH-LH-S$_1$ (about 7900 IU LH/mg).

In starch gel immunoelectrophoresis preparation HK 27 B showed one precipitation line against an anti-HCG serum. No precipitation line was observed against an anti-FSH serum. Polyacrylamide gel electrophoresis revealed no discrete bands as were found by Peckham (16) but merely colored material from the site of application up to the position of FSH. HK 27 B must therefore contain LH material physicochemically different from the LH isolated by Peckham et al. (17). Furthermore it is not entirely free from immunochemical FSH activity, indicating that the anti-HCG serum used for immunochromatography adsorbed some FSH.

It can therefore be concluced that by a combination of conventional and immunochromatographic methods, it is possible to isolate urinary LH with a biological potency equal to that of pituitary LH. Gel electrophoresis indicates, however, that the nature of the urinary material differs from that of the pituitary material.

ACKNOWLEDGMENT

I thank Mr. J. Kouwenberg, who performed the bioassays, and Mr. A. Delver for the statistical treatment of the results and the helpful discussions on this matter. I am also indebted to Dr. B. C. Goverde and Mr. F. J. N. Veenkamp for the NANA determinations. Moreover my thanks are due to Mr. J. I. J. van Casteren, Mr. D. M. Dijkhuizen, and Mr. J. I. van Lieshout for their skilled and devoted technical assistance.

REFERENCES

1. Donini, P., D. Puzzuoli, I. D'Alessio, G. Bergesi, and S. Donini, in W. R. Butt, A. C. Crooke, and M. Ryle, Gonadotrophins and Ovarian Development, E. & S. Livingstone, Edinburgh, 1971, p. 39.

2. Donini, S., and P. Donini, Acta Endocrinol (Kbh) 63(Suppl. 142):263, 1969.

3. van Hell, H., R. Matthijsen, and G. A. Overbeek, Acta Endocrinol (Kbh) 47:409, 1964.

4. Steelman, S. L., and F. M. Pohley, Endocrinology 53:604, 1953.

5. den Hollander, F. C., and A. H. W. M. Schuurs, in press, 1971.

6. van Hell, H., R. Matthijsen, and J. D. H. Homan, Acta Endocrinol (Kbh) 59:89, 1968.

7. Akroyd, P., Anal Biochem 19:399, 1967.

8. Slater, R. J., Arch Biochem 59:33, 1955.

9. Goverde, B. C., F. J. N. Veenkamp, and J. D. H. Homan, Acta Endocrinol (Kbh) 59:105, 1968.

10. Schuurs, A. H. W. M., E. de Jager, and J. D. H. Homan, Acta Endocrinol (Kbh) 59:120, 1968.

11. Wide, L., Acta Endocrinol (Kbh) 63(Suppl. 142):207, 1969.

12. Axén, R., J. Porath, and S. Ernback, Nature (London) 214:1302, 1967.

13. Porath, J., and H. Bennich, Arch Biochem, Suppl. 1 152: 1962.

14. Roos, P., Acta Endocrinol (Kbh) 59(Suppl. 131); 1968.

15. Reichert, L. E., R. H. Kathan, and R. J. Ryan, Endocrinology 82:109, 1968.

16. Peckham, W. D., and A. F. Parlow, Endocrinology 84:953, 1969.

17. Peckham, W. D., and A. F. Parlow, Endocrinology 85:618, 1969.

17. Studies on the Primary Structure of HCG and its Relationship to other Glycoprotein Hormones

Om. P. Bahl

Human chorionic gonadotropin (HCG) is a glycoprotein hormone produced by the placenta during pregnancy. Recently a great deal of progress has been made in the understanding of the chemistry of HCG and other glycoprotein hormones including luteinizing (LH) and follicle stimulating hormones (FSH), and thyrotropin (TSH). Based on their physicochemical and biological properties and on their primary structures a picture indicating close structural relationships has emerged. All of them contain covalently bonded carbohydrate moiety which forms approximately 15 to 35% of the molecule. The size of the protein moiety is similar and consequently the differences in their molecular weights are probably due to variation in their carbohydrate content. Some of the general characteristics of these hormones are described in Table I.

The carbohydrate moiety of HCG as well as of the other glycoprotein hormones is made up of sialic acid, L-fucose, D-galactose, D-mannose, 2-acetamido-2-deoxy-D-glucose, and 2-acetamido-2-deoxy-D-galactose. The proportion of individual monosaccharide not only varies with the hormone but also with the animal species. The carbohydrate compositions shown in Table II clearly indicate that human LH (1-3), FSH (4, 5), and TSH (6) have much less sialic acid and galactose compared with HCG (7, 8). Similarly, bovine (9) and ovine LH (10, 11) have even lesser amounts of these monosaccharides than the human hormones. Of all of the above hormones HCG has the highest amount of carbohydrate.

TABLE I. Some general characteristics of HCG, LH, FSH, and TSH

Hormone	Molecular weight	$S_{20,w}$	Isoelectric point	Carbohydrate (%)	Number of subunits	Number of complex carb. units		Reference
						α	β	
HCG	40,660 ± 3000[a] 36,000[b]	2.89	2.95	30-33	2	2	2	(7, 8, 25)
Human LH	26,750	2.71	5.4	13.9	2			(1)
Ovine LH	27,400	2.68	7.3	14.4	2	2	1	(10, 22)
Human FSH	31,000	2.89	4.25	15.3	2			(4, 5, 30)
Ovine FSH	32,095	2.5	4.4	20.1	2			(31)
Bovine TSH	28,300	2.76	>7.0	21.4	2	2	1	(19)

[a]Data from Bahl (7), except that the value for partial specific volume used was 0.6⁣9 obtained from the chemical composition.
[b]From the chemical composition data; Swaminathan and Bahl (12).

201

TABLE II. Carbohydrate compositions of HCG, human LH, TSH and FSH
(residues 28,000 molecular)

Carbohydrate	HCG Bahl (7)	LH Braikevitch and Hartree (2)	TSH Shome et al. (3)	FSH Saxena and Rathnam (4)
Fucose	1	1.7	1.3	
Mannose	9	7.0	7.4	10.5
Galactose	9	3.0	2.0	
Glucosamine	11	9.5	8.8	7.3
Galactosamine	3	1.6	2.2	
Sialic acid	8	n.d	1.7	4.8

HCG as well as other glycoprotein hormones, as indicated by their amino acid compositions in Table III, have a high content of proline and half-cystine. None of them has any free sulfhydryl group. Obviously HCG (7) is much closer to human LH (2) than to FSH (4, 10) or TSH (6) in their amino acid compositions. Although the amino acid compositions of HCG, FSH, LH, and TSH show striking differences, their relative proportions follow a similar pattern. The presence of tryptophan needs to be further substantiated by structural studies.

HCG has been dissociated into two nonidentical subunits, designated as α and β, by incubation with 8M urea (12). The subunits are easily separable by chromatography on DEAE-Sephadex. The method is simple and well-suited for a large-scale preparation of the subunits, often required for structural investigation. Also, the method seems to be of general application with some modification of the chromatographic conditions depending on the hormone and recently has been successfully applied to human FSH (4) and LH (13). It is simpler than the one based on countercurrent distribution, which has been employed in the preparation of the subunits of bovine (9, 14, 15) and ovine LH (16, 17), human (14) and bovine TSH (18), and ovine FSH (15). The subunits of ovine FSH, obtained by countercurrent distribution, could not be reconstituted to give back biological activity. On the other hand, human FSH subunits prepared by dissociation with urea (4) could be reassociated to recover about 50% of the activity. It may be due to the low pH used in the countercurrent distribution procedure which might cause some hydrolysis of the labile ketosidic bonds of sialic acid.

Both α and β subunits of HCG can be reassociated by incubation in an equimolar proportion (approximately 1 : 1 w/w) in 0.04M sodium phosphate buffer, pH 7.5. The reconstituted HCG is similar to native HCG in biological and

TABLE III. Amino acid compositions of HCG, human LH, TSH, and FSH

Amino acid	HCG Bahl (7)	LH Hartree (24)	TSII Shome et al. (3)	FSH Saxena and Rathnam (4)
Lysine	7	6.8	12.2	13
Histidine	3	4.4	5.5	6
Arginine	11	10.6	7.9	9
Aspartic acid	12	10.8	14.4	15
Threonine	12	12.6	17.7	20
Serine	16	12.0	13.0	19
Glutamic acid	13	15.8	16.9	23
Proline	20	17.1	15.0	16
Glycine	9	10.8	9.9	11
Alanine	9	8.0	10.2	12
Half-cystine	14	14.9	16.9	21
Valine	13	14.2	12.9	16
Methionine	3	3.3	4.4	13
Isoleucine	4	5.0	9.0	7
Leucine	10	10.5	11.3	15
Tyrosine	4	4.8	11.8	11
Phenylalanine	4	4.8	8.1	8
Tryptophan	1	1 4		1

physicochemical behavior, such as electrophoretic mobility in polyacrylamide gel (19). The α subunit of HCG can be substituted by the α subunit of LH or TSH indicating that the α subunits in all are identical or similar in structure. Recent studies on the primary structures of α HCG (20), α-TSH (21), and α-LH (22, 23), confirm the conclusions reached by hybridization studies. The β subunit is the one which confers hormonal specificity and is, therefore, referred as hormone specific subunit.

The amino acid compositions of the α and β subunits of HCG show striking differences (Table IV). The α-HCG is rich in lysine, histidine, glutamic acid, half-cystine, methionine, tyrosine, and phenylalanine. The β subunit has higher amounts of arginine, proline, and isoleucine (12). The α and β subunits of HCG (Table IV) resemble closely those of human LH (24). They also show (Table V) a great deal of similarity with the subunits of bovine (9) and ovine LH (16). The amino acid composition of the subunits of human (4) and ovine FSH (15) show similarity and so do the human (14) and bovine TSH subunits (18).

The carbohydrate compositions of the α and β subunits of HCG are quite different. The β subunit has a much higher content of sialic acid and galactose

TABLE IV. Amino acid compositions of the α and β subunits of HCG, human FSH, LH, and TSH (residues/100 residues of protein)

Amino acid	HCG[a] α	HCG[a] β	FSH[b] α	FSH[b] β	LH[c] α	LH[c] β	TSH[d] α	TSH[d] β
Lysine	6.8	2.9	5.2	5.9	6.0	2.3	6.0	6.2
Histidine	3.1	0.8	2.8	1.4	–	–	3.2	2.4
Arginine	3.0	7.3	3.1	2.3	4.4	8.5	3.4	4.9
Aspartic acid	7.0	8.2	8.9	8.6	6.0	6.8	6.0	9.5
Threonine	8.0	6.8	7.2	7.7	8.3	6.2	8.2	9.1
Serine	9.3	9.6	6.6	5.3	7.8	5.8	7.6	4.6
Glutamic acid	10.8	7.3	10.6	10.0	10.2	7.5	9.5	6.6
Proline	7.9	15.0	8.8	11.8	9.2	13.9	7.3	6.7
Glycine	4.9	6.2	6.2	3.9	5.4	7.1	4.8	3.8
Alanine	5.0	5.8	7.4	6.8	4.6	4.8	4.5	5.5
Half-cystine	10.2	7.7	5.8	13.2	9.8	10.1	11.0	10.0
Valine	7.9	7.1	6.9	6.5	7.9	10.0	7.6	4.0
Methionine	2.5	0.7	5.9	1.1	2.5	1.5	3.4	1.6
Isoleucine	0.9	2.8	3.7	4.1	1.6	3.9	1.9	7.9
Leucine	3.9	2.9	5.0	5.1	5.1	7.6	5.0	5.3
Tyrosine	3.9	1.9	1.3	3.1	3.6	2.0	5.2	8.4
Phenylalanine[e]	4.2	1.6	4.5	3.2	4.4	1.9	5.3	3.8

[a]Swaminathan and Bahl (12).

[b]Saxena and Rathnam (4).

[c]Hartree (24).

[d]Pierce et al. (19).

[e]Tryptophan was not determined.

than the α subunit (Table VI). Similarly, the carbohydrate compositions of the α and β subunits of bovine (9) and ovine LH (16), ovine FSH (15), and bovine TSH (14), are different from each other.

Each carbohydrate moiety consists of one or more multibranched carbohydrate units of varying molecular sizes. For example, the α and β subunits of HCG have two bulky carbohydrate units each, in other words, four such units in all in the intact molecule (25). The structures of these complex carbohydrate units have been investigated with specific glycosidases and have been found similar to the other plasma glycoproteins such as α_1-glycoprotein (26) and fetuin (27). The α subunits of ovine LH (22, 23) and bovine TSH (21) have two carbohydrate units while the β subunits of bovine TSH and ovine LH (22, 28) have only one. The carbohydrate units of HCG, ovine LH, and bovine TSH are located closer to their carboxy terminals and the carbohydrate unit(s) in the β

TABLE V. Amino acid compositions of the α and β subunits of bovine and ovine LH, bovine TSH, and ovine FSH (residues/100 residues of protein)

Amino acid	Bovine LH[a]		Ovine LH[b]		Ovine FSH[b]		Bovine TSH[c]	
	α	β	α	β	α	β	α	β
Lysine	9.9	2.1	9.6	1.9	10.5	7.8	10.7	8.2
Histidine	3.3	2.3	2.9	2.8	3.2	3.1	3.0	2.5
Arginine	3.3	5.2	2.9	6.6	4.5	4.0	3.3	3.7
Aspartic acid	6.2	4.2	6.7	4.7	11.2	10.0	6.5	8.5
Threonine	8.4	6.1	9.6	4.7	6.2	9.5	8.9	9.4
Serine	4.8	6.1	5.8	4.7	5.7	7.5	5.7	4.1
Glutamic acid	7.9	6.3	9.6	5.7	12.6	11.0	8.4	6.3
Proline	8.0	18.0	7.7	18.9	5.6	6.7	7.3	6.3
Glycine	4.7	7.0	4.8	5.7	4.7	4.9	4.3	3.6
Alanine	9.2	7.6	7.7	6.6	8.3	8.3	7.4	5.3
Half-cystine	9.4	8.5	9.6	9.4	4.9	8.0	10.3	10.6
Valine	6.2	7.1	5.8	7.6	5.5	6.3	5.3	4.9
Methionine	4.2	2.2	3.9	1.9	0.3	0.3	4.1	3.8
Isoleucine	2.3	3.6	1.9	3.8	2.7	3.6	2.1	5.5
Leucine	3.6	9.8	1.9	11.3	9.0	4.8	2.2	3.8
Tyrosine	4.8	1.3	4.8	0.9	2.7	3.8	5.5	9.7
Phenylalanine	3.6	2.5	4.8	2.8	4.2	3.8	4.9	3.8

[a]Reichert et al. (9).

[b]Papkoff and Ekbald (15).

[c]Pierce et al.(19).

subunits are located near the amino terminals suggesting that in the intact hormones the C terminal of one subunit is in close proximity to the N terminal of the other. The complex carbohydrate units in HCG have been found to be linked to the polypeptide chains by N-acetylglucoaminyl-asparagine linkages (25). Most likely, similar linkages are present in other glycoprotein hormones. HCG, in addition, seems to have from the indirect evidence so far, short oligosaccharide chains of mucin-type which may be attached to the polypeptide chains by N-acetylgalactosaminyl-serine bonds. The presence of both types of linkages in the same molecule are not unique to HCG; other examples, though few, are also known (29).

Recently rapid progress has been made in establishing the amino acid sequences in HCG (20), bovine TSH (21), and ovine LH (22, 23, 28). The α subunits of bovine and ovine LH are identical and show a great deal of similarity with the α subunit of HCG (21). The β subunits of HCG and LH show even

TABLE VI. Carbohydrate compositions of the α and β subunits of HCG, bovine and ovine LH, ovine FSH, and bovine TSH

Carbohydrate	HCG[a]		Bovine LH[b]		Ovine LH[c]		Ovine FSH[d]		Bovine TSH[e]	
	α	β	α	β	α	β	α	β	α	β
Fucose	0.36	1.30	0.80	0.92					0.54	1.04
Galactose	1.52	7.50			7.2	4.0	2.8	13.8	0.26	3.21
Mannose	5.40	4.80	9.17	3.19					7.46	
Glucosamine	8.55	7.40	4.72	3.03	7.7	4.9	2.3	7.1	8.13	3.93
Galactosamine	0.19	2.00	1.67	1.33					3.16	1.18
Sialic acid	3.9	10.20					0.8	3.7		

[a]Swaminathan and Bahl (12).
[b]Reichert et al. (9).
[c]Papkoff and Ananthasamy (16).
[d]Papkoff and Ekbald (15).
[e]Pierce et al. (19).

HCG β	Ser-Lys	(N-terminal)
	1 2	
LH β	Ser-Arg	

HCG β   Pro-Ileu-Asp(CHO)-Ala-Thr-Leu-Ala-Val-Glu-Lys-Gly-Cys-Pro-Val-Cys-Ileu
          11   27
LH β   Pro-Ileu-Asp(CHO)-Ala-Thr-Leu-Ala-Ala-Glu-Lys-Ala-Cys-Pro-Val-Cys-Ileu

HCG β   Thr-Ser-Thr-Ileu-Cys-Ala-Gly-Tyr

LH β   Thr-Thr-Ser-Ileu-Cys-Ala-Gly-Tyr

HCG β	Met-Lys-Arg
	41 43
LH β	Met-Lys-Arg

HCG β   Asp-Val-Arg-Phe-Glu-Ser-Ileu-Arg-Leu-Pro-Gly-Cys-Pro-Pro
       62   75
LH β   Glu-Leu-Arg-Phe-Ala-Ser-Val-Arg-Leu-Pro-Gly-Cys-Pro-Pro

HCG β   Gly-Val-Asp-Pro-Val-Val-Ser-Tyr-Ala-Val-Ala-Leu
       76   87
LH β   Gly-Val-Asp-Pro-Met-Val-Ser-Phe-Pro-Ala-Ala-Leu

HCG β	Ser-Thr-Thr-Asp
	97 100
LH β	Ser-Ser-Thr-Asp

HCG β	Gly-Pro-Gly-Lys
	102 105
LH β	Gly-Pro-Gly-Arg

HCG β	Cys-Asp-His-Pro
	112 114
LH β	Cys-Asp-His-Pro

HCG β	Pro-Asp	(C-terminal)
	117 118	
LH β	Pro-Asp	

FIG. 1. Comparison of amino acid sequences in HCG and ovine LH.

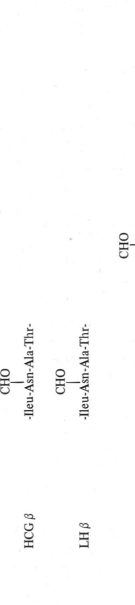

HCG β
CHO
|
-Ileu-Asn-Ala-Thr-

LH β
CHO
|
-Ileu-Asn-Ala-Thr-

CHO
HCG β -Glu-Gly-Cys-Pro-Val-Cys-Ileu-Asn-Val-Thr-Ser-Thr-Ileu-Cys-Ala-Gly-Tyr-Thr-Pro-Met-Arg
21   42
LH β -Glu-Ala-Cys-Pro-Val-Cys-Ileu-Thr-Phen-Thr-Thr-Ser-Ileu-Cys-Ala-Gly-Tyr-Cys-Pro-Ser-Met-Lys

FIG. 2.   Glycopeptides of HCG β and ovine LH β.

greater similarity as indicated in Fig. 1. The β subunit of HCG has two carbohydrate units as opposed to LH which has only one. The sequence of the amino acids near the carbohydrate unit of the first glycopeptide of β-HCG is identical with that of the LH β (Fig. 2). The sequence of the amino acids near the second carbohydrate of β-HCG is almost identical with another peptide in LH β (residues 21 to 42), in which threonine (residue 28) has been replaced by asparagine, giving the sequence -Asn-X-Thr-, hence the second carbohydrate unit of HCG. Although TSH is functionally unrelated to LH or HCG, its β subunit shows some identical sequences with their hormone specific subunits (Fig. 3). These regions may represent the regions involved in the binding of the α and β subunits. However, further work is necessary to confirm this observation.

HCG β Ileu-Asn(CHO)-Ala-Thr
            12   15

LH β Ileu-Asn(CHO)-Ala-Thr
            22   25

TSH β Ileu-Asn(CHO)-Thr-Thr

HCG β Ileu-Cys-Ala-Gly-Tyr
            33   37

LH β Ileu-Cys-Ala-Gly-Tyr
            26   30

TSH β Val-Cys-Ala-Gly-Tyr

HCG β Val-Ser-Tyr-Ala-Val-Ala-Leu-Ser
            81   88

LH β Val-Ser-Phe-Pro-Val-Ala-Leu-Ser
            75   82

TSH β Phe-Ser-Tyr-Pro-Val-Ala-Ileu-Ser

FIG. 3. Common sequences in HCG β, ovine LH β and bovine TSH β.

ACKNOWLEDGMENT

Supported by NIH grant AM-10273.

REFERENCES

1. Rathnam, P., and B. B. Saxena, J Biol Chem 245:3725, 1970.
2. Braikevitch, M., and A. S. Hartree, in W. R. Butt, A. C. Crooke, and M. Ryle, Gonadotrophins and Ovarian Development, E. & H. Livingstone, Edinburgh, 1970, p. 131.
3. Shome, B., D. M. Brown, S. M. Howard, and J. G. Pierce, Arch Biochem Biophys 126:456, 1968.

4. Saxena, B. B., and P. Rathnam, J Biol Chem 246:3540, 1971.

5. Papkoff, H., L. J. Mahlmann, and C. H. Li, Biochem 6:3976, 1967.

6. Shome, B., A. F. Parlow, U. D. Ramirez, H. Elrick, and J. G. Pierce, Arch Biochem Biophys 103:444, 1968.

7. Bahl, O. P., J Biol Chem 244:567, 1969.

8. Got, R., Europ Rev Endocrinol Suppl I:191, 1965.

9. Reichert, L. E., Jr., M. R. Rasco, D. N. Ward, G. D. Niswender, and A. R. Midgley, Jr., J Biol Chem 244:5110, 1969.

10. Papkoff, H., D. Gospodarowicz, A. Candiotti, and C. H. Li, Arch Biochem Biophys 111:431, 1965.

11. Walborg, E. F., Jr., and D. N. Ward, Biochim Biophys Acta 78:305, 1963.

12. Swaminathan, N., and O. P. Bahl, Biochem Biophys Res Commun 40:422, 1970.

13. Rathnam, P., and B. B. Saxena, J Biol Chem 246:7087, 1971.

14. Pierce, J. G., T. H. Liao, S. M. Howard, B. Shome, and J. S. Cornell, Rec Progr Horm Res 27:000, 1971 (in press).

15. Papkoff, H., and M. Ekbald, Biochem Biophys Res Comm 40:614, 1970.

16. Papkoff, H., and T. S. Anathasamy, Biochim Biophys Acta 147:175, 1967.

17. Lamkin, W. M., M. Fujino, J. D. Mayfield, G. N. Holcomb, and D. N. Ward, Biochim Biophys Acta 214:290, 1970.

18. Liao, T. H., G. Hennen, S. M. Howard, B. Shome, and J. G. Pierce, J Biol Chem 244:6458, 1969.

19. Pierce, J. G., O. P. Bahl, J. S. Cornell, and N. Swaminathan, J Biol Chem 246:2321, 1970.

20. Bahl, O. P., unpublished results, 1971.

21. Liao, T. H., and J. G. Pierce, J Biol Chem 246:850, 1971.

22. Papkoff, H., M. R. Sairam, and C. H. Li, J Amer Chem Soc 93:1531, 1971.

23. Liu, W. K., H. S. Nahm, C. M. Sweeney, H. N. Baker, W. H. Lamkin, and D. N. Ward, Res Commun Chem Pathol Pharmacol 2:168, 1971.

24. Hartree, A. S., Rec Prog Hormone Res 27:000, 1971 (in press)

25. Bahl, O. P., J Biol Chem 244:575, 1969.

26. Wagh, P. V., I. Bornstein, and R. J. Winzler, J Biol Chem 244:658, 1969.

27. Spiro, R. G., J Biol Chem 237:382, 1962.

28. Liu, W. K., C. M. Sweeney, H. S. Nahm, G. N. Holcomb, and D. N. Ward, Res Commun Pathol Pharmacol 1:463, 1970.

29. Spiro, R. G., Ann Rev Biochem 39:599, 1970.

30. Barker, S. A., G. J. Gray, J. F. Kennedy, and W. R. Butt, J Endocr 45, 275, 1969.

31. Cahil, C. L., M. R. Shetlar, R. W. Payne, B. Endecott, and Y. T. Li, Biochim Biophys Acta 154, 40, 1968.

18. Studies on the Structure and Activity of HCG

Francis J. Morgan, Sandra Kammerman, and Robert E. Canfield

The demonstration that pregnancy human chorionic gonadotropin (HCG), like the other gonadotropic glycoprotein hormones, possesses two nonidentical subunits (1) which can readily be separated from reduced alkylated HCG (1, 2) and from native HCG (2, 3) provides a powerful and simple approach for the study of this hormone. The fact that recombination of native subunits leads to the formation of a molecule with high biological activity (2) gives us a method for assembling molecules whose subunits have been selectively modified and whose activity can easily be measured. A simple procedure that has proved helpful in the study of the hormone is SDS-polyacrylamide gel electrophoresis (2, 4). We can now demonstrate the presence of two nonidentical subunits in the native molecule by this method (2) and we can easily monitor the purity of the subunit fractions and localize modifications to one or the other of the subunit. This communication deals with experiments that have been conducted on these lines.

MATERIALS AND METHODS

HCG was purified from commercial HCG as previously described (5). The subunits were separated by chromatography on DEAE-Sephadex (2). Recombination of the subunits was performed as described for luteinizing hormone (2, 6). SDS-polyacrylamide disc gel immunoelectrophoresis was performed essentially as described by Weber and Osborn (4) in 5% acrylamide gels. Asialo derivatives were prepared by treatment with neuraminidase (8). Iodination of HCG was performed by the method of Greenwood et al. (7). In vivo ovarian uptake of iodinated HCG and competitive binding studies were performed in mice by iv tail vein injection of labeled hormone and subsequent counting of the excised ovaries (5, 9).

RESULTS AND DISCUSSION

It has been shown that the subunits of LH can be recombined with moderate but significant restoration of activity (6). Recombination of the HCG subunits in a 1 : 1 ratio by weight by the method used for recombination of the LH subunits, resulted in a product that contained about 9000 IU/mg in the ventral prostate weight assay. The α subunit possessed no significant activity and the β subunit about 400 to 800 IU/mg (2). The starting material assayed at 13,000 IU/mg. We became aware that the β subunit was significantly larger than the α, and a maximal regaining of activity to 12,000 IU/mg was obtained when the subunits were mixed in a ratio of 1 : 1.4. Excess of either subunit did not inhibit activity. The restoration of activity is particularly high. Under ideal conditions it may be possible to obtain higher potency than the starting product, as the subunit separation in effect provides a further step in the purification process. The ratio of subunits for optimum recombination was consistent with the molecular weight differences estimated from their relative migration in SDS-gel electrophoresis. It is also consistent with the molar extinction coefficient for each subunit. The $E_{1\ cm}$ for the α subunit is 0.401 and for the β 0.262. The $E_{1\ cm}$ for the HCG preparation is 0.388, which corresponds closely the figure reported by Bahl (10), but is lower than that reported by Got (11).

The subunits can be dissociated by incubation in 10M urea at 40 C for 1 hr, and can be separated by chromatography on DEAE-Sephadex in 8M urea. It is clear from these experiments that exposure to urea under rigorous conditions has no harmful effect on the hormone preparation. The use of cyanate-free urea and buffers containing amines, together with minimum duration of exposure are important considerations.

A constant finding has been that the β subunit of HCG possesses a small amount of biological activity. It was of interest to see if the question of intrinsic activity in the subunits could be resolved. The isolated β subunit of LH seems to possess some activity.

In addition to the routine bioassay there is some further evidence that our HCG β subunit might possess some activity from studies with an in vivo competitive binding system using mouse ovaries as the target organ (5, 9). [125] I-HCG given by iv injection is concentrated in mouse ovarian tissue (5) as had been shown by Eshkol and Lunenfeld (11); this label can be readily displaced by cold native HCG in very small doses; LH in larger doses also displaced the label, but asialo HCG is relatively inefficient in displacing the label. However, our preparations of β subunit were consistently able to displace significant amounts of label, whereas the α subunit was inactive. This work on the ovarian binding of HCG in vivo has recently been extended to studies of the uptake of iodinated HCG by intact viable porcine granulosa cells in vitro in order to characterize the structural requirements of the tropic hormone for binding to receptors independent of the processes involved in vivo in biological halflife and clearance. In collaboration with Dr. Cornelia Channing (University of Pittsburgh), Dr. Sandra Kammerman of our laboratory has found that unlabeled HCG and human LH have virtually identical ability to displace iodinated HCG from these granulosa cells. In addition, asialo HCG also behaved indistinguishably from intact HCG in vitro, whereas in vivo it has both reduced biological activity and binding to ovaries. The β subunit of HCG had modest receptor affinity, whereas the α subunit was inactive. FSH did not appear to bind to the receptors that have a high affinity for HCG and LH in these granulosa cells. Neither of these experiments, however, settled the question of small contamination with undissociated hormone. We were also interested in the observation of Van Hall et al. (8) that desialylation up to about 25% produced a moderate fall in activity, followed by a more rapid loss as desialylation was increased to 62%; the small residual activity was not affected by further loss of sialic acid. The relative sialic acid content of the subunits ($\beta : \alpha = 2:1$) suggested that selective loss from one or the other subunit might explain this phenomenon.

Individual subunits were desialylated by neuraminidase as described by Van Hall et al. (8) and recombined as shown in Table I. All combinations of asialo and native subunit result in a dimeric product as demonstrated by gel filtration; all have activities in the range of asialo HCG. Complete absence of sialic acid

TABLE I. Gel filtration of asialo HCG recombinations

Experiment	Description	V_e	V_e/V_o
1	asialo $\beta + \alpha$	203.9 (major)	1.361
		261.3 (minor)	1.961
2	β + asialo α	198.9	1.416
		292.5	2.083
3	$\alpha + \beta$	183.3	1.305
4	asialo α + asialo β	202.8 (major)	1.405
		276.9 (minor)	1.918
5	α	267.4	1.891
6	β	194.0	1.428
7	asialo α	284.7	1.973
8	asialo β	230.1	1.594
9	HCG	180.4	1.242
10	asialo HCG	198.9	1.416

from either subunit alone produces on recombination an HCG whose activity is consistent with that of desialylated HCG. Thus the combination asialo α plus native β, which contains approximately 70% of the sialic content of the native HCG. Random removal of 30% of the sialic acid from native HCG results in the retention of a significantly larger degree of activity (8).

One further point concerning the differences between the subunits merits consideration. SDS-gel electrophoresis presents a very convenient method for monitoring selective modifications to the subunits. ^{125}I-HCG prepared by the method of Hunter and Greenwood retained 80% of its biological activity (9) in confirmation of earlier reports (12, 13). HCG is somewhat unusual in the degree of biological activity retained after iodination by the Chloramine-T method. When the subunits of the material are separated by SDS-gel electrophoresis and the gels scanned for radioactivity after slicing, it is found that virtually all the label resides in the α subunit. The iodine is presumably on tyrosine residues, although this has not been demonstrated, and suggests that the tyrosines of the α subunit, and perhaps the α subunit itself is more accessible. Further, the lack of modification in the β subunit might explain the high activity in the iodinated HCG if the β subunit is important for activity. This finding, of course, also raises some further questions, and indicates that a somewhat more complex approach for investigating the metabolism and action of the hormone is needed. If iodine-labeled HCG is used for studies of the mechanism of action of the hormone, localization of the label does not serve to localize the hormone itself, merely the α subunit. The absence of a label indicates absence of the hormone, or more precisely, of the β subunit. It seems clear that differentially labeled hormone formed from recombination of the subunits possessing different labels will provide a powerful tool in the study of the localization of the hormone and its individual subunits, and of their individual roles in its mode of action.

ACKNOWLEDGMENT

We are grateful to Dr. G. Ross and his colleagues for helpful discussions, and for performing bioassays. Dr. Vaitukaitis performed the desialylation of the separated subunits. Supported by research grants from the National Institutes of Health (AM 09579 and TIAM 05397), from the Population Council of New York and by NIH contract (70-2251).

REFERENCES

1. Canfield, R. E., G. M. Agosto, and J. J. Bell, in W. R. Butt, A. C. Crooke, and M. Ryle (Eds.), Gonadotrophins and Ovarian Development, E. & S. Livingstone, Edinburgh, in press, 1970.
2. Morgan, F. J., and R. E. Canfield, Endocrinology 88:1045, 1971.
3. Swaminathan, N., and O. P. Bahl, Biochem Biophys Res Commun 40:422, 1970.

4. Weber, K., and M. Osborn, J. Biol Chem 244:4406, 1969.

5. Canfield, R. E., F. J. Morgan, S. Kammerman, J. J. Bell, and G. M. Agosto, Rec. Prog Hormone Res 27:121, 1971.

6. Reichert, L. E., Jr., M. A. Rasco, D. N. Ward, G. D. Niswender, and A. R. Midgley, J Biol Chem 244:5110, 1969.

7. Greenwood, F. C., W. M. Hunter, and J. S. Glover, Biochem J 89:114, 1963.

8. Van Hall, E. V., J. L. Vaitukaitis, G. T. Ross, J. W. Hickman, and G. Ashwell, Endocrinology 88:456, 1971.

9. Kammerman, S., and R. E. Canfield, submitted for publication.

10. Bahl, O. P., J Biol Chem 244:567, 1969.

11. Got, R., and R. Bourrillon, Biochim Biophys Acta 39:241, 1960.

12. Lunenfeld, B., and A. Eshkol, Vitamins Hormones 25:137, 1967.

13. Midgley, A. R., Jr., Endocrinology 79:10, 1966.

DISCUSSION

W. R. BUTT. Notable work on human FSH has come from the laboratories of Roos, Peckham and Parlow, Ryan, Saxena, Reichert, Li, and Papkoff. I would like to present our own recent experience in this field. A stable preparation of gonadotropin (CP1) in dry form is obtained by a method described earlier (W. R. Butt, A. C. Crooke, and F. J. Cunningham, Biochem J 81:596, 1961). Following chromatography on CM-cellulose, calcium phosphate, and DEAE-cellulose, the product, precipitated by ethanol, contains 7 to 800 IU FSH/mg and 100 IU LH/mg. Such material is useful as a laboratory standard and for clinical applications (A. C. Crooke, W. R. Butt, and P. V. Bertrand, Acta Endocrinol Suppl 111, 1966). Further chromatography on DEAE-cellulose (W. R. Butt, S. S. Lynch, and J. F. Kennedy, 2nd Int Symp on Protein and Polypeptide Hormones, Liege, in press 1971) yields a fraction, which in the batches produced so far, contains on average about 8500 IU FSH/mg. The calculated yield per acetone-preserved pituitary is 44 IU FSH. Purified preparations have been stored in solution at -20 C for up to 12 months without loss of potency. On calibrated Sephadex G-100 columns the Stokes radius of FSH was calculated to be 31.3Å with a minor component of 23Å. Earlier work demonstrated that smaller molecular weight species are observed in IM NaCl solution (C. J. Gray, Nature 216:112, 1967). There appears to be a reversible dissociation to the monomer (molecular wt 16,000), dimer (32,000) and tetramer (64,000). More recently we have shown reversible dissociation in sodium dodecyl sulfate. In work of this nature, where the biological activity of the smaller fragments is low, the in vitro technique is very useful [M. Ryle, M. F. Chaplin, C. J. Gray, and J. F. Kennedy, in W. R. Butt, A. C. Crooke, and M. Ryle (Eds.), Gonadotrophins and Ovarian Development, E. & S. Livingstone, Edinburgh, 1971, p. 98]. The fragments are frequently extremely active in stimulating follicular growth and increasing the incorporation of ^{3}H-thymidine into ovarian DNA in vitro. This test is used routinely in parallel with bioassay and radioimmunoassay.

In our experiments to date we have failed to produce subunits of FSH by use of 1M-propionic acid as used by Papkoff and Ekblad for ovine FSH (Biochem Biophys Res Commun 40:614, 1970). There has been irreversible loss of biological activity which is consistent with our other studies which demonstrate the lability of FSH to acid media.

O. D. SHERWOOD. I will present four slides which show recent results obtained in the laboratory of Dr. W. H. McShan at the University of Wisconsin. The experiments conducted with ovine LH confirm and extend observations made by Squire and Jutisz about ten years ago. LH obtained from ovine anterior pituitary

216

glands consists of a microheterogeneous population of biologically active molecules. This microheterogeneity suggests that the concept of a single chemical structure for sheep LH should be accepted with caution (Fig. 1). (O. D. Sherwood, H. J. Grimek, and W. H. McShan, Biochim Biophys Acta 221:87, 1970). A highly purified preparation of ovine LH designated CM_2 and containing approximately 2 U NIH-LH-Sl/mg dry wt was obtained by ion exchange chromatography on CM-Sephadex. This LH preparation was layered on a column of hydroxylapatite equilibrated with 0.005M sodium phosphate at pH 6.8. When a linear gradient of sodium phosphate was applied, protein was eluted over the range of 0.06 to 0.15M. Bioassay in intact male rats demonstrated that LH activity was located throughout the eluted protein. Three fractions corresponding to the centers of the three most clearly distinguishable protein peaks observed on the chromatograph were pooled to form fraction 1 (Fr 1), fraction 2 (Fr 2), and fraction 3 (Fr 3). When these three LH fractions were individually rechromatographed on hydroxylapatite, each fraction was eluted over the same sodium phosphate concentration range originally required for elution. Physicochemical analyses of the three LH fractions were conducted. Dissimilarity in molecular size and immunological specificity were not detected with the techniques employed. However, differences among the three LH fractions were clearly detected with acrylamide disc gel electrophoresis and isoelectrofocusing. Moreover, amino acid analyses suggested differences in certain amino acids.

NH$_2$-terminal amino acid analyses have now been conducted on these three LH fractions by Lloyd and Nuti by a quantitative dansyl chloride procedure. Serine and phenylalanine are the predominant NH$_2$-terminal amino acids of Fr 3. Although the microheterogeneity of glycoproteins may be caused by a combination of factors such as proteolytic enzyme degradation, variations in carbohydrate composition, variations in amino acid composition and partial oxidation of methionine residues. The results shown in Table I indicate that differences in NH$_2$-terminal amino acids may contribute to the microheterogeneity of ovine LH. Microheterogeneity is also observed with anterior pituitary LH obtained from other species. Figure 2 shows electrofocusing results obtained with highly purified equine LH (W. E. Braselton, Jr., and W. H. McShan, Arch Biochem Biophys 139:45, 1970). Biological assays showed LH activity was spread over a range of at least 4 pH U. A different approach to this problem suggests that rat anterior pituitary LH is also microheterogenous (D. R. Hodges, and W. H. McShan, Acta Endocrinol 63:378, 1970). Anterior pituitary secretory granules were extracted and then analyzed by means of analytical acrylamide disk gel electrophoresis at pH 8.9. Figure 3 diagramatically summarizes the location of stained protein and biological activities. LH activity was found in two gel segments and could not be correlated with a stained protein band.

D. N. WARD. I should point out that I stressed in my presentation the corrections of our LH β subunit sequence. This was the addition of threonine plus the elucidation of the C-terminal heterogeneity. We are not the only

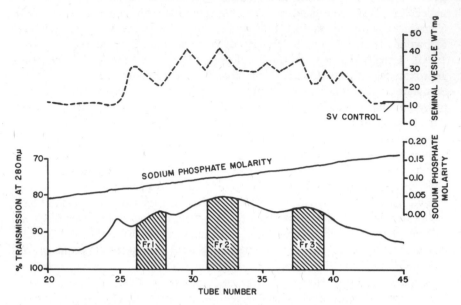

FIG. 1. Chromatography of the purified LH preparation CM 3 (150 mg protein) on a 2.8 × 40 cm column of hydroxylapatite at 25 C. LH activity was located by administering a constant volume from each tube to immature male rats and measuring the weights of the seminal vesicles. Reproduced by permission of Elsevier Publishing Company.

laboratory that has made corrections of the sequence. The report in 1969 from Dr. Li's laboratory (T. S. A. Samy, H. Papkoff, and C. H. Li, Arch Biochem Biophys 130:679, 1969) had 101 amino acids for this subunit and since that time, they have added 19.

O. P. BAHL. I think I would agree with Dr. Ward on this and if you look at all the other proteins which have been sequenced, papain is a clear example. The first reported sequence invariably had to be corrected. Its sequence was started some time in the late fifties and has been corrected and completed only recently with the help of x-ray diffraction studies. Another example which may be cited here is that of ribonuclease. Its original sequence was later corrected by Sanford and Moore. It is not an easy task and obviously mistakes are possible.

I have a question for Dr. Nureddin. Have you noticed any heterogeneity in your preparation of LH? If so, how did it affect the sequence studies with your automatic sequenator?

A. NUREDDIN. We have not observed any heterogeneity in the determination of the sequence of the α subunit. Only one NH₂-terminal residue is detected, namely valine. In this respect it is interesting to note Dr. Ward's comments on the heterogeneity observed in the α subunit of ovine LH. This heterogeneity is

observed in the peptide comprising the first seven amino acid residues from the
NH_2-terminal end of the molecule. This heptapeptide is missing in the human
subunit.

TABLE I. NH_2-terminal amino acids isolated as dansyl derivatives from ovine
luteinizing hormone

Preparation or fraction	CM 3	Fr 1	Fr2	Fr 3
Amino acid[a]				
Serine	0.32 (0.69)[b]	0.26 (0.46)	0.28 (0.62)	0.36 (0.78)
Threonine	0.23 (0.37)	0.06 (0.10)	0.15 (0.25)	0.37 (0.61)
Phenylalanine	0.13 (0.21)	0.34 (0.55)	0.18 (0.29)	0.06 (0.11)
Glycine	0.12 (0.21)	0.08 (0.14)	0.18 (0.31)	0.06 (0.11)
Aspartic acid	0.08 (0.14)	0.07 (0.12)	0.07 (0.13)	0.02 (0.03)
Glutamic acid	0.02 (0.04)	0.01 (0.02)	0.01 (0.02)	0.01 (0.01)
Lysine	0.01 (0.01)	0.03 (0.02)	0.02 (0.01)	0.01 (0.01)

[a]Values expressed as nanomoles of amino acid/nanomole of LH (molecular weight of
30,000). These data are the average of four determinations.

[b]Values in parentheses are corrected for destruction during hydrolysis and recovery from
the thin layer plates. NH_2-terminal analysis of bovine insulin yielded 0.50 (0.81) and 0.48
(0.84) nm of phenylalanine and glycine/nanomole of insulin, respectively.

P. ROOS. Roos, Nyberg, and Gemzell have developed a procedure for the
isolation of human pituitary LH from whole frozen pituitaries. Four biologically
active components were obtained (two major, II and III, and two minor, I and
IV). The procedure involved extraction of homogenized pituitaries, ammonium
sulfate fractionation, chromatography on DEAE-cellulose, Sephadex G-100, and
SE-Sephadex C-50 and polyacrylamide gel electrophoresis.

The yield of each of the major components was in the range of 0.2 to 0.3
mg/100 g pituitary tissue with biological potencies of about 7000 IU of LH
activity/mg. The four components of LH were all homogenous when examined
by polyacrylamide gel electrophoresis, that is in a sieving medium, and by free
zone electrophoresis, a nonsieving medium. No heterogeneity was observed when
the components were studied in the ultracentrifuge by sedimentation equilibrium technique. All the components had molecular weights of about 40,000.
Sedimentation velocity experiments with component II and III revealed in each
case one boundary. The sedimentation coefficients were 3.2 S and 3.5 S,
respectively.

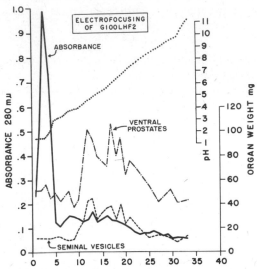

FIG. 2. Elctrofocusing of LH fraction G100LHF2 in a 1% solution of pH 3 to 10 ampholytes. An LKB 8101 electrofocusing column was used. The cathode, at the top, consisted of 2% (v/v) ethylenediamine and the anode, at the bottom, consisted of 0.2 ml H_3PO_4, 14 ml H_2O, and 12 g sucrose. A potential of 340 V was applied for 36 hr, the current having stabilized at 0.9 mA after a total of 20 hr. The sample contained 2 mg protein. Aliquots from each tube were assayed at a dose level of 5-g equivalents of fresh tissue in intact immature male rats.

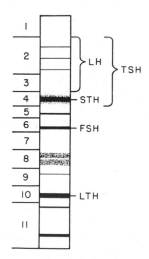

FIG. 3. Diagram of the staining pattern following electrophoresis of extracts of rat anterior pituitary secretory granules. The separate segments cut and assayed are numbered on the left and the active zones are indicated on the right. The anode is at the bottom.

220

In immunodiffusion using antiserum to a pituitary LH preparation, components II and III showed identity. Only one precipitation line was obtained between antiserum and each of the components. Component 1 gave one weak precipitation line indicating partial identity with components II and III. The existence of a precipitation line between component IV and the antiserum could not be definitely established.

Amino acid analysis of components II and III indicated 265 and 277 residues/mole, respectively. No significant difference in the composition was observed. The molecular weights of the protein moieties were calculated to be 30,400 and 31,500, respectively. The carbohydrate composition of the two components was determined by gas chromatography. Values of 10,600 (component II) and 12,800 (component III) were calculated for the molecular weights of the carbohydrate moieties. The data suggest a difference in carbohydrate composition.

From the analysis data, the molecular weights of components II and III were consequently 41,000 and 44,300 in good agreement with the ultracentrifugation data.

H. VAN HELL. In 1969 we subjected a urinary FSH preparation of a biological potency of 3300 IU/mg to isoelectric focusing. We found FSH and LH focused at about the same pH values of the ampholine as the Hamburg group reported here. The most potent FSH isolated had a potency of about 1200 IU. It struck me that your best material had the same FSH potency as ours. This data was presented in Birmingham in 1969 (W. R. Butt, A. C. Crooke, and M. Ryle (Eds.), Gonadotrophins and Ovarian Development, E. & S. Livingstone, Edinburgh, 1970).

A. R. MIDGLEY. I think Dr. Rathnam and Dr. Nureddin each indicated that the sedimentation coefficient decreased with decreasing concentrations. This has been interpreted as being the result of dissociation. In particular the results presented by Dr. Rathnam indicated the relationship to be linear on an arithmetic plot. However, the lowest concentrations tested were far greater, by many orders of magnitude, than those found in serum. Does anyone have good data to indicate the state of aggregation/dissociation in serum? Do components of serum affect these properties? It would seem unlikely that subunits could exist in circulation in a completely dissociated state.

B. B. SAXENA. The sedimentation rates of FSH and LH are dependent on the protein concentration. The FSH is not completely dissociated into its subunits by dilution alone. It would appear from the data that FSH dissociates into its monomeric form at higher dilution and into subunits by digestion with 8M urea. Highly active FSH preparations are assayed in rats at concentrations as low as $6 \times 10^{-5}\%$ (0.6 μg/ml), hence it is possible that FSH may exist in the circulation in its monomeric and biologically active form.

J. A. COPPOLA. Please excuse what may appear to be a naive question, but I am confused on sialic acid. Perhaps Dr. Reichert can clarify one point of interest. Earlier you said removal of sialic acid decreases biological potency and increases immunoreactivity by unmasking a site. Dr. Graesslin stated that there appears to be only one mole of sialic acid/mole/molecule of LH so that by removing one molecule of sialic acid from one molecule of LH you decrease biological potency and increase immunoreactivity. Is this a common mechanism and does the unmasking of this one site do both these things?

G. T. ROSS. In answering your question, there are at least four points I would like to emphasize. First, the sialic acid content of different preprations of HLH is variable, some containing more, some containing less than others. Second, the apparent amount of change in both immunologic and biologic properties following removal of sialic acid varies with the methods used to examine these properties. Third, gonadotropins are not the only glycoproteins whose properties have been studied before and after desialation. Removal of a single sialic acid residue from some glycoprotein molecules profoundly alters the rate at which these substances disappear from plasma. Finally, the immunogenicity of some of these nonhormonal glycoproteins has been shown to increase following desialylation.

A. NUREDDIN. In relation to the dissociation of LH and the change in the behavior of the sedimentation coefficient as a function of protein concentration, we have purposely avoided extrapolating to zero concentration because we do not know what happens at that concentration, since in the ultracentrifuge the peak at the lower concentrations would be very broad and would not give accurate data. However, I believe that LH exists in equilibrium with its subunits. Upon storage of LH, disc gel electrophoresis indicates the presence of bands with mobilities equivalent to those of the subunits. Furthermore, the association-dissociation equilibrium seems to be a function of the ionic strength of the medium. At an ionic strength of 0.2, the equilibrium is shifted to lower concentration of the hormone. Thus at an ionic strength of 0.1, the equilibrium is established at a concentration of 0.4 g/100ml, while at an ionic strength of 0.2, this equilibrium is reached at 0.25 g/100ml.

P. J. CZYGAN. May I briefly present some data on the preparation of highly purified HCG. The crude material supplied by Dr. van Hell from Organon, containing 3000 IU/mg was applied to a column of CM-Sephadex C-50, using sodium potassium phosphate buffer of pH 5.2 of increasing molarity. Four distinct peaks were separated (Fig. 4). The third fraction, representing 15% of starting protein, showed the highest biological activity; approximately, 3 times that of the crude material. In analytical disc electrophoresis at pH of 8.9, purified HCG migrated as a broad protein zone as found by other investigators (Fig. 5a). In analytical flat gel isoelectric focusing, however, six distinct protein bands became obvious (Fig. 5b). Fraction 3 from CM-Sephadex showed only two narrow protein zones on a preparative slab with ampholine of pH range of 3 to 6. These bands were dissected from unstained gel and the proteins extracted. The ampholines were removed and the material lyophilized. Analytical refocus-

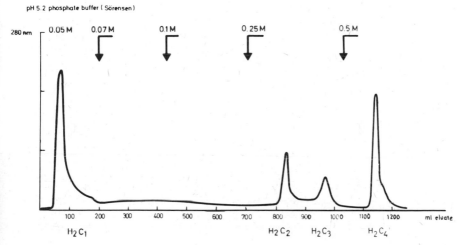

FIG. 4.

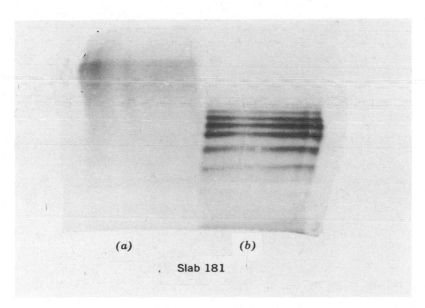

(a)   *(b)*

Slab 181

FIG. 5.

ing and gel filtration on Sephadex G-100 demonstrated homogeneity of these fractions. Figure 6 shows the superiority of the gel electrofocusing procedure over the disc electrophoresis as used in the purification of HCG. On the left is shown a disc electrophoretic pattern of HCG in polyacrylamide gel. On the right is shown the isoelectric refocusing pattern of single bands compared with the pattern of the starting material. The second band revealed 14,000 IU/mg in bioassay and 17,500 IU/mg by radioimmunoassay, an isoelectric point of 4.3 and a sialic acid content of 8.8%.

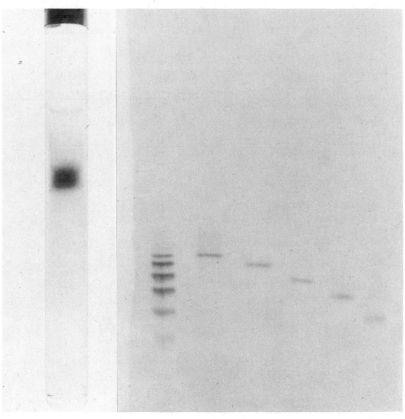

FIG. 6.

Mechanism of Action
of Gonadotropins

19.   Interaction of LH with the Ovary

Patricia Coulson, Tsui-Chu Liu, Paul Morris, Jack Gorski

The term receptor, according to Jensen (1), refers to a hypothetical entity capable of receiving and binding a chemical agent thus initiating a physiological or pharmacological response. Broadly defined, many categories of such receptors exist, each having a specific affinity for their ligands but differing in the consequences of their interactions. For example, there are receptors on enzymes and antibodies for holding their substrates, there are storage receptors, silent receptors, and serum-carrier or transport receptors (1).

Experimentally, receptors have several measurable criteria. Receptors for hormones are assumed to have a finite number of sites within their "target" tissue and therefore are saturable. These sites exhibit high specificity for their specific ligands as demonstrated by competitive inhibition studies. The binding affinity of the tissue receptors for their ligands by necessity must be greater than that of other potential receptors, such as blood-carrier proteins and nonspecific storage receptors, in order that the hormone at low circulating concentrations can be preferentially concentrated.

As other papers in this symposium illustrate, researchers are beginning to understand the structure and biological effects of the gonadotropin, LH. Little is currently known, however, about receptor sites for gonadotropins or large protein hormones in general. The LH molecule has a molecular weight of about 30,000 and is composed of two nonidentical subunits (2, 3). Similar subunit structures have been found with other protein hormones including the placental hormone, HCG (4), TSH (5), and FSH (6). The subunits of LH can be separated and characterized, but are completely inactive as single chains. Under carefully controlled conditions the subunits can be recombined for renewed activity (7-12). LH and HCG are both glycoproteins which appear to have multiple and

227

heterogeneous carbohydrate groups on each molecule (7, 13). Segments of the LH subunits have amino acid sequences in common with other hormones including HCG, TSH, and FSH (4, 5, 14). The short serum halflife of either endogeneous or isotopically labeled LH is approximately 10 to 20 min (15-18).

Target tissue responses of the ovary to LH have been studied extensively. The hormone is known to affect the circulation (19, 20); steroid and sterol synthesis patterns (21-23); DNA, RNA, and protein synthesis rates (24, 25); mito-chondrial cytochromes (26); and other cellular metabolic activities (27-29). At very short time periods following stimulation, LH has been shown to change the cellular levels or activities of several molecules such as adenyl cyclase (30-33), prostaglandins (34, 35), or histamine (36). Such findings have given rise to the possibility of an obligatory role for these "secondary mediators."

The biological function or necessity of the double-stranded form of LH is still an enigma. One hypothesis suggests that the configuration of the two chains facilitates the penetration of the target issue, but both chains may not be necessary for interaction at the receptor level. It is not yet known whether the large protein hormones actually enter the target cells to interact with their effector sites. Some large molecules, however, have been shown to penetrate cell membranes intact but these usually suffer variable metabolic destruction rates later within the host cell (37, 38).

Mounting evidence for a "multiple action" theory for protein hormones may reconcile much current conflicting data on sites of action (39). Such a model, utilizing separate active sites for different discrete functions (40) could explain external binding to the plasma membrane versus separate internal effector sites. It could also explain short-term versus long-term effects on the tissue or multiple hormonal effects (LH, +FSH, +TSH) of the same purified hormonal preparation.

Studies in this laboratory on preovulatory rabbit ovarian tissue exposed to LH in vitro have demonstrated a stimulatory effect on steroid synthesis (41). By developing a procedure for maintaining short-term cultures of free ovarian cells, we have eliminated some of the problems of tissue permeability and extracellular space. In this system a hormone dose-response curve (Fig. 1) showed that the ovarian cells were sensitive to in vitro stimulation at concentrations less than 3.3 $\times 10^{-11}$M, approximately 0.001 μg LH/ml (42).

From published data on the circulating levels of LH in mature cycling rats just prior to the ovulatory surge, the concentration of hormone was calculated to be about 10^{-10}M, with the ovulatory surge increasing the concentration briefly tenfold (15, 43). These low concentrations of LH either present in the blood or necessary to stimulate steroidogenesis must be taken into account in studying the interaction of LH with its target tissue.

TRACER STUDIES WITH LABELED GONADOTROPINS

Radioactive tracer techniques offer many advantages for separating the effects of LH into its initial interaction and its subsequent magnification steps. Isotopic

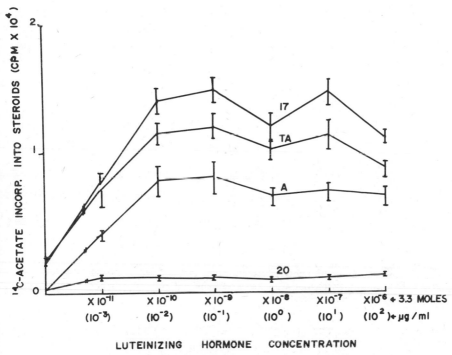

LUTEINIZING   HORMONE   CONCENTRATION

FIG. 1. Effects of LH concentrations on the incorporation of 2-¹⁴C-acetate into steroids (42). One ml of cell suspension (13 µg of DNA) was incubated at 37 C with 2-¹⁴C-acetate with or without LH for 4 hr. Steroid extracts were first paper chromatographed. The eluates of the uv absorbing radioactive areas were then acetylated and rechromatographed on the thin layer plates. Each point represents the mean ± SE (vertical bars) of 3 or 4 determinations. 17 = 17-Hydroxyprogesterone; TA = testosterone acetate; A = androstene-dione; 20 = 20d-hydroxypregn-4-en-one. Reproduced by permission of J. B. Lippincott Company.

labeling allows direct study of the possible presence of receptor sites within ovarian tissue with the ability of specifically accumulating gonadotropic hormone. Tracer studies would allow investigation at very low concentration, such as those found in the circulation in vivo. The molecular concentrations and the molecular forms of protein hormones in their target cells or tissues, however, have yet to be demonstrated. This is an important point to ascertain in order to illuminate the mechanism of hormonal function at the cellular level.

Any labeled compound used for tracer studies must satisfy several important criteria. It must be stable at biological pH and have a high specific activity. At the same time it should retain its original biological and immunological activities, as well as its original in vivo metabolic function and half-life in the circulation (44).

Some of the first reports of specific gonadotropic hormone uptake by the ovary with appropriate controls were published by Eshkol and Lunenfeld (45, 46), and by Kazeto and Hreshchyshyn (47). Both groups showed that blood levels fell rapidly after a single IV injection of labeled HCG (Fig. 2), but that the

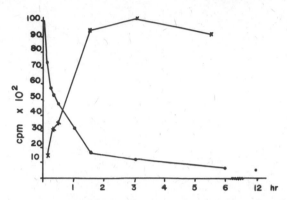

FIG. 2. Concentration of radioactivity in blood (●,expressed as%) and in ovaries (x in cpm × 10^2/100 mg tissue) following a single IV injection of labeled HCG (46). Reproduced by permission of Plenum Press.

cpm/mg tissue which accumulated in the ovary continued to increase with time and reached a peak 5 times blood levels (cpm/$\mu\ell$) by 2 to 4 hr after injection (Fig. 3).

Espeland et al., (48) recently reported a 6-8-fold increase in ^{125}I-HCG uptake by the ovaries of mature, estrogen +PMS-primed female rats. The competitive inhibition studies suggested the presence of a common receptor for most of the gonadotropic hormones tested in proportion to their LH-like biological activities (49-51). Beals and Midgley (52) reported a blood to ovarian tissue ration for ^{131}I-HCG uptake in untreated female rats as 1.56 and up to 22.9 in rats prepared for the Parlow ovarian ascorbic acid depletion (OAAD) assay.

LABELING LH WITH Na^{125}I

Iodination with Na^{125}I (isotopic activity, 1.72 x 10^4 Ci/g I) was chosen for labeling in our studies because the procedure (53, 54) is fast, gentle (pH 7.5) and results in a product with extremely high specific activity (S A = 100 μCi/μg or approximately 1 ± 0.5 ^{125}I molecules/LH molecule). Figure 4a shows the pattern of a labeled LH preparation (ovine LH, LER-777-3 with 1.43 x NIH-LH-S1 (55) or 84 IU 2nd-IRP (56) potency) after it was desalted to remove any unreacted ^{125}I and electrophoresed on acrylamide gel. A comparison with labeled single-chain LH (Fig. 4b) indicates that our labeled ^{125}I-LH product (Fig. 4a) is still in its native (double-stranded) form and that little or no labeled single-chain LH is present (see arrow in Fig. 4a).

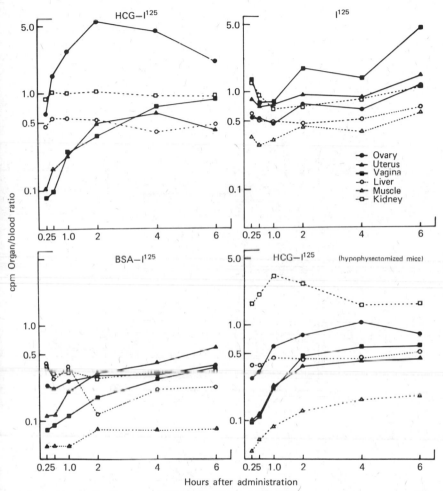

FIG. 3. Tissue distribution of ^{125}I-HCG, ^{125}I, and ^{125}I-BSA, expressed as cpm organ/blood ratio in intact and hypophysectomized mice (47). Reproduced by permission of The C. V. Mosby Company.

Bioassays of LH using the OAAD procedure and labeled with 1 to 2 I/molecule have shown that the biological activity was not destroyed by iodination (Tables I and II). This is in agreement with other hormone studies where preparations with 1 to 2 I/protein molecule have retained their biological (16, 30, 45) and immunological activity (57, 58). This is an extremely important check as it is known that higher levels of iodination (greater than 5 to 10 I/molecule) or other stronger chemical treatments can easily reduce the biological activity of pituitary hormones to zero (49, 58).

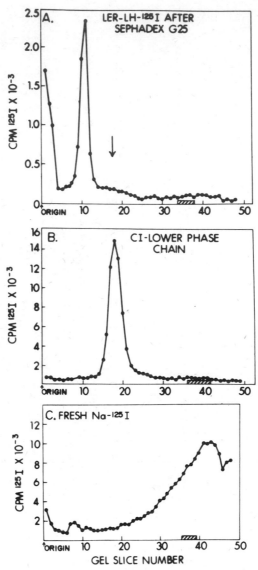

FIG. 4. Polyacrylamide electrophoresis of labeled LH. ^{125}I-LH is shown in Fig. (a) in the native form after desalting with Diaflo ultrafiltration followed by a Sephadex G-25 column. Fig. (b) Separation of LH from a preparation of its subunit, LH-CI (both LH CI and CII electrophorese together in this system). A 10% acrylamide gel was used in pH 9.5, Tris acetate buffer, following the procedure of Summers et al. (89) with 0.5 M urea, 0.1% sodium dodecyl sulfate, and 0.1% mercaptoethanol in the gel mixture. Fig. (c) Fresh ^{125}I-Na oxidized and reduced via the labeling procedure. Gels a, b, and c were coelectrophoresed at 3 mA/tube for 5.5 hr with bromophenyl blue as the tracking dye (▨).

TABLE I. OAAD assay of iodinated NIH-LH-S11[a]

Group	Dose	Ascorbic acid mean ± SE (μg/100 mg ovary)	LH Recovered (μg)	LH Recovered (%)	Significance by students "t" test
1	BSA 3 mg/0.5 ml (CRYS)	93.37 ± 2.77			1 vs 2, p = 0.950
2	0.2 μg NIH-LH-S11	82.21 ± 0.95			2 vs 3, p = 0.990
3	1.0 μg NIH-LH-S11	58.02 ± 3.05			3 vs 4, p = 0.950
4	5.0 μg NIH-LH-S11	41.49 ± 1.60			
5	0.2 μg Oxidized LH	88.10 ± 2.06	∿ 0.132	66.1	5 vs 6, p = N.S.
6	0.2 μg ^{125}I-LH	87.33 ± 2.48	∿ 0.142	71.1	1 vs 5 or 6, p = 0.800
7	2.5 μg Oxidized LH	62.01 ± 2.79	∿ 1.05	42.2	7 vs 8, p = N.S.
8	2.5 μg ^{125}I-LH	58.33 ± 3.30	∿ 1.27	50.8	1 vs 7 or 8, p = 0.995

[a]4 to 5 rats were used/group; 2 determinations/rat.

TABLE II. OAAD assay of iodinated LER-LH-777-3[a]

Group	Dose	Ascorbic acid mean ± SE (μg/100 mg ovary)	LH Recovered (μg)	LH Recovered (%)	Significance by students "t" test
1	Saline	80.46 ± 1.39			1 vs 2, p = 0.950
2	0.1 μg LER-LH	72.40 ± 1.12			2 vs 3, p = 0.950
3	0.5 μg LER-LH	63.71 ± 1.36			3 vs 4, p = 0.950
4	2.5 μg LER-LH	53.39 ± 2.32			
5	0.1 μg oxidized LER-LH	75.59 ± 3.27	$\sim$ 0.069	69.0	5 vs 6, p = N.S.
6	0.1 μg ^{125}I-LER-LH	75.95 ± 2.27	$\sim$ 0.065	65.0	1 vs 5 or 6, p = 0.750
7	2.5 μg oxidized LER-LH	54.78 ± 3.23	$\sim$ 2.35	93.5	7 vs 8, p = N.S.
8	2.5 μg ^{125}I-LER-LH	55.84 ± 1.039	$\sim$ 2.22	89.0	1 vs 7 or 8, p = 0.995

[a]4 to 5 rats were used/group; 2 determinations/rat.

IN VIVO STUDIES ON ^{125}I-LH

Using ^{125}I-LH (LER 777-3, ovine) in rats luteinized by a modification of the Parlow pretreatment, we found that ovarian tissue showed a dramatically different retention-time pattern from other control tissue (59). The results presented in Fig. 5 give the ratio of cpm/100 mg wet wt of tissue versus cpm/0.1

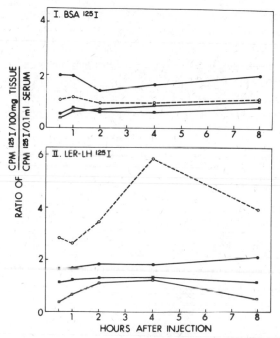

FIG. 5. In vivo ^{125}I-LH versus ^{125}I-BSA distribution in rats. Group (a) was injected intravenously with 0.0247 ug ^{125}I-BSA (SA = 22.7 uCi/ug). Group (b) was injected IV with 0.0053 μg ^{125}I-LH (SA = 68 uCi/ug). Each point represents the tissue from 3 rats: ovary (○), liver (●), adrenal (■) and uterus (□).

ml rat serum. Theoretically, a ratio of 1 or less would suggest no active accumulation above blood levels, while a constant value for any one tissue would indicate that the tissue counts are following the decline in blood values with time. The tissue to serum ratio (T/S ratio) using ^{125}I-BSA for ovary and control tissues were low, fairly constant, and focused around a value of 1 (Fig. 5a).The T/S ratio was about 1 in the ^{125}I-LH experiments for the control tissues, adrenal, and uterus, while the ovary showed a peak at 4 hr with a ratio of 6. Liver in both the ^{125}I-BSA and the ^{125}I-LH groups gave a fairly constant ratio of 2. These results were in good agreement with the HCG versus BSA studies of Kazeto et al. (47).

It has been demonstrated by Ellis (19) and others that rat ovaries under hormonal stimulation exhibit linear hyperemic responses to LH stimulation at doses of 0.5 to 2.0 μg LH/0.2 ml/rat. This increased vascularity or imbibition of fluid could be demonstrated by an increased uptake of dye or a labeled protein such as BSA. Although our experiments were run at concentrations well below those in the Ellis bioassay, further clarification of the separate roles of hyperemia versus specific hormone uptake was necessary.

Follicularized ovaries were prepared by the procedure of Espeland et al. (51), which eliminated the use of HCG priming. The retention of label in ovary or thymus tissue was measured after a single IV injection of one of three test solutions: ^{125}I-LH, ^{125}I-LH + LH or ^{125}I-BSA + LH. The ratio of labeled to unlabeled hormone was 1 : 100. All injections were made in a 1 : 10 dilution of fresh egg white to prevent competition from potential BSA hormone contamination (60).

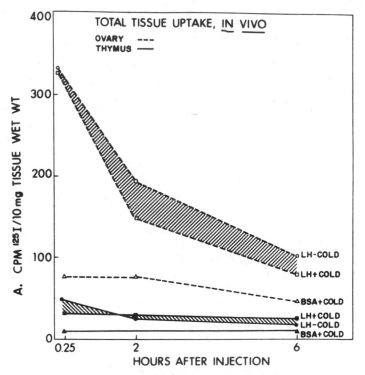

FIG. 6a. In vivo competition studies with ^{125}I-LH. Retention of label by ovarian (_ _ _ _ _) and thymus (_____) tissue was studied at 1/4, 2, and 6 hr after IV. Three test solutions were: (1) LH + Cold (○ & ●), 0.072 μg ^{125}I-LH (SA = 62.5 μCi/μg); (2) LH + Cold (□ & ■), 0.072 μg ^{125}I-LH + 7.0 μg unlabeled LH; or(3) BSA + Cold (△ & ▲), 0.02 μg ^{125}I-BSA (SA = 22.7 μCi/μg) + 7 μg unlabeled LH. Injection vol was 0.5 ml/rat with tissues from 4 rats pooled per point. Total uptake expressed on a wet weight basis.

Figure 6a shows the decrease in hormone retained in the tissue with time. The T/S ratio in thymus control tissue for either ^{125}I-BSA or ^{125}I-LH was consistently below 1, indicating no active concentration above blood levels (Fig. 6b). The

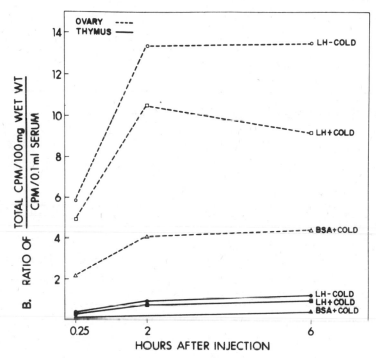

FIG. 6b. In vivo competition studies. For symbols see Fig. 6a. Data are expressed as ratio of tissue counts to serum counts.

^{125}I-BSA uptake by ovarian tissue in the presence of 7.0 μg of LH/rat (BSA + unlabeled or cold) reached a maximum ratio of 4 after 6 hr, suggesting that the presence of unlabeled hormone did influence ovarian tissue vascularity. However, this factor alone will not explain the even greater ratio obtained when only ^{125}I-LH (LH-cold) was used as shown at 2 and 6 hr (Fig. 6b). If vascularity changes were solely responsible for increased uptake, the ^{125}I-LH + 7μg of LH might be expected to show greater uptake than ^{125}I-LH alone.

The fact that cold LH only partially decreased the uptake of ^{125}I-LH by ovarian tissue (Fig. 6a) even at extremely high ratios of unlabeled to labeled LH, suggests that the specific binding sites for LH represent a smaller percentage of the total uptake than do the nonspecific sites. Apparently the specific sites were being saturated by the levels of hormones used and a large excess of hormone was spilling over into the nonspecific sites. The results in Fig. 6 show that a minimum of 25% of the total hormone bound could be specifically displaced with unlabeled competitive LH. Further work is necessary to prove conclusively that the effect of unlabeled LH is to compete for specific binding sites versus nonspecific sites; however, this appears to be the most likely explanation.

Studies with the ACTH receptor in adrenal tissue suggest that there are two orders of binding for the adrenal hormone with apparent association constants of 10^{12} and 10^7, respectively. The high affinity sites represented about 0.1% of the total ACTH receptor population in these studies (61). This dual set of receptors may agree with the suggestion of the presence of two binding sites in ^{131}I-insulin systems by Garrett (62) termed active (high affinity) and storage (low affinity) sites.

SUBCELLULAR DISTRIBUTION OF ^{125}I-LH

To investigate subcellular distribution of accumulated hormone, ovarian and thymus tissues were fractionated by ultracentrifugation in 0.22M sucrose. The uptake of ^{125}I-LH by the 800 × g pellet, the mitochondrial-microsomal fraction and the 100,000 × g supernatant or cytosol is shown in Fig. 7.

In addition an attempt was made to extract the labeled hormone from the 800 × g pellet with 2.0M urea, pH 9.5, at 4 C. This is insufficient urea to separate the two LH subunits. Since most of the ^{125}I in the 800 × g pellet could be solublized with this procedure, the possibility is very small that strong disulfide or peptide bonds are involved in the retention of hormone in the membraneous ovarian fraction.

The labeled hormone recovered was 90% precipitable by 10% cold TCA indicating the isotope was still bound to at least a large peptide structure. However, its relationship to the original native hormone should be further investigated. Preliminary work on LH, insulin (62, 63), and other protein hormones suggests that they may be metabolized consiserably by their target tissues in contrast to such steroid hormones as estradiol and aldosterone (64, 65), which have been shown to exhibit little or no chemical alteration during and after interaction with their receptor sites.

Considerable controversy exists as to which, if any, cell types preferentially concentrate gonadotropic hormones during ovarian stimulation. Autoradiographic studies at low magnification, have shown iodine-labeled HCG to be concentrated preferentially in the follicular envelopes, theca cells, and stroma of the ovary (46). De Kretser et al (66, 67) have shown that ^{125}I-LH binds in the testis to rat interstitial cells but not germinal cells. Castro et al. (68) have shown preferential localization of ferritin-labeled LH in male rats in the vesicles and dense bodies of the Leydig cells. The decrease in LH metabolized or bound by ovaries treated with contraceptive steroids, such as Ovulen or Ortho-Novum, also suggests that the ovarian uptake of hormone involves only certain cell types in specific stages of the female cycle (69). Rencently Cons and Kragt (70) have shown that pretreatment with HCG caused a decrease in the circulating half-life of labeled FSH. These reports indicate a correlation between utilization or degradation of the hormone and the physiological state of the animal and its target tissue.

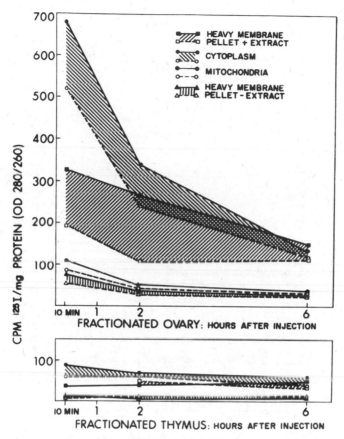

FIG. 7. In vivo competition studies in fractionated tissue. Tissue distributions are expressed as cpm/mg fractionated protein, (O.D. 280/260. Solid lines or solid symbols represent ^{125}I-LH (LH – cold) and open symbols or dashed lines represent ^{125}I-LH + unlabeled LH (LH + cold). Difference due to unlabeled LH competition is shaded. Symbols represent 800 × g pellet (heavy membrane fraction, □ and ■), 100,000 × g pellet (mitochondrial ⊥ microsomal fraction, ○ and ●), cytosol (○ and ●), and 800 × g pellet after extraction with 2.0M urea (△ and ▲).

IN VITRO STUDIES ON ^{125}I-LH

Rabbit ovarian tissue chunks incubated in vitro were also able to concentrate LH from the labeled media. Figure 8 illustrates uptake of ^{125}I-LH with or without a 1000-fold excess of unlabeled LH. The uptake of ^{125}I-LH in the presence of unlabeled LH (20 µg/flask) was reduced by 15 to 20% after 2 to 3 hr incubation. The heavy membrane fraction, 800 × g pellet, and the cytosol fraction contained most of the TCA-precipitable radioactivity. Those fractions also accounted for most of the specifically bound LH as demonstrated by the decreases due to competition with unlabeled hormone.

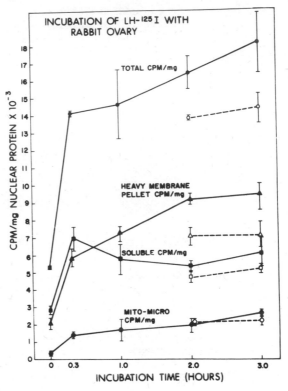

FIG. 8. In vitro uptake of ^{125}I-LH. Rabbit ovarian tissue chunks incubated at 37 C under an atmosphere of 95% O_2 + 5% CO_2 in Eagles's medium in 0.02 μg ^{125}I-LH in 2 ml/flask (o—o) or 0.02 μg ^{125}I-LH (SA = 52.5 μCi/μg) + 20 μg cold LH in 2 ml/flask (o---o). Zero time samples kept at 4 C for 3 hr. Tissue chunks washed, homogenized in 0.3M sucrose, and fractionated as in Fig. 7. Fractions were precipitated with 10% TCA, counted, and the protein was measured by the Lowry procedure. Data are expressed as the mean ± range with 2 flasks/group.

An in vivo experiment demonstrating the difference in the distribution of ^{125}I-LH in ovarian tissue versus adrenal tissue is shown in Fig. 9. Between 40 to 60% of the total labeled hormone is taken up by the heavy pellet fraction of ovarian tissue compared to less than 15% by the same adrenal fraction at all three times studied. Control ^{125}I-BSA uptake showed less than 15% of the total counts in the heavy pellet fraction for both the ovarian and the adrenal tissues.

The presence of specific binding for LH in both fractions may be real, but the possibility of contamination of one fraction by another during homogenization cannot be ruled out. This is particularily a problem if receptor sites are membrane bound rather than soluble (71).

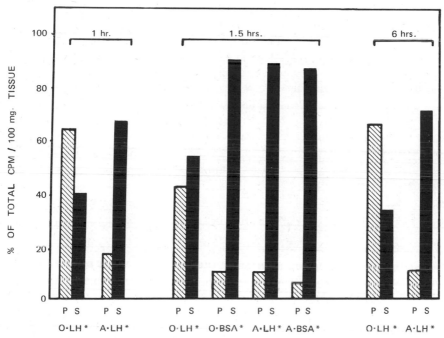

FIG. 9. Distribution of ^{125}I-LH in vivo. ^{125}I-LH fractionated into an 800 X g pellet and supernatant portion following a single iv injection. The histograms represent pooled adrenal (A) and ovarian (O) tissue from 6 or 7 rats homogenized in 0.04M Tris, 0.1M KCl, pH 7.5, and fractionated into 800 X g pellet

(P = ▨) and soluble (S = ■) fractions. Groups 1 and 2, 7 and 8, were injected with 0.001 μg ^{125}I-LH (LH*) in 0.5 ml/rat (SA = 50 μCi/μg) for 1 and 6 hr, respectively. Groups 3 to 6 were injected with 0.062 μg ^{125}I-LH (LH*) in 0.5 ml/rat (SA = 136 μCi/μg) or 0.107 μg ^{125}I-BSA (BSA*) in 0.5 ml/rat (SA = 26 μCi/μg) for 1-1/2 hr each. The 100% cpm/gm averages for groups 1 to 8 respectively were: (1) 3306; (2) 2335; (3) 32,298; (4) 10,190; (5) 17,429; and (6) 9914.

Studies with ^{131}I-insulin in rat diaphragm (63) and with ^{3}H-ACTH in rat adrenals (72) or ^{125}I-ACTH in mice adrenals (61) showed that the majority of the binding was in the heavy 700 x g cell debris fraction. The specific hormone binding sites demonstrated by competition with unlabeled hormone were primarily in the 100,000 x g supernatant for both the ^{131}I-insulin (63) and the ^{125}I-ACTH (61) studies.

The chemical nature of the proposed receptors for protein hormones is essentially unknown at present. Preliminary studies on ^{131}I-insulin specific binding suggest that it is combined with a component of higher molecular weight than the hormone (63). Studies on fat cells indicate that receptors for lipolytic hormones are trypsin-sensitive and therefore at least partly protein in nature (73). Much more work needs to be done on assays for receptor sites before the receptors themselves can be characterized chemically.

Our studies on LH, as well as work by others on protein hormones, suggest that the hormone may, in whole or in part, interact with the mitochondria (74), the nuclei (72), or other intracellular components (30). Other workers, using hormones bound to large inert molecules and other techniques, have argued that ACTH (61, 75), insulin (76), and lipolytic hormones (73, 77) can work without entering their target cells. Other studies show hormones which require intact cells or plasma membranes for in vitro stimulation (78). Current views support the possibility that certain protein hormones have multiple active sites and multiple cellular functions located both inside the cell and at the plasma membrane surface (39, 40, 65, 79-84).

LEVELS OF LH SPECIFICALLY BOUND

Data from the binding experiments such as those described can be used to calculate the number of LH molecules bound/cell, and thus give estimates of the maximum number of receptor sites involved. By using the specific activity of the labeled hormone preparation, the isotopic abundance of ^{125}I and thus its specific activity, it is possible to calculate the actual number of LH molecules bound with and without the presence of unlabeled, competitive hormone. Using an empirically determined estimate of 10^8 cells/100 mg wt for rat ovarian tissue, calculations can then be made on the in vivo data (Fig. 6) and expressed as LH molecules bound/ovarian cell (Table III).

At 2 hr after tail vein injection the decrease in uptake of ^{125}I-LH due to competitor was 24.1% of the total (1.937×10^3 cpm/100 mg wet wt) counts or equivalent to 3.77 molecules of LH/cell. At 6 hr the decrease in label due to competitor was 23.3% of the total (1.013×10^3 cpm/100 mg wet wt) counts or equivalent to 1.89 molecules of LH/cell.

Data from an in vitro binding experiment using the free rabbit ovarian cell suspension described above were utilized for similar calculations. The suspensions, as opposed to tissue chunks, allowed further reduction of the variability due to extracellular tissue space, diffusion rates in large tissue pieces, and nonspecific uptake of proteins due to the broken and dead cells present in tissue chunks (85). This suspension system yielded cells with a 92.4% viability as determined by nigrosin dye exclusion and showed very little cell debris under

TABLE III. Calculations for LH binding

	In vivo - 2 hr	In vitro - 2 hr
Ovarian cells	10^8 cells/100 mg tissue	1.73×10^7 free cells/ml
SA ^{125}I-LH	62.5 μCi/μg	43.0 μc/g
Dose	0.073 μg LH/rat	3.82×10^6 dpm[a]
Ratio ^{125}I-LH : LH	1 : 100	1 : 250
Total counts bound	10.5×10^3 dpm/100 mg tissue	3.47×10^4 dpm
Total LH/cell	15.6 molecules	360 molecules
Competition decrease	2,536 dpm/100 mg tissue	544 dpm
Sp. bound LH/cell	3.77 molecules	5.63 molecules

[a]Dpm corrected for decay and counting efficiency.

440 to 1000 magnification with a phase contrast microscope. With a free cell population of 1.73×10^7 cells/ml/tube and 0.04 μg of ^{125}I-LH, SA of 43 μCi/μg, the incubation medium contained 6.82×10^{11} molecules of LH/tube or 3.95×10^4 potential molecules of LH/cell, if all the hormone was bound.

After 2 hr incubation with labeled LH and thorough washing, about 1% of the hormone in the media was bound to the whole cell pellet. This represented approximately 3.6×10^2 molecules of LH/ovarian cell. When unlabeled LH was added simultaneously with the labeled hormone in a ratio of 1 : 250, a small decrease was observed representing approximately 5.63 molecules of LH/ovarian cell (Table III).

The small number of specific receptor sites/ovarian cell in vitro is in good agreement with our estimates from the in vivo experiments described above. Both in vivo and in vitro calculations suggest that further experiments should be made at 10 to 100-fold lower dose levels. In general, the total ^{125}I-LH bound in the in vitro system was 10 to 20-fold greater per cell than in vivo, and showed a smaller percentage decrease due to cold competitor. This indicates greater nonspecific binding in vitro but indicates comparable values for the specific receptors in vivo and in vitro.

The above calculations were made on the basis of total cell population, while it is probable that only some fractional number of the total ovarian cells are actually responding to LH. If only 10% of the total cell population in either the in vivo or the in vitro was actually involved in the specific hormone uptake, as autoradiographic studies suggest, that is still somewhat less than 100 specific hormone receptors/active ovarian cell.

A comparison of the LH binding results with steroid hormone binding using estradiol which has been estimated to have 16,000 to 20,000 specific receptors/rat uterine cell and a binding constant of 7×10^{-10}M (86-88) or aldosterone (64) which has been estimated to have about 1000 to 2000 specific receptors/rat kidney cell shows a 100 to 1000-fold lower receptor concentration/cell for LH than for the steroid hormones (Table IV). If protein hormones do function with tens of receptor sites/cell instead of thousands/cell, they may well require a different type of control sequence than the steroid hormones.

TABLE IV. Comparison of LH and estrogen hormone

	Estradiol in uterus	Ref.	LH in ovary	Ref.
In vivo competition	↓ 71%	(90)	↓ 25%	
Labeled : unlabeled	1:100	(90)	1:100	(59)
Binding constant	7×10^{-10} M	(87)	10^{-11} M	(2)
Receptor sites/cell	20,000	(88)	10-100	(59)

Since there is no reason, a priori, for protein receptors to follow the same pattern as steroid hormone receptors, it is important to consider alternative explanations for the data obtained in these experiments. If the LH molecules were altered during the hormone-receptor interaction, all or portions of the hormone could be released in an inactive or modified form. Alternatively, any brief interaction of the hormone and receptor resulting in a conformational change of the receptor only and the release of an intact hormone would be undetected in this system. The strong binding constant theoretically needed to concentrate hormone from serum concentration of 10^{-11}M also suggest a very slow hormone release after receptor-hormone contact. However, the metabolic fate of the labeled hormone after interaction with its target cell deserves much more study. Even if most of the hormone in the target tissue is found to be degraded, there may be an important difference in the metabolic fate of the bound hormone versus the unbound hormone.

SUMMARY

Experiments to investigate the distribution of ^{125}I-LH after a single exposure in vivo or in vitro indicated that the hormone was definitely taken up by its target tissue and retained at greater concentrations than in other tissues. This is in agreement with recent studies in two different laboratories on the uptake of ^{131}I-HCG (45, 46, 63). Experiments using labeled albumin indicated that simple vascular characteristics of various tissues could not account for the retention differences as shown by tissue to blood ratios. However, uptake of label in itself is not evidence for a physiological interaction of the labeled hormone with a target tissue.

Displacement studies using large amounts of unlabeled hormone showed a small, discrete number of specific LH receptor sites. Calculations on the number of receptor sites per ovarian cell in both in vivo and in vitro studies indicate less than 10 sites/ovarian cell (Table III). After fractionation of subcellular particles by differential centrifugation, the label was primarily in the cytoplasmic fraction, cytosol, and in the 800 × g pellet, crude nuclear-membraneous pellet.

A comparison of current research on steroid hormone receptor sites suggests that the two classes of hormones are not only structurally different but probably function through different mechanisms due primarily to the dissimilarity of their cellular receptor concentrations (Table IV).

ACKNOWLEDGMENT

Supported by grants from the Population Council (M68.714) and the National Institutes of Health (AM 06327).

REFERENCES

1. Jensen, E. V., Science 159:1261, 1968.
2. Squire, P. G., and C. H. Li, J Biol Chem 234:520, 1959.
3. Ward, D. N., Fajino, M., and W. M. Lamkin, Fed Proc 25:348, 1966.
4. Morgan, F. J., and R. E. Canfield, Endocrinology, 88:1045, 1971.
5. Liao, T-H., and P. G. Pierce, J Biol Chem 245:3275, 1970.
6. Papkoff, H., and M. Ekblad, Biochem Biophys Res Commun 40:614, 1970.
7. Reichert, L. E., M. Rasco, D. Ward, G. Niswender, and A. R. Midgley, J Biol Chem 244:5110, 1969.
8. Papkoff, H., and T. Samy, Biochim Biophys Acta 147:175, 1967.
9. Liao, T-H., G. Hennen, S. M. Haward, B. Shone, and P. Pierce, J Biol Chem 244:6458, 1969.
10. Pierce, P. G., O. Bahl, J. S. Cornell, and N. Swaminathan, J Biol Chem 246:2321, 1971.
11. Llosa, P., and M. Jutisz, Biochim Biophys Acta 181:426, 1969.
12. Samy, T. S., H. Papkoff, and C. H. Li, Arch Biochem Biophys 130:674, 1969.
13. Bahl, O. P., J Biol Chem 244:567, 1969.
14. Howard, S. M., and J. G. Pierce, J Biol Chem 244:6468, 1968.
15. Gay, V. L., A. R. Midgley, and G. D. Niswender, Fed Proc 29:1880, 1970.
16. Kohler, P. O., J. M. Phang, W. W. Tullener, G. T. Ross, and W. D. Odell, J Clin Endocrinol 28:613, 1968.
17. Kohler, P. O., G. T. Ross, and W. D. Odell, J Clin Invest 47:38, 1968.
18. Yen, S., O. Llerena, A. Little, and O. Pearson, J Clin Endocrinol Metab 28:1763, 1968.
19. Ellis, S., Endocrinology 68:334, 1961.
20. Wurtman, R. J., Endocrinology 75:927, 1964.
21. Marsh, J. M., and K. Savard, J Reprod Fert, Suppl 1:113, 1966.
22. Hall, P., and E. G. Young, Endocrinology 82:449, 1968.

23. Armstrong, D. T., Rec Prog Hormone Res 24:255, 1968.
24. Villee, D. B., Science 158:652, 1967.
25. Reel, J. R., and J. Gorski, Endocrinology 83:1083, 1968.
26. Cooper, J. M., and P. Thomas, Biochem J 117:24P, 1970.
27. Armstrong, D. T., R. Kilpatrick, and R. O. Greep, Endocrinology 73:165, 1963.
28. Gorski, J., and D. Padnos, Arch Biochem Biophys 113:100, 1966.
29. Kobayaski, Y., J. Kupelian, and D. Maudsley, Science 172:379, 1971.
30. Lefkowitz, R. J., J. Roth, W. Pricer, and I. Pastan, Proc Natl Acad Sci 65:745, 1970.
31. Pastan, I., J. Blanchette-Mackie, and W. Pricer, in press, 1971.
32. Murad, F., B. Strauch, and M. Vaughan, Biochim Biophys Acta 177:591, 1969.
33. Birnbaumer, L., and M. Rodbell, J Biol Chem 244:3477, 1969.
34. Kuehl, F., J. L. Humer, J. Farnoff, V. Cirillo, and E. H. Ham, Science 169:883, 1970.
35. Anderson, G. G., and L. Speroff, Science 171:502, 1971.
36. Szego, C. M., Fed Proc 24:1343, 1965.
37. Ryser, J. J-P., in Proceedings 4th International Congress Pharmacology Vol. III, Schwabe und Co., Basel-Stuttgart, 1970, p. 96.
38. Ryser, J. J-P., in Oak Ridge Symposium on Membranes and the Coordination of Cellular Activity, Biomembranes, in press, 1971.
39. Paiva, M. P., Arch Biol Med Expler 6:89, 1969.
40. Fellows, R. E., J. Kostyo, and H. Goodman, Excerpta Med Abst ICE Series #157, 1968.
41. Gorski, J., D. Padnos, and N. Nelson, Life Science 4:713, 1965.
42. Liu, T-C, and J. Gorski, Endocrinology 88:419, 1971.
43. Daane, T. Z., and A. F. Parlow, Endocrinology 88:653, 1971.
44. Sonenberg, M., and W. L. Money, Rec Prog Hormone Res 11:43, 1955.
45. Lunenfeld, B., and A. Eshkol, Vitamins and Hormones, 25:137, 1967.
46. Eshkol, A., and B. Lunenfeld, Adv Exper Med Biol 2:223, 1968.
47. Kazeto, S., and M. M. Hreshchyshyn, Amer J Obst Gyn 106:1229, 1970.
48. Espeland, D., F. Naftolin, and C. Paulsen, in E. Rosemberg (Ed.), op cit., 1968, p. 177.
49. Izzo, J., J. W. Bartlett, A. Ronconi, M. Izzo and W. F. Bole, J Biol Chem 242:2343, 1967.
50. Espeland, D. H., and C. A. Paulsen, manuscript in preparation, 1971.
51. Espeland, D. H., and C. A. Paulsen, Clin Res Conf, p. 121 (abst), 1970.
52. Beals, T. F., and A. R. Midgley, Soc Study Reprod 2:3 (abst), 1969.
53. Greenwood, F. C., W. M. Hunter, and J. S. Glover, Biochem J 89:114, 1963.
54. Greenwood, F. C., and W. M. Hunter, Biochem J 91:42, 1963.
55. Niswender, G., A. R. Midgley, S. Monroe, and L. E. Reichert, Proc Soc Exper Biol Med 128:807, 1968.
56. Rosemberg, E., in E. Rosemberg (Ed.), Gonadotropins 1968, Geron-X Inc., Los Altos, 1968, p. 387.
57. Wilde, E. E., A. H. Orr, and K. D. Bagshawe, J Endocrinol 35:iii, 1966.
58. Midgley, A. R., Endocrinology 79:10, 1966.
59. Coulson, P., and J. Gorski, in press, 1971.
60. Midgley, A. R., in E. Rosemberg (Ed.), op cit., 1968, p. 78.
61. Lefkowitz, R. J., J. Roth, and I. Pastan, Science 170:633, 1970.
62. Garratt, C. J., R. J. Jarrett and H. Keen, Biochim Biophys Acta 121:143, 1966.

63. Brush, J. S. and A. E. Kitabchi, Biochem Biophys Acta 215:134, 1970.

64. Swaneck, G., L. Chu, and I. W. Edelman, J Biol Chem 245:5382, 1970.

65. Munck, A., Rec Adv Endocrinol 8:139, 1968.

66. de Kretser, D. M., K. J. Catt, and C. A. Paulsen, Endocrinology 88:332, 1971.

67. de Kretser, D. M., K. J. Catt, H. Burger, and G. Smith, J Endocrinol 43:105, 1969.

68. Castro, A. E., A. C- Seiguer, and R. E. Mancini, Proc Soc Exper Biol Med 133:582, 1970.

69. Llerena, L. A., A. Guevara, J. Lobotsky, C. Lloyd, and J. Weiss, J Clin Endocrinol 29:1083, 1969.

70. Cons, J., and C. L. Kragt, The Endocrine Society, Abstract 3, 1970.

71. Himms-Hagen, J., Fed Proc 29:1388, 1970.

72. Scriba, P. C., O. Mueller, in M. Margoulies (Ed.), Protein and Polypeptide Hormones, Proc Internat Symp ICS 161, Excerpta Medica, Amsterdam, 1969, p. 939.

73. Rodbell, M., L. Birnbaumer and S. L. Pohl, J Biol Chem 245:718, 1970.

74. Koritz, S. B., and A. M. Kumar, J Biol Chem 245:152, 1970.

75. Schimmer, B. P., K. Ueda, and G. H. Sato, Biochem Biophys Res Commun 32:806, 1968.

76. Cuatrecasas, P., Proc Natl Acad Sci 63:450, 1969.

77. Rodbell, M., L. Birnbaumer, and S. Pohl, J Biol Chem 244:3478; 245:718, 1970.

78. Pandian, M. R., S. L. Gupta, and G. P. Talwar, Endocrinology 88:928, 1971.

79. Brovetto-Cruz, J., C. H. Li, and T. A. Bewley, Biochemistry 8:4695, 1969.

80. Kono, T., Fed Proc 27:495, 1968.

81. Hamashige, S., and M. Astor, Fert Sterility 20:1029, 1969.

82. Rudman, D. L., L. Garcia, and A. Del Rio, Biochemistry 7:1875, 1969.

83. Nutting, D., J. Kostyo, H. Goodman, Endocrinology 86:179, 1970.

84. Tong, W., E. Knopp, and V. Stolc, The Endocrine Society/Program, Abstract 18, 1970.

85. Ryser, H. J P., Science 159:390, 1968.

86. Gorski, J., D. Toft, G. Shyamala, D. Smith, and A. Notides, Rec. Prog Hormone Res 24:45, 1968.

87. Gorski, J., and A. Notides, in R. Baserga (Ed.), Biochemistry of Cell Division, Charles C. Thomas, Springfield, Ill., 1969, p. 57.

88. Gorski, J., G. Shyamala, and D. Toft, in J. F. Danielli, J. F. Moran, and D. J. Friggle (Eds.), Fundamental Concepts in Drug-Receptor Interactions, Academic, New York, 1970, p. 215.

89. Summers, D. F., J. Maizel, and J. E. Darnell, Proc Natl Acad Sci 54:505, 1965.

90. Noteboom, W. D., and J. Gorski, Arch Biochem Biophys 111:559, 1965.

20. Gonadotropin Binding to Frozen Sections of Ovarian Tissue

A. Reese Midgley, Jr.[1]

A number of studies have now been reported which indicate that radioiodinated gonadotropic hormones may be taken up and bound by components of gonadal tissues (1-7). Autoradiographic analysis of bound radiolabeled gonadotropins have suggested that preferential binding occurs to restricted cell types within the gonad (1, 3, 5, 7).

Unfortunately it is difficult with autoradiographic studies to determine if the reduced grains of silver represent the localization of intact hormone or metabolites of the hormones and whether the localization represents that of bound or free hormone. Interpretation of some of the reported autoradiographic studies is further complicated by the use of radiolabeled hormone of rather low purity. As a consequence, it is difficult to be certain that the localized radioactivity is due to the hormone and not to labeled impurities.

Previous studies in our laboratory indicated that large amounts of unlabeled or labeled HCG injected intravenously, can be taken up by and bound to luteinized cells in ovaries of immature, hormonally induced pseudopregnant rats (4). Other studies have indicated that radioiodinated HCG (8) and prolactin (9) can bind in vitro to sedimentable components of luteinized rat and sheep ovarian tissues. These observations raised the possibility that the binding components might persist in unfixed frozen tissue sections of ovary. If this were true, it should be possible to apply hormone directly to the tissue section and then localize the bound hormone. The problem of translocation of hormone during

[1]Career Development Awardee of National Institute of Child Health and Human Development.

tissue preparation procedures would be minimized by such a method as would the possibility of metabolic transformation of the added hormone. The following study was designed to determine if radioiodinated gonadotropins would bind to unfixed frozen sections of ovarian tissue and to determine if the binding sites would be localized to specific ovarian structures.

MATERIALS AND METHODS

The majority of these studies utilized ovaries from immature female rats which had been injected with 50 IU of pregnant mare serum gonadotropin (PMS) on day 25, 30 IU of HCG on day 27, and twice daily injections of 10 μg of estradiol benzoate (E2) in oil beginning on day 29 (10). Rats treated in this fashion (PMS-HCG-E2) are suitable for the ovarian ascorbic acid depletion (OAAD) bioassay for LH or HCG at anytime over a 1-month period, and possess ovaries with multiple corpora lutea. Some studies were done with adult female rats at different times during the estrous cycle (day estimated from vaginal smear data, and presence or absence of tubal ova and uterine ballooning), or rats at the eighth day of pregnancy. All rats were killed by decapitation. The ovaries were promptly dissected, placed in an aluminum foil boat containing 1% egg white in 0.01M phosphate buffered (pH 7.0) 0.14M sodium chloride (PBS), and frozen by partial immersion of the boat and contained tissue in a mixture of dry ice and ethanol. The resulting block was stored at -70 C until time for study.

Hormones used in this study included: HCG (11), ovine prolactin (LER-866-2, 26 NIH-FSH-S1 U/mg), ovine LH (LER-777-3, 1.43 NIH-LH-S1 U/mg), human FSH (LER-1114, highly purified, immunochemical grade FSH which after iodination, gave a single band on polyacrylamide gel electrophoretic analysis), human growth hormone (HGH, HS 1395, highly purified immunochemical grade GH), and human chorionic somatomammotropin (HPL, purified placental protein, Lederle lot No. 717340). These hormones, and crystalline bovine serum albumin (BSA) were iodinated with ^{131}I or ^{125}I using procedures described previously (11-14).

Resulting specific activities ranged from 150 to 250 μCi/μg. The labeled hormones were diluted in 1% egg white in PBS, such that for most experiments, a 50-μl aliquot contained approximately 0.2 ng of hormone. The labeled hormones were stored at 4 C.

Serial sections of the frozen ovarian tissue were cut at either 6 or 10 μ, applied to glass slides or narrow cover slips, and placed in a moist chamber at room temperature until a sufficient number of sections could be accumulated for study. A small wax ring was drawn around each tissue and 30μl of an appropriate labeled hormone were placed on top of each section. The tissue sections, covered by these small droplets of labeled hormone, were placed in a warm (37 C) moist atmosphere for 60 min or as described otherwise below. The sections were washed for 5 min in each of three changes of PBS at 4 C. They were then dipped in water and allowed to dry. The washed and air-dried sections were coated with Kodak NTB-3 liquid dipping emulsion in a dark room, allowed to dry, and exposed for 1 to 2 months. Washed, air-dried cover slips were placed in tubes and counted by γ-ray spectroscopy to determine the radioactivity associated with bound hormone. Results were expressed as a percent of the total hormone added to each section.

TABLE I. Binding of 0.15 ng ^{131}I-proteins by 10-μ frozen sections (37 C, 30 min, 50 μl)

| ^{131}I-protein | Total ^{131}I-protein bound (%) | | | |
	Glass	Skeletal muscle	Lymph node	Ovary[a]
HCG	0.2	0.2	0.3	5.9
HPL	1.4	5.4	10.4	6.1
O-Prol.	1.8	6.4	8.9	10.3
HGH	1.7	1.4	4.8	16.6
OLH	0.4		0.5	0.9
BSA	0.4		0.4	0.4

[a]Immature rat, primed with PMS-HCG and maintained with estradiol benzoate.

TABLE II. Binding of 0.15 ng ^{131}I-hormones by 10-μ frozen tissue sections (37 C, 30 min, 50 μl)

| Tissue | ^{131}I-hormone | Unlabeled HCG (μg) | Total ^{131}I-hormone bound (%) | |
			pH 7.0	pH 3.6
None	^{131}I-HCG		0.3	
None	^{131}I-HCG	25	0.3	
Lymph node	^{131}I-HCG		0.5	
Lymph node	^{131}I-HCG	25	0.4	
Ovary[a]	^{131}I-HCG		17.5	1.1
Ovary[a]	^{131}I-HCG	25	0.3	
Ovary[a]	^{131}I-O-Prol		26.6	27.1
Ovary[a]	^{131}I-HFSH		0.9	1.6

[a]Immature rat, primed with PMS-HCG and maintained with estradiol benzoate.

RESULTS

As shown in Table I, the binding of HCG was relatively specific for ovarian tissue since no significant binding occurred to sections of skeletal muscle or lymph node. Labeled human chorionic somatomammotropin (HPL) and ovine prolactin bound well to all three tissues, whereas human growth hormone showed

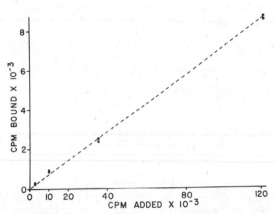

FIG. 1. The effect of concentration of ^{131}I-HCG on binding to 10 μ serial frozen sections of an ovary from a rat treated with PMS-HCG-E2.

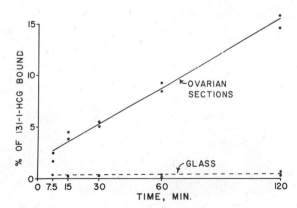

FIG. 2. Effect of incubation time at 37 C on binding of 0.15 ng of ^{131}I-HCG to serial frozen sections of an ovary from a rat treated with PMS-HCG-E2, compared with the binding observed to a comparable region of bare glass under similar conditions.

preferential binding to ovarian tissue sections and lesser binding to lymph node. Ovine LH and bovine serum albumin did not bind to the tissues studied. As indicated in Fig. 1 and 2, over the range of conditions studied, the binding of labeled HCG was a direct function of concentration and time. Over the course of a 1-hr reaction time, the binding was greatest at 37 C and lowest at 4 C for both HCG and ovine prolactin. Unlabeled HCG, added in excess, was capable of inhibiting the binding of labeled HCG (Table II). The latter bound well at pH 7.0 and poorly at pH 3.6 while ovine prolactin bound equally well at pH 3.6 and pH 7.0.

Autoradiographic analysis of tissue sections incubated with either HCG, ovine FSH, or ovine prolactin, each labeled with ^{125} I, revealed the presence of highly specific binding to different tissue components. As shown in Fig. 3a, labeled HCG and ovine prolactin bound to all corpora lutea in sections of ovaries from immature rats primed with PMS-HCG-E2. Labeled HCG also bound slightly to some interstitial connective tissue structures (Fig. 3b). It was not possible to demonstrate binding of FSH in these sections.

On the eighth day of pregnancy, as in the PMS-HCG-E2 pseudopregnant rat, prolactin bound exclusively and well to all demonstrable corpora lutea (Fig. 4a).

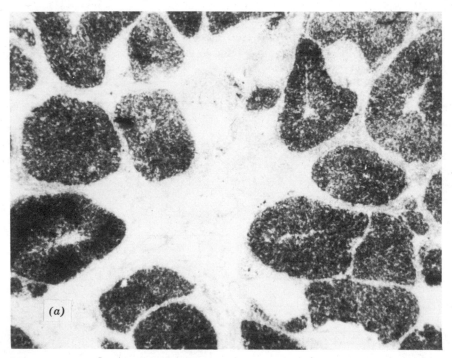

FIG. 3. Autoradiogram of two unstained serial sections from an ovary of an immature rat treated with PMS-HCG-E2. (a) Localization of applied ^{125}I-ovine prolactin.

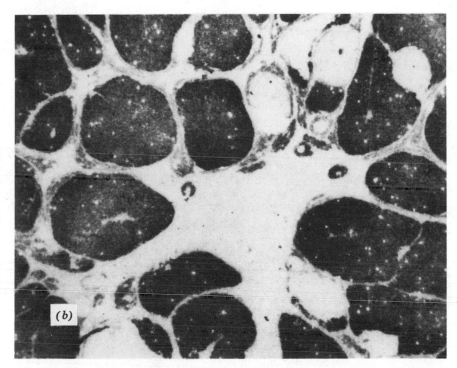

FIG. 3 (<u>continued</u>). Autoradiogram of two unstained serial sections from an ovary of an immature rat treated with PMS-HCG-E2. (b) Localization of applied ^{125}I HCG. Note that all corpora lutea have bound each of these two hormones, but additional interstitial components have bound labeled HCG as well.

HCG also bound to all corpora lutea and to interstitial structures. In addition, HCG bound to peripheral granulosa cells of occasional large follicles (Fig. 4b).

In contrast to the consistent binding of HCG to corpora lutea of pregnancy and hormonally induced pseudopregnancy, HCG binding to corpora lutea from rats at various stages of the estrous cycle showed great variation (Figs. 5b and 6b). Some of the corpora lutea exhibited a strong affinity for labeled HCG, while others either failed to bind this hormone or showed weak affinity. The pattern of HCG binding in the latter situation suggested that HCG is binding to individual, isolated cells in the corpora lutea (Fig. 5b). Prolactin did not exhibit this variability in binding. As in pregnancy and hormonally induced pseudo-pregnancy prolactin bound consistently and well to all corpora lutea (Figs. 5a and 6a). The interstitial structures, observed to bind HCG but not prolactin on the eighth day of pregnancy, bound both hormones consistently and well at all stages of the estrous cycle which have been studied.

Granulosa cells within most, but not all, moderately large to large follicles bound FSH well (Figs. 5c and 7b), and, to a small extent, prolactin (Fig. 5a).

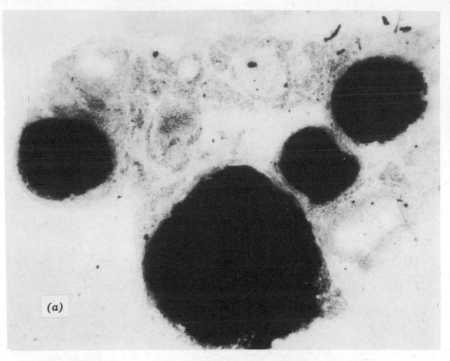

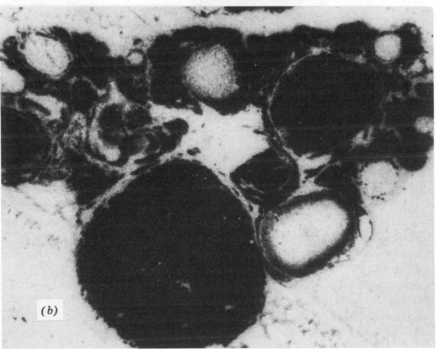

FIG. 4. Autoradiograms of two adjacent serial sections from an ovary of a rat on the eighth day of pregnancy. (a) ^{125}I-ovine prolactin, applied to this section, appears to be localized almost exclusively to 4 corpora lutea. (b) ^{125}I-HCG, applied to this section, appears to have been bound by the same corpora lutea as well as a large number of interstitial structures and the outer granulosa cells of one follicle (lower right). Although not shown in this figure, the inner granulosa cells of this same follicle in the next adjacent serial section bound labeled ovine FSH.

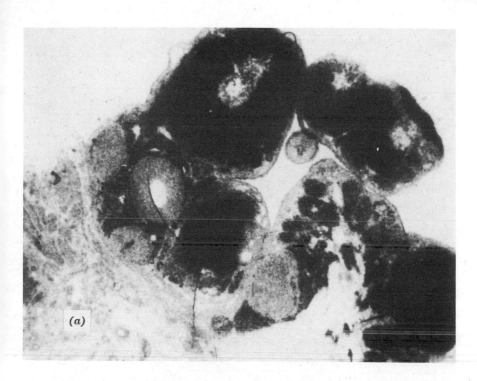

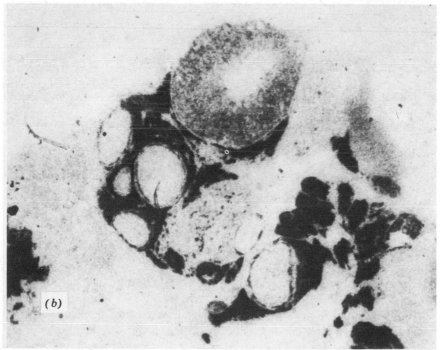

FIG. 5. Three adjacent, unstained serial sections of an ovary from a rat on the first day of diestrus. (a) Illustrates the localization of labeled ovine prolactin. (b) Localization of labeled HCG.

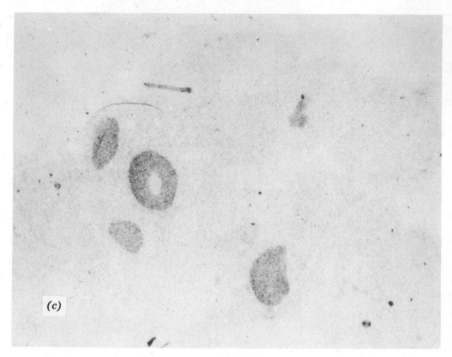

FIG. 5 (continued). Three adjacent, unstained serial sections of an ovary from a rat on the first day of diestrus. (c) Localization of labeled FSH. Note the presence of bound prolactin in all corpora lutea and interstitial structures plus a lesser degree of binding to the granulosa cells of the follicle. HCG was bound most strongly to the interstitial structures, and the thecal cells surrounding the follicle, and, to a variable extent, to the corpora lutea. FSH was bound exclusively to the granulosa cell.

HCG bound to thecal cells surrounding follicles (Figs. 5b, 6b, and 7b), and, in addition, HCG bound to the outer granulosa cells of an occasional follicle (Fig. 7a). It is not apparent why such differences in hormone-binding activity exist for granulosa cells in morphologically similar follicles.

DISCUSSION

These preliminary observations on the binding of labeled gonadotropic hormones to rat tissue sections confirm earlier results (8, 9) which indicated: (1) that radioiodinated gonadotropins bind to sedimentable components in tissue homogenates; (2) that binding can be affected by pH, incubation time, temperature and hormone concentration; and (3) that there is hormone-organ and hormone-tissue specificity. Although binding to soluble components will not be revealed with the use of washed tissue sections nor will binding of low

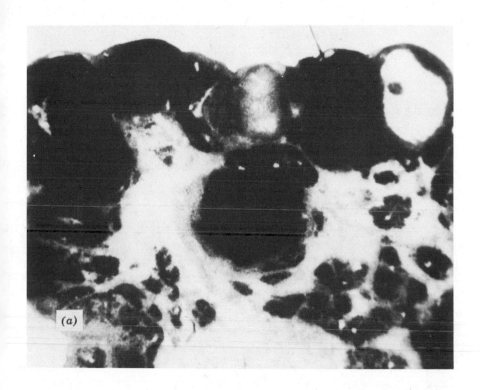

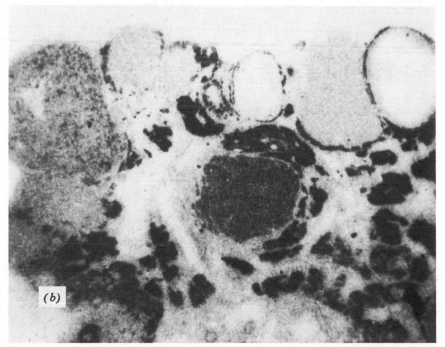

FIG. 6. Two adjacent, unfixed serial sections from an ovary of a rat on the second day of diestrus. (a) Represents a section incubated with labeled prolactin while (b) represents a section incubated with labeled HCG. The results are similar to those shown in Fig. 5, except the HCG shows more pronounced variability in binding to the corpora lutea.

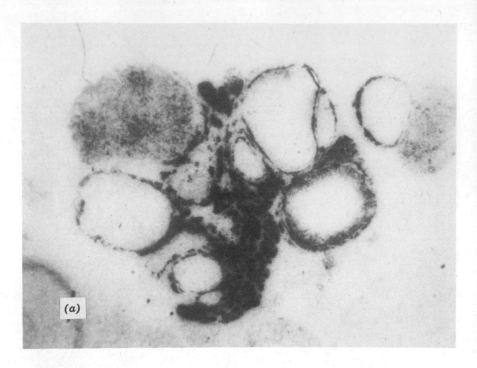

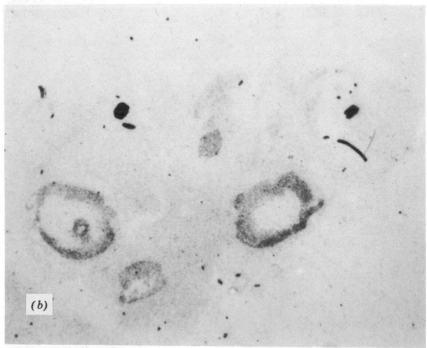

FIG. 7. Two adjacent unstained sections from an ovary of a rat on the day of proestrus. (a) Illustrates a section incubated with HCG while (b) illustrates a section treated with labeled FSH. Note that two large follicles (upper right) did not bind FSH but their surrounding thecal cells did bind HCG. Note the presence of FSH binding to the cumulus oophorus cells in the follicle at left. The outer granulosa cells of the follicle at the lower right bound HCG while granulosa cells in the other follicles did not.

affinity, the similarities of results obtained suggested that many of the sedimentable hormone-binding components persist in washed, nonfixed frozen tissue sections. Failure to observe significant binding of LH to frozen sections may be related to low affinity, perhaps as a result of iodination-induced hormone alteration.

Although it is impossible to draw many conclusions from the preliminary autoradiographic studies completed to date, three labeled hormones (HCG, prolactin, and FSH) showed individual intraovarian localization patterns which varied during different functional states in the rat. These results suggest that the extent of binding, or characteristics of specific binding components, change with the functional state of ovarian tissues and cells. If this is true, it is possible that protein hormone-binding components may be able to regulate the responsiveness of a tissue to hormonal stimulation. Specific developmental processes may well depend on the maturation or activation of hormone-binding components.

Further discussion of the implications deriving from knowledge of structure-specific, intraovarian hormone binding would seem to be premature prior to demonstrating the functional importance of such binding. Use of this technique in conjunction with enzymatic and immunohistochemical studies should be of considerable help in the identification of target tissues and in working out certain aspects concerning the mechanism of hormone action. Such information may be of importance to our understanding of intraovarian mechanisms such as regulation of follicular development, ovulation, steroidogenesis and structural maintenance of corpora lutea.

In addition to studying the binding of hormones, tissue section binding analysis should find applicability to the study of other biologically active substances such as drugs and inhibitors. Although negative results may be of little significance, the procedure is simple and positive results can reveal the existence of unsuspected interactions.

ACKNOWLEDGMENT

The author wishes to acknowledge the technical assistance of Mrs. S. Pletcher, the criticisms and suggestions of Dr. J. S. Hunter and Dr. T. F. Beals, the gift from Dr. L. E. Reichert of the protein hormones bearing the prefix "LER" , and the gift of human growth hormone from Dr. A. E. Wilhelmi supported in part by USPHS Program Project in Reproductive Endocrinology, NIH HD-05318, and by a grant from the Population Council.

REFERENCES

1. Sonnenberg, M., W. L. Money, A. S. Keston, P. J. Fitzgerald, and J. T. Godwin, Endocrinology 49:709, 1951.
2. Eshkol, A., and B. Lunenfeld, in E. Rosemberg (Ed.), Gonadotropins 1968. Geron-X Inc., Los Altos, 1968, p. 184.

3. Espeland, D. H., F. Naftolin, and C. A. Paulsen, in E. Rosemberg (Ed.), Gonadotropins 1968, Geron-X Inc., Los Altos, 1968, p. 177.

4. Beals, T. F., and A. R. Midgley, Jr., Program of the 2nd Meeting of the Society for Study of Reproduction, 1969, p. 3.

5. DeKretser, D. M., K. J. Catt, H. G. Burger, and G. C. Smith, J Endocrinol 43:105, 1969.

6. Figarova, V., J. Presl, V. Wagner, and J. Horsky, Experientia 26:1017, 1970.

7. Rajaniem, H., P. Tuohimaa, and M. Niemi, Histochemie 23:342, 1970.

8. Danzo, B. J., A. R. Midgley, Jr., and L. J. Kleinsmith, Fed Proc 30:420, 1971.

9. Sheth, A. R., A. R. Midgley, Jr., and G. D. Niswender, Biol Reprod submitted for publication.

10. Bogdanove, E. M., and V. L. Gay, Endocrinology 81:1104, 1967.

11. Midgley, A. R., Jr., Endocrinology 79:10, 1966.

12. Midgley, A. R., Jr., J Clin Endocrinol 27:295, 1967.

13. Niswender, G. D., L. E. Reichert, Jr., A. R. Midgley, Jr., and A. V. Nalbandanov, Endocrinology 84:1166, 1969.

14. Davis, S. L., L. E. Reichert, Jr., and G. D. Niswender, Biol Repro, in press, 1971.

21. Subcellular Distribution of HCG in the Rat Corpus Luteum

CH. V. Rao, B. B. Saxena [1] and Hortense M. Gandy

Gonadotropins stimulate steroid, nucleic acid, and protein synthesis, and enzyme induction in ovarian cells (1-4). There is evidence that gonadotropins stimulate adenyl cyclase system in plasma membranes without inhibiting phosphodiesterase activity (5). Cyclic AMP has been shown to mimic the effect of LH on steroidogenesis (6). However, little is known about gonadotropin interaction with receptors. The present study provides evidence that HCG enters luteal cells to mediate its action and that plasma membranes of luteal cells contain a specific receptor for HCG.

MATERIALS AND METHODS

Highly purified HCG (13,000 to 15,000 IU/mg) was a gift from Dr. S. Kammerman. HCG antisera was purchased from Research Plus Laboratories, New York. Ten micrograms of HCG was labeled with ^{131}I or ^{125}I (7). Iodinated HCG was purified by gel filtration on a column of Sephadex G-100 using physiological saline containing 1% bovine serum albumin (BSA) as the eluant. The radiation damage and binding ability of the iodinated HCG was examined by chromatoelectrophoresis (8). The specific activity of HCG ranged from 50 to 100 $\mu Ci/\mu g$.

Twenty-five-day-old female rats (Holtzman Company, Madison, Wisconsin) were superovulated (9). Each rat received 0.6 μg of labeled HCG in 0.5 ml physiological saline containing 1% BSA by tail vein injection. The animals were sacrificed by cervical dislocation after 90 to 120 min; ovaries, liver, kidney,

[1]Career Scientist Awardee, Health Research Council, City of New York, Contract No. 1-621.

261

rectus muscle, and an aliquot of blood were obtained. Ovaries and kidneys were minced, suspended in 0.01M Tris-HCl buffer of pH 7.4 containing 0.32M sucrose and 1mM $MgCl_2$ and homogenized by 10 to 15 strokes in a glass-teflon Potter-Elvehjem homogenizer at 4 C. The homogenates were adjusted to a 1 : 10 dilution and filtered through four layers of cheese cloth; the filtrate was centrifuged at 2000 X g for 10 min. The supernate was centrifuged at 10,000 X g for 15 min to obtain mitochondrial fraction. The remaining supernate was centrifuged again at 109,000 X g for 60 min to obtain cytosol and microsomal fractions. The 2000 X g pellet was washed and divided into two equal portions for purification of plasma membranes and nuclei (10-12). Subcellular fractions were washed 6 times with 0.05M phosphate buffer of pH 7.4. Proteins in an aliquot of each subcellular fraction were precipitated by the addition of chilled 10% trichloroacetic acid. The tubes were centrifuged at 4800 X g for 20 min. The supernates were decanted and the precipitates counted in a Packard Autogamma Counter (Model 5219, Packard Instrument Company, Inc. Downers Grove, Illinois).

An aliquot of each subcellular fraction was diluted with 0.1N NaOH containing 1 mg/ml sodium dodecyl sulfate and heated in boiling water for 30 min; an aliquot was then taken for protein determination (13). Five milligrams of protein aliquots of mitochondrial and microsomal fractions were incubated with labeled HCG and BSA in 1 ml of 0.05M phosphate buffer of pH 7.4 for 60 min at 37 C in a Dubanoff shaker. The incubated mitochondrial and microsomal fractions were centrifuged at 10,000 X g for 15 min and at 109,000 X g for 30 min, respectively. The supernates as well as the pellets representing mitochondria and microsomes were counted.

Aliquots of plasma membrane fractions containing 100 μg protein were incubated with labeled HCG at different pH, temperatures, and length of time as indicated in Fig. 1. A plasma membrane fraction containing 100 μg protein was incubated with labeled and unlabeled HCG in 1 ml of Tris HCl buffer of pH 7 for 6 hr at 36 C. The incubates were centrifuged at 4800 X g for 20 min and supernates were decanted; the pellet was washed once with Tris HCl buffer and then counted. Blanks consisted of incubation of labeled HCG in Tris HCl buffer. The percent radioactivity remaining in the blank tube was subtracted from those of plasma membranes.

RESULTS AND DISCUSSION

Ovarian uptake of labeled HCG was maximum between 90 to 120 min. Administration of potassium thiocyanate to rats did not influence ovarian uptake of labeled HCG. The ovarian uptake of radioactive iodine or iodinated BSA was insignificant. The ovarian uptake of labeled HCG was sevenfold greater in superovulated rats than in normal rats; however, renal and hepatic uptake remained unchanged (Table I).

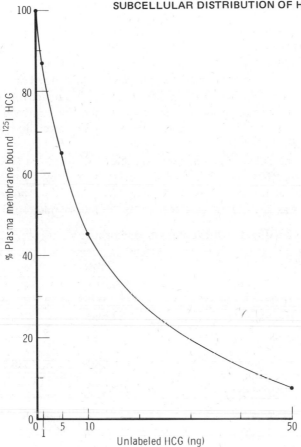

FIG. 1.

TABLE I. Ratio of radioactivity after ^{131}I-HCG injection

	Normal	Superovulated
Ovary/blood	4.62 ± 1.08[a]	34.0 ± 8.36
Ovary/muscle	58.6 ± 9.27	197.86 ± 74.54
Kidney/blood	2.42 ± 0.26	1.93 ± 0.2
Liver/blood	0.31 ± 0.03	0.21 ± 0.01

[a]Mean ± SE.

The ovarian homogenate contained 87,666 cpm/mg protein, whereas kidney homogenate contained 2660 cpm/mg protein. The presence of labeled HCG in all subcellular fractions suggested the entry of HCG into the luteal cells. These observations are consistent with those of others reported earlier (14-16), (Table II).

The relative distribution of labeled HCG in subcellular fractions of ovaries and kidney of superovulated rats is illustrated in Table III. The crude nuclear pellet contained the highest radioactivity. The pellet was furrther purified by discontinuous sucrose gradient centrifugation to yield purified nuclei and plasma membranes. Approximately 15 and 2% of the total radioactivity was found in plasma membranes and purified nuclei, respectively. The relative distribution of radioactivity was higher in ovarian microsomes and lower in cytosol than in similar fractions of kidney.

When the subcellular fractions were incubated with labeled HCG and BSA, a greater incorporation of the former was demonstrated by ovarian and kidney mitochondria and microsomes. It is of interest that the uptake by ovarian microsomes was significantly greater than that of kidney microsomes.

TABLE II. Distribution of Radioactivity

Fraction	Protein (cpm/mg)	
	Ovary	Kidney
Homogenate	87,660	2660
Crude nuclei	62,340	2490
Mitochondria	130,780	3380
Microsomes	126,030	1020
Cytosol	17,930	2030
Plasma membranes	54,520	2130

Greater than 92% of the radioactivity was present in trichloroacetic acid precipitate of ovarian subcellular fractions, whereas 48 to 77% radioactivity was precipitable in similar fractions of kidney (Table IV). Greater than 90% radioactivity was lost following four washings from kidney subcellular fractions. Similar treatment resulted in 18 to 30% loss of radioactivity from ovarian subcellular fractions (Table V). Simultaneous administration of labeled HCG and HCG antisera resulted in a decrease of radioactivity of both ovarian and kidney subcellular fractions.

As shown in Fig. 1, addition of increasing amounts of unlabeled HCG quantitatively displaced ^{125}I-HCG from the ovarian plasma membranes. The addition of 0.05 ml of HCG antisera in a dilution of 1 : 100 at the beginning of incubation also decreased the plasma membrane binding markedly. These data suggest that radioactivity found in ovarian and kidney subcellular fractions represented labeled HCG and the uptake by ovarian subcellular fractions was of significantly greater magnitude and specificity than those of kidney; and further suggest the presence of a specific receptor for HCG in ovarian plasma

TABLE III. Distribution of radioactivity and protein in subcellular fractions

Fraction	Ovary		Kidney	
	Radioactivity (%)	Protein (%)	Radioactivity (%)	Protein (%)
Homogenate	100.0	100.0	100.0	100.0
Crude nuclei	53.9 ± 4.6[a]	33.6 ± 3.1	51.7 ± 3.9	38.6 ± 3.7
Mitochondria	16.9 ± 1.5	7.6 ± 0.5	14.5 ± 2.4	8.0 ± 1.6
Microsomes	16.5 ± 0.4	11.3 ± 0.8	4.9 ± 0.7	10.9 ± 1.1
Cytosol	9.5 ± 0.9	39.9 ± 1.9	25.4 ± 1.3	34.4 ± 2.6
Plasma membranes	2.5 ± 2.2	2.9 ± 0.2	4.2 ± 1.8	4.2 ± 0.7

[a]Mean ± SE.

265

TABLE IV. Percent TCA-precipitable radioactive material
after ^{131}I-HCG injection

Fraction	Ovary	Kidney
Homogenate	97.6 ± 0.2[a]	63.2 ± 2.1
Crude nuclei	97.5 ± 0.3	73.1 ± 1.6
Mitochondria	95.3 ± 0.4	68.3 ± 4.8
Microsomes	97.7 ± 0.6	77.6 ± 2.1
Cytosol	92.0 ± 1.5	48.4 ± 1.8
Plasma membranes	93.7 ± 1.9	59.6 ± 5.0

[a]Mean ± SE.

TABLE V. Percent radioactivity in washed[a] fractions

Fraction	Ovary	Kidney
Crude nuclei	75.5 ± 3.1[b]	4.8 ± 0.8
Plasma membranes	75.3 ± 2.6	4.5 ± 1.0
Mitochondria	70.3 ± 1.7	11.0
Purified nuclei	81.5	4.7

[a]Washed four times.
[b]Mean ± SE.

membranes. Renal plasma membranes failed to bind ^{125}I-HCG. As shown in Fig. 2, optimal binding of ^{125}I-HCG by ovarian plasma membranes was obtained at 36 C after 6 hr incubation at pH 7 suggesting configurational requirement of the receptor for binding. It is of interest that plasma membrane fraction obtained from superovulated rat ovary could be frozen for at least 4 weeks without loss of binding to labeled HCG. The use of such receptors may provide a specific and sensitive radioligand assay for HCG similar to those suggested for ACTH and prolactin (17, 18).

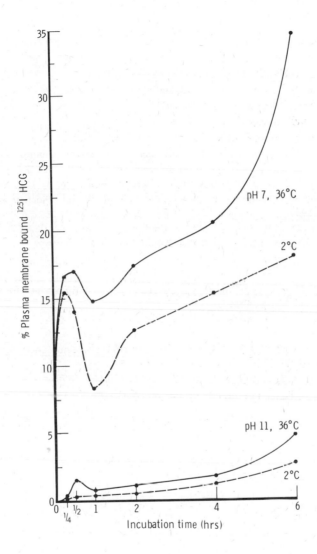

FIG. 2.

ACKNOWLEDGMENT

This work was supported by grants M71.26 from the Population Council, New York City and AM-11187, R01-HD 04173 from the National Institutes of Health, Bethesda, Maryland, and 70-2140 from the Ford Foundation. We thank Dr. Sandra Kammerman for a gift of purified HCG and Dr. K. S. Raghavan for assistance with some experiments.

REFERENCES

1. Mason, N. R., J. M. Marsh, and K. Savard, J Biol Chem 237:1801, 1962.
2. Reel, J. R., and J. Gorski, Endocrinology 83:1092, 1968.
3. Reel, J. R., and J. Gorski, Endocrinology 83:1083, 1968.
4. Kobayashi, Y., J. Kupelian, and D. V. Maudsley, Science 172:379, 1971.
5. Marsh, J. M., J Biol Chem 245:1596, 1970.
6. Marsh, J. M., and K. Savard, Steroids 8:133, 1966.
7. Hunter, W. M., and F. C. Greenwood Nature 194:495, 1962.
8. Saxena, B. B., H. Demura, H. M. Gandy, and R. E. Peterson, J Clin Endocrinol 28:519, 1968.
9. Major, P. W., D. T. Armstrong, and R. O. Greep, Endocrinology 81:19, 1967.
10. Emmelot, P. C., J. Bos, E. L. Benedetti, and P. H. Rumke, Biochem Biophys Acta 90:126, 1964.
11. Hofmann, K., W. Wingender, and F. M. Finn, Proc Natl Acad Sci USA 67:829, 1970.
12. Fang, S., K. M. Anderson, and S. Liao, J Biol Chem 244:6584, 1969.
13. Lowry, O. H., H. J. Rosebrough, A. L. Farr, and R. J. Randall, J Biol Chem 193:265, 1951.
14. Beals, T. F., and A. R. Midgley, Jr., Program of the 1969 Society for the Study of Reproduction, Davis, Calif.
15. Danzo, B. J., A. R. Midgley, Jr., and L. J. Kleinsmith, Fed Proc 30:2 Abstract No. 1248, 1971.
16. Lee, C. Y., and R. J. Ryan, Program of the 1971 Endocrine Society Meetings, San Francisco, Calif.
17. Lefkowitz, R. J., J. Roth, and I. Pastan, Science 170:633, 1970.
18. Turkington, R. W., J Clin Invest 50:94a 1971.

22. Dynamic Aspects of Ovarian Cholesterol Metabolism: Regulation by Gonadotropins

A. P. F. Flint and David T. Armstrong

The important, if not obligatory, role of cholesterol as an intermediate in the biosynthesis of ovarian steroid hormones has been well established. A great deal of research has been focused on the enzymes involved in the conversion of cholesterol to these hormones, and on the role of gonadotropins, particularly LH, in the regulation of this conversion. Less is known of the factors which determine the availability of cholesterol as a substrate to the enzymes involved in steroidogenesis. Some of these factors will be discussed in the present paper particularly the central question of the immediate source of the cholesterol utilized for hormone biosynthesis. At least three sources are possible: (a) cholesterol synthesized de novo within the steroidogenic cell; (b) that obtained from the circulation, and (c) that stored in the cell.

CHOLESTEROL SYNTHESIS IN OVARIAN CELLS

Control by Gonadotropins

The ability of various types of steroidogenic cells to synthesize cholesterol de novo is known (1-3); the biosynthetic pathway appears to be essentially the same as that in the liver (4-6). The possibility has been raised that the ability of LH to increase steroid production in the corpus luteum may result in part from an increased flow through this pathway (7). An important argument in support of this suggestion is that stimulation of steroidogenesis in tissue-slice preparations incubated with ^{14}C-acetate by LH is accompanied by increased incorporation of ^{14}C into steroids, frequently causing an increase in the specific radioactivity of the steroids produced (7, 8). However, it was subsequently demonstrated that under similar conditions, the specific activity and total ^{14}C content of cholesterol isolated from tissue slices is considerably decreased as a result of the action of LH (9-12), an observation difficult to reconcile with a stimulatory action upon cholesterol biosynthesis. Studies in which an inhibitor of cholesterol biosynthesis (AY 9944) was employed, have demonstrated fairly conclusively that de novo cholesterol synthesis is not essential for the stimulation of steroid production by LH in acute in vitro experiments with bovine corpus luteum or rabbit ovarian interstitial tissue slices (9, 13).

Compartmentation of Steroidogenic Cholesterol

The effect of LH in decreasing the apparent incorporation of ^{14}C from acetate into cholesterol and concomitantly increasing its incorporation into progesterone has been explained by the suggestion that cholesterol synthesized from labeled precursor is preferentially converted to progesterone without equilibrating with the total intracellular cholesterol and that LH enhances this conversion. The observation that the specific activity (SA) of progesterone is invariably higher than that of sterols synthesized from ^{14}C acetate (10, 11, 14) is consistent with this hypothesis. The following experiments have been conducted in our laboratory recently in attempts to place this hypothesis on a firmer experimental foundation.

Since the final steps in cholesterol biosynthesis were believed to occur in the smooth endoplasmic reticulum (15), this was considered to be the most likely intracellular localization of the steroidogenic pool of cholesterol. Accordingly, luteinized rat ovaries were incubated with 1-^{14}C-acetate in vitro under conditions previously shown to result in the production of steroids with a considerably higher specific activity than that of cholesterol. At the end of incubation, the slices were homogenized in buffered 0.25M sucrose and separated into microsomal, mitochondrial, and cytoplasmic fractions by differential centrifugation. Free and esterified cholesterol were extracted from each of these fractions and purified as 5,6-dibromocholestanol prior to determination of SA as described previously (16). As summarized in Table I, the SA of free cholesterol in the microsomal fraction is 3- to 4-fold higher than that in either of the other fractions and approaches that of the steroids synthesized during the incubation of the slices (6150 ± 707 dpm/μmole). These findings provide the first evidence of a morphological basis for the postulated compartmentation of intracellular cholesterol.

The question of whether LH causes a decrease in the rate of synthesis of cholesterol in addition to the proposed stimulation of conversion of recently synthesized cholesterol to steroids remains unanswered. An alternative explanation is that the decreased incorporation of ^{14}C from acetate into cholesterol is

TABLE I. Specific radioactivities of nonesterified and esterified cholesterol in subcellular fractions prepared from slices of luteinized rat ovary incubated with 1-^{14}C-acetate.

	Specific activity of cholesterol (dpm/μmole)	
Subcellular fraction	Nonesterified	Esterified
Cytosol	1220 ± 374	600 ± 91
Microsomal fraction	4020 ± 443	760 ± 74
Mitochondria	1510 ± 254	700 ± 134

Note: Slices were incubated for 3 hr in 10 ml bicarbonate-buffered medium containing glucose (1 mg/ml) and 1 mM- 1-^{14}C-acetate (2 μCi/ml). After incubation the slices were removed from the incubation medium and homogenized in triethanolamine-buffered 0.25M sucrose before differential centrifugation to prepare the fractions listed. Specific activities of cholesterol were subsequently determined after saponification, bromination, and debromination (16); values are expressed as dpm/μmole of cholesterol (mean ± SE of 6 determinations in each case).

the result of dilution of the ^{14}C-acetyl CoA pool with ^{12}C-acetyl CoA, arising in increased amounts from endogenous sources. This possibly results from an increase in the rate of β oxidation, utilizing cholesterol ester-fatty acid, liberated as a result of the LH-stimulated increase in cholesterol esterase activity (17, 18). It is unlikely to be caused by increased metabolism of 4-methylpentanoate, liberated on LH stimulation of the rate of cholesterol side-chain cleavage, since the oxidation of acetyl CoA derived from 4-methylpentanoate probably accounts for less than 3% of the total rate of oxidation of acetyl CoA in luteinized rat ovary slices incubated in vitro [calculated from the data of Flint and Denton, (17, 19)]. The increased rate of glucose metabolism observed in preparations of ovaries from LH-treated animals is unlikely to contribute significantly to the dilution of the label in the acetyl CoA pool, since LH has no effect on the proportion of the O$_2$ consumption, accounted for by the oxidation of glucose carbon and since negligible amounts of glucose carbon are incorporated into lipids derived from acetyl CoA, either in animals treated with LH or in controls (19). Whatever the mechanism of the decreased acetate incorporation, it apparently occurs in the absence of any increase in the rate of oxygen consumption (19, 20).28.

Intracellular Location of Cholesterol Side-Chain Cleavage Enzyme

The demonstration that cholesterol synthesized from acetate in the endoplasmic reticulum can be converted to steroids, without equilibration with less highly labeled cholesterol in other compartments, is somewhat difficult to reconcile with the generally accepted mitochondrial site of cholesterol side-chain cleavage enzyme. If this enzyme system is located on the inner mitochondrial membrane, as suggested by the recent investigation of a mouse Leydig cell tumor (21), it would be necessary to postulate a rather complicated mechanism in order to explain the transfer of cholesterol from the endoplasmic reticulum to this site, without at least some mixing with mitochondrial cholesterol. On the other hand, Bartosik and Romanoff (22) have suggested the existence of two compartmentalized cholesterol side-chain cleavage enzymes on the basis of rates of incorporation of ^{14}C-acetate and ^{3}H-cholesterol into steroids by perfused luteal bovine ovaries. To obtain evidence for an alternative hypothesis, we have investigated the possibility that there may be cholesterol side-chain cleavage activity associated with the endoplasmic reticulum.

Evidence for the existence of a microsomal cholesterol side-chain cleavage enzyme is presented in Table II. Mitochondria and microsomes were isolated from homogenates of luteinized rat ovary and bovine corpus luteum in buffered isotonic sucrose by differential centrifugation. Cholesterol side-chain cleavage enzyme and cytochrome P-450, a component of the cholesterol side-chain cleavage enzyme complex (23, 24), were found in both mitochondria and microsomes. Analysis of the cytochrome (a + a$_3$) and glutamate dehydrogenase contents of these fractions indicated that these microsomes were free of measurable mitochondrial contamination.

Although this demonstration of a second site of cholesterol side-chain cleavage enzyme is of considerable interest and appears to shed some light on the previously unexplained phenomenon of nonequilibration of cholesterol from various sources, its quantitative importance may not be great. The studies referred to above (9, 13, 14), in which it was demonstrated that progesterone production was relatively unchanged by an inhibitor of cholesterol biosynthesis, would appear to relegate cholesterol synthesized in situ to a minor role in the provision of carbon for steroidogenesis. However, the stimulatory effect of LH on steroid synthesis occurs concomitantly with a decrease in the specific activity of whole-tissue cholesterol formed from ^{14}C-acetete. This implies that the microsomal cholesterol side-chain cleavage enzyme may be activated by LH treatment and may explain the failure of previous investigators (25, 26) to observe a stimulatory effect of LH or cyclic-3′,5′-AMP on the mitochondrial enzyme. It will be of interest to determine whether this can be confirmed by direct experimentation.

STEROIDOGENESIS FROM PLASMA CHOLESTEROL

Uptake of Cholesterol from Plasma

Chronic investigations of adrenal steroidogenesis by Morris and Chaikoff (27) have demonstrated that dietary (i.e., plasma) cholesterol is the source of more

TABLE II. Enzyme and cytochrome activity in mitochondria and microsomes from corpora lutea of cow and rat

Enzyme or Cytochrome	Cow		Rat	
	Mitochondria	Microsomes	Mitochondria	Microsomes
Cholesterol side-chain cleavage enzyme	660 ± 58 (9)	1230 ± 110 (9)	8460 ± 890 (9)	2130 ± 650 (9)
Cytochrome P-450	350 ± 43 (11)	50 ± 5 (6)	290 ± 10 (6)	130 ± 13 (5)
Cytochrome $(a + a_3)$	950 ± 120 (9)	<30 (5)	350 ± 27 (6)	<50 (5)
Glutamate dehydrogenase	18 ± 0.6 (4)	<1.7 (4)	56 ± 6 (4)	<0.25 (4)

Mitochondria and microsomes were prepared from whole bovine corpora lutea or luteinized rat ovaries by homogenization in buffered 0.25M-sucrose and differential centrifugation. Cholesterol side-chain cleavage enzyme was assayed by the method of Raggatt and Whitehouse (55); 26-^{14}C-cholesterol (0.05μCi) was added in dimethylformamide (0.05ml) and tissue fractions were incubated for 2 hr in 50mM potassium phosphate containing 10mM $MgCl_2$ and 1mM NADPH, pH 7.3. Non-incubated control values have been subtracted. Rates were linear with respect to both time and enzyme concentration under the conditions used. Values are expressed as dpm incorporated in to 4-methyl-pentanoate/hr/mg of protein. Cytochromes P-450 and $(a+a_3)$ were assayed by the methods of Omura and Sato (56) and Cammer and Estabrook (57); activities are expressed as nmole/g protein. Glutamate dehydrogenase was determined as described by Flint and Denton (58); activities are expressed as U/g protein (measured at 25C). Values are means ± SE of the number of determinations in parenthesis. Data from Flint and Armstrong (59).

than 90% of the corticoids produced in the rat and 40% of the androgen carbon; and Werbin and Chaikoff (28) demonstrated that it accounted for 60% of the corticoids and 13% of the androgens in the guinea pig. Apparently, no similar studies have been reported for ovarian tissues. However, the investigations of Solod, Armstrong, and Greep (29), and of Major, Armstrong, and Greep (16) have revealed that rabbit ovarian interstitial tissue and rat lutein tissue take up cholesterol from plasma and convert it to steroids. We have examined the kinetics of uptake of plasma cholesterol by rat lutein tissue in detail and have measured the rate of its esterification and conversion to steroids (30). As shown in Fig. 1, the iv administration of 4-^{14}C-cholesterol to rats with luteinized ovaries results in labeling of the ovarian cholesterol. The SA of ovarian free cholesterol reaches a maximum at 1 to 2 hr following the administration of label; isotopic equilibration between free and esterified cholesterol occurs at about 8 hr. At all times measured, the specific activities of progesterone and 20α-hydroxypregn-4-en-3-one in the tissue were equal to that of the free cholesterol. Three conclusions can be drawn from this experiment: (1) plasma cholesterol is utilized for steroid synthesis; (2) the substrate for cholesterol

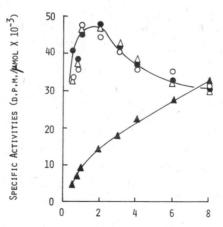

TIME AFTER ADMINISTRATION OF (^{14}C)CHOLESTEROL (HR)

FIG. 1. Effect of time after administration on the specific activities of nonesterified cholesterol (o), esterified cholesterol (▲), progesterone (△), and 20α-hydroxypregn-4-en-3-one (●), in the luteinized ovaries of rats given an iv injection of 4-^{14}C-cholesterol. Ovaries removed after the administration of 2μCi cholesterol and lipids extracted in chloroform-methanol (2:1, v/v) by homogenization. Specific activities of esterified and free cholesterol were determined in each ovary; those of the steroids were determined in pooled fractions from each pair of ovaries. Thus the values for cholesterol specific activities (both free and esterified) are means of six or more determinations; those of the steroids are means of three or more values.

side-chain cleavage enzyme is either unesterified cholesterol or a related compound, in isotopic equilibrium with unesterified cholesterol; and (3) operationally, the free cholesterol in the tissue constitutes a single pool. The fact that labeled cholesterol delivered to the tissue in the blood apparently equilibrates with endogenous cholesterol rapidly, whereas that generated in situ from ^{14}C-acetate does not (see Table I), further indicates that the pool of steroidogenic cholesterol associated with the endoplasmic reticulum and the rate of its conversion to steroid must be relatively small.

It is not known whether cholesterol from the plasma enters the ovarian cells by simple diffusion or whether some form of facilitated uptake is involved. It remains to be determined whether gonadotropins have any direct effect on cholesterol uptake. Pretreatment with LH has been found to increase uptake of ^{3}H-cholesterol from plasma by luteinized rat ovaries and to partially reverse the decrease in uptake observed on hypophysectomy (13); perfusion of luteal phase bovine ovaries with LH causes a decrease in the arteriovenous difference of ^{3}H-cholesterol added to the perfusate (22). However, these findings cannot be attributed to direct effects on cholesterol transport because of the possibility that they may be influenced by changes in the activity of cholesterol ester synthetase. The possibility cannot be excluded, however, that gonadotropins stimulate cholesterol transport directly. Such an action has recently been reported for ACTH on the adrenal cortex (31), based on the rate of uptake of ^{3}H-cholesterol administered iv; however, these data take no account of possible effects of ACTH on the rate of equilibration of plasma and tissue free cholesterol.

Loss of Cholesterol from Tissue to Plasma

A growing body of evidence is accumulating that suggests part of the ovarian free cholesterol may be lost, under some conditions, to the plasma. Thus measurement of ovarian cholesterol concentration and steroid synthesis before and after LH treatment of rabbit ovarian interstitial tissue indicates that only a fraction of the cholesterol ester that disappears is converted to steroids and lost from the tissue as such (29). This implies loss from the gland of unconverted cholesterol, on LH stimulation. On the other hand, Bartosik and Romanoff (22) have shown that LH decreases the rate of cholesterol discharge from the perfused luteal phase bovine ovary, as indicated by a decrease in the arteriovenous difference with respect to ^{3}H-cholesterol added to the perfusate. There is also evidence that a similar phenomenon may occur in vitro: Flint and Denton (17) found an unaccountable deesterification of cholesterol ester in slices of rat lutein tissue during 4-hr incubations and attributed it to loss, not of Lieberman-Burchard positive cholesterol ester, but of free cholesterol derived from cholesterol ester. Although the physiological importance of this loss is difficult to assess, it does indicate the possibility of a rapid rate of recirculation of cholesterol between tissue and blood.

STORAGE OF CHOLESTEROL

Evidence for Storage of Cholesterol Ester in Lipid Droplets

Cholesterol, free and esterified, accounts for up to one-fifth of the dry weight of some ovarian tissues. In most species, the majority of this sterol is in the form of the long-chain acyl 3β-esters of cholesterol (16, 32, 33), which are presumably located intracellularly in lipid droplets or lipid granules, and which undergo hydrolysis on gonadotropic stimulation (33, 34). The evidence for the storage of cholesterol esters in lipid droplets in ovarian tissues is as follows: (1) histochemical evidence indicates that almost all the cholesterol in rabbit ovary is envacuolated (35); (2) the cholesterol ester content of the tissue and both the size (35-37) and the number (35, 38) of the droplets in the tissue, as determined microscopically, decrease in parallel under conditions of high secretory activity; and (3) the droplet and the cholesterol ester contents of the tissue rise in parallel towards the end of the estrous cycle and approaching luteolysis in corpora lutea (38, 39).

Rate of Turnover of Stored Cholesterol

Although the use of isotopes has allowed the determination of fractional turnover rates for the intracellular storage forms of a variety of substances, this technique has not been applied to ovarian cholesterol stores. There is some circumstantial evidence to suggest, however, that the turnover of these stores is rapid. The rate of accumulation of cholesterol ester following either LH-stimulated depletion of luteinized rat ovaries (13) or in vivo treatment with aminoglutethimide phosphate (40) suggests that esterification can occur at a rate of up to 6.7 μmole/g wet wt/hr. Net deesterification has been observed at rates of 4.1 μmole/g/hr on LH stimulation of luteinized rat ovaries (13), and of 61 μmole/g/hr., shortly (30 min) after stimulation of luteinized ovaries from aminoglutethimide phosphate-treated rats (40).

The rates of esterification and deesterification, which in a steady-state situation must be equal, can be calculated for unstimulated rat lutein tissue from data of the sort given in Fig. 1. Calculation of the fractional turnover rate for cholesterol ester in vivo, on the basis of the rate of change of specific activities of the free and esterified cholesterol pools following administration of ^{14}C-cholesterol, yields for control animals a value of 0.27/hr (Fig. 2), assuming the model shown in Fig. 3. Thus if the tissue contains 30 μmole/g wet wt of cholesterol ester, the rate of esterification and deesterification calculated from these data would be approximately 8.1 μmole/g wet wt/hr in the "resting" state (which for the short-term purposes of this experiment probably represents a steady-state condition). The corresponding value for cholesterol ester in the ovaries of LH-treated animals is 0.18/hr. Since these ovaries contain little cholesterol ester (approximately 4 μmole/g) the rates of esterification and deesterification are considerably less under these conditions (approximately 0.72 μmole/g/hr.). This effect of chronic LH treatment in vivo is consistent with the

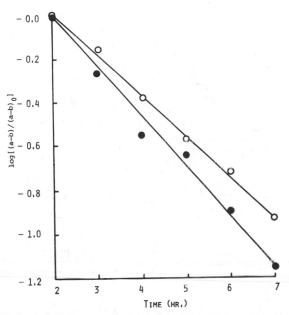

FIG. 2. Calculation of fractional turnover rate of cholesterol ester in vivo, from data obtained as described in legend to Fig. 1. The expression $\log [(a - b)/(a - b)_0]$ is plotted against time after administration of label; $(a - b)$ equals the difference between specific activities of whole tissue free and esterfied cholesterol at time t, and $(a - b)_0$ is the difference at time 0, which is taken for the purposes of the calculation as 2 hr after administration of the labeled cholesterol. The slope of this line $(-k)$ is related to the fractional turnover rate by a factor of 2.303/2. Luteinized ovaries were from controls (•) and "chronically" LH-treated (50 µg daily for 4 days) rats (○).

inhibitory effect of this regimen on the prolactin induced maintenance of cholesterol ester synthetase observed by Behrman. These rates are clearly comparable to those suggested by the changes in cholesterol ester concentration following LH stimulation. There are at present no available data on the fractional turnover rate of ovarian free cholesterol.

Formation and Mobilization of Lipid-Storage Droplets

The rapid rates of synthesis and removal of ovarian cholesterol ester leads to the related problems of how it is formed into lipid droplets and mobilized from them. The only evidence as to the nature of the processes leading to the formation of lipid-storage droplets comes from the electron microscopic studies of Bjersing (41), who observed such droplets surrounded by a layer apparently continuous with the endoplasmic reticulum, and concluded that this represented the formation of a lipid droplet from the endoplasmic reticulum by a pinching-off process. Such a process would appear to be similar morphologically

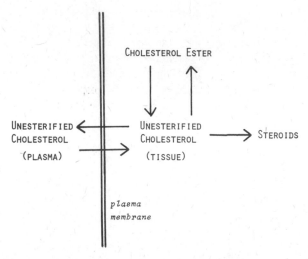

FIG. 3. Model for uptake and esterification of cholesterol used in calculating the fractional turnover rate of esterified cholesterol. It is assumed that 1) in a steady-state situation the rate of esterification equals that of deesterification; 2) the rate of uptake of free cholesterol from the plasma equals the rate of loss from the gland; 3) the rate of uptake from the plasma greatly exceeds that of esterification; 4) the rates of both these processes far exceed the rate of steroid synthesis; 5) the esterified cholesterol in the gland does not equilibrate with that in the plasma; and 6) the rate of isotopic exchange catalysed by cholesterol ester synthetase in the absence of flow is relatively small. Experimental evidence has been found in support of assumptions 1 to 5. It should be emphasized that the values for the fractional turnover rate of cholesterol ester arrived at are maximum values. In particular, the rate of possible isotopic exchange reactions, catalyzed by cholesterol ester synthetase and sterol hydrolase, are difficult to correct for. This is unlikely to lead to large errors, however, since both these steps are probably essentially irreversible; the esterase is, at least in vitro (18).

to that believed to occur during the formation of storage granules in other endocrine tissues; it is apparently unconfirmed. Several workers in this field have been led to believe that lipid-storage droplets may be surrounded by a shell or membrane (42, 43). Such a shell would be expected were droplets to arise by a pinching off from the endoplasmic reticulum of segments containing large amounts of cholesterol ester.

There is no electron microscopic evidence directly relating to the mobilization of cholesterol esters from storage droplets, although the whorls of smooth endoplasmic reticulum often found surrounding these droplets in rapidly secreting ovarian tissues (38, 42, 44, 45) have been said to reflect this process (38).

Two lines of biochemical investigation have provided indications of the nature of the storage and mobilization process. Examination of the intracellular locations of cholesterol esterase and of cholesterol ester synthetase by Behrman and his colleagues (18, 46) has revealed that the ester synthesizing enzyme (assayed with exogenous 1-^{14}C-palmitoyl CoA and endogenous cholesterol) is located mostly in the microsomes prepared by differential centrifugation from homogenates of rat lutein tissue. Similar studies by these authors have shown the esterase to be a soluble enzyme, although the work of Coutts and Stansfield (47), using both bovine corpora lutea and rat lutein tissue, suggested that it may be more generally distributed throughout the cell, with most of the activity in a fraction sedimented by centrifugation for an unspecified time at 5000 g. A microsomal location for the sterol ester synthetase is consistent with the mode of formation of lipid storage droplets proposed by Bjersing (38).

The question of whether the droplets are surrounded by a sheath or membrane has been investigated in our laboratory by a serial washing technique. Droplets prepared by centrifugal flotation from homogenates of rat lutein tissue were resuspended and reisolated in a serial washing procedure repeated up to four times. Assays of protein, phospholipid, nucleotide phosphatase, and cholesterol ester in portions of the washed droplet suspensions indicated that these components remained associated with cholesterol throughout the washing procedure (Table III). Although the nucleotide phosphatase was assayed with ATPMg^{2-}, it also catalyzed the liberation P$_i$ from ADP, AMP, UTP, CTP, GTP, and ITP, in the presence of Mg^{2+}. Approximately 30% of the droplets were lost at each successive wash; the suspensions were free of contaminating cytoplasmic enzymes after the first wash. The ratio of protein to phospholipid found in this

TABLE III. Effect of serial washing on protein, phospholipid, ctyoplasmic enzymes, and ATPase associated with lipid-containing droplets

After wash number	Lipid-soluble phosphorus	Protein	Activities of Enzymes			ATPase activity
			G-6-PDH	LDH	ME	
0	0.035 ± 0.004	65 ± 5.6	1.10	1.35	1.90	7.3
1	0.037 ± 0.005	61 ± 19.6	-	-	-	4.4
2	0.047 ± 0.005	61 ± 8.6	-	-	-	3.3
3	0.036 ± 0.006	75 ± 11.8	-	-	-	4.2
4	0.034 ± 0.003	67 ± 15.4	-	-	-	4.2

Lipid-containing droplets were prepared by centrifugal flotation from homogenates of luteinized rat ovary, and were washed by resuspension in the homogenization medium and re-flotation. After each successive wash, a portion of the resuspended droplets was taken for analysis. Lipid-soluble phosphorus (μg/μmole cholesterol ester), cytoplasic enzymes (% activity in droplet preparations as percent that in cytosol, v/v), protein (μg/μmole cholesterol ester) and ATPase (pmole ATP hydrolyzed/20 min/μmole cholesterol ester) were assayed by standard methods and are expressed in the terms given in parentheses. Values are means ± SE, where applicable of 4 determinations). G-6-PDH μ glucose 6-phosphate dehydrogenase; LDH = lactate dehydrogenase; ME = malic enzyme; -, not detectable.

study (1.9 : 1.0 w/w) is comparable to that found in naturally occurring membranes (48). The presence of a nucleotide phosphatase associated with the droplets is of interest, not only because it verifies the presence of protein in the droplets, but also because ATPases are common constituents of storage granules from other endocrine tissues (49, 50). It is tempting to speculate that this enzyme may play a role in the release of cholesterol from the droplets.

The problem of whether this adhering shell or membrane represents a biological membrane in the generally accepted sense, or is a randomly absorbed layer of material, has not been approached experimentally.

Regulation of Ovarian Cholesterol Storage and Mobilization by Gonadotropins

Evidence for an increased net mobilization and hydrolysis of cholesterol caused by LH has been presented, based on the net rate of disappearance of the sterol ester from stimulated tissue. This effect of LH has been separated from that on cholesterol side-chain cleavage enzyme by the use of aminoglutethimide phosphate, a cholesterol side-chain cleavage enzyme inhibitor. Using this compound, Behrman and his colleagues (40) have been able to demonstrate a stimulation of the net deesterification of cholesterol by LH in the absence of any cholesterol side-chain cleavage activity. It appears therefore that LH has two separable effects on the steroidogenic pathway, one at cholesterol esterase and one at cholesterol side-chain cleavage enzyme. The evidence for an effect on cholesterol side-chain cleavage enzyme, however, cannot be regarded as conclusive, since it is largely derived from cell free preparations. It is not known whether cholesterol side-chain cleavage enzyme is rate limiting in steroid synthesis in whole cells or whether flow through it is influenced by substrate, in other words, cholesterol, concentration (51).

There is no evidence from studies of whole-cell preparations to suggest that this depletion of cholesterol ester is due to a stimulation of the rate of deesterification. In view of the rapid rate of turnover of stored cholesterol ester discussed earlier, the depletion may, a priori, be due either to an increased rate of hydrolysis or to a decrease in the rate of esterification. The rate of depletion appears to be too high to be accounted for solely on the basis of the esterase activity estimates of Behrman and Armstrong (18), although as discussed below, such estimates are difficult to make. LH, which has previously been shown to decrease the rate of in vitro incorporation of ^{14}C-acetate into sterol esters in rabbit ovarian interstitial tissue (9), rat corpora lutea (11), and bovine corpora lutea (10), has been observed to decrease the rate of incorporation of labeled long-chain fatty acids into sterol esters by slices of rabbit ovarian interstitial tissue whether injected in vivo 12 hr before removal of ovaries for incubation (52) or added directly to incubation media (Table IV). This effect cannot be explained by the decreased incorporation into the cholesterol moiety of the ester of ^{14}C-acetate derived by β oxidation from the labeled oleate added as substrate and therefore appears to be a reliable reflection of decreased esterification.

TABLE IV. Effect of LH in vitro on incorporation of ^{14}C from oleate and acetate into sterol esters and other lipids by slices of rabbit ovarian interstitial tissue

Substrate	In vitro treatment	^{14}C Incorporated (dpm/mg tissue) into:			
		Sterol ester-sterol	Sterol ester-fatty acid	Triglyceride	Phospholipid
1-^{14}C-oleate	None	15 ± 2	690 ± 131	218 ± 64	672 ± 83
1-^{14}C-oleate	+LH	6 ± 3	207 ± 34	164 ± 58	529 ± 72
1-^{14}C-acetate	None	201 ± 59	499 ± 152	67 ± 14	84 ± 21
1-^{14}C-acetate	+LH	47 ± 15	77 ± 8	48 ± 14	99 ± 28

Slices of rabbit ovarian interstitial tissue were incubated for 2 hr in a bicarbonate-buffered medium containing glucose (1 mg/ml) and either 0.5 mM 1-^{14}C-acetate (1 μCi/ml) or 16.6 mM 1-^{14}C-oleate (1 μCi/ml), with or without LH (NIH-LH-S15, 1 μg/ml). Incorporation of ^{14}C into the lipid fractions listed was determined after separation by TLC and saponification. Values are means ± SE of 7 determinations. Tissue slices from the ovaries of each rabbit were distributed between each of the 4 treatment groups used; each flask contained tissue from only one animal.

281

Prolactin, in contrast to LH, stimulates the storage of cholesterol esters (11, 13, 53, 54). Both free and esterified cholesterol accumulate under the influence of prolactin, in both corpora lutea and ovarian interstitial tissue. Whether this results solely from an increase in the rate of synthesis from acetate is unknown, although prolactin administration in vivo has been found to increase the rate of incorporation of acetate carbon into cholesterol observed in vitro in both tissues (11, 54). Whether the increased storage of cholesterol esters is a consequence of an increased rate of esterification or of a decreased rate of deesterification has, as in the case of LH-stimulated depletion of cholesterol esters, not been measured directly in whole-cell preparations.

Properties and Gonadotropic Regulation of Ovarian Cholesterol Esterase and Sterol Ester Synthetase

Two enzymes apparently connected with the storage and utilization of cholesterol esters have been partially purified from ovarian sources by Behrman and his colleagues (18, 46). These enzymes, sterol ester hydrolase (EC 3.1.1.13, cholesterol esterase) and acyl CoA:3β-hydroxysterol acyltransferase, (EC 2.3.1, cholesterol ester synthetase) have been mentioned above in connection with their intracellular distribution. It is possible but unconfirmed that a third enzyme, a phosphatidylcholine:3β - hydroxysterol acyltransferase (EC 2.3.1) is involved in ovarian cholesterol esterification. Possible evidence for the involvement of this enzyme is indicated by the lack of a sufficiently high total activity of assayable cholesterol ester synthetase to account for the rates of esterification of cholesterol which have been demonstrated to occur.

The control of the total activity of the sterol esterase and microsomal cholesterol ester synthetase by gonadotropins has been investigated by Behrman and co-workers (18, 46). It was found initially that LH administered in vivo to immature rats with luteinized ovaries increased the total activity of cholesterol esterase in the tissue by about 25% (18). This effect was cited in explanation of the effect of LH in depleting the tissue of cholesterol esters. However, the measured activity of this enzyme (0.17 mU/g, at 37 C) (18) is insufficient to account for the maximum apparent flow through it (61 μmole/g/hr) (40) during LH-stimulated cholesterol ester depletion. It follows, therefore, that either the enzyme was not measured under conditions of maximum activity, which is likely since the assay of enzymes with lipid-soluble substrates is notoriously difficult, or activity was lost on extraction of the tissue. In either case, failure to assay the enzyme at maximum activity may lead to a misleading interpretation of the apparent stimulatory effect of LH on it. It may be that either the activity was limited in the ovaries from LH-treated rats by factors other than the enzyme activity and that the stimulatory effect of LH was in reality higher than that observed, or that the stimulatory effect was unrelated to the total enzyme activity, being a consequence of some other effect of LH. Subsequently, it was found that cholesterol esterase activity was maintained in the luteinized ovaries of hypophysectomized rats by prolactin (46).

Similar factors are unlikely to invalidate the assay of microsomal cholesterol ester synthetase (46) since the added labeled substrate in the assay of this enzyme, palmitoyl CoA, is watersoluble. Measurements of this enzyme in luteinized ovaries from hypophysectomized rats (46) have indicated that the decline in activity associated with hypophysectomy can be prevented by prolactin therapy, but not by LH. However, similar limitations apply in the case of the assay of this enzyme because, as with the sterol esterase, measured activity (1 mU/g measured at 37 C) (46) cannot account for the maximum observed flow through the step (6.7 μmole/g/hr) (40). This has been cited above as possible evidence for the existence of a separate cholesterol esterifying system.

The effects of LH and prolactin on net disappearance and accumulation of cholesterol ester can be accounted for, at least qualitatively, in view of the demonstration of its rapid turnover, by the effects of these gonadotropins on the enzymes presently believed to catalyze cholesterol ester hydrolysis and esterification. Perturbation of the cyclic esterification and deesterification process so as to cause net deesterification would be expected to result from the stimulatory effect of LH on cholesterol esterase and its inhibitory effect on the esterifying enzyme (18, 46). Net esterification may be caused by the pronounced effect prolactin has in stimulating the esterifying enzyme (46), together with a mass-action effect resulting from the higher total tissue free cholesterol concentrations observed in tissues from prolactin-treated animals (11, 13).

CONCLUSIONS AND SUMMARY

Evidence has been presented relating (1) to the compartmentation of steroidogenic cholesterol arising as a result of biosynthesis from acetate; (2) to the utilization of plasma cholesterol for steroid synthesis; and (3) to the storage and mobilization of cholesterol ester in ovarian tissues.

The biosynthesis of cholesterol from ^{14}C-acetate has been shown to result in the formation of ^{14}C-cholesterol associated with the endoplasmic reticulum. The metabolism of this cholesterol by a cholesterol side-chain cleavage enzyme shown to be located in the endoplasmic reticulum may explain the preferential utilization of "recently formed" cholesterol previously observed in ovarian tissues. It can be concluded, however, that the production of steroids from this pool of cholesterol accounts for a small proportion of the total rate of steroidogenesis. The effects of LH in stimulating steroid synthesis and concomitantly decreasing the specific activity of whole-tissue cholesterol formed in incubations in the presence of ^{14}C-acetate have been discussed in terms of the control of a cholesterol side-chain cleavage enzyme located in the endoplasmic reticulum.

The utilization of plasma cholesterol for steroid synthesis has been investigated following the intravenous administration of ^{14}C-cholesterol to rats with luteinized ovaries. At various times prior to the equilibration of isotope between free and esterified cholesterol, the specific activities of the tissue steroids equal that of the free cholesterol and exceed that of the esterified cholesterol. It has been inferred, using this technique, that plasma cholesterol equilibrates with that in the ovaries, that free cholesterol is the substrate for side-chain cleavage, and that the free cholesterol in the tissue appears at least operationally to constitute a single pool. The fractional turnover rate has been calculated from the data obtained in this type of experiment, and the resulting values (0.27 hr $^{-1}$ for control animals and 0.18 hr $^{-1}$ for animals treated chronically with LH) has been discussed in connection with the activities of sterol ester hydrolase (EC 3.1.1.13) and cholesterol ester synthetase reported in the literature. It is concluded that the steady-state rate of esterification and deesterification of cholesterol ester (8.1 μmole/g/hr. for control animals and 0.72 μmole/g/hr. for ovaries of LH-treated animals) calculated from the fractional turnover rate is comparable to the rate of accumulation and mobilization of cholesterol esters observed in vivo, but not with the activities of the enzymes apparently catalyzing these steps. The measured rates exceed the enzyme activities by factors of 130 to 800. Independent evidence is also presented to suggest that LH reduces the rate of esterification in vitro.

Finally, it has been found that serial washing of suspensions of lipid-storage droplets prepared from rat lutein tissue results in no loss of the protein, phospholipid, and nucleotide phosphatase activity associated with them. This chemical evidence for the existence of membrane-delimited lipid-storage droplets is discussed in relation to electron microscopic investigations of the nature of the cholesterol ester mobilization and accumulation processes and to similarities between these lipid-storage droplets and the storage granules of other endocrine tissues.

ACKNOWLEDGMENT

This work was supported by NIH contract 69-2165 and Medical Research of Canada grant MA 3372.

REFERENCES

1. Srere, P. A., I. L. Chaikoff, and W. G. Dauben, J Biol Chem 176:829, 1948.
2. Zaffaroni, A., O. Hechter, and G. J. Pincus, J Amer Chem Soc 73:1390, 1951.
3. Werthessen, N. T., E. Schwenk, and C. Baker, Science 117:380, 1953.
4. Caspi, E., R. I. Dorfman, B. T. Kahn, G. Rosenfeld, and W. Schmid, J Biol Chem 237:2085, 1962.
5. Billiar, R. B., A. Oriol Bosch, and K. B. Eik-Nes, Biochemistry 4:457, 1965.
6. Salokangas, R. A., H. C. Rilling, and L. T. Samuels, Biochemistry 4:1606, 1965.
7. Savard, K., and P. J. Casey, Endocrinology 74:599, 1964.
8. Savard, K., J. M. Marsh, and B. F. Rice, Rec Prog Hormone Res 21:285, 1965.

9. Armstrong, D. T., Nature 213:633, 1967.

10. Armstrong, D. T., and D. L. Black, Can J Biochem 46:1137, 1968.

11. Armstrong, D. T., L. S. Miller, and K. A. Knudsen, Endocrinology 85:393, 1969.

12. Armstrong, D. T., T. M. Jackanicz, and P. L. Keyes, in K. W. McKerns (Ed.), The Gonads 1969, Appleton-Century-Crofts, New York, 1969, p. 3.

13. Armstrong, D. T., Rec Prog Hormone Res 24:255, 1968.

14. Armstrong, D. T., T. P. Lee, and L. S. Miller, Biol Reprod 2:29, 1970.

15. Siekevitz, P., Ann Rev Physiol 25:15, 1963.

16. Major, P. W., D. T. Armstrong, and R. O. Greep, Endocrinology 81:19, 1967.

17. Flint, A. P. F., and R. M. Denton, Biochem J 116:79, 1970.

18. Behrman, H. R., and D. T. Armstrong, Endocrinology 85:474, 1969.

19. Flint, A. P. F., and R. M. Denton, Biochem J 112:243, 1969.

20. Channing, C. P., and C. A. Villee, Biochem Biophys Acta 115:205, 1966.

21. Moyle, W. R., Ph. D. Thesis, Harvard University, Cambridge, Mass. 1970.

22. Bartosik, D. B., and E. B. Romanoff, in K. W. McKerns (Ed.), The Gonads 1969, Appleton-Century-Crofts, New York, 1969, p. 211.

23. Koritz, S. B., Biochem Biophys Res Commun 23:485, 1966.

24. Simpson, E. R., and G. S. Boyd, Biochem Biophys Res Commun 24:10, 1966.

25. Jackanicz, T. M., and D. T. Armstrong, Endocrinology 83:769, 1968.

26. Yago, N., M. S. Nightingale, R. I. Dorfman, and E. Forchielli, J Biochem 62:274, 1967.

27. Morris, M. D., and I. L. Chaikoff, J Biol Chem 234:1095, 1959.

28. Werbin, H., and I. L. Chaikoff, Arch Biochem Biophys 93:476, 1961.

29. Solod, E. A., D. T. Armstrong, and R. O. Greep, Steroids 7:607, 1966.

30. Flint, A. P. F., and D. T. Armstrong, Biochem J 123:143, 1971.

31. Dexter, R. N., L. M. Fishman, and R. L. Ney, Endocrinology 87:836, 1970.

32. Claesson, L., E. Diczfalusy, N. Hillarp, and B. Hojberg, Acta Physiol Scand 16:183, 1948.

33. Herbst, A. L., Endocrinology 81:54, 1967.

34. Armstrong, D. T., J. O'Brien, and R. O. Greep, Endocrinology 75:488, 1964.

35. Claesson, L. Acta Physiol Scand 31:Suppl. 113, 53, 1954.

36. Barker, W. L., Endocrinology 48:772, 1951.

37. Deane, H. W., and A. M. Seligman, Vitamins Hormones 11:173, 1953.

38. Bjersing, L., Z Zellforsch Mikrosk Anat 82:187, 1967.

39. Everett, J. W., Amer J Anat 77:293, 1945.

40. Behrman, H. R., D. T. Armstrong, and R. O. Greep, Can J Biochem 48:881, 1970.

41. Bjersing, L., Z Zellforsch Mikrosk Anat 82:173, 1967.

42. Blanchette, E. J., J Cell Biol 31:517, 1966.

43. Christensen, A. K., and S. W. Gillim, in K. W. McKerns (Ed.), The Gonads 1969, Appleton-Century-Crofts, New York, 1969, p. 415.

44. Enders, A. L., and W. R. Lyons, J Cell Biol 22:127, 1964.

45. Belt, W. D., L. F. Cavazos, L. L. Anderson, and R. R. Kraeling, Biol Reprod 2:98, 1970.

46. Behrman, H. R., G. P. Orczyk, G. J. Macdonald, and R. O. Greep, Endocrinology 87:1251, 1970.

47. Coutts, J. R. T., and D. A. Stansfield, J Lipid Res 9:647, 1968.

48. Korn, E. D., Ann Rev Biochem 38:263, 1969.

49. Winkler, W. H., H. Hortnagl, H. Hortnagl, and A. D. Smith, Biochem J 118:303, 1970.

50. Woodin, A. M., and A. A. Wieneke, Biochem J 90:498, 1964.

51. Newsholme, E. A., and W. Gevers, Vitamins Hormones 25:1, 1967.

52. Armstrong, D. T., and J. M. Price, Anat Rec 160:309, 1968.

53. Zarrow, M. X., and J. H. Clark, Endocrinology 84:340, 1969.

54. Armstrong, D. T., K. A. Knudsen, and L. S. Miller, Endocrinology 86:634, 1970.

55. Raggatt, P. R., and M. W. Whitehouse, Biochem J 101:819, 1966.

56. Omura, T., and R. Sato, J Biol Chem, 239:2270, 1964.

57. Cammer, W., and R. W. Estabrook, Arch Biochem Biophys 112:735, 1967.

58. Flint, A. P. F., and R. M. Denton, Biochem J 117:73, 1970.

59. Flint, A. P. F., and D. T. Armstrong, Nature 231:60, 1971.

23. Effect of Cyclic 3', 5'-Adenosine Monophosphate on Gonadal Diphosphopyridine and Triphosphopyridine Nucleotide Linked Dehydrogenases

Sorel Sulimovici and Bruno Lunenfeld

Experimental evidence supports the contention that cyclic 3',5'-adenosine monophosphate (cyclic-AMP) is the intracellular mediator of ACTH-induced steroidogenesis in adrenal cortex (1) and of LH in ovarian tissue (2). It is believed that these tropic hormones stimulate steroidogenesis in adrenal cortex and gonads through activation of adenyl cyclase, a membrane bound enzyme which catalyzes the cyclization of ATP to cyclic-AMP. The stimulatory effect of ACTH on the adrenal adenyl cyclase (1) and of LH on ovarian (3) and testicular (4) adenyl cyclase have been demonstrated. The increased levels of cyclic-AMP will in turn enhance the mitochondrial conversion of cholesterol (cholest-5-en-3β-ol) to pregnenolone (3β-hydroxy-Δ^5-pregnen-20-one) the rate-limiting step in steroidogenesis (5). On the contrary cyclic-AMP was found to inhibit the conversion of pregnenolone to progesterone (6-8). This latter action is catalyzed in steroidogenic tissue by a consecutive action of a NAD$^+$ dependent Δ^5,3β-hydroxysteroid dehydrogenase, and a Δ^5, Δ^4, 3-ketosteroid isomerase. These enzymes were found to be related to both micochrondria and microsomal fractions (7, 8).

In the present report we wish to summarize experiments conducted in our

287

laboratory dealing with the effect of cyclic-AMP on some NAD^+- and $NADP^+$-dependent steroid dehydrogenases and on certain pyridine nucleotide-dependent dehydrogenases of gonadal origin, which might produce reducing equivalent to the system.

EFFECT OF CYCLIC-AMP ON THE CHOLESTEROL SIDE CHAIN CLEAVAGE ENZYMES

The complex of enzymes involved in the side-chain cleavage of cholesterol have been studied in mitochondria isolated from ovaries of immature rats pretreated with pregnant mare's serum gonadotropin (PMSG) and human chorionic gonadotropin (HCG) (9). Using 4-^{14}C-cholesterol as substrate and a NADPH generating system, the main product obtained was progesterone (pregn-4-ene-3,20-dione) together with small amounts of pregnenolone and 20α-hydroxy pregn-4-en-3-one. The failure of pregnenolone to accumulate suggested   either that the mitochondrial preparations were contaminated to a significant degree with microsomes which contained a very active Δ^5,3β-hydroxysteroid dehydrogenase (10) or that this subparticulate fraction contained this enzyme. Electron microscopy of such a mitochondrial preparation revealed little evidence of contamination with microsomes and incubation with pregnenolone as substrate and NAD^+ demonstrated the presence of the enzymes which transform pregnenolone to progesterone in rat ovarian mitochondria (9).

The effect of cyclic-AMP on the cholesterol side-chain cleavage enzymes in rat ovarian mitochondria is shown in Fig. 1. The cyclic nucleotide at concentrations of 1 to 10 μmoles/ml incubation increased the conversion of cholesterol to pregnenolone and decreased progesterone synthesis. However, the over-all side-chain cleavage reaction (pregnenolone + progesterone) was not affected at this concentration of cyclic-AMP. At higher concentration, 15 μmoles/ml, due to a marked decrease in progesterone synthesis, the over-all side-chain cleavage activity was decreased. Similar results were reported for rat adrenal mitochondria (11).

The enhancement of pregnenolone accumulation in this system by cyclic-AMP might be ascribed to stimulation of the cholesterol side-chain cleavage enzymes and to the inhibition of the further conversion of pregnenolone to progesterone. The accumulation of pregnenolone from cholesterol by cyclic-AMP confirmed the hypothesis that the cyclic nucleotide as well as a tropic hormone might stimulate steroidogenesis at the same rate limiting step, in other words, the conversion of cholesterol to pregnenolone (5). These results also suggested an inhibitory effect of cyclic-AMP on the conversion of pregnenolone to progesterone and the accumulation of pregnenolone is not due to increased synthesis but rather to an inhibition of its transformation to progesterone. These observations prompted us to investigate the effect of cyclic-AMP on the conversion of Δ^5-3β-hydroxysteroids to Δ^4-3-ketosteroids.

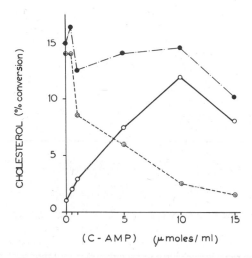

FIG. 1. Effect of cyclic-AMP on the mitochondrial conversion of 4-^{14}C-cholesterol to 4-^{14}C-pregnenolone (o) 4-^{14}C-progesterone (--o--) and total conversion (●). The mitochondrial incubation mixture contained 15 mg protein in 0.1M phosphate buffer pH 7.3, 50 μMoles magnesium sulphate, 5 μMoles NADP$^+$, 40 μMoles D-glucose-6-phosphate, 1.0 IU D-glucose-6-phosphate dehydrogenase 0.2 μCi 4-^{14}C-cholesterol and different amounts of cyclic AMP. The final volume was 5 ml and incubations were carried out at 37 C for 60 min in air. Data adapted from Sulimovici and Boyd (12).

EFFECT OF CYCLIC-AMP ON $\Delta^5,3\beta$-HYDROXYSTEROID DEHYDRO-GENASE AND $\Delta^5,\Delta^4$3-KETOSTEROID ISOMERASE IN IMMATURE RAT OVARIAN TISSUE PRETREATED WITH PMSG

Mitochondria and microsomal fractions were isolated from immature rat ovarian tissue pretreated with PMSG (7). The enzymes were solubilized following ultrasonication and freeze-drying of the subparticulate fractions. Figure 2 shows that cyclic-AMP inhibits the $\Delta^5,3\beta$-hydroxysteroid dehydrogenase in a soluble mitochondrial and microsomal preparations from luteinized rat ovarian tissue. The inhibitory effect of cyclic-AMP on the conversion of pregnenolone to progesterone was found to be very specific since other nucleotides related in structure to cyclic-AMP such as AMP, ADP, ATP, 2',3'-AMP were found not to influence the $\Delta^5,3\beta$-hydroxysteroids dehydrogenase activity. The cyclic nucleotide was apparently a noncompetitive inhibitor of the dehydrogenase-isomerase system in ovarian mitochondria whereas the inhibition of the microsomal $\Delta^5,3\beta$-hydroxysteroid dehydrogenase by cyclic-AMP was released by increasing the concentrations of exogenous NAD$^+$ suggesting a competitive inhibitory effect (Fig. 3).

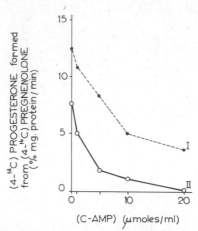

FIG. 2. Effect of cyclic-AMP on the conversion of 4-^{14}C-pregnenolone to 4-^{14}C-progesterone in a 105,000 × g supernatant from lyophilized rat ovarian mitochondria (I) and lyophylized microsomes (II). The mitochondrial incubation mixture contained 0.5 mg protein in 0.1M phosphate buffer pH 7.4, 50 μMoles magnesium sulphate, 0.75 μMoles NAD$^+$, 0.05 μCi 4-^{14}C-pregnenolone and different concentrations of cyclic-AMP to a total volume of 4 ml. The lyophilized rat ovarian microsomal incubation mixture contained 0.5 mg protein in 0.1M phosphate buffer pH 7.4, 50 μMoles magnesium sulphate, 75 mμMoles NAD$^+$, 0.05 μCi 4-^{14}C-pregnenolone and different concentrations of cyclic-AMP. The total volume was 4 ml and the incubations were carried out at 37 C for 15 min in air. Data from Sulimovici and Boyd (7).

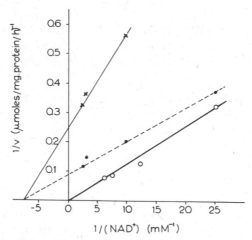

FIG. 3. Effect of NAD$^+$ on the mitochondrial (x) and microsomal (o) conversion of 4-^{14}C-pregnenolone to 4-^{14}C-progesterone in the presence of cyclic-AMP. (•) control; (x) mitochondrial 6 μMoles cycle-AMP/ml; (o) microsomes 6 μMoles cyclic-AMP/ml. The velocity is expressed as percentage conversion of 4-^{14}C-pregnenolone to 4-^{14}C-progesterone. Data from Sulimovici and Boyd (7).

290

THE EFFECT OF CYCLIC-AMP AND OF N⁶-2'-O-DIBUTYRYL CYCLIC 3',5'-ADENOSINEMONOPHOSPHATE (DBC) ON THE MOUSE OVARIAN $\Delta^5,3\beta$-HYDROXYSTEROID DEHYDROGENASE

For a better understanding of the inhibitory effect of cyclic-AMP described in mitochondrial and microsomal fractions isolated from luteinized rat ovarian tissue, the action of the cyclic nucleotide was further examined in an ovarian preparation devoid of corpora lutea. Immature female Swiss albino mice were used in this experiment. The animals varied in age from 21 to 25 days and in weight from 10 to 13 g at the commencement of the experiment. Histological examination of ovaries of animals of this age showed no signs of ovulation. The $\Delta^5,3\beta$-hydroxysteroid dehydrogenase and $\Delta^5,\Delta^4,3$-ketosteroid isomerase were examined in a 40,000 × g supernatant of ovarian homogenate employing two substrates: pregnenolone and dehydroepiandrosterone (3β-hydroxy-5-adrosten-17β-ol). The effect of cyclic-AMP and DBC was tested on the dehydrogenase-isomerase system in experiments in vitro and after administration of nucleotides in vivo (12).

Incubations of the 40,000 × g supernatant of mouse ovarian homogenate in the presence of 0.2-5 μmoles/ml cyclic-AMP inhibited the conversion of pregnenolone to progesterone (Fig. 4) and of dehydroepiandrosterone to Δ^4-androstenedione (androst-4-ene-3,17-dione) (Fig. 5). The dibutyryl analog

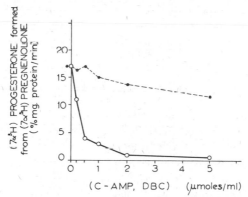

(C – AMP, DBC)   (μmoles/ml)

FIG. 4. Effect of cyclic-AMP (o) and DBC (●) on the conversion of 7α-³H-pregnenolone to $7\alpha^3$ H-progesterone in a 40,000 × g supernatant from immature mouse ovarian tissue. Incubation mixture 1 mg protein enzyme in 0.1M phosphate buffer pH 7.4, 50 μMoles magnesium sulphate 2 μM NAD⁺, 0.1 μCi 7α-³H-pregnenolone, and different concentrations of cyclic-AMP and DBC. Incubations were carried out at 37 C for 2 min in air.

employed in concentrations of up to 5 μmoles/ml did not inhibit the reaction (Figs. 4 and 5.) The concentrations of cyclic-AMP used in the present experiments to produce inhibition in vitro on the dehydrogenase system (0.2

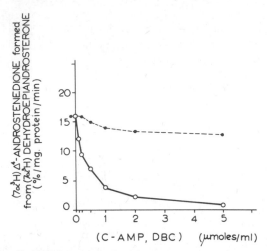

FIG. 5. Effect of cyclic-AMP (o) and DBC (•) on the conversion of 7 α-³H-dehydroepian-drosterone to 7 α-³H-Δ⁴-androstenedione in a 40,000 × g supernatant from immature mouse ovarian tissue. The incubation mixture contained 1 mg protein enzyme in 0.1M phosphate buffer pH 7.4, 50 μMoles magnesium sulphate, 2 μM NAD⁺, 0.1 μCi 7 α-³H-dehydroepian-drosterone, and different concentrations of cyclic-AMP and DBC to a total vol of 2 ml. Incubations were carried out in air at 37 C for 2 min.

mM) were smaller than that employed in luteinized rat ovarian tissue. Nevertheless, these concentrations appeared to be much higher than that found endogenously in the adrenal gland (13) and corpora lutea (14). The inhibition of $\Delta^5,3\beta$-hydroxysteroid dehydrogenase by cyclic-AMP was released by increasing the concentrations of exogenous NAD⁺ which suggested a competitive relationship between NAD⁺ and cyclic-AMP in this system. It also indicated that the inhibition had occurred at the dehydrogenase rather than the isomerase site since the latter enzyme does not require coenzyme for its activity. These observations confirmed our previous results and the findings of other investigations employing homogenates and subparticulate fractions of rat adrenal gland (6, 8). All these reports support the view that cyclic-AMP may influence steroidogenesis by inhibiting the NAD⁺ dependent dehydrogenases. In the present experiments DBC used at the same concentrations as the natural nucleotide was found to have no effect on the enzymic conversion of pregnenolone to progesterone and of dehydroepiandrosterone to Δ⁴-androstenedione (Figs. 4 and 5). These results were rather unexpected, since the dibutyryl analog has been observed in a number of experimental situations to be more effective than cyclic-AMP (15, 16). This added activity of the dibutyryl derivative was attributed to its increased penetration of the cell membrane and to its resistance to hydrolysis by phosphodiesterase enzyme (15).

In the phosphorylase activation system it has been reported that DBC has to be activated by removal of the butyryl group from the ribosyl residue before it becomes effective (15). Activation was attributed to a soluble esterase present in the liver that removed the 2'-O-acyl group. It might be possible that this esterase is not present in the 40,000 × g supernatant of the ovarian homogenate and this might explain the failure of the derivative to produce an effect. In addition it was demonstrated that DBC decomposed in buffers commonly used for the incubations of biological material (17).

For in vivo studies four groups of 40 mice each were used (12). Group I received cyclic-AMP (2 mg/animal/day); Group II, DBC (2 mg/animal/day); Group III, HCG (8 IU/animal/day); and Group IV, 0.85% NaCl. The nucleotides, HCG, and 0.85% NaCl were injected into animals in equally divided doses twice a day for four days. The preparations were dissolved in 0.85% NaCl and injected subcutaneously in a volume of 0.5 ml/animal. On the fifth day, the daily dose was administered in a single injection and the animals were sacrificed 5 hr later, after which the ovaries of each group were weighed and homogenized in 0.1M phosphate buffer. The 40,000 × g supernatant of the ovarian homogenates were incubated with pregnenolone or dehydroepiandrosterone together with NAD$^+$ The administration of either cyclic-AMP or DBC did not increase ovarian and uterine weight. Table I shows that cyclic-AMP and its dibutyryl analog injected in vivo had no effect on the ovarian conversion of pregnenolone to progesterone. On the other hand the transformation of exogenously added dehydroepiandro-

TABLE I. Effect of cyclic-AMP, DBC, and HCG injected subcutaneously to female mice on the conversion of 7α-^{3}H-pregnenolone to 7α-^{3}H-progesterone and $7\alpha^3$H-dehydroepiandrosterone to 7α-^{3}H-Δ^4-androstenedione by a 40,000 × g supernatant of ovarian homogenate.

Treatment	Ovaries	40,000 × g super-natant of ovarian homogenate mg protein/ovary	7α-^{3}H progesterone (%/mg protein/min)[a]	7α-^{3}H Δ^4-androstenedione (%/mg protein/min)[a]
Saline	72	0.083	14.20 ± 0.65	18.40 ± 0.50
Cyclic-AMP	76	0.078	13.80 ± 0.63	4.50 ± 0.67
DBC	74	0.081	12.50 ± 0.41	13.90 ± 0.50[b]
HCG	40	0.210	23.70 ± 0.84	31.40 ± 1.07

[a]Results are presented as the mean and standard deviation of five determinations.

[b]$p<0.001$ for difference between this value and corresponding control.

The cyclic nucleotides and the HCG were administered as described in the text. Each incubation flask contained, in addition to 0.1 μCi 7α-^{3}H-pregnenolone or 0.1 μCi 7α-^{3}H-dehydroepiandrosterone, 1 mg protein enzyme of 40,000 × g supernatant in 0.1M phosphate buffer pH 7.4, 50μmoles magnesium sulfate, and 2 μM NAD$^+$, to a total volume of 2 ml. Incubations were carried out for 2 min in air.

sterone to Δ^4-androstenedione was inhibited in the ovaries obtained from cyclic-AMP treated mice and was only slightly affected in the ovaries obtained from the DBC treated group. When a total of 8 IU HCG/animal/day was injected for a period of five days an increase in ovarian and uterine weight was noted. The protein content of the 40,000 × g supernatant was increased in the HCG treated animals, and the conversion of pregnenolone to progesterone and of dehydroepiandrosterone to Δ^4-androstenedione was significantly stimulated (Table I). This confirmed the observation that long-term administration of gonadotropic hormones was followed by an increase in Δ^5, 3β-hydroxysteroid dehydrogenase activity (18).

The results obtained after in vivo administration of the cyclic nucleotides might suggest the existence of two different Δ^5,3β-hydroxysteroid dehydrogenases in the mouse ovary. This possibility was reported previously (7, 19). Available evidence suggests the existence of separate isomerase and dehydrogenase enzymes in several steroid-producing endocrine tissues (20, 21). A single Δ^5,3β-hydroxysteroid dehydrogenase seems to occur in each of these tissues (21, 22). In contrast, several substrate specific steroid isomerase enzymes have been noted in bovine adrenal preparations (23, 24). One theoretical possibility is that cyclic-AMP might indirectly influence these reactions at the isomerase level, since the stimulation of Δ^5,Δ^4,3-ketosteroid isomerase in rat adrenal microsomes by NAD^+ and NADH was inhibited by cyclic-AMP (25).

The increase in Δ^5,3β-hydroxysteroid dehydrogenase activity by HCG, may be due to the fact that HCG, like LH stimulates the ovarian adenyl cyclase enzyme (3). This would result in an increase of endogenous cyclic-AMP so that the stimulation of the ovarian Δ^5,3β-hydroxysteroid dehydrogenase may be related to the elevated amounts of the cyclic nucleotide. If this were the case, the inhibition of Δ^5,3β-hydroxysteroid dehydrogenase in experiments in vitro or after the administration of the cyclic nucleotide in vivo could be attributed to the large and nonphysiological concentrations of cyclic-AMP.

EFFECT OF CYCLIC-AMP ON 17β-HYDROXYSTEROID DEHYDRO-GENASE IN RAT TESTIS

The above investigations revealed that cyclic-AMP inhibits the conversion of Δ^5-3β-hydroxysteroids to Δ^4-3-ketosteroids. The inhibition was apparently localized at the dehydrogenase step and seems to be affected by competition of the cyclic nucleotide for the NAD^+ binding site.

It was therefore found relevant to investigate the effect of the cyclic-AMP on another steroid dehydrogenase not mainly NAD^+ dependent. To this end 17β-hydroxysteroid dehydrogenase was studied in rat testis; this enzyme interconverts Δ^4-androstenedione to testeosterone (17β-hydroxyandrost-4-en-3-one). Mature male Charles River rats about 300 g body wt, 2 to 3 months old, were used in this experiment. After killing the rats their testis were removed, decapsulated and then homogenized in 0.25M sucrose, and mitochondrial and microsomal fractions isolated following differential centrifugation. The C_{19}-17β-hydroxysteroid dehydrogenase activity was found to be present in both subparticulate fractions with the dehydrogenase activity greater in microsomes. For the reduction of Δ^4-androstenedione to testosterone NADPH was the electron donor whereas the oxidation of testosterone to Δ^4-androstenedione utilized $NADP^+$ as well as NAD^+ as electron acceptors, the activity being higher when $NADP^+$ was the cofactor. The cyclic nucleotide and its dibutyryl analog were found to have neither an effect on the mitochondrial and microsomal conversion of Δ^4-androstenedione to testosterone in the presence of NADPH nor on the reverse conversion of testosterone to Δ^4-androstenedione when $NADP^+$ was employed as cofactor. However, the transformation of testosterone to Δ^4-androstenedione in the presence of NAD^+ was inhibited in both subparticulate fractions by cyclic-AMP whereas DBC had no effect on this conversion (Fig. 6). Increasing the concentrations of exogenous NAD^+ the inhibitory effect of

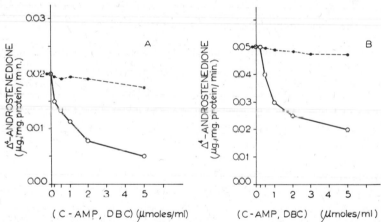

FIG. 6. Effect of cyclic-AMP (o) and DBC (•) on the conversion of testosterone to Δ^4-androstenedione from rat testis mitochondria (a) and microsomes (b). The mitochondrial incubation mixture contained 5 mg protein 0.1M phosphate buffer pH 7.4, 0.2 μMoles NAD^+ 50 μMoles magnesium sulphate, 50 μg testosterone, and different amounts of cyclic-AMP and DBC to a total volume of 3 ml. The microsomal incubations mixture contained 5 mg protein in 0.1M phosphate buffer pH 7.4, 0.2 μMoles NAD^+, 50 μMoles magnesium sulphate, 50 μg testosterone, and different amounts of cyclic-AMP and DBC to a total volume of 3 ml. In both subparticulate fractions incubations were carried out at 34 C in air for 60 min.

cyclic-AMP was counteracted in both subparticulate fractions (Fig. 7). Thus the cyclic-AMP binds to the cofactor site and selectively inhibits the NAD^+- and not the $NADP^+$-dependent conversion of testosterone to Δ^4-androstenedione.

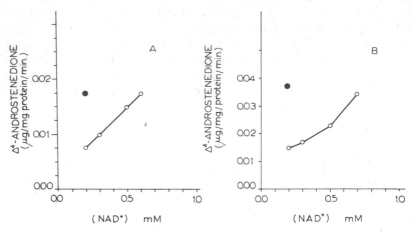

FIG. 7. Effect of increasing the amounts of NAD$^+$ on the conversion of testosterone to Δ^4-androstenedione in the presence of a constant amount of cyclic-AMP1 μMoles/ml in rat testis mitochondria (a) and microsome (b). The incubation mixtures; 5 mg mitochondrial (a) or microsomal protein (b) in 0.1M phosphate buffer pH 7.4, 50 μMoles magnesium sulphate 50 μg testosterone in the absence of cyclic-AMP ($\bullet$) and in the presence of 1 μMoles/ml cyclic-AMP (o). The final volume was 3 ml and the incubations were carried out at 34 C in air for 60 min.

EFFECT OF CYCLIC-AMP ON CERTAIN MITOCHONDRIAL AND SOLUBLE PYRIDINE NUCLEOTIDE DEPENDENT DEHYDRO-GENASES IN RAT TESTIS

The generation of cytoplasmic NADPH may take place by oxidation of glucose via the hexose monophosphate pathway, by oxidation of isocitrate and malate as well as by pyridine nucleotide transhydrogenation. The observation that bovine and human corpora lutea are very rich in glucose-6-phosphate dehydrogenase (G-6-PD) (26) indicated that hexosomonophosphate oxidation constitutes a dominant metabolic pathway in ovarian tissue and that G-6-PD activity is of prime importance. In contrast superovulated rat ovarian tissue has been shown to contain higher amounts of NADP$^+$ malate dehydrogenase (MDH) and NADP$^+$ isocitrate dehydrogenase (ICD) than G-6-PD (27). This indicates that the citric cycle enzymes play an important role in the formation of NADPH. The role of these and other possible reactions for the supply of NADPH in testicular tissue and the influence of cyclic-AMP on these processes has not been established. A study was therefore undertaken to determine the effect of cyclic-AMP on some pyridine nucleotide linked dehydrogenases in rat testis. Several NADP$^+$-linked dehydrogenases were estimated in high-speed supernatant of testicular homo-genates and NAD$^+$-linked dehydrogenases were assayed in mitochondria of rat testis. The results and the respective methods employed for these estimations are listed in Tables II and III respectively.

TABLE II. Effect of c-AMP on certain NADP$^+$-linked dehydrogenases in high speed supernatant (105,000 × g) of rat testis[a]

	G-6-PD[b]	6-PGD[c]	ICD[d]	MDH[e]
Control	10.5 ± 1.29	19.2 ± 1.30	21.0 ± 1.30	30.5 ± 2.07
c-AMP 0.2 mM	11.5 ± 1.91	18.6 ± 1.10	21.4 ± 0.89	30.7 ± 0.95
c-AMP 0.5 mM	10.0 ± 1.15	18.0 ± 1.20	20.4 ± 1.05	31.4 ± 1.15
c-AMP 1.0 mM	9.5 ± 0.51	18.7 ± 0.70	21.5 ± 1.20	29.2 ± 0.90
c-AMP 2.0 mM	10.4 ± 1.04	18.4 ± 0.85	20.4 ± 1.67	29.0 ± 0.81

[a]Results are expressed as means ± SD of five determinations. Activities are calculated as mμmoles product formed/mg protein/min.

[b]G-6-PD: glucose-6-phosphate dehydrogenase EC 1.1.1.49 Glock and McLean (28).

[c]6-PGD: 6-phosphogluconate dehydrogenase EC 1.1.1.44 Glock and McLean (28).

[d]ICD: NADP$^+$ isocitrate dehydrogenase EC 1.1.1.42 Ochoa (29).

[e]MDH: NADP$^+$ malate dehydrogenase (malic enzyme) EC 1.1.1.40 Ochoa (30).

TABLE III. Effect of c-AMP on certain NAD$^+$ linked dehydrogenases in rat testis mitrochondria.

	ICD[b]	MDH[c]
Control	17.6 ± 0.89	1706 ± 24.4
c-AMP 0.2 mM	16.4 ± 0.89	1654 ± 48.9
c-AMP 0.5 mM	12.0 ± 1.05	1248 ± 30.0
c-AMP 1.0 mM	11.0 ± 1.00	1117 ± 40.0
c-AMP 2.0 mM	8.0 ± 0.81	842 ± 43.5

[a]Results are expressed as means ± SD of five determinations. Activities are calculated as mμmoles product formed/mg protein/min.

[b]ICD: NAD$^+$ isocitrate dehydrogenase EC 1.1.1.41 Plaut (31).

[c]MDH: NAD$^+$ malate dehydrogenase EC 1.1.1.37 Kitto (32).

All the methods used were based on the measurement of the increase in optical density at 340 mμ due to the reduction of NADP$^+$ or NAD$^+$ in the presence of enzyme and an adequate substrate. In the case of NAD$^+$ malate dehydrogenase the rate of oxidation of NADH at 340 mμ was recorded since the equilibrium position of this reaction markedly favors the reduction of oxalocetate to malate. Isocitrate may be oxidized by a $NADP^+$-dependent isocitric dehydrogenase which is mainly a supernatant enzyme and by a NAD^+ isocitric dehydrogenase which is located in mitochondria (33). For the estimation of NAD^+ isicitric dehydrogenase, mitochondria were depleted of endogenous pyridine nucleotide by preincubation at 30 C in a medium containing 0.25M sucrose and 0.05M phosphate. This treatment leads to loss of mitochondrial pyridine nucleotides in general and in particular of mitochondrial NAD^+ (34). It was assumed that endogenous $NADP^+$ was also destroyed under these conditions since these mitochondria did not decolorize 2,6-dichloro-phenolindophenol in the presence of isocitrate unless a catalytic amount of $NADP^+$ was added.

The results illustrated in Tables II and III confirm previous data (35) and demonstrate the presence in testicular tissue of higher amounts of $NADP^+$ isocitric dehydrogenase and malic enzyme than that of G-6-PD and 6-phospho-gluconate dehydrogenase (6-PGD). Also it shows that isocitrate may be oxidized in rat testis mitochondria by NAD^+-dependent isocitric dehydrogenase and that the mitochondrion contains large amounts of NAD^+ malate dehydrogenase.

Cyclic-AMP used at concentrations of 0.2 to 2.0 mM had no effect on $NADP^+$-linked dehydrogenases (Table II) whereas the mitochondrial NAD^+-linked dehydrogenases (isocitrate and malate) were inhibited by cyclic-AMP. (Table III) As in the case of NAD^+ dependent steroid dehydrogenase the cyclic nucleotide inhibited the NAD^+-dependent dehydrogenase of the citric acid and had no effect on $NADP^+$-linked dehydrogenases tested. The inhibitory effect on NAD^+ malate dehydrogenase might be of some physiological importance since malate and oxaloacetate might act as carriers of hydrogen equivalent between mitochondria and cytoplasm. NADH in one compartment is taken to react with oxaloacetate; the malate formed traverses the mitochondrial membrane and reacts in other compartments with NAD^+ to generate NADH and oxaloacetate. Since cyclic-AMP inhibits the NAD^+ malate dehydrogenase, the malate available in the cytoplasm might be decarboxylated by the malic enzyme and this reaction will generate NADPH. This will increase the formation of NADPH at the expense of NADH and this increase in NADPH biosynthesis could be used in steroidogenesis. An inhibitory effect by cyclic-AMP on the oxidation of NADH in bovine adrenal cortex was recently demonstrated (36). This observation as well as the present findings might indicate a role of this nucleotide in controlling the cellular levels of pyridine nucleotides.

ACKNOWLEDGMENT

This investigation was supported by Ford Foundation grant 670-0470. The technical assistance of Mrs. M. Kaufman and Mrs. V. Rotary is gratefully acknowledged.

REFERENCES

1. Grahame-Smith, D. G., R. W. Butcher, R. L. Ney, and E. W. Sutherland, J Biol Chem 242:5535, 1967.

2. Marsh, J. M., and K. Savard, Steroids 8:133, 1966.

3. Dorrington, J. H., and B. Baggett, Endocrinology 84:989, 1969.

4. Murad, F., B. S. Strauch, and M. Vaughan, Biochim Biophys Acta 177:591, 1969.

5. Karaboyas, G. C., and S. B. Koritz, Biochemistry 4:462, 1965.

6. Koritz, S. B., J. Yun, and J. J. Ferguson, Jr., Endocrinology 82:620, 1968.

7. Sulimovici, S., and G. S. Boyd, Eur J Biochem 7:549, 1969.

8. McCune, R. W., S. Roberts, and P. L. Young, J Biol Chem 245:3859, 1970.

9. Sulimovici, S., and G. S. Boyd, Eur J. Biochem 3:332, 1968.

10. Beyer, K. F., and L. T. Samuels, J Biol Chem 219:69, 1956.

11. Roberts, S., R. W. McCune, J. E. Creange, and P. L. Young, Science 158:372, 1967.

12. Sulimovici, S., and B. Lunenfeld, Hormone Metab Res 3:114, 1971.

13. Haynes, R. C., Jr., E. W. Sutherland, and T. W. Rall, Rec. Prog Hormone Res 16:121, 1960.

14. Marsh, J. M., R. W. Butcher, K. Savard, and E. W. Sutherland, J Biol Chem 241:5436, 1966.

15. Posternak, Th., E. W. Sutherland, and W. F. Henion, Biochim Biophys Acta 65:558, 1962.

16. Butcher, R. W., R. J. Ho, H. C. Meng, and E. W. Sutherland, J Biol Chem 240:4515, 1965.

17. Swislocki, N. I., Anal Biochem 38:260, 1970.

18. Samuels, L. T., and M. L. Helmreich, Endocrinology 58:435, 1956.

19. Handler, R. P., and E. D. Bransome, Jr., J. Clin Endocrinol 29:1117, 1969.

20. Ewald, W., H. Werbin, and I. L. Chaikoff, Steroids 4:759, 1964.

21. Cheatum, S. G., and J. C. Warren, Biochim Biophys Acta 122:1, 1966.

22. Neville, A. M., J. C. Orr, and L. L. Engel, J Endocrinol 43:599, 1969.

23. Kruskemper, H. L., E. Forchielli, and H. G. Ringold, Steroids 3:295, 1964.

24. Ewald, W., H. Werbin, and I. L. Chaikoff, Biochim Biophys Acta 111:306, 1965.

25. Oleinick, N. L., and S. B. Koritz, Biochemistry 5:715, 1966.

26. Savard, K., J. M. Marsh, and D. S. Howel, Endocrinology 73:554, 1963.

27. Flint A. P. F., and R. M. Denton, Biochem J 117:73, 1970.

28. Glock, G. E., and P. McLean, Biochem J 55:400, 1953.

29. Ochoa, S., in S. P. Colowick, and N. O. Kaplan (Eds.), Methods in Enzymology, Vol. I, Academic, New York, 1955, p. 699.

30. Ochoa, S., in S. P. Colowick, and N. O. Kaplan (Eds.), Methods in Enzymology, Vol. I, Academic, New York, 1955, p. 739.

31. Plaut, G. W. E., in S. P. Colowick, N. O. Kaplan, and J. M. Lowenstein (Eds.), Methods in Enzymology, Vol. XIII, Academic, New York and London, 1969, p. 34.

32. Kitto, G. B., in S. P. Colowick, N. O. Kaplan, and J. M. Lowenstein (Eds.), Methods in Enzymology, Vol. XIII, Academic, New York and London, 1969, p. 106.

33. Goebell, H., and M. Klingenberg, Biochem Biophys Res Commun 13:209, 1963.

34. Ernster, L., and A. J. Glasky, Biochem Biophys Acta 38:168, 1960.

35. Lunaas, T., R. L. Baldwin, and P. T. Cupps, J Reprod Fert 17:177, 1968.
36. Akhtar, M., D. P. Bloxham, and P. C. Poat, Int J Biochem 1:381, 1970.

24. Stimulation by Gonadotropins and their Subunits of a Multiple Receptor Adenyl Cyclase from an Adrenocortical Cancer

Immanuel Schorr, P. Rathnam, B. B. Saxena[1] and Robert L. Ney

ACTH stimulates adenyl cyclase activity in normal rat adrenals, while other hormones are without effect. Studies of the properties of the adenyl cyclase of a corticosterone-producing rat adrenocortical carcinoma revealed that it responded not only to ACTH, but unexpectedly to TSH, epinephrine, and norepinephrine as well (1). The tumor cyclase was not stimulated by a number of other polypeptide hormones, including glucagon, vasopressin, thyrocalcitonin, and parathyroid hormone. Preparations of LH and FSH derived from bovine, ovine, and porcine pituitaries increased the activity of the tumor cyclase (1). However, these gonadotropin preparations contained contaminating TSH in sufficient quantities to make it uncertain whether the tumor responses were due to the gonadotropins or to TSH. We have, therefore, tested the effects of highly purified preparations of human pituitary LH and FSH (2, 3). These hormones are each composed of 2 chains (4, 5), designated as α and β subunits. The α subunit is homologous for the two hormones, while the β subunit is hormone specific (6). In addition to studying the parent hormones, we have examined effects of these subunits on the adrenocortical cancer adenyl cyclase.

[1]Career Scientist Awardee, Health Research Council of the City of New York, Contract I-621.

MATERIALS AND METHODS

Rat adrenocortical carcinoma 494, originally found by Snell and Stewart, was maintained by transplantation in male Sprague-Dawley rats as described before (7). The tumor has been shown to produce corticosterone (8).

The tissue was homogenized in a buffer composed of Tris (hydroxymethyl)-aminomethane (HCl) 62.2mM and theophylline 15.5mM at pH 7.4. The homogenate was centrifuged at 1000 × g for 10 min. The sediment, resuspended in the buffer, was then used for the adenyl cyclase assay. This 1000 × g particulate fraction has previously been shown to possess the highest cyclase activity of any fraction obtained by differential centrifugation (1). The vessel with the tissue preparation was maintained at 4 C throughout these steps.

The adenyl cyclase assay was based on the conversion of α-^{32}P-ATP to ^{32}P-cyclic-AMP. Cyclic-AMP uniformly labeled with tritium was added to the reaction mixture to allow correction for losses during the assay. The details of the assay have been described in a previous publication (1). Adenyl cyclase activity is expressed as picomoles cyclic-AMP formed/mg protein/20 min. Protein concentrations were determined by the method of Lowry et al. (9).

Purified LH and FSH and their α and β subunits were prepared by previously described methods (2-5) from human pituitaries provided by the National Pituitary Agency. The preparations were assayed for LH activity by the ovarian ascorbic acid depletion method (10) and for FSH activity by the ovarian augmentation assay (11). The units of activity in Tables I and II are based on the standards NIH-LH-Sl and NIH-FSH-Sl.[2] In testing the compounds in the adenyl cyclase assay, starting hormone concentrations of known weight and potency, as determined in the FSH and LH bioassays, were diluted tenfold serially. Each hormone concentration was not tested for potency in the LH and FSH bioassays; values listed in Tables I and II were calculated from the known potency of the starting compound. Each concentration of the hormones, however, was tested for effects on the adrenocortical cancer adenyl cyclase.

RESULTS

Human pituitary LH and its β subunit clearly stimulated the adenyl cyclase of the adrenocortical cancer whereas the α subunit had a lesser effect (Fig. 1). Table I summarizes the results of these experiments. Hormone concentrations are shown as the actual w/v ratios employed, as well as in approximate moles/l. The latter was calculated using a molecular weight of approximately 28,000 for LH, which is close to current estimates for this hormone in the human (3). Molecular weight of half this amount were used in calculating subunit concentrations in moles/l (13). The table shows the LH activity which would be

[2]In the FSH assay, one NIH-FSH-Sl Unit equals 26.5 IU 2nd IRP-HMG. In the LH assay, one NIH-LH-Sl equals 588 IU of 2nd IRP-HMG (12).

TABLE I. Effects of preparations of LH and its subunits on the adrenocortical cancer adenyl cyclase

Compound tested	mg/ml	moles/l[a]	LH activity U/ml[b]	Adenyl cyclase pmoles cyclic AMP/mg protein/20 min[c]
None	0	0	0	489
LH	0.00035	10^{-8}	0.0035	554
LH	0.0035	10^{-7}	0.035	483
LH	0.035	10^{-6}	0.35	1102
LH	0.35	10^{-5}	3.5	1558
α subunit	0.0035	2×10^{-7}	0.0027	425
α subunit	0.035	2×10^{-6}	0.027	434
α subunit	0.35	2×10^{-5}	0.27	644
β subunit	0.0035	2×10^{-7}	0.0074	380
β subunit	0.035	2×10^{-6}	0.074	418
β subunit	0.35	2×10^{-5}	0.74	1134

[a]Moles/l calculated assuming mol wt of LH of 30,000 and 15,000 for each subunit.

[b]One U NIH-LH-S1 equals 588 IU 2nd IRP-HMG by ovarian ascorbic acid depletion assay (12).

[c]Mean of duplicates not deviating more than 5% from the mean.

present at each concentration of each preparation, calculated from the known potency of the compounds employed. Finally the table shows the tumor adenyl cyclase activity which was observed at each hormone concentration. It can be seen that the lowest active concentration of LH in stimulating tumor cyclase was about 10^{-6} moles/l, similar to the lowest active concentrations of ACTH, TSH, epinephrine, and norepinephrine (1). The β subunit of LH was considerably less potent both in LH activity and in the tumor cyclase assay, although a clear stimulation in the latter was seen at about 2×10^{-5} moles/l. The α subunit produced only a small stimulatory effect at this concentration.

Human pituitary FSH also stimulated the tumor adenyl cyclase (Fig. 2), although the magnitude of the effect was less than that seen with comparable quantities of LH. The enzyme activity was increased by the β subunit of FSH, but only at the highest concentrations tested (Fig. 2). The α subunit was not stimulatory at any concentration, and was actually inhibitory at the highest concentration. The data for FSH and its subunits are summarized in Table II. In calculating the hormone concentrations on a moles/liter basis, a molecular weight for human FSH of 32,000 has been used (14). Calculations of concentrations of the FSH subunits on a moles/l basis have been arbitrarily

TABLE II. Effects of preparations of FSH and its subunits on the adrenocortical cancer adenyl cyclase

Compound tested	mg/ml	moles/l[a]	FSH activity U/ml[b]	Adenyl cyclase pmoles cyclic AMP/mg protein/20 min[c]
None	0	0	0	435
FSH	0.000015	0.5×10^{-9}	0.0023	478
FSH	0.00015	0.5×10^{-8}	0.023	488
FSH	0.0015	0.5×10^{-7}	0.23	456
FSH	0.015	0.5×10^{-6}	2.3	577
FSH	0.15	0.5×10^{-5}	23.0	618
α subunit	0.003	2×10^{-7}	0.009	317
α subunit	0.03	2×10^{-6}	0.09	353
α subunit	0.3	2×10^{-5}	0.9	44
β subunit	0.003	2×10^{-7}	0.036	344
β subunit	0.03	2×10^{-6}	0.36	391
β subunit	0.3	2×10^{-5}	3.6	667

[a]Moles/liter calculated assuming mol wt of FSH of 30,000 and 15,000 for each subunit.

[b]One U NIH-FSH-S1 equals 26.5 IU 2nd IRP-HMG by ovarian augmentation assay (12).

[c]Mean of duplicates not deviating more than 5% from the mean.

based on molecular weights half that of the parent hormone. The lowest active concentration of FSH in stimulating tumor adenyl cyclase activity was about 0.5×10^{-6} moles/l, similar to the concentrations of ACTH, TSH, catecholamines, and LH which stimulate the tumor enzyme. The β subunit which was much less active in the FSH bioassay, was also less potent in the tumor cyclase assay.

DISCUSSION

Previous studies showed that the adenyl cyclase of a transplanted corticosterone-producing rat adrenal carcinoma was stimulated by TSH, epinephrine, and norepinephrine, as well as by ACTH (1). In addition, preparations of LH and FSH derived from bovine, ovine, and porcine pituitaries stimulated the tumor cyclase. The tumor response was not completely without specificity, however, since there was no effect of vasopressin, thyrocalcitonin, parathyroid hormone, glucagon, and several other polypeptide hormones. Other than ACTH, no hormone preparation even at high concentrations stimulated normal adrenal adenyl cyclase. It is therefore highly unlikely that any of the stimulatory effects of the hormones on the tumor cyclase can be ascribed to contamination by ACTH.

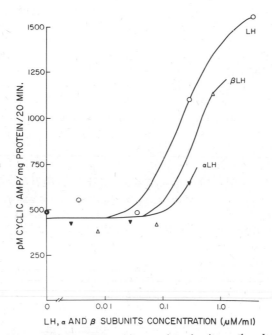

FIG. 1. Effects of human pituitary LH and its α and β subunits on the adrenocortical cancer adenyl cyclase. Hormone concentration is shown on a log scale on the abscissa and adenyl cyclase activity is shown on the ordinate.

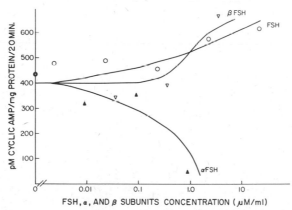

FIG. 2. Effects of human pituitary FSH and its α and β subunits on the adrenocortical cancer adenyl cyclase. Hormone concentration is shown on a log scale on the abscissa and adenyl cyclase activity is shown on the ordinate.

305

More recent evidence suggests that the tumor adenyl cyclase does not possess a single degenerate adenyl cyclase hormone receptor which responds to many substances, but rather that it possesses multiple specific hormone receptors (15). For example, the effects of the catecholamines are inhibited by propranolol but not by phentolamine. Propranolol does not interfere with the stimulatory effects of ACTH, TSH, LH, or FSH on the tumor cyclase. It thus appears that the tumor possesses a specific β-adrenergic receptor.

Since the LH and FSH preparations used in our initial studies contained considerable quantities of contaminating TSH (1), we could not exclude the possibility that the responses to the gonadotropin preparations were due to the TSH contained in them. The present studies were therefore undertaken employing highly purified human pituitary LH and FSH and their α and β subunits. LH produced marked increases in tumor cyclase activity. Its β subunit was also active, although it was less potent in the LH bioassay and the adrenal tumor adenyl cyclase assay than the parent hormone. The α subunit possessed less activity than the β subunit in both assays. It is noteworthy that the lowest active concentration of LH was approximately 10^{-6} moles/l, similar to that observed for ACTH, TSH, epinephrine, and norepinephrine (1). The high degree of purity of the LH preparations (3) supports the concept that their effects on the tumor cyclase are intrinsic to LH and not due to hormone contaminants.

FSH also stimulated the tumor cyclase, although to a lesser extent than LH. The β subunit of FSH stimulated the cyclase, but only at the highest concentration tested. For reasons that are not clear at present, the α subunit at high concentrations repeatedly inhibited the tumor cyclase. Once again, it is to be noted that the lowest active concentration of FSH, about 10^{-6} moles/l, was similar to that noted for the other hormones which stimulate the tumor cyclase. The high degree of purity of the FSH preparations (2) suggests that the observed responses are intrinsic to FSH, and not due to contaminants.

The possibility of cross-contamination of the different subunit preparations might be raised. For example, the small amount of activity noted in the α subunit of LH could be due to a small amount of contamination by the β subunit of LH. It is probable, however, that the activities of the β subunits of LH and FSH can not be ascribed to contamination by their corresponding α subunits which possess little or no stimulatory activity in the adrenal tumor adenyl cyclase assay. In fact the divergent effects of the subunits of FSH (stimulation by the β subunit and inhibition by the α subunit) makes the possibility of any significant cross-contamination unlikely.

The present results taken together with those of earlier experiments (1) suggest that the tumor cyclase possesses receptors for ACTH, TSH, LH, FSH, and catecholamines with β-adrenergic activity. Since the effects of these hormones are not additive (1, 15), the different hormone receptors probably regulate a common cyclase catalytic unit.

Current evidence suggests that in a given species the β subunit of LH and the β subunit of FSH are hormone specific, while the α subunit of LH is homologous to the α subunit of FSH (6). In addition, the α subunit of LH has been shown to be homologous to the α subunit of TSH (16). It is of interest that the activity of the gonadotropins in stimulating the adrenal tumor adenyl cyclase appears to be associated predominantly with the β subunit of each hormone. These results are in keeping with the concept that different receptors are involved for the different gonadotropins, rather than a common receptor which interacts with a homologous α subunit of LH and FSH. It is noteworthy, that while LH has been found to stimulate adenyl cyclase in homogenates of the ovary (17), FSH has been inactive in these preparations.

The physiological significance of the responses of the tumor adenyl cyclase to hormones other than ACTH remains to be determined. For example, although corticosterone produced by the tumor suppresses ACTH secretion in tumor-bearing animals (7), it is possible that the other hormones might regulate tumor cyclic-AMP levels and thereby control steroidogenesis.

ACKNOWLEDGMENT

These investigations were supported by the following grants: P-537 from the American Cancer Society; CA-10408 from the National Institutes of Health; 5T01 AM 05574 from the National Institutes of Health; IN 15-L from the American Cancer Society; and M-70.13 from The Population Council, Rockefeller University, New York.

REFERENCES

1. Schon, I., and R. L. Ney, J Clin Invest 50:1295, 1971.
2. Saxena, B. B., and P. Rathnam, J Biol Chem 242:3769, 1967.
3. Rathnam, P., and B. B. Saxena, J Biol Chem 245:3725, 1970.
4. Saxena, B. B., and P. Rathnam, Fed Proc 30:473, 1971.
5. Saxena, B. B., and P. Rathnam, J Biol Chem 246:3549, 1971.
6. Saxena, B. B., and P. Rathnam, Second International Symposium on Protein and Polypeptide Hormones, Liege, Belgium, in press, 1971.
7. Ney, R. L., N. J. Hochella, D. G. Grahame-Smith, R. N. Dexter, and R. W. Butcher, J Clin Invest 48:1733, 1969.
8. Johnson, D. F., K. C. Snell, D. Francois, and E. Heftmann, Acta Endocrinol 37:329, 1961.
9. Lowry, O. H., N. J. Rosenbrough, A. L. Farr, and R. J. Randall, J Biol Chem 193:265, 1951.
10. Parlow, A. F., in A. Albert (Ed.), Human Pituitary Gonadotropins, Charles C Thomas, Springfield, Ill., 1961, p. 300.
11. Steelman, S. L., and F. M. Pohley, Endocrinology 53:604, 1953.
12. Rosemberg, E., in E. Rosemberg (Ed.), Gonadotropins, Geron-X, Inc., Los Altos, 1968, p. 387.
13. Reichert, L. E., Jr., M. A. Rasco, D. N. Ward, G. D. Niswender, and A. R. Midgley, Jr., J Biol Chem 244:5110, 1969.

14. Odell, W. D., R. W. Swain, and M. Nydick, J Clin Endocrinol 24:1266, 1964.
15. Schorr, I., B. B. Saxena, and R. L. Ney, in preparation.
16. Pierce, J. G., T. H. Liao, R. B. Carlsen, and T. Reimo, J Biol Chem 246:866, 1971.
17. Dorrington, J. H., and B. Baggett, Endocrinology 84:989, 1969.

25. Effects of Gonadotropins on Placental Steroidogenesis

Claude A. Villee and Steven G. Gabbe

The placenta is unique among endocrine glands in that it both produces a gonadotropin and also may serve as a possible target organ of that hormone. Luteinizing hormone has been shown to regulate steroidogenesis in the ovaries (1). The placenta plays a key role in steroidogenesis in the pregnant woman and it would seem reasonable to suppose that one or more aspects of the process of steroidogenesis in the placenta may be regulated by the chorionic gonadotropin synthesized by the placenta. It has been demonstrated that the placenta has the entire complement of enzymes needed to synthesize progesterone from acetate or mevalonate (2, 3). It lacks the 17, 20 desmolase (4) and therefore cannot convert C_{21} steroids to C_{19} steroids, but it does have a remarkably effective aromatization system for the production of C_{18} estrogens from C_{19} androgens (5).

Attempts to demonstrate an effect of HCG on some aspect of placental metabolism have given conflicting results. These may be due to varying amounts of endogenous HCG present in the placenta at the beginning of the experiment or to varying amounts of HCG synthesized by the placenta in the course of an experiment, especially if the placenta is perfused over a long time. The circulatory system on the fetal side of the placenta is closed anatomically and can be readily cannulated through the umbilical artery and vein. This makes the placenta particularly suitable for perfusion experiments. The perfusion of the maternal side of the placenta is a much more difficult operation but has been accomplished successfully by perfusion systems such as that of Krantz (6). In Sweden, Cassmer (7) and Diczfalusy (8) have perfused human placentas through

309

the umbilical artery and vein while it is still in its normal place in the uterus. These experiments were conducted after the fetus had been removed in the course of a legal abortion.

In experiments with the perfused placenta at term Levitz and his co-workers (9) found that neither HCG nor ACTH had any effect on the conversion of ^{14}C-mevalonate to squalene or lanosterol. Villee, van Leusden, and Zeleswki (10) carried out a series of incubations of minced term placenta with ^{14}-acetate and found that they recovered less ^{14}C-cholesterol from those incubations that contained HCG than from paired incubations to which no HCG had been added (Table I). This finding led to the inference that HCG stimulates the conversion of cholesterol to products such as pregnenolone and progesterone and was consistent with the finding of Levitz and others that HCG is without effect on the synthesis of sterols from mevalonate.

TABLE I. Incorporation of ^{14}C from 1-^{14}C-acetate into total sterols and cholesterol by minced human placenta[a]

| | | Percent 1-^{14}C-acetate incorporated | | |
| | | | Cholesterol | |
1-^{14}C-acetate added	IU HCG added	Total sterols	I	II
Initially	0	0.118	0.005	0.004
Initially	250	0.091	0.005	0.004
30 min intervals	0	0.136	0.003	0.003
30 min intervals	250	0.118	0.002	0.002

[a]Incubation of 10 g minced placenta in 10 ml of incubation medium for 2 hr (I) or 2.5 hr (II) with 500 μCi 1-^{14}C-acetate added either at the beginning of incubation or in four equal amounts at 0, 30, 60, and 90 min. 7α-^{3}H-Cholesterol was added after incubation.

There are several isolated clinical observations which are consistent with this hypothesis. It is known for example that the concentration of HCG in the serum and in the placenta is greatest during the ninth and tenth weeks of pregnancy (11). Subsequently the concentration of HCG in both placenta and blood decreases. It is at this same time in gestation that the concentration of progesterone in the placenta reaches its peak (11). During dilation of the cervix prior to a therapeutic abortion in the first trimester of pregnancy the concentrations of both HCG and progesterone in the blood increase. Fylling (12) has suggested that an increase in HCG production that occurs secondarily to a release of oxytocin or vasopressin might stimulate the synthesis of progesterone in the placenta.

In their early experiments Levitz, Condon, and Dancis (13) perfused isolated cotyledons of term placentas. Subsequently Troen (14) and Cedard (15) have perfused entire term or early placentas. Cedard has carried out an extensive series of placental perfusions. In her initial perfusion experiments she found that when estradiol and chorionic gonadotropin were added to the perfusion fluid a substance was released into the fluid which resembled estriol. When the steroid extract of the perfusion mixture was subjected to countercurrent distribution, the peak of fluorescence had a partition coefficient identical with that of estriol. The addition of 20 mg of estrone or estradiol to the perfusion fluid increased the amount of estriol obtained subsequently from the perfusions. When 20,000 IU HCG was added in addition to the estradiol a fivefold increase in the estriol content of the perfusion fluid was observed. The addition of HCG without estradiol did not increase the amount of estriol recovered. Certain findings in these investigations deserve a thorough critical review. The amount of estriol in the presence of estradiol and HCG is only slightly more than that found during the fourth hour of a controlled perfusion to which no hormones have been added. Only 5% of the estrogens in the perfusion fluid are estriol. This value is quite different from the percentage found in the urine of a pregnant woman, in which some 95% of the estrogens are estriol. Bolté and co-workers (16) could find no evidence for 16-hydroxylation after in situ perfusion of placentas of 17 to 20 weeks gestation with estradiol. They could find no evidence for conversion of estradiol to estriol. In unpublished experiments from our own laboratory carried out some ten years ago, we found no evidence for 16-hydroxylation of estradiol by placental minces or homogenates from term or young placentas. Bolté and his colleagues were unable to demonstrate any stimulatory effects of chorionic gonadotropin on the metabolism of their 17- to 20-week placentas perfused for short periods in situ.

In another series of experiments Cedard et al. (17) found a large conversion of 16α-hydroxyestrone to estriol by perfused placenta. In the same series of experiments 16α-hydroxyandrostenedione or 16α-hydroxytestosterone added to the perfusion liquid resulted in the appearance of large amounts of estriol. The conversion of precursor to estriol was much greater in those perfusions to which human chorionic gonadotropin was added at zero time, than in paired perfusions to which no HCG was added. The sixteen hydroxylations of the neutral steroids that serve as precursors of estrogens have been clearly shown to occur in the fetal adrenal by D. B. Villee and her associates (18).

In further perfusion experiments Cedard (19) has found that 19-hydroxy-androstenedione is a much more effective precursor of estrogens than was testosterone or androstendione. Dehydroepiandrosterone was nearly as effective a precursor as 19-hydroxyandrostendione and was converted to estrogen as nearly twice as fast as testosterone. The amount of estrone and estradiol isolated from the perfusion fluid increased linearly with the amount of dehydroepian-drosterone added as substrate. Although the addition of 20,000 IU HCG to the perfusion fluid increased the very small conversion of androstenedione or androstenediol to estrogens found in control perfusions, it had only a minimal effect on the conversion of dehydroepiandrosterone and no effect at all on the conversion of 19-hydroxy-Δ^4-androstenedione. This finding led Cedard to infer that HCG has an effect on the hydroxylation of androstenedione at carbon 19 and that it may do this by some effect on the generation of TPNH, the cofactor required for hydroxylation. This theory then parallels the suggestion that ACTH regulates the hydroxylation in cholesterol in the adrenal and LH regulates the initial hydroxylation of cholesterol in the ovary. The action of these tropic hormones at this point would explain the increased production of progesterone which follows.

In continuing her investigations Cedard et al. showed that either bovine or human LH would increase the transformation of labeled testosterone into estrone and estradiol. Thus in perfused term placentas either HCG or LH will increase the aromatization of androgens to estrogens. This effect of LH or HCG could be observed with small placentas obtained from first trimester gestations as well as with term placentas. Her perfusion experiments also enabled her to demonstrate an effect of LH or HCG on glycogenolysis (21). This effect again parallels reports (22) that LH increases the phosphorylase activity in luteinized ovaries and thus increases the rate of glycogenolysis. The addition of 50 mg of 3'5'-cyclicAMP to the perfusion increased the production of estrogens from testosterone and also produced a transitory but significant rise in the concentration of glucose in the perfusion fluid. These experiments thus suggest that the effect of LH on the ovary and the stimulation of estrogen production by HCG in the perfused placenta may involve an increase in adenyl cyclase activity and the production of cyclic AMP.

There is a discrepancy in the literature between the investigators who, on the one hand, have looked specifically for 16-hydroxylase activity in the placenta and have been unable to find it, and investigators such as Troen (14) and Cedard et al. (15) who report that when they add estradiol to a perfused placenta there is an increase in estriol in the perfusion fluid. This discrepancy may be more apparent than real as the experiments by Troen (14) and Cedard et al. (15) were carried out with unlabeled materials and their experiments did not necessarily imply that the estriol found in the perfusion fluid came from the estradiol added to the perfusion fluid. There is a large amount of estriol present in placental tissue at term and it is possible that adding estrone or estradiol to the perfusion fluid simply displaces some estriol from receptor proteins present in the placenta. In contrast, in the experiments with 16-hydroxylated neutral steroids, the precursors were labeled. There was clear evidence of conversion of 16-hydroxyandrostenedione to estriol by the perfused placenta and the addition of HCG had a definite stimulatory effect on this reaction.

The effect of HCG on the aromatizing system of the placenta may be compared to the demonstration by Channing (23) that LH stimulates the ovarian aromatizing enzymes when ovarian cells are grown in tissue culture. Another interesting parallel between the effect of HCG on the placenta and of LH on the ovary is the effect on glycogenolysis. This has been shown in the ovary by

Stansfield and Robinson (24), Marsh (22), and Channing and Villee (25), and in the perfused placenta by Cedard et al. (26). In the latter system, Cedard was able to demonstrate that cyclic AMP and theophylline have effects that parallel those of HCG. Thus it seems likely that at least part of the effect of HCG may be mediated by a stimulation of adenyl cyclase to produce cyclic AMP. This in turn increases the activity of placental glycogen phosphorylase and perhaps of other enzymes.

Although isolated placental mitochondria readily convert cholesterol to pregnenolone and progesterone, neither Ryan (27) nor our own laboratory (28) was able to demonstrate any effect of HCG on the rate of cholesterol metabolism by the mitochondrial system. Other studies in our laboratory showed that the conversion of pregnenolone to progesterone by placental homogenates was not influenced by the addition of HCG. The lack of effect of HCG on these cell-free systems is paralleled by the general lack of effect of LH on cell-free systems in the ovary. The positive effects of LH have been observed with minced ovaries or with ovarian cells in tissue culture. The C_{20}-hydroxylation of cholesterol appears to be rate limiting in the conversion of cholesterol to pregnenolone, FSH, LH, and HCG have been shown to increase the activity of these enzymes in preparations from bovine corpora lutea or immature rat testes. Thus if HCG affects placental progesterone synthesis, it seems likely that it would do so by accelerating the conversion of cholesterol to pregnenolone rather than the conversion of pregnenolone to progesterone.

This question has been taken up most recently in our laboratory employing organ culture methods (29) which have been found of use in studying placental metabolism. Placental villi are cultured for 24 hr in the presence of HCG and homogenized and incubated for 1 hr with either 7α-^{3}H-cholesterol or 7α-^{3}H-pregnenolone and added HCG. Preliminary investigations had shown no effect of HCG on the metabolism of either cholesterol (Table II) or pregnenolone (Table III) by homogenized placentas from early pregnancies or term pregnancies. Similarly HCG had no demonstrable effect on the conversion of pregnenolone to progesterone by placental villi in organ culture (Table IV). However, the conversion of cholesterol to pregnenolone and progesterone by term villi was stimulated 25 to 100% when HCG (1 IU/ml) was added to the culture medium and HCG 2.5 IU/ml was added to the incubation medium (Table V).

Thus, in summary, there are very strong parallels between the effects of HCG on placental metabolism and the effects of LH on ovarian metabolism. In both tissues the gonadotropin increases the activity of glycogen phosphorylase, increases the conversion of cholesterol to pregnenolone, and increases the aromatization of C_{19} precursors. In the placenta there is suggestive evidence that this increase in aromatization is restricted to the initial hydroxylation at carbon 19 and that HCG is not effective on any of the steps after the initial hydroxylation. It is possible that the HCG has some effect on hydroxylation processes in general. Both the 20-hydroxylation of cholesterol and the 19-hydroxylation of testosterone or androstenedione require TPNH as cofactor.

TABLE II. Conversion of cholesterol to pregnenolone and progesterone by placental homogenates

Placental homogenate	Controls			HCG added (2.5 IU/ml)		
	Pregnenolone	Progesterone	Total	Pregnenolone	Progesterone	Total
Term	0.466	0.146	0.612 ± 0.189[a]	0.572	0.157	0.729 ± 0.197[a]
11 Weeks	0.435	0.159	0.594 ± 0.174	0.360	0.130	0.490 ± 0.192

[a]Mean ± SE of 3 incubations.

Note: Values are expressed as percent of 7α-^{3}H-cholesterol recovered as each of the products. Homogenates were incubated for 1 hr at 37 C.

TABLE III. Conversion of pregnenolone to progesterone by placental homogenates

Placental homogenate	Controls	HCG added[a]
Term	1.84 ± 0.35[b]	1.52 ± 0.44
16 Week	2.22 ± 0.28	2.64 ± 0.64

[a]25 IU/ml.
[b]Mean ± SE.

Note: 100 μg of pregnenolone was added to each incubation flask. Values are
expressed as percent of 7α-^{3}H-pregnenolone recovered as progesterone. Homogenates incubated 1 hr at 37 C.

TABLE IV. Conversion of pregnenolone to progesterone by placental villi maintained in organ culture 24 hr and incubated for 1 hr

Placental villi	Controls	HCG added[a]
Term	2.13 ± 0.22[b]	1.87 ± 0.36
16 week	2.46 ± 0.31	2.35 ± 0.51

[a]1 IU/ml added to culture medium and 25 IU/ml added to incubation media.
[b]Mean ± SE.

Note: 100 μg of unlabeled pregnenolone was added to each incubation flask.
Tissues were incubated for 1 hr at 37 C. Values are expressed as percent of
7α-^{3}H-pregnenolone.

It is tempting to suppose that the increased TPNH results from increased
dehydrogenation of glucose-6-phosphate, produced in turn by an increased
glycogenolysis resulting from the stimulation of the adenyl cyclase system.
However, there is so little glycogen in either the term placenta or the ovary
that this does not seem very probable. Thus we must look for some other
effect of HCG on the generation of TPNH.

TABLE V. Conversion of cholesterol to pregnenolone and progesterone by placental villi maintained in organ culture 24 hr

	Control			HCG		
	Pregnenolone	Progesterone	Total	Pregnenolone	Progesterone	Total
Term	0.301	0.128	0.429 ± 0.015[a]	0.564	0.167	0.731 ± 0.150[a]

[a]Mean ± SE.

Note: 1 IU/ml HCG in culture medium; 2.5 IU/ml HCG in incubation medium. Tissues were incubated with 7α-^{3}H-cholesterol for 2 hr at 37 C.

REFERENCES

1. Savard, K., J. M. Marsh, and R. L. Howell, Endocrinology 73:554, 1963.
2. Villee, C. A., and S. L. Tsai, in A. Pecile C. Finzy (Eds.), The Foeto-Placental Unit, Excerpta Medica Foundation, Amsterdam, p. 10, 1969.
3. Zelewski, L., and C. A. Villee, Biochemistry 5:1805, 1966.
4. Sobrevilla, L., D. D. Hagerman, and C. A. Villee, Biochim Biophys Acta, 93:665, 1964.
5. Ryan, K. J., J Biol Chem 234:2006, 1959.
6. Krantz, K. E., Proceedings of the 3rd Rochester Trophoblast Conference, 1965, p. 298.
7. Cassmer, O. Acta Endocrinol (Kbh), Suppl 45, 1959.
8. Mikhail, G., N. Wiqvist, and E. Diczfalusy, Acta Endocrinol 42:519, 1963.
9. Levitz, M., G. P. Condon, and J. Dancis, Endocrinology 58:376, 1956.
10. Villee, C. A., H. van Leusden, and L. Zelewski, Advances in Enzyme Regulation, Vol. IV, in G. Weber (Ed.), Pergamon, Oxford and New York, 1966, p. 161.
11. Diczfalusy, E., and P. Troen, Vitamins Hormones 19:229, 1961.
12. Fylling, P., and N. Norman, Acta Endocrinol (Kbh), 65:293, 1970.
13. Levitz, M., G. P. Condon, and J. Dancis, Fed Proc 14:245, 1955.
14. Troen, P., J Clin Endocrinol 21:895, 1961.
15. Cedard, L., J. Varangot, and S. Yannotti, C R Acad Sci 254:1870, 1962.
16. Varangot, J., L. Cedard, and S. Yannotti, Amer J Obst Gyn 92:534, 1965.
17. Villee, D. B., L. L. Engel, J. M. Loring, and C. A. Villee, Endocrinology 69:354, 1961.
18. Cedard, L., J. Varangot, and S. Yannotti, C R Acad Sci 258:3769, 1964.
19. Cedard, L., E. Alsat, C. Ego, and J. Varangot, Steroids 11:179, 1968.
20. Cedard, L., E. Alsat, M. J. Urtasun, and J. Varangot, in A. Pecile and C. Finzy (Eds.), The Foeto-Placental Unit, Excerpta Medica Foundation, Amsterdam, 1969, p. 207.
21. Marsh, J. M., R. W. Butcher, K. Savard, and E. N. Sutherland, J Biol Chem, 241:5436, 1966.
22. Channing, C. P., J Endocrinol 43:415, 1969.
23. Stansfield, D. A., and I. W. Robinson, Endocrinology 76:390, 1965.
24. Channing, C. P., and C. A. Villee, Biochim Biophys Acta 115:205, 1965.
25. Cedard, L., E. Alsat, M. J. Urtasun, and J. Varangot, Steroids 16:361, 1970.
26. Ryan, K. J., R. A. Meigs, and Z. Petro, Amer J Obst Gyn 96:675, 1966.
27. Villee, C. A., C. P. Channing, B. Eckstein, and V. Sulovic, in K. W. McKerns, (Ed.), The Gonads, Appleton-Century-Crofts, New York, 1969, p. 285.
28. Gabbe, S., and C. A. Villee Amer J Obst Gyn, 111:31, 1971.

DISCUSSION

A. ESHKOL. It was encouraging to see Dr. Midgley's interesting autoradiographs with labeled FSH. This hormone is usually neglected in uptake studies. In the past we have had difficulty showing retention of labeled FSH in immature mouse ovaries. On the basis of some studies of the mechanism of action of FSH, mainly on DNA synthesis, we think that we have found some of the reasons for this.

TABLE I. Ovary/plasma ratios of cpm following IV injection of ^{125}I-FSH

Pretreatment	Anti FSH	Time after ^{125}I-FSH injection (min)			
		45	90	180	360
–	–	0.80	0.72	1.27	0.63
HMG (2d)	–	1.40	1.75	1.86	ND[a]
HMG (2d)	+	ND	ND	0.23	ND[a]

[a]ND = not determined.

Table I shows the uptake of labeled FSH in intact 21-day-old mice, expressed as the ratio of ovary/plasma counts. In the nonpretreated animals the ratios were rather low. However, when they received HMG 2 days prior to the ^{125}I-FSH injection, ovarian concentration of radioactivity was significantly higher. The specificity of the uptake was proven by its inhibition by an antiserum to FSH resulting in a ratio as low as 0.23. When HMG was administered only 90 min prior to the administration of labeled FSH, ovarian uptake was also higher than without pretreatment (Table II). However, the uptake was low compared to that observed following the injection of labeled HCG.

TABLE II. Organ/plasma ratios of cpm 90 min after injection

	Ovary	Liver	Gall bladder	Kidney
^{125}I-FSH	1.01	1.67	2.70	4.87
^{125}I-HCG	4.65	0.25	0.33	2.30

A striking difference was also observed in the concentration of radioactive material in the liver which was high after injection of ^{125}I-FSH and low after ^{125}I-HCG. The latter observations might reflect the role of carbohydrates and sialic acid in the metabolism of these gonadotropic hormones.

Autoradiographs of the ovaries showed that FSH was localized in granulosa cells while HCG was found in theca and interstitial cells [A. Eshkol and B. Lunenfeld (Eds.), Protein and Polypeptide Hormones, Plenum, 1968].

P. DONINI. We are also studying the distribution of iodinated FSH in immature rats. I think that it would be interesting to give some specifications on the labeled FSH which was used in these experiments by both ourselves and the group at the Institute of Endocrinology, Tel-Hashomer, Israel. When labeled protein hormones are to be used for physiological studies, the damage due to oxidation and/or radiation should be as low as possible. In our labeling procedure, the percent of utilization of iodine was 76.8%. The SA of the entire protein peak obtained by gel filtration on a Sephadex G-25 column, was 17.1 μCi/μg of FSH; the iodine incorporated was 0.27 atoms/protein molecule, assuming a molecular weight of 30,000. Even though approximately one-third of the injected molecules were labeled, I would like to report the results of the bioassay of ^{125}I-FSH. Unlabeled and labeled hormones were assayed by the Steelman-Pohley method. A 2 + 2 bioassay design and 4 rats/dose were used. Following gel filtration, a 90% recovery of labeled protein and 20% radiation damage was achieved. Assuming a potency of 900 IU/mg (2nd IRP-HMG) for the unlabeled FSH, we injected total doses of 4 or 8 IU FSH plus 40 IU HCG/rat. The animals were killed 72 hr after the first injection. The ovaries of each rat were carefully cleaned and weighed and the incorporated radioactivity was counted. The relative potency of the labeled FSH was found to be 0.80. The dose-response curves did not deviate from parallelism and the precision index was 0.23. The ovarian weight and radioactivity are shown in Table III.

TABLE III. Immunoreactivity of ^{125}I-FSH extracted from rat ovaries

Materials	cpm/tube	cpm bound to antiserum	Binding (%)	Immunoreactivity
^{125}I-FSH for bioassay	3855	1277	33.1	
^{125}I-FSH from ovaries of rats injected with 4 IU	1192	230	19.3	58.4
^{125}I-FSH from ovaries of rats injected with 8 IU	3311	446	13.5	40.7

Furthermore, it was interesting to compare the immunoreactivity of the labeled FSH to that of the ^{125}I-FSH extracted from the ovaries of the animals injected. Aliquots of the labeled FSH solution used for the bioassay and supernatants obtained by centrifuging the ovarian homogenates were incubated with a suitable amount of polymerized anti-FSH serum. The immunoassayable FSH extracted from the ovaries is shown in Table IV. I would like to point out that the immunoreactivity of the labeled FSH extracted from ovaries was about 50% of that obtained from the labeled FSH injected.

TABLE IV. Radioactivity in the ovaries of rats following injection with ^{125}I-FSH

Material injected	Rat no.	Ovarian wt (mg)	Total cpm in ovaries	(cpm/mg) ovarian tissue
4 IU ^{125}I-FSH	1	81.8	4930	60.2
(5.55 μg = 98.2 μCi)	2	32.8	8501	102.7
+ 40 IU HCG	3	63.5	5192	81.8
	4	91.5	5240	57.4
8 IU ^{125}I-FSH	1	202.8	18177	89.6
(11.11 μg = 196 μCi)	2	121.9	15672	128.6
+ 40 IU HCG	3	106.6	13439	126.1
	4	80.6	10312	127.9

R. N. MOUDGAL. I would like to present some data by Dr. Moyle and me relevant to the first three papers presented this morning. Cell suspensions of Leydig tumor cells were exposed to different concentrations of S-LH for a period of 15 min and were then exhaustively washed to remove any nonspecifically bound LH. Incubation of these cells led to steroid synthesis, the amount of steroid formed increasing with time (Fig. 1). Addition of a specific antiserum to S-LH to the incubation flasks led to a drastic reduction in the amount of progesterone synthesized. This suggested that S-LH was retained by the tumor cells even though they had been exhaustively washed and that retention of S-LH was an essential prerequisite for the cells to make steroids. The dilution achieved by washing was of the order of 1 : 100,000 or more and in the absence of binding, this would have put the LH levels well below that essential for eliciting a steroid response. The specific binding of LH to the cells was demonstrated by the use of radioimmunoassay. Thus we were able to show that the Leydig tumor cells in contrast to red blood cells and thymocytes, which were used as controls, retained LH specifically and this capacity could not be removed by dilution. Figure 2 shows the ability of the cells to synthesize testosterone with an excellent correlation between LH binding and the amount of testosterone synthesized. Finally, differential centrifugation of homogenates of cells, exhaustively washed after exposure to LH, showed that 80 to 90% of the LH was specifically retained in the 600 $\times$ g pellet.

D. M. DE KRETSER. I think that in considering the mechanism of action of gonadotropins we should not entirely neglect the male. We have been interested

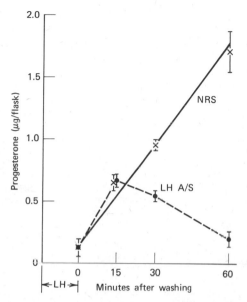

FIG.1. Progesterone synthesis as a function of time. Small clumps of Leydig tumor cells were incubated with 0.5 μg LH/ml at 37 C. After 15 min LH was removed from the tumor cells by centrifugation in 0.9% saline. Duplicate flasks of cells were then reincubated in normal rabbit serum (NRS) or antiserum to LH (LH-A/S) for the time periods indicated. Progesterone was measured by thin layer chromatography and gas chromatography. The vertical bars extent to the values of the SD.

in studying the action of LH and its binding to the interstitial cells of the testis. It has been somewhat complicated because the volume of interstitial cells composes such a small percentage of total testicular volume. Consequently we moved to a system in the rat where the seminiferous tubules were separated by dissection from the interstitial cells; the interstitial cells were incubated with radioactively labeled LH. The localization of labeled LH in the interstitial cells of the testis is clearly seen, especially at higher magnification. Most of this localization is cytoplasmic in nature, the nucleus being entirely free. We are looking at a smear of a cell and the cell membrane covers the nucleus. This area is still relatively free of radioactivity suggesting that the localization of the labeled material is not on the plasma membrane but is probably intracytoplasmic.

Labeled FSH could not be localized to the interstitial cells in a similar system. When the whole testis is homogenized it binds ^{131}I-labeled LH. Unlabeled LH displaces labeled LH and furthermore a nonreactive tissue such as muscle does not bind labeled LH.

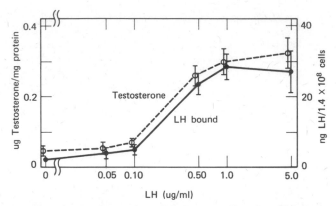

FIG. 2. Testosterone production and LH binding as a function of LH concentration. Testosterone: small pieces of Leydig cell tumors were incubated to triplicate in Krebs-Ringer bicarbonate buffer at 37 C. After 2 hr the tissue was extracted with $CHCl_3$:CH_3OH (2:1) and lipids separated and analyzed by thin layer and gas chromatography. Vertical bars extend to the limits of the SD for triplicate determinations. LH binding: Leydig tumor cells were incubated with varying concentrations of LH in Krebs-Ringer bicarbonate buffer at 37 C. After 15 min the cells were washed by centrifugation in 0.9% saline to remove unbound LH. LH bound to the cells was quantitated by radioimmunoassay. Vertical bars extend to the limits of the SD for triplicate determinations in two experiments averaged at each LH concentration.

E. M. COUTINHO. It may be of interest to those studying the interaction of gonadotropins with the ovary that we have observed and recorded changes in human intraovarian pressure following gonadotropin stimulation. We suspect that one of the earliest effects of these hormones is intumescence of the ovarian follicles.

In some cases fluctuations or rapid changes in pressure have also been recorded suggesting contractile activity, which seem to be correlated with distention of the reticular fibrils surrounding the follicles. A balloon tipped catheter inserted into the ovarian mass was used to measure these pressure changes. The increase in pressure was recorded following the injection of either HCG or HMG. The time interval between injection and the response was found to be 2 to 8 min and the duration 5 to 30 min depending on the dose and whether the injection was intramuscular or intravenous.

CH. V. RAO. I have two questions for Dr. Midgley. Using peroxidase labeled antibody technique, you showed that HCG was present in the cytoplasm of luteal cells. Is the microscopic resolution high enough to say whether HCG is in mitochondria and microsomes? You mentioned that the plasma membranes did not seem to have a specific receptor. Would you please comment on this observation?

A. R. MIDGLEY. I do not mean to imply that the plasma membrane does not have specific receptors. I have only stated that there does not appear to be a differential concentration at the plasma membrane. My personal view at the moment is that the receptors are membrane-bound and that the membrane system on the outside of the cell is continuous with that on the inside of the cell. I tend to believe that the hormone does get inside the cell in an immunologically recognizable form and, once inside, the hormone is probably bound to some of the internal cell membranes as well. I think the same conclusion can be made for the studies shown by Dr. de Kretser. We have not attempted yet to localize the hormone at the subcellular level by ultrastructural examination. We have studied the binding to subcellular components and it is clear from these studies that there is binding to both microsomal and mitochondrial fractions.

M. JUTISZ. I would like to report some results concerning the role of "regulating protein" and molecular oxygen in the mechanism of action of LH. Dr. Hermier and Mr. Combarnous are studying in my laboratory the mechanism of action of ovine LH on the biosynthesis of progesterone in the rat corpus lutea. They used as experimental models ovaries of pseudopregnant rats obtained according to Parlow's technique. The ovaries are sliced and incubated in a Krebs-Ringer-bicarbonate buffer containing 0.2% glucose and 0.5% serum albumin. After 15 to 30 min of preincubation and changing the medium, incubation was carried out for time periods varying from 15 min to 5 hr. At the end of the incubation, tissues were homogenized and total progesterone was assayed.

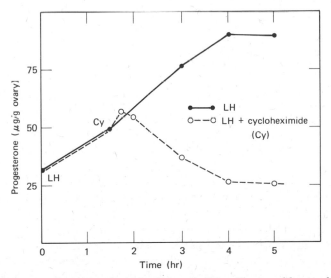

FIG. 3. Comparative kinetics of the action of LH with or without addition of cycloheximide during incubation period. (C. Hermier and M. Jutiz, Biochem Biophys Acta, in press 1971). Reproduced by permission of Elsevier Publishing Company.

Figure 3 shows the kinetics of the synthesis of progesterone in a normally oxygenated medium of 93% O_2 and 7% CO_2. In this experiment LH was added to all media at zero time and cycloheximide into one set of flasks 90 min later. Fifteen to 30 min after the addition of antibiotic, a decrease of progesterone was observed. The decrease might correspond to cessation of synthesis of progesterone and/or to its transformation. Consequently, the synthesis of progesterone depends on the presence of a rapid turnover rate of protein as already shown by Marsh and Savard. The same results were obtained when cyclic AMP was used instead of LH.

Figure 4 shows the result of an experiment in which 2 sets of sliced ovaries were incubated. The same amount of LH was added to all media. Starting from zero time continuous oxygenation was supplied by bubbling a mixture of O_2 and CO_2 in one set of flasks. The second set of flasks, which contained sliced ovaries,

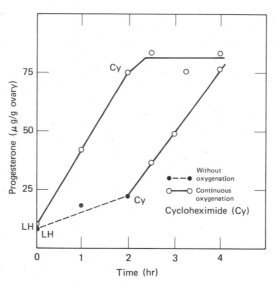

FIG. 4. Comparative kinetics of the action of LH in the presence of cycloheximide in oxygenated or nonoxygenated KRB media. (C. Hermier and M. Jutiz, Biochem Biophys Acta, in press 1971). Reproduced by permission of Elsevier Publishing Company.

was incubated in a nonoxygenated Krebs-Ringer media. After 2 hr incubation, cycloheximide was added to both sets of flasks and continuous oxygenation was established. The results obtained showed that deficiency of O_2 inhibits the synthesis of progesterone in the presence of LH, and that the inhibitory effect of cyclohexamide on the synthesis of progesterone in the presence of LH is suppressed when the antibiotic is added after the tissues have been incubated with LH in a nonoxygenated medium. Identical results were obtained with cyclic AMP instead of LH.

Taking into account all that we know about the mechanism of action of LH and ACTH from the work of others, the following hypothesis on the action of LH may be postulated: LH acts on the adenyl cyclase system producing cyclic AMP which stimulates the synthesis of a protein with a rapid turnover rate and a halflife time of about 8 to 10 min. This step does not require molecular O_2. The "regulating protein" stimulates in some way the interaction between cholesterol and mitochondrial 20α-hydroxylase. This last step requires molecular O_2. It seems that molecular O_2 is also necessary for intramitochondrial reactions leading to the synthesis of progesterone.

F. C. GREENWOOD. Do you know which subunit you are labeling? Is it possible to dissociate LH, label both subunits with iodine, and then recombine?

A. R. MIDGLEY. I don't know. We have attempted to label subunits of HCG kindly supplied by Dr. Bahl with iodine and we have been unable to demonstrate any significant uptake. However, this may only indicate that we have iodination damage and not that the subunits are incapable of binding. It may be worth mentioning that the β subunits of LH, at least, contain only 2 tyrosine moieties. If these tyrosine residues are required for biological activity, the chance of demonstrating β subunit binding might be very low.

J. WEISZ. In addition to concentrating gonadotropins, the ovary appears also to utilize or metabolize these hormones. This is suggested by our findings in 18 normal women of lower levels of LH in ovarian than in peripheral venous blood. Similar findings have been reported by Naftolin and Paulsen. In women receiving contraceptives, on the other hand, there were no differences between the ovarian and peripheral LH levels, suggesting that the utilization of gonadotropins by the ovary depends on its functional and structural state. The situation with respect to FSH is different and intriguing. Although we did not have a sufficient number of samples to be sure, there was a suggestion of cyclic changes in the utilization of FSH by the ovaries.

I have talked with Dr. Midgley about the difficulty of studying uptake of gonadotropins by ovaries that have been taken from an environment that already contained gonadotropins. I wonder, for instance, whether the patchy uptake of labeled gonadotropins by the follicles which appears to be at about the same stage of development, might not be because some perfectly good receptor sites are occupied by endogenous gonadotropins. One way of finding out would be to compare sections prepared with labeled antibody with those prepared with labeled gonadotropin.

H. VAN HELL. I want to ask a question about the first paper after the intermission. One slide showed the effect of LH β and LH α subunits on the amino cyclase. I noticed that the curve of LH β subunit went straight up at a certain dose, the curve of LH α subunit only went up slightly. Are there any more data to show the curve of LH α subunits at higher doses? If the curve of LHα subunit continues to go up a higher doses, the difference between LHα and LHβ subunits is only a factor 10.

I. SCHORR. We did not test these at higher concentrations because we were limited as to the amounts of subunits available. I presume that the subunits were pure. However, there is a slight possibility that the α subunit had some cross-contamination with the β subunit and this could have caused a slight and insignificant rise in the cyclase activity. I think that Dr. Saxena might have some additional comments.

B. B. SAXENA. The subunits used by Dr. Schorr were not purified on Sephadex G-100. However, I doubt that minor contamination, if present, would have affected the results obtained by Dr. Schorr.

F. LEINENBERGER. We have been studying the differential binding of α and β subunits of HCG and bovine LH to rat testicular homogenates and also to interstitial tissue. Labeling the α and β subunits with the Greenwood-Hunter method, we found a difference in uptake of the α and β subunits. The β subunits bound 10 to 20 times better to both tissues than the α subunits. The β subunits also bound significantly better than LH or HCG.

P. TROEN. I am very pleased to hear the discussion of the placenta as an autoregulatory organ with regard to steroidogenesis, a concept which may have great significance. In addition to the areas of action of HCG discussed by Dr. Villee this morning, it is worth emphasizing the role of HCG on hydroxylation mechanisms in the human placenta. We reported in 1959 and 1961 that HCG stimulated formation of ^{14}C-estriol from ^{14}C-estradiol. Despite negative reports from some laboratories, others have subsequently confirmed the presence of 16α-hydroxylation in the human placenta (Jungmann and Schweppe, 1966 and 1967; Slaunwhite et al. 1965). We have also been able to show that 6-hydroxyestradiol is formed and that this substance was not mistaken as estriol in the report by Alonso and Troen, 1966. More recently, Tabei and I (1969) reported stimulation by HCG of 6β-hydroxylation ^{14}C-progesterone by the human placenta.

Antibodies to Gonadotropins

26. Application of Immunologic Techniques to the Study of Gonadotropin Action

Kenneth A. Laurence, K. Loewitt, R. Monastirsky, S. Badawy, H. Hassouna and S. Kim

The role played by the anterior pituitary and its gonadotropins in the reproductive processes has been recognized, documented, and accepted for several decades. Even though there have been some minor differences in opinion as to the mode of action of the gonadotropins, it has been generally accepted that, in the female, FSH brings about the maturation of egg-bearing ovarian follicles and the subsequent growth of the ovary (1). In the male, most studies have indicated that FSH promotes an increase in size of the seminiferous tubules and stimulates spermatogenic activity (2).

It has been similarly accepted that LH in the female promotes the secretion of estrogen, stimulates ovulation, and converts the follicle into a luteinized body (1). In the male, LH promotes maintenance of the interstitial tissue and the subsequent production of androgen by this tissue (1, 3).

These gonadotropin activities have been delineated by studies in which intact immature or adult hypophysectomized animals have been the test animals. Obviously, the use of immature animals for evaluation and discrimination of gonadotrophic activity cannot discount the effects of endogenous hormones nor can the removal of the entire pituitary gland be counted upon to distinguish absolutely the interrelationship of one gonadotropin to another and to the other hormones known to exist in this gland, or to assess the total possible physiologic effect on the reproductive and nonreproductive organs.

The ability to recognize the physiological effects of a single trophic hormone in an intact mature animal requires a special technique with known specificity. The tools and technique of immunology, whose very foundation as a science are

329

dependent upon such specificity of biologic and chemical reactions, should fill this niche.

Immunotechnique, however, have only recently been systematically applied to the study of endocrinology. The development of immunoendocrinology had to await the development of the physicochemical sciences and the ability to separate and purify the hormonal and antigenic molecules of the gonadotropins.

Some progress has been made in the last decade which now permits immunologic procedures to be applied to the entire process of reproduction. With the knowledge and understanding that the pituitary hormones are not yet immunologically homogeneous antigens, studies are now underway which have been designed to verify assumptions made earlier, and to open up new avenues of study on the mode of action of the gonadotropins in relation to reproduction.

The following is an attempt to demonstrate those specific steps of reproduction that have recently been studied immunologically through which, in the future, the mode of action of gonadotropins may be determined.

PHYSIOLOGIC EFFECTS OF IMMUNOLOGIC NEUTRALIZATION OF THE GONADOTROPINS IN THE MALE

The active immunization of the adult male rabbit and rat with ovine or bovine LH in Freund's adjuvant results in serologically detectable antibodies to the hormone (4, 5). Concomitant with the rise in antibovine LH levels, a series of events occur in the donor animals which lend support to the concept that LH is the gonadotropin responsible for maintenance and repair of the interstitial tissue of the testes and maintenance of the libido. The most dramatic biologic effect of the production of anti-LH was the rapid diminution of the sexual appetite of the immunized rabbit. Within 3 to 5 weeks of the initial immunization, every male so immunized failed to service an artificial vagina which it had previously served thrice weekly. Histological examination of the testes at this time revealed a change in the appearance of the interstitial tissue. Instead of compact islands of Leydig cells, the interstitial tissue was seen to be extensively fibroblastic in character. The alteration of morphology and function of this tissue was to be expected, for it has long been assumed and demonstrated that the interstitial tissue is under the influence of this hormone. What was not expected, however, was the uniform exfoliation of germinal elements and longstanding interruption of spermatogenesis. The testes weight was generally one-tenth the weight of adjuvant control. It became apparent that the neutralization of endogenous LH by the antibody to bovine LH reduced the activity of the Δ^5-3β-hydroxy steroid dehydrogenase (Δ^5-3β-OHSDH) and, as a result, androgen production was held to a minimum. Accompanying the loss of enzyme activity was the occurrence of Sudan IV positive droplets within the tubules. In addition, an abnormally large PAS positive zone could be visualized.

These observations suggested that antibody neutralization of endogenous LH prevented the synthesis of at least one enzyme system responsible for androgen production, which in turn adversely affected the libido and subsequently spermatogenesis.

More surprising, however, is the fact that extensive immunization of the male with FSH does not result in the termination of spermatogenesis. One might explain this lack of effectiveness of anti—FSH in respect to the inability of the antibody to sufficiently sequester all of the FSH released by the pituitary and thereby not interfere with spermatogenesis. To study this phenomenon further, our laboratory shifted its attention to the possibilities of examining the role of the gonadotropins in terms of their biologic effect on the maturation of the gonads and what influence specific antibodies to either FSH or LH would have on delaying puberty.

This was accomplished by creating a condition of immunologic unresponsiveness to rabbit anti-LH or rabbit anti-FSH in newborn male and female rats (6). By preventing the recipients from producing antibody to the passively administered antiserum, it was possible to neutralize, on a daily basis, the biologic activity of the endogenous gonadotropins as they are released from the pituitary for as long as desired.

The results of administering either anti-LH or anti-FSH over a period of 35 consecutive days indicated that the anti-LH, but not anti-FSH, prevented spermatogenesis. The testes of anti-LH treated male rats remained infantile, weighing about 0.2 g, with only spermatogonia present. The Δ^5-3β-OHSDH activity, if any, remained minimal and generally below threshold levels of detection (7). On the other hand, the anti-FSH did not affect Δ^5-3β-OHSDH, or spermatogenesis. The testes were, however, somewhat smaller than those control animals which had received normal rabbit serum in the same amount and quantity. As might be expected, pituitary weights of males treated with anti-LH and anti-FSH after five weeks of treatment were enlarged as compared to the controls. The weight of the pituitaries approached the pituitary weight of animals castrated at birth.

This study would thus suggest that LH is the predominant gonadotropin required for testes maturation, spermatogenesis, and the development of the adrenal glands, probably through its stimulation of the interstitial tissue and its subsequent production of androgens.

PHYSIOLOGIC EFFECTS OF ANTIGONADOTROPINS IN THE FEMALE

It has been well documented that antigonadotropins, particularly anti-LH, can prevent the continuation of the estrus cycle in the rat, prevent ovulation, delay implantation, and cause total fetal resorption before day 14 of pregnancy (8, 9). These studies have implicated the anti-LH in preventing the synthesis and release of the steroids necessary for ovum implantation and pregnancy maintenance. In relation to estrogen production, which is known to be important for implantation, Chang and Laurence (10) found that in rats treated for 9 consecutive days with antibovine LH, beginning day 1 of pregnancy, nidation was delayed for as long as 17 days. Based upon the day of parturition, spontaneous implantation occurred on day 14 or on day 17 in about 60% of the treated animals. In the remainder, implantation failed to occur with or without exogenously administered estrogen if given after day 20 of pregnancy.

This study implies that estrogen synthesis and release was affected by the anti-LH treatment but progesterone synthesis was not, based upon the viability of the blastocyst which remained free within the uterine cavity.

It can be assumed that estrogen synthesis and release were affected by the anti-LH treatment for variable periods of time or until the neutralizing effect of the antiserum had dissipated. The immunologically delayed nidation is not unlike the delayed implantation phenomena which occurs in ovariectomized but progesterone-maintained pregnant rats (11).

The effects of anti-LH in post-implantation phenomena, however, appear to implicate a reduction in progesterone synthesis. Loewitt and Laurence (9), Loewitt, Badawy, and Laurence (12), and Madhwa Raj and Moudgal (13) have all found that the administration of anti-LH between days 7 to 12 of pregnancy in the rat terminates the pregnancy by causing total fetal resorption. Progesterone concomitantly administered with the anti-LH prevented the resorption process and maintained the pregnancy.

Within the 24 to 48 hr after anti-LH treatment an alteration in the normal ovarian steroidogenic pathway occurs. It will be recalled that the Δ^5-3β- OHSDH enzymes responsible for the synthesis of progesterone and 20α-progesterone, can both be demonstrated histochemically during the preimplantation period of pregnancy. During most of the postimplantation period 20α-hydroxy steroid dehydrogenase (20α-OHSDH) activity cannot be demonstrated, while Δ^5-3β-OHSDH remains at high and constant levels. With anti-LH treatment, the termination of pregnancy results in a rapid return of 20α-OHSDH to the luteal tissue. This is not unlike the studies of Wiest (14) who demonstrated the reappearance of the 20α-OHSDH after placental dislocation. Thus it must be ascertained whether the reappearance of 20α-OHSDH activity after anti-LH treatment is due to direct action of the antibody on the ovary or whether the anti-LH affects placental function which is subsequently reflected in the deterred activity in the corpus luteum.

In an attempt to answer this question, traumatized pseudopregnant animals were treated with anti-LH to observe the effect of the antibody on the decidual response and the relationship of the Δ^5-3β-OHSDH to the maintenance of the pseudopregnant condition.

Interestingly, anti-LH administered either on or before traumatization (days 1 to 4) or after traumatization (days 5 to 8) significantly reduced the expected decidual response. Only with the administration of both progesterone (4 mg/day) and estrone (1 ug/day) for 8 consecutive days was the inhibitory capacity of the anti-LH overcome with the decidual response achieving normal weight. Histochemical demonstration of Δ^5-3β- and 20α-OHSDH revealed a significant difference from that which occurs in pregnancy. The levels of both of the dehydrogenases were demonstrable throughout the period of pseudopregnancy, whether treated with anti-LH or not. The continuous demonstration of the 20α-OHSDH activity tends to indicate that in pregnancy the fetal placental unit has direct control of the steroidogenic pathway rather than the pituitary itself. Further studies must be carried out to verify this assumption and to clarify the steroidogenic mechanisms involved.

That the effects of the anti-LH are of short duration is indicated by the recent observations of Hassouna and Laurence (15). These investigators have shown that a single injection of anti-LH on day 10 of pregnancy terminates the pregnancy within 24 to 48 hr and that the treated female rat returns to normal estrus within 7 days of the treatment. Further, it has been shown that three pregnancies in the same animals were terminated within 43 days.

CONCLUSIONS

There is no longer any question that immunologic technique can supply some answers to some of the perplexing questions as to the mode of action of the gonadotropins during the process of reproduction. It might be expected that immunology will not only verify some of the outstanding studies of some years ago, but might also be expected to shake some of the traditional and cherished foundations of endocrinology, which we have so long accepted. Whether or not the tools of immunology will continue to advance the knowledge of reproductive physiology must await further developments of the biochemists in making pure and crystalline protein hormones available for the immunologist to study.

REFERENCES

1. Greep, R. O., in W. C. Young (Ed.), Sex and Internal Secretions 1961, Williams & Wilkins, Baltimore, 1961, p. 240.
2. Simpson, M. E., C. H. Li, and H. M. Evans, Endocrinology 48:370, 1951.
3. Monastirsky, R., K. A. Laurence, and E. Tovar, Fert Steril 22:318, 1971.
4. Talaat, M., and K. A. Laurence, Fert Steril 22:113, 1971.
5. Pineda, M. H., D. C. Lueku, L. C. Faulkner, and M. L. Hopwood, Proc Soc Exp Biol Med 125:665, 1967.
6. Weigle, W. O., Natural and Acquired Immunologic Unresponsiveness, World, Cleveland, 1968.
7. Monastirsky, R., K. A. Laurence, and E. Tovar, Endocrinology, submitted for publication.
8. Laurence, K. A., and S. Ichikawa, Endocrinology 82:1190, 1968.
9. Loewit, K. K., and K. A. Laurence, Fert Steril 20:679, 1969.
10. Chang, C. C., and K. A. Laurence, Biol Reprod, in press, 1971.
11. Nutting, E. F., and R. K. Meyer, in A. C. Enders (Ed.), Delayed Implantation, Univ. Chicago Press, Chicago, 1963, p. 233.

12. Loewit, K. K., S. Badawy, and K. A. Laurence, Endocrinology 84:244, 1969.
13. Madhwa Raj, H. G., and N. R. Moudgal, Endocrinology 96:874, 1970.
14. Wiest, W. G., W. R. Kedwell, and K. Balogh, Jr. Endocrinology 82:844, 1968.
15. Hassouna, H., and K. A. Laurence, Fert Steril, in press, 1971.

27. Gonadotropic Regulation of Ovarian Development in Mice During Infancy

Aliza Eshkol and Bruno Lunenfeld

The mouse ovary of some strains is, at birth, a solid organ comprised mainly of oocytes which occupy most of the ovarian cortex, and of the central core containing stroma cells (1, 2). During the first week the ovary enlarges and by 7 days some of the oocytes have begun to grow and are already surrounded by one or two rows of granulosa cells. At this time an early development of the theca can also be observed. In other strains follicular development starts in the prenatal period and at birth follicles with a complete ring of up to 20 or more cells/section of granulosa cells are seen in the center of the ovary.

During the second week of life oocytes continue to grow, follicles develop and, at 14 days, are surrounded by 3 or more rows of follicular cells. These follicles are enveloped by a theca layer consisting of several rows of disc-like cells. There is also some indication that during the second week the ovary produces hormones which cause an increase in uterine weight. When rats were spayed at 2 days of age and killed at 8 days, normal uterine weights were recorded. However, when the animals were allowed to survive to 14 days, the weights of the uteri of the spayed females were distinctly lower than normal (3).

Control mechanisms which are involved in early development have only partially been elucidated. In these regulatory mechanisms genetic control, hormonal regulation, and environmental factors are interrelated.

In this study an attempt was made to determine the role of gonadotropic hormones, namely whether structural and functional development of the ovary during the first two weeks of life is dependent on gonadotropic stimulation and if so which of the processes are regulated by FSH and which developmental changes require both FSH and LH.

Administration of pituitary extracts or gonadotropic preparations was shown to accelerate ovarian development of 10- to 14-day-old rats (1, 4-6) and mice (7, 8). According to Greep (6) and Hertz (1) ovaries become sensitive to gonadotropic stimulation when antrum formation begins and they conclude that up to this stage follicular development is independent of gonadotropins. There are, however, some indications pointing to earlier effects. Follicular development was advanced in rats killed at 9 days of age after having been treated with equine gonadotropins from day of birth (9). Ovarian weights of rats injected with equine gonadotropins between the ages of 4 and 10 days increased by 60% but differed histologically from the controls only in respect to the theca which was increased in width and contained far more numerous mitoses in the experimental animals (10). The uteri of the injected females were increased 82% in weight, indicating the secretion of sex steroids (10). Belterman and Stegner (11) demonstrated in electron microscopic studies, that human pituitary gonadotropins administered to newborn mice induced the formation of interstitial cells within 24 hr which were normally observed only in 9 day old animals. Selye and Collip (12), and Picon (13) postulated that stimulation of interstitial tissue and of estrogen secretion becomes evident before an effect on the follicles is discernible. These findings would tempt one to conclude that the follicular cells become responsive to exogenous gonadotropins at a later stage than the theca and interstitial cells. It is, however, possible that an effect on the latter cell types can be observed since they change in appearance and organelle composition, while an effect on granulosa cells can be assessed only on the basis of either their quantitative evaluation or measurement of synthetic activity such as DNA synthesis. Furthermore, Pedersen (14) demonstrated that the doubling time of granulosa cells in medium sized follicles in ovaries of 7 day old animals is significantly shorter than in prepubertal animals (38 vs 84 hr). Thus it is possible that the growth of these follicles can indeed not be accelerated since it is already maximal.

Irrespective of the effects of exogenous gonadotropins on the infantile ovary, the question whether the structural and functional differentiations are independent of endogenous gonadotropic stimulation remains to be answered.

To elucidate the existence of an interrelationship between an organ and a hormonal control center, the two have to be dissociated and, under such conditions, persistence or cessation of organized growth and development has to be analyzed.

Walker et al. (15) studied the effects of hypophysectomy in rats at 6 days of age. They found that ovarian and uterine development was markedly inhibited when examined 54 days later. It should be noted that in this experiment the autopsy was carried out at the age of 60 days, at a time when gonadal dependency on gonadotropins has been clearly established. In other similar studies, the hypophysectomy has been performed at later "gonadotropin-dependent" ages.

Organ culture of whole ovaries yielded contradictory results. Francke (16) obtained growth and differentiation in ovaries of rats 0 to 7 days old. Similar results were reported by Pavic (17). Lostroh (18) on the other hand cultivated ovaries from 4-day-old mice and observed atrophy of the follicular and thecal cells and a general loss of the organization of the ovary; the primordial follicles were not maintained and their maturation was arrested. Some or all of these degenerative changes were prevented when estrogens, HCG or LH, were added to the medium.

On the basis of the evidence that antihormone treatment is effective in counteracting the action of circulating pituitary gonadotropins (19), this approach was chosen in the present study. Unlike hypophysectomy, antiserum administration can be initiated even in newborn rodents. Since the purpose was to deprive the animals of their own gonadotropins and also to study the effects of human FSH and FSH + LH in such animals, an antiserum, neutralizing mouse gonadotropins but not reacting with human gonadotropins, had to be employed. Antiserum to sheep gonadotropins or to bovine gonadotropins were inappropriate due to their broad spectrum of cross reactions. Antiserum to rat pituitary gonadotropins (aRG) as prepared and characterized by Lunenfeld et al. (19) seemed therefore to be a suitable tool for the present study.

Ovarian development was studied in mice deprived of endogenous gonadotropic stimulation from birth by daily administration of aRG. As substitution, either biologically pure FSH (20) or HMG were administered daily, half an hour following the aRG injection. The quantitative evaluation (21) of follicular development was performed using the classification proposed by Pederson and Peters (22). In the strain of mice used in this study significant progress in follicular development could be observed during the first 5 days of life. During this period granulosa cell proliferation advanced markedly. This was also observed in animals deprived of endogenous gonadotropins (Table I). It thus becomes evident that granulosa cell proliferation can take place in the absence of gonadotropins. However, the fact that gonadotropins have a stimulatory effect on follicular growth prior to this age, is indicated by the findings that, although the total number of growing follicles was identical in both groups, the number of follicles with 10 to 20 granulosa cells/largest cross-section (LCS) was larger in the aRG treated animals ($p < 0.025$), whereas the number of follicles with more than 21 granulosa cells per LCS was smaller than in the controls) $p < 0.025$). The ratio of the smaller to the larger follicles was 0.8 in controls and 1.4 in gonadotropin-deprived animals. It therefore seems that prior to 5 days, gonadotropic stimulation accelerates follicular growth beyond the stage of 10 to 20 granulosa cells/LCS while up to this stage follicular growth is not affected by the absence of gonadotropins. The fact that more such follicles are seen in the aRG-treated animals can be explained by the diminution in development to the next stage. Light microscopic inspection of control and gonadotropin-deprived

TABLE I. Mean number of follicles in newborn and 5 day old mice

	Number of granulosa cells on LCS			
	10-20	21-40	41-60	Total
Day of birth	91.5 (27.6)[b]	12.5 (2.1)	0	104.0 (25.4)
Day 5—control	75.6 (10.2)	88.2 (7.6)	7.2 (10.2)	171.0 (13.1)
Day 5—aRG	100.8[c] (5.1)	70.2[c] (2.5)	0	171.0 (2.5)

[a]( ) = SD.

[b]p < 0.025 as compared to day 5 control.

mice did not reveal any differences in their appearance. The differences in the stage of follicular development were revealed only on the basis of differential follicular counts in serial sections of the ovaries.

The ovaries of 7-day-old, aRG-treated mice were smaller and follicles did not reach a similar developmental stage as the normal controls. Follicles with more than 41 cells/LCS, but not exceeding 50, were seen only occasionally, whereas in the normal 7-day-old mice some follicles had 61 to 100 cells and infrequently even more (Table II). Follicular development did not progress beyond the 40-cell stage, similar to newborns, but the number of follicles reaching the 21- to 40-cell stage was significantly higher (12 and 90 respectively) (Tables I and II). The nuclei of granulosa cells in aRG-treated animals were close to each other and appeared crowded; they were not organized into well-defined layers. There seemed to be less disc-like cells around the basal membrane and thus an appearance of empty spaces between adjacent follicles and the surrounding tissue was produced. Also the vascular system did not reach the same stage as that in the ovary of the normal 7 day old mouse.

The partial arrest of follicular development observed in gonadotropin-deprived animals was prevented by substitution with FSH. Differential counts revealed that the total number of growing follicles was even larger in the FSH-treated animals than in the untreated controls (248 and 166 respectively; see Table II). The number of follicles with 41 to 60 cells, practically absent in the aRG-treated mice, was similar to that of the controls (47 and 41 respectively). The same was also true for follicles with more than 60 cells. The number of small follicles with 10 to 40 granulosa cells was significantly higher (p < 0.0125) in the FSH-treated animals than in the controls and was similar to that of the aRG-treated animals. Their number was 105 in the ovaries of controls, 172 in aRG-treated animals, and 187 in aRG + FSH-treated animals.

TABLE II. Mean number of follicles in ovaries of the various experimental groups at the age of 7 days

		Number of granulosa cells on LCS					
		10-20	21-40	41-60	61-100	> 100	Total
1	Control	42.5 (9.3)[a]	62.6 (28.7)	41.0 (18.3)	16.6 (7.5)	2.9	165.6 (57.5)
2	aRG	81.3 (28.6)	90.5 (17.8)	2.0 (2.8)	0	0	173.8 (21.5)
3	aRG + FSH	68.4 (10.2)	118.8 (14.8)	46.8 (10.2)	14.4 (5.1)	0	248.4 (30.5)
4	aRG + HMG	61.2 (10.2)	122.4 (15.3)	55.8 (2.5)	16.2 (2.5)	0	255.5 (25.7)

[a]( ) = SD.

Note: Total number of follicles in group 2 did not differ from that in group 1 ($p > 0.40$) and group 4 was not different from group 3 ($p > 0.40$). Number of follicles in ovaries of mice receiving substitution therapy (group 3 and 4) was significantly different ($p < 0.005$) from controls and aRG treated (Group 1 and 2) animals.

Histologic investigation showed the presence of follicles with several layers of regularly arranged granulosa cells. The nuclei were not crowded as after aRG injection but were spaced similarly to those in ovaries of control animals. Many mitoses among the granulosa cells of the growing follicles were noted. Around the granulosa layers, thin elongated theca cells were seen. Also the vascular system in the FSH-treated animals was more developed than in the gonado-tropin-deprived animals.

When gonadotropin-deprived mice received substitution therapy with FSH + LH (HMG), the appearance of the ovary in 7-day-old animals seemed similar to those receiving FSH alone. In addition, the differential counts of the follicles in these two groups were similar (Table II). The deficient ovarian vascularization observed in the gonadotropin deprived mice, was restituted by substitution with HMG. Since neither thecal nor vascular development were fully restored by FSH alone, it can be concluded that normal ovarian development at this age is both FSH- and LH-dependent.

With the advancement of age the dependency of normal ovarian development became more evident. Retardation and alteration of such development was more pronounced in animals deprived of endogenous gonadotropins for 14 days than in those examined in an earlier age. This is in agreement with investigations of

TABLE III. Mean number of follicles in ovaries of the various experimental groups at the age of 14 days

| | Number of granulosa cells on LCS | | | | | |
	10-20	21-40	41-60	61-100	>100	Total
Control	40.8 (22.3)[a]	54.9 (18.9)	50.4 (5.1)	61.5 (25.2)	27 (16.2)	234.6 (48.6)
aRG	33.3 (15.6)	69.3 (5.4)	38.7 (9.5)	21.6 (2.8)	0	163.5 (21.5)
aRG + FSH	77.4 (28.0)	99.0 (15.3)	81 (12.7)	102.6 (7.6)	16.2 (2.5)	356.2[c] (25.7)
aRG + HMG	59.4 (2.5)	57.6 (10.2)	66.6(3.6)[b] (7.6)	82.8(10.8)[b] (20.4)	14.4(3.6)[b] (15.3)	280.0 (10.2)

[a]( ) SD.

[b]Follicles with antra.

[c]Significantly different from the control (p < 0.025) and from the aRG treated mice (p < 0.0005).

serum levels of gonadotropins in normal female rats. LH increased after 7 days of age and highest values were reached in 14-day-old animals. During this period also the pituitary content of LH rose and paralleled the FSH pattern (23).

The ovaries of the animals deprived of gonadotropins for the first two weeks of life were considerably smaller than ovaries of normal animals. Whereas, in comparison to the controls, no significant deviation in the number of follicles with 10 to 60 granulosa cells/LCS was observed ($p > 0.40$), the number of follicles with 61 to 100 granulosa cells/LCS was significantly lower ($p < 0.025$). Follicles with over 101 granulosa cells/LCS were practically absent in ovaries of gonadotropin-deprived mice (Table III). Whether granulosa cell proliferation is diminished because fewer granulosa cells actively proliferate and/or because the generation time of the individual proliferating cell is lengthened, has not been investigated. The disturbance in the development of the individual granulosa cells is characterized by an apparently abnormal development of the cytoplasm, their tendency to crowd together, and the lack of spaces between cells. Crowding of the nuclei seems to suggest that the cytoplasm is diminished. This might be due to impairment of metabolic processes dependent on gonadotropic stimulation. However, the growth of oocytes seems undisturbed. In normal animals oocytes reach a diameter of about 60 μ in follicles with more than 100 granulosa cells/LCS (Fig. 1); however in the gonadotropin-deprived animals, oocytes of this size were found in follicles which had only up to 40 granulosa

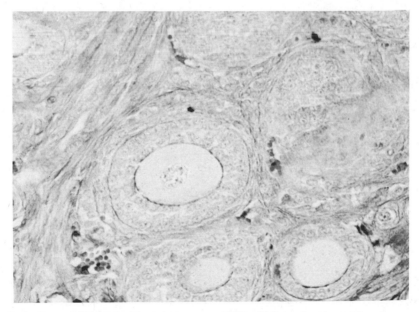

FIG. 1. Ovary of 14-day-old control mouse (X40). Well-developed granulosa layer and basement membrane. Theca layer with many cells (Azan stain).

cells/LCS (Fig. 2). Such a disproportionate growth of oocytes was also observed in some ovarian explants from 4-day-old rats cultivated in vitro for 5 days (24). The fact that granulosa cell proliferation does not seem to keep in step with apparently normal oocyte growth suggests that these two processes are not governed by the same stimuli. Oocyte growth does not seem to be dependent on either gonadotropins or normal granulosa cell proliferation. However, whether a growing occyte residing in an abnormal follicle envelope is functionally competent cannot be decided by these experiments.

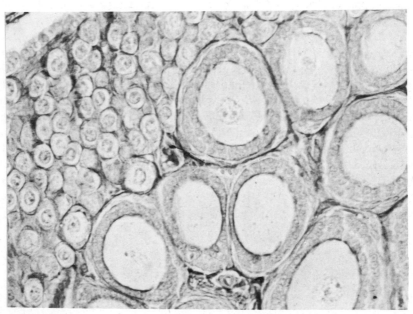

FIG. 2. Ovary of 14-day-old aRG treated mouse (X40). Narrow granulosa layer. Poorly defined basement membrane. Empty space in undeveloped theca layer (Azan stain).

In control animals the zona pellucida forms a continuous band around the oocyte but in the gonadotropin-deprived mice the zona pellucida around most of the oocytes was discontinuous or disrupted (Fig. 2). Histological examination showed an abnormal appearance of the granulosa cells and the theca layer, as well as the stroma. The nuclei of the granulosa cells of aRG-injected animals were densely packed together with little cytoplasm and no spaces between them. This forms a shell around the oocyte which is narrower than the envelope of a normal follicle containing the same number of granulosa cells (Figs. 1 and 2). The basement membrane was poorly defined and in some follicles partially or even totally absent. In the theca layer only a few poorly developed cells were seen which were irregularly arranged with empty spaces between them. The periphery of the thecal layer was delineated by fibrous material simulating a membrane. Between the granulosa cells and this membrane-like structure a space was left containing only a few thin (probably theca) cells (Fig. 2). Red blood cells were not seen in these spaces. The small oocytes appeared closely packed with only a few cells between them. The vascular system and the stroma appeared poorly developed.

Daily simultaneous administration of 0.5 IU FSH and aRG for 14 days caused a considerable change in the development of the ovary as compared to the ovaries of gonadotropin-deprived animals. The over-all microscopic appearance of the ovary was similar to that of the control animals. The granulosa cells appeared normal and were arranged in concentric layers around the oocyte. They had ample cytoplasm and spaces were noted between them. The basement membrane seemed intact but the theca layer was uneven in thickness and thinner than in the controls (Fig. 3). The membrane-like structure limiting the thecal

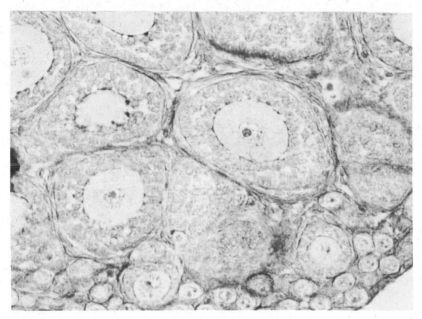

FIG. 3. Ovary of 14-day-old aRG + FSH treated mouse (X40). Granulosa layer well developed. Theca layer thin (Azan stain).

space in the aRG-injected animals was not seen in the aRG + FSH-injected animals (compare Figs. 2 and 3). The cortex appeared similar to that of control ovaries with well-spaced small oocytes and many cells between them. However, the capillary system still seemed poorly developed. Differential counts of follicles revealed that deprivation of endogenous gonadotropins could be totally overcome by the administration of FSH (Table III). Moreover, the total number of growing follicles was larger in the FSH-treated animals than in either the controls or the aRG-treated animals (Table III). The number of follicles in the aRG-treated animals with more than 60 cells/LCS was only 22, while in the FSH-treated animals, it was 119. The number of follicles with 10 to 60 cells/ LCS, which in control and aRG-treated animals was similar (146 and 141 respectively), was increased in the FSH-treated animals to 212 (Table III).

When HMG was administered for 14 days simultaneously with the aRG., follicular growth was not significantly different from that of the animals which received FSH. However, many of the growing follicles had antra of different sizes. Antrum development was not observed in the control litter mates. The basement membrane was complete and the theca layer was wider and seemed to contain more cells. Red blood cells were seen within the theca layer (Fig. 4). A large number of groups of irregularly shaped pale cells described as 'cloudy areas' in the control animals were seen between the follicles. The center of the organ, which in the normal 14-day-old mouse is solid, showed in the aRG- and HMG-injected mice the beginnings of a 'lace-like appearance'. The capillary system was well developed with vessels of irregular shape and dilatation, a development seen in the normal animal only during the third week of life.

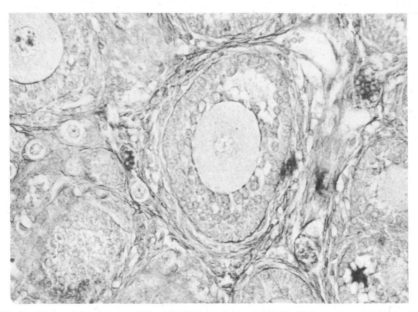

FIG. 4. Ovary of 14-day-old aRG + HMG treated mouse (X40). Well-developed follicle with beginning of antrum formation. Theca layer consists of several rows of cells (Azan stain).

These results indicate that gonadotropins are indispensable for normal organization and spacing of granulosa cells, the integrity of the basement membrane, the development or maintenance of the thecal cells, and the development of the vascular system. Granulosa cell proliferation can be stimulated during the first two weeks of life by FSH and the absence of gonadotropins diminishes their proliferation significantly but does not prevent it completely. The dependence on gonadotropins in itself demonstrates the existence of ovarian target receptors to gonadotropins. This was further confirmed by the observation that their administration could prevent the alterations and retardation of ovarian development caused by their absence. FSH was found to be primarily responsible for the stimulation of granulosa cell proliferation and organization. The addition of LH to FSH initiated secretory activity of granulosa cells, antrum formation, enrichment and maintenance of the theca layer, an increase in the amount of interfollicular tissue, and development of the vascular system. The restoration of thecal development might be due either to the direct effect of gonadotropins on these cells or the result of the normalization of granulosa cell development which in turn might have influenced the thecal development. Such cellular interrelationship has been postulated by Dubreuil (25-27) and Hisaw (28). According to these authors the granulosa produces an inductor substance which causes the differentiation of the theca. The effects observed in animals which received FSH and LH as compared with those which received only FSH, cannot be attributed to the direct action of LH alone. The combined effect of both hormones on their respective receptors, and the structural and metabolic interrelationship of the various ovarian components must be taken into consideration.

ACKNOWLEDGMENT

This investigation (thesis of E.A.) was supported by Ford Foundation grant 670-0470. The expert technical assistance of Mrs. Juliana Ben-Zimra is sincerely appreciated.

REFERENCES

1. Hertz, R., in H. G. Grady, and D. E. Smith (Eds.), The Ovary, & Wilkins, Baltimore, 1963, p.120.
2. Peters, H., Acta Endocrinol 62:98, 1969.
3. Price, D., Anat Record 97:519, 1947.
4. Corey, E. L., Anat Record 41:40, 1928.
5. Ben-Or, S., Embryol Exper Morphol 11:1, 1963.
6. Greep, R. P., in H. G. Grady, and D. E. Smith (Eds.), The Ovary, Williams & Wilkins, Baltimore, 1963, p.48.
7. Pfeiffer, C. A., and C. W. Hooker, Anat Record 84:311, 1952.
8. Zarrow, M. X., and E. D. Wilson, Endocrinology 69:851, 1969.
9. Eayrs, J. T., J Endocrinol 7:271, 1951.
10. Price, D., and E. Ortiz, Endocrinology 34:215, 1944.

11. Belterman, R., and H. E. Stegner, Acta Endocrinol 57:279, 1968.

12. Selye, H., and J. B. Collip, Proc Soc Exper Biol Med 30:647, 1933.

13. Picon, L. Arch Anat Microscop 45:311, 1956.

14. Pedersen, T., presented at the Workshop Conference on the Developments of the Ovary in Infancy, Birmingham, 1969.

15. Walker, D. G., M. E. Simpson, C. W. Asling, and H. M. Evans, Anat Record 106:539, 1950.

16. Francke, C., Endocrinology 39:430, 1946.

17. Pavic, D., J Endocrinol 26:531, 1963.

18. Lostroh, A. J., Endocrinology 65:124, 1959.

19. Lunenfeld, B., A. Eshkol, G. Baldratti, and G. K. Suchowsky, Acta Endocrinol 54:311, 1967.

20. Eshkol, A., and B. Lunenfeld, Acta Endocrinol 54:91, 1967.

21. Zuckerman, S., Rec. Prog. Hormone Res 6:63, 1961.

22. Pedersen, T., and H. Peters, J Reprod Fertil 17:555, 1968.

23. Weisz, J., and M. Ferin, presented at the Workshop Conference on the Development of the Ovary in Infancy, Birmingham, 1969.

24. Fainstat, T., Fert Steril 19:317, 1968.

25. Dubreuil, G., Ann Endocrinol 3:179, 1942.

26. Dubreuil, G., Ann Endocrinol 9:436, 1948.

27. Dubreuil, G. Gyn Obst 49:282, 1950.

28. Hisaw, F. L., Physiol Rev 27:95, 1947.

28.   Actions of LH—Antisera on Corpus Luteum Function

Harold R. Behrman, N. Raghuveer Moudgal[1], and Roy O. Greep

A new avenue of research which opened with the advent of specific antisera is neutralization of gonadotropins in vivo. This method permits selective removal of individual hormones and thus allows for a study of their mechanism of action in vivo. Moudgal and co-workers (1-3) used luteinizing hormone antisera (LH-A/S) to demonstrate that neutralization of LH terminated pregnancy in the rat when administered in the first half of gestation.

The regulation of corpus luteum function has been shown to involve LH insofar as the acute stimulation of progesterone synthesis is concerned (4) and we have shown that a direct action of LH is to activate the hydrolysis of cholesterol esters (5). The enzymes controlling synthesis and hydrolysis of cholesterol esters are regulated by gonadotropins (6) and we have proposed that steroidogenesis is, in part, regulated by the availability of cholesterol for oxidative side-chain cleavage.

The studies reported herein are centered around the role of LH determined by in vivo neutralization with A/S, on the regulation of ovarian progestin output, sterol levels, and enzyme activity associated with cholesterol ester turnover in the pregnant and pseudopregnant rat.

MATERIALS AND METHODS

Animals

Pregnant rats were purchased from Holtzman Company, Madison, Wisconsin and the day of spermatozoa detection in the vaginal lavage was termed day 1 of

---

[1]Visiting Associate Professor, Department of Anatomy, Harvard Medical School. Present Address: Department of Biochemistry, Indian Institute of Science, Bangalore 12, India.

pregnancy. Immature female rats were purchased from the same source and in some experiments were treated with 50 IU pregnant mare serum (PMS) at 28 days of age, followed 60 to 70 hr later with 25 IU HCG to induce highly luteinized ovaries. In other experiments, immature rats were treated with 4 IU PMS and made pseudopregnant 72 hr later by stimulating the cervix. The animals were provided with food and water ad libitum and 14 hr light each day.

Preparation of LH-A/S

NIH-LH-S16 was injected into New Zealand white rabbits to produce antibodies as described earlier (7); absorption and characterization of the A/S was carried out using procedures previously reported (3). The amount of A/S administered was based on the minimum effective dose given subcutaneously which caused vaginal bleeding and resorption in day 8 pregnant rats (0.3 to 0.4 ml). Normal rabbit serum (NRS) was used as the control treatment.

Chemical and Surgical Procedures

Ovarian venous blood was collected from pregnant animals and stored frozen. The contralateral ovary from the side used to collect blood was analyzed for sterol content. Peripheral blood from pseudopregnant rats was collected after decapitation and the blood from 3 animals was pooled for each analysis. Incubation of ovarian tissue slices to determine progesterone output in vitro was identical to the procedure reported earlier (8).

Steroid levels in blood, serum, and incubated slices of ovarian tissue were determined by gas-liquid chromatography after isolation by thin layer chromatography (9). Cholesterol and cholesterol ester were quantitated as described earlier (10), and cholesterol ester synthetase and cholesterol esterase were assayed in extracts of homogenized luteal tissue (5, 6).

RESULTS

From the data in Fig. 1, it is evident that treatment 24 hr earlier with LH-A/S produced a significant decline ($p < 0.005$) in ovarian progesterone secretion of about 80% in the day 8 pregnant rat. On the other hand, 20α-hydroxypregn-4-en-3-one (20α-ol) secretion was markedly enhanced ($p < 0.01$), increasing by almost 8-fold within 24 hr. At the time of collection, vaginal bleeding and resorption was evident in day 8 pregnant animals treated with LH-A/S. Conversely, LH-A/S did not produce abortion when administered to day 15 pregnant rats. In these animals a less marked reduction in progesterone secretion was evident (25%; $p < 0.10$) and in contrast to the day 8 pregnant animals, 20α-ol secretion was reduced by 46% ($p < 0.10$).

The corpora lutea from the day 8 and day 15 pregnant rats were whitish in color after treatment in vivo with LH-AS. This effect we have generally found to indicate lipid accumulation, and a two fold increase in cholesterol ester content (p < 0.01) was observed. Free cholesterol also increased but to a smaller extent (Fig. 2).

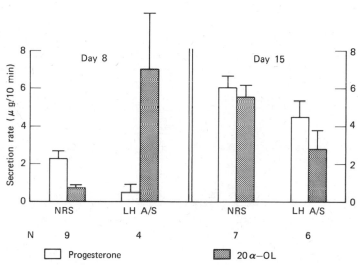

FIG. 1. Effect of LH-A/S (24 hr) on progesterone and 20α-ol secretion in the day 8 and day 15 pregnant rat (mean ⊥ SE).

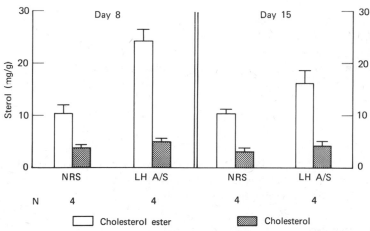

FIG. 2. Effect of LH-A/S (24 hr) on ovarian sterol content in day 8 and day 15 pregnant rats (mean ± SE).

It was considered of interest to examine the effect of LH-A/S in the pseudopregnant animal in order to remove effects which the gravid uterus may produce on luteal function. In Fig. 3 the effect of LH-A/S administered to superovulated rats 12 hr before sacrifice is shown. Both progesterone and 20α-ol levels in peripheral serum were reduced by 50% (p < 0.10), an effect similar to that produced in the day 15 pregnant rat.

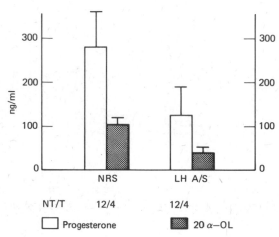

FIG. 3. Effect of LH-A/S (12 hr) on peripheral serum levels of progesterone and 20α-ol in superovulated rats (mean ± SE).

When LH-A/S was administered to pseudopregnant rats 24 hr before sacrifice and the ovaries removed, sliced, and incubated in vitro, the output of progesterone was found to increase almost two fold (p < 0.10) while 20α-ol output remained unchanged (Fig. 4). In these animals, the ovarian content of cholesterol ester increased by 2.5-fold (p < 0.001) and free cholesterol increased 1.4-fold (p < 0.01).

Analysis of the enzymes controlling cholesterol ester turnover reveal that LH-A/S decreased cholesterol esterase activity by almost 90% (p < 0.001) within 24 hr (Fig. 5). On the other hand, cholesterol ester synthetase activity was elevated 1.6-fold (p < 0.001) in the same interval. The net effect on the activity of these enzymes points to the probable mechanism for increased cholesterol ester accumulation following the administration of LH-A/S.

DISCUSSION

Neutralization of LH with specific antisera reduced progesterone output in vivo both in the pregnant and pseudopregnant animal. Associated with this response

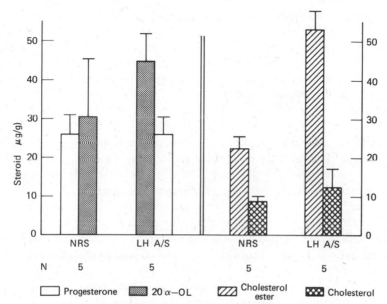

FIG. 4. Effect of LH-A/S (24 hr) on progesterone and 20α-ol levels in incubated slices of ovarian tissue and ovarian sterol levels in pseudopregnant rats (mean ± SE).

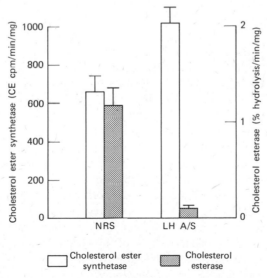

FIG. 5. Effect of LH-A/S (24 hr) on cholesterol ester synthetase and cholesterol esterase activity in luteinized ovaries (mean ± SE).

was a marked accumulation of cholesterol ester produced by an inhibition of cholesterol esterase and enhanced cholesterol ester synthetase activity. However, when ovaries were incubated in vitro following LH-A/S treatment in vivo, a stimulation of progesterone output was observed. The opposite effect of LH-A/S on ovarian progesterone output measured in vivo and in vitro is puzzling but may be due to the availability of cholesterol for steroidogenesis. Free cholesterol levels in the ovary were elevated by LH-A/S treatment and when incubated in vitro this excess cholesterol may become more available and increase steroidogenesis through a mass-action effect. For example, a similar observation was made by Wilks et al. (10) after treatment in vivo with aminoglutethimide (a reversible inhibitor of steroidogenesis). In their hands, the tissues which had been exposed to the inhibitor in vivo actually produced more steroid in vitro than the control tissue. This inhibitor increases ovarial cholesterol levels (9, 10) and the enhanced steroidogenesis in vitro may have arisen from the increased availability of cholesterol after the inhibitor had been removed by washing.

The marked decrease in cholesterol esterase activity produced by LH-A/S confirms our earlier observation where LH was shown to increase cholesterol esterase activity within 1 hr of treatment in vivo (5). In the presence of decreased activity of this enzyme, hydrolysis of cholesterol esters would be reduced and also the availability of cholesterol for conversion to steroids. In earlier studies, we observed that chronic LH treatment was detrimental to the ability of prolactin to maintain ovarian cholesterol ester synthetase activity in hypophysectomized animals (6). The present data confirm this observation since neutralization of LH increased the activity of cholesterol ester synthetase. Thus LH appears to regulate ovarian cholesterol ester turnover by inhibiting the synthetase enzyme and activating the hydrolytic enzyme, effects which are directly related to the action of LH to increase progesterone biosynthesis.

The large increase in ovarian 20α-ol secretion in the day 8 pregnant rat indicates that active luteolysis (11) was induced by neutralization of circulating LH. However, this effect was not produced by LH-A/S when administered to the day 15 pregnant or the pseudopregnant rat. In addition, progesterone output in vitro was enhanced after 24 hr exposure to LH-A/S in vivo. These latter data argue that the ability of the corpus luteum to convert cholesterol to progesterone was not impaired by loss of LH and further imply that steroidogenesis can, under acute conditions, proceed in the absence of LH (i.e., in vivo neutralization followed by rinsing of the tissue before incubation) providing cholesterol is available. The effect of LH-A/S to decrease progesterone synthesis in vivo (presumably because of cholesterol esterase inhibition) appears to be the mechanism for termination of pregnancy in the day 8 pregnant rat. The appearance of a large 20α-ol secretion observed under these conditions probably reflects a secondary effect of LH-A/S produced by a decrease in progesterone secretion which was insufficient to maintain pregnancy. For example, placental dislocation was shown by Wiest et al. (11). to increase 20α-ol secretion.

ACKNOWLEDGMENT

The authors express their appreciation to Miss Karen Thode and Mrs. Nancy DeLancey for their skillful technical assistance, and to the Endocrine Study Section, NIH for the generous gifts of pituitary hormones. This work was supported by grants from The Ford Foundation, NIH HD-03736, and NIH 69-2214.

REFERENCES

1. Madhwa Raj, H. G., M. R. Sairam, and N. R. Moudgal, J Reprod Fert 17:335, 1968.

2. Moudgal, N. R., H. G. Madhwa Raj, A. Jagannadha Rao, and M. R. Sairam, Ind J Exp Biol 7:45, 1969.

3. Madhwa Raj, H. G., and N. R. Moudgal, Endocrinology 86:874, 1970.

4. Armstrong, D. T., J. O'Brien, and R. O. Greep, Endocrinology 75:488, 1964.

5. Behrman, H. R., and D. T. Armstrong, Endocrinology 85:474, 1969.

6. Behrman, H. R., G. P. Orczyk, G. J. Macdonald. and R. O. Greep, Endocrinology 87:1251, 1970.

7. Moudgal, N. R., and C. H. Li, Arch Biochem Biophys 95:93, 1961.

8. Behrman, H. R., K. Yoshinaga, and R. O. Greep, Amer J Physiol 221:16, 1971.

9. Behrman, H. R., D. T. Armstrong, and R. O. Greep, Can J Biochem 48:881, 1970.

10. Wilks, J. W., G. B. Fuller, and W. Hansel, Endocrinology 87:581, 1970.

11. Wiest, W. G., W. R. Kidwell, and K. Balogh, Endocrinology 82:844, 1968.

DISCUSSION

CH. V. RAO. We have investigated HCG antibody binding both in vivo and in vitro. Preliminary data strongly suggests that HCG antibody does not combine with HCG already bound to luteal cell membranes. Conversely, luteal cell membranes do not bind HCG, which has already combined with its antibody. Our experiments have shown that luteal cell membranes or antibody, whichever is exposed to HCG first, will bind and the binding seems to be relatively strong. Therefore, it appears that HCG antibody neutralizes free HCG, but does not have any effect at receptor level. Dr. Behrman, do you have any data as to whether this is so with LH antibodies?

H. R. BEHRMAN. No, but perhaps Dr. Moudgal does.

R. N. MOUDGAL. Dr. Moyle and I observed in our in vitro Leydig tumor cell incubation studies that it takes some time for the antiserum to be effective in reducing steroidogenesis which takes place under LH stimulation. This can either be due to the time it takes for the antibody to pull the LH off its binding site or the time it takes for the already available substrate to be exhausted. I think it is difficult to demonstrate by actual measurement that LH cannot be removed once it is bound.

E. ROSEMBERG. Dr. Laurence, you have described very interesting effects of LH antisera in the male in two species, the rat and the rabbit. Would you assume that the same effect could be obtained in the human?

G. T. ROSS. I will answer for Dr. Laurence. The answer is no.

I. ROTHCHILD. I have a question in relation to the last paper on the difference in the effect of the anti-LH between the pregnant rat and the pseudopregnant rat. The point was made that the anti-LH reduced the progesterone secretion in the pregnant rat by 80% or more, while in the pseudopregnant rat the reduction was about 50%. The pregnant state is different from the pseudopregnant state. The peripheral blood level of progesterone in the rat on the 6th to 12th day of pregnancy is 50 to 100% higher than during pseudopregnancy, and this is probably caused by placental secretion. If LH is important in the regulation of progesterone secretion, why does LH antiserum, which would affect only the action of LH and not that of the placental hormone, have a greater reducing effect on the progesterone secretion in pregnancy than in pseudopregnancy?

H. R. BEHRMAN. In the pregnant animal, we measured ovarian secretion rate

354

of progesterone; in the pseudopregnant animal we measured progesterone concentration in peripheral serum. The concentration of progestins in ovarian venous blood is much higher than in peripheral serum. Thus because of the two methods used to determine the effect of LH antiserum on progestin output in the pregnant and pseudopregnant animal, the magnitude of effect of LH antiserum cannot be compared on a quantitative basis. However, a magnified effect of LH antiserum on progesterone secretion would be expected over that produced on peripheral serum progesterone because the concentration in serum is influenced by many secondary factors.

I. ROTHCHILD. This only accentuates the difference I am talking about, because one would expect that the level of progesterone in peripheral blood after treatment of the pregnant rat with LH antiserum would probably be 90 to 95% less than in the untreated animal. So I would like to ask again: Why does the antiserum have this effect in the pregnant state and not in the pseudopregnant state? I think there must be some change in the activity of the corpus luteum induced by the placental hormone that makes it more sensitive to removal of LH by antiserum and I am raising the question of the nature of the interaction between LH and the placental hormone that could produce this effect.

H. R. BEHRMAN. On the basis of our available data I can't answer that question.

R. N. MOUDGAL. At the present moment, we cannot exclude the possibility of placental hormones contributing to the luteotropic pool. In addition to what Dr. Behrman mentioned, I would like to point out that the day 8 corpus luteum of a pregnant rat is not directly comparable to the day 5 corpus luteum of a pseudopregnant rat. The progesterone synthesis capacity of the pseudopregnant rat ovary reaches its maximum by day 5 and this could be compared to the ovary of day 12 to 14, but not to the ovary of day 8 pregnant rat. Thus once corpora lutea reach their maximal capacity to synthesize steroids, under any given situation, they seem to become less sensitive to the lack of LH.

H. VAN HELL. I would like to ask a question related to the first paper because the conclusion of the first paper strikes at the basis of our belief in the action of gonadotropins. One of the conclusions was that anti-FSH has no effect on spermatogenesis, suggesting that the FSH has no action on growth of the testis. Is there any more evidence for a specific anti-FSH activity of the antiserum?

K. A. LAURENCE. I think that you missed a couple of points. Anti-FSH kept the weight of the gonad down to about half of what it should have been, even though there was no interference with the spermatogenesis. This anti-FSH can combine with FSH in vitro and inhibit FSH. In addition, FSH is antigenic and can indeed cause a rise in antibodies, which influence the outcome of follicular development and ovulation. I might add that there are a few other things in a paper which we recently published. When we immunized newborn male and female rabbits with LH and FSH at 3 and 4 weeks of age and then permitted the animals to go to 7 months of age (sexual puberty), the LH-immunized rabbits had no adrenal glands to speak of but only infantile testes. The FSH-immunized male rabbits had complete spermatogenesis and normal size adrenal glands.

I. ROTHCHILD. I have a question for Dr. Eshkol. There seems to be an interesting difference between the results you obtained with the antiserum in the newborns and the effects of hypophysectomy in older rats. In the latter case the animals obviously are completely deprived of both FSH and LH and yet follicles not only developed up to the antrum stage, but there seemed to be no difference in the rate of transformation of primordial to primary follicles or in the rate of growth of the primary follicles up to the point of development of the antrum. Included with this is a fairly good development of the theca interna. I would be interested in explanations you may have for this difference. Presumably what you are looking at also is the independence of the ovary from the pituitary in the development of follicles up to the point where the antrum and the theca are formed.

A. ESHKOL. We did not administer this antiserum to weanling mice, so we cannot make any comparison with hypophysectomized weanling rats. We did, however, inject antigonadotropins from birth until the age of 21 days. The ovaries of these animals disclosed further development as reflected by the increase in follicular size, but antrum formation was not observed. One possible explanation for the presence of follicles with antra in surgically hypophysectomized rats could be due to some residual cells secreting gonadotropins. This has been demonstrated by Dr. A. Lostrob (1963) who showed that administration of antigonadotropin serum to male rats following hypophysectomy resulted in severe regression in spermatogenesis.

U. K. BANIK. Dr. Laurence, have you checked the fertility of these males 2 to 3 months after immunization?

K. A. LAURENCE. We are checking the fertility activity now but we have no definitive data up to this point.

R. N. MOUDGAL. It is common practice among physiologists and biochemists to use specific inhibitors as tools to study the mode of action of biologically active substances. It is increasingly realized that antisera raised to hormones and characterized for specificity can be effectively used to "dehormonize" a system. However, a number of limitations in the use of these reagents exist and these must be appreciated.

Firstly, the pituitary gonadotropins commonly used as immunogens are only relatively pure and it is sometimes observed that hyperimmunization of animals with any one of these preparations leads to the formation of antibodies to contaminating hormone proteins. In addition to contaminating hormones, structural and antigenic similarities in the subunits of the glycoprotein hormones complicate the production of specific antisera even when highly purified preparations are used as immunogen. In some instances, antibodies to contaminants can be removed by selective absorption with the contaminating hormone proteins, leaving a specific antiserum.

Secondly, the specificity of the antibody must be checked by as many methods as possible, these ranging from the simple agar-gel diffusion studies to radiolabeled hormone binding tests and bioassay to determine whether the antiserum neutralizes gonadotropins other than that to which it has been raised. In addition, when the antiserum has been raised to a heterologous hormone, the efficacy of the antiserum in neutralizing the endogenous hormone of the test species must be determined.

Finally, in order to effectively use the antiserum as a specific inhibitor of a hormone, it is advisable to use minimal effective doses of a well-characterized high-titer antiserum. A high-titer antiserum makes repetitive testing in large numbers of animals possible.

Several investigators have been using active immunization to study the physiological effect of neutralizing LH or FSH. In view of the several precautions detailed above which have to be taken to insure the specificity of the antibodies produced, it is simpler to use passive immunization rather than active immunization techniques to study the physiological and biochemical mode of action of hormones.

Radioimmunoassay of Gonadotropins and Evidence of Specificity

29.   The Gonadotropins: Radioimmunoassay Technique and Physiologic Evidence of Specificity

Paul Franchimont, J. C. Hendrick, A. Reuter, and J. J. Legros

The radioimmunoassays of FSH and LH were first developed in 1966 and have since been widely used to study the secretion of the gonadotropins under normal and pathologic conditions.

In this paper we should like to consider certain aspects of the radioimmunoassay technique, although we shall not go into the classical literature on the subject (1-3). We shall also present results establishing the specificity of the FSH and LH assays.

RADIOIMMUNOASSAY TECHNIQUE

Damaged Hormone

The presence of damaged labeled hormone makes it impossible to perform an accurate radioimmunoassay. In particular, sensitivity drops and the inhibition slopes become flatter. Any damaged hormone present must thus be detected and eliminated..

FSH

The extent of damage may be determined by starch gel electrophoresis according to Ferguson and Wallace (4), since undamaged labeled FSH (FSH*) migrates with the post-albumins (5) while the damaged fractions remain at the site of application or migrate with various proteins such as the albumins, the slow α_2 globulins and the α blobulins. Damage may also be estimated by determining the percentage of labeled hormone which fails to be bound by an excess of antibody (6).

Elimination of the damaged FSH can be achieved by electrophoresis in starch gel (5-9) or in polyacrylamide gel (10, 11). However, the damaged hormone can be more easily removed by filtration on Sephadex G-100 (6, 12) or by chromatography on DEAE-cellulose (5-8). For this latter technique, the current practice is to apply the preparation of FSH* to a 20 X 1 cm column of DEAE-cellulose equilibrated with 0.01M K_2HPO_4. Unlike the undamaged hormone, the degraded molecules and any labeled contaminants present of the albumin or α_1 globulin type will not be retained by the ion exchanger. The undamaged FSH is eluted with 0.05M K_2HOP_4, as shown by immunoelectrophoretic and biologic analysis of the eluate.

There have been recent proposals (13, 14) to purify FSH* by adsorption chromatography on cellulose. Although undamaged FSH* appears to bind less well to cellulose than other hormones such as insulin, growth hormone, and LH (15), this purification technique can nevertheless be used for FSH.

LH

Some LH may be damaged during iodination. In addition, the hormone may undergo degradation during storage. For example, after 10 days storage with bovine albumin at 18, 4, and -20 C, the immunoreactivity of a preparation of LH* decreases by 44, 30, and 25% respectively.

The degree of LH* degradation may be estimated with a number of different techniques. Aluminum silicate (kaolin) adsorbs undamaged LH* but not the damaged hormone. This technique has also been applied to human growth hormone (16). Similarly, undamaged LH* adsorbs to charcoal while the undamaged hormone remains in liquid phase. Both the charcoal and the kaolin methods are rapid and easy. Damaged LH* fails to adsorb to cellulose and can be detected by determining the percentage of radioactivity which, in the absence of antibody, leaves the region of the cellulose strip to which it had been applied during chromatoelectrophoresis. The extent of damage may also be determined by measuring the percentage of LH* which remains unbound in the presence of an excess of antibody (6). Starch gel electrophoresis is not suitable for LH since this hormone migrates with the lipoproteins and the slow α_2 globulins to the same zone as some of the degradation products (17).

The damaged LH* may successfully be removed by filtration on Sephadex G-75 (18, 19), G-100 (6), or G-200 (5-8). With Sephadex G-200 the hormone preparation is applied to a 50 X 1 cm column. Elution is performed with 0.05M Sorensen phosphate buffer pH 7.5 containing 0.1% bovine albumin and 0.9% NaCl.

Adsorption chromatography on cellulose may also be employed for purifying

LH after iodination (13-15) and for separating the damaged LH* from the undamaged hormone. The procedure described by Jeffcoate (13) consists of applying the LH* to the top of a 10-ml column of powdered cellulose (Whatman CF 11) packed in 0.1M phosphate buffer pH 7.4. The damaged hormone is eluted by washing with 20 to 30 ml of the same buffer while the undamaged LH* is eluted with 50% horse serum. Saxena (14) has recently proposed a similar technique that has the advantage of being easier to perform. A small (2.5 cm) column of cellulose (Whatman CF 11) is formed in a 5-ml plastic syringe. The crude iodination mixture is applied to the top of the column and the column is then washed with 0.05M phosphate buffer pH 7.5. The radioactive iodinated radicals and the damaged LH are eliminated during this first step. The undamaged LII* is then eluted with 5 ml of 0.05M phosphate buffer, pH 7.5, containing 5% fresh bovine or human albumin and 10% acetone. In our hands this method gives very good results.

Verification of Antiserum Specificity

The specificity of FSH and LH antisera must be verified rigorously because of the partial cross-reaction between the glycoprotein hormones. Antiserum raised against one of the gonadotropins may contain antibody capable of reacting indistinctly with all the glycoprotein hormones.

SPECIFIC ANTI-FSH

FSH possesses antigenic groups common to the four glycoprotein hormones (FSH, LH, HCG, TSH) as well as antigenic sites specific to it alone (5-8, 10-12, 20). As a result, any FSH antiserum may contain nonspecific antibodies that react with LII, IICG, and TSII. To neutralize these antibodies, the antisera must be incubated with HCG, whose immunochemical structure is very close to that of LH. If desired, the exact amount of HCG to be added may be calculated by determining the smallest amount of hormone that produces a maximum reduction in the percentage of FSH* bound by antibody. In practice, however, an excess of HCG is simply incubated with the anti-FSH (5, 8, 9) or added extemporaneously to each incubation tube (10, 11, 21).

SPECIFIC ANTI-LH AND ANTI-HCG

Few workers use anti-LH in the LH radioimmunoassay (22, 23). Most (5-8, 19, 24-29) employ HCG antisera in view of the highly similar antigenic structures of LH and HCG. However, LH and HCG also possess antigenic groups common to TSH and FSH; preparations used for immunization may be contaminated by these glycoprotein hormones. Thus it is imperative to verify the specificity of LH and HCG antisera.

Control procedures have disclosed that many HCG antisera are not suitable for assaying either LH or HCG, as they contain nonspecific antibodies which react with all the glycoprotein hormones. These antibodies seem to be directed against the common portion of the glycoproteins since incubation of the antiserum with pure FSH eliminates the cross-reaction with TSH (Fig. 1). In practice, however, the rarity of pure FSH makes it impossible to neutralize these nonspecific antibodies.

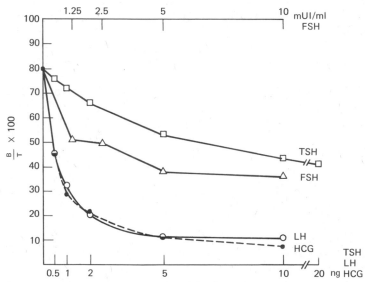

FIG. 1. Displacement of bound labeled LH by FSH (Medical Research Council Standard A), LH (7500 IU/mg preparation of Dr. Hartree), HCG (14,000 IU/mg, Organon) and TSH (4 IU/mg) using an antiserum to HCG. Note the partial cross-reaction with TSH and FSH, and the total cross-reaction between LH and HCG. LH* = 0.1 ng; anti HCG serum = 1/720,000.

Certain LH and HCG antisera, in contrast, contain no antibody capable of reacting with FSH or TSH at the dilutions at which they bind LH* and HCG* adequately for purposes of radioimmunoassay (17, 30). The specificity of these antisera is demonstrated on the one hand by their inability to bind either TSH* or FSH* and on the other hand by the fact that unlabeled TSH and FSH fail to produce a significant reduction in the percentage of LH* bound, in contrast to unlabeled LH and increasing volumes of human menopausal serum. Such antisera may therefore be employed in the LH radioimmunoassay with no risk of interference by FSH or TSH.

When anti-HCG is used for assaying LH, it must be borne in mind that the cross-reaction between HCG and LH is only partial; each of these hormones possesses its own specific antigenic determinants (17, 31, 32). Anti-HCG may contain antibody directed specifically against HCG and unable to react with LH (17) (Fig. 2). Furthermore, highly dissimilar inhibition slopes for HCG* are obtained depending on whether LH or HCG is utilized as the reference preparation. In assay systems using HCG antisera, therefore, LH should always be employed as both tracer and standard (Fig. 3).

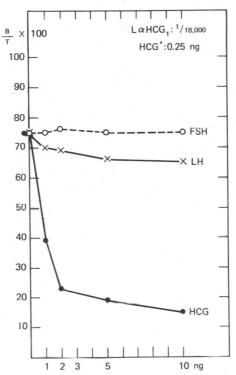

FIG. 2. Effects of unlabeled FSH, LH, and HCG on the percentage of labeled HCG bound by antibody. This is a relatively specific radioimmunoassay for HCG since unlabeled FSH and LH do not modify the percentage bound (17). Reproduced by permission of Springer Verlag.

Choice of Reference Preparation

Metabolic transformations of the gonadotropins within the body alter their immunochemical structure. For example, the pituitary FSH molecule apparently possesses antigenic groups which are lost during metabolism, since they are no longer present on the urinary FSH molecule (20, 21). In addition, during metabolism there appear to be changes in tertiary structure. As a result, some antigenic sites which were hidden on the pituitary molecule may be unmasked on the urinary molecule and thus become capable of inducing the formation of antibody specific to the urinary hormone. Such is the case for FSH (Fig. 4) (33).

In view of these differences in immunologic behavior depending on the biologic fluid from which the gonadotropins are extracted, it is highly desirable to employ homogeneous assay systems. For example, in assaying urinary FSH it

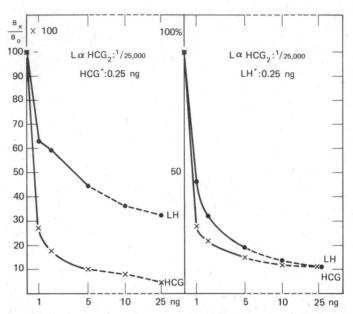

FIG. 3. Displacement of bound labeled urinary FSH by urinary FSH (FSH$_u$) and pituitary FSH (FSH$_p$) using an antiserum to urinary FSH. At equal doses a flatter curve was obtained with FSH$_p$) than with FSH$_u$, and at doses equal to or greater than 2 mIU the percentage bound was stabilized at a markedly higher level with FSH$_p$ (33). Reproduced by permission of J. B. Lippincott Company.

is best to use urinary FSH as both tracer and standard as well as an antiserum raised against urinary FSH. Similarly, the radioimmunoassay of serum FSH should ideally be performed with labeled and unlabled FSH of pituitary origin and antiserum to pituitary FSH. When such homogeneous systems are used, the results obtained by radioimmunoassay and bioassay are concordant (10, 11, 20-22, 34-37).

Separation Methods

Many methods have been proposed for separating the free molecules from the antigen-antibody complexes in radioimmunoassay. Those applicable to the gonadotropins include chromatoelectrophoresis (38, 39), starch gel electrophoresis (5), the double antibody system (6, 9-12, 21, 22, 24, 28), polymerized antisera (40), chemical precipitation with organic solvents such as dioxane (29), solid-phase antibody (27), and immunosorbents (41, 42).

The double antibody system is the most widely used technique and is very practical. Its sensitivity within 95% confidence limits ranges from 1 to 10 pg.

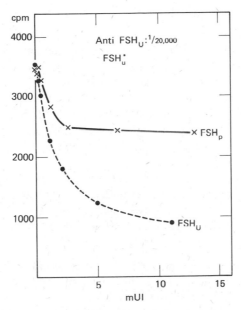

FIG. 4. Displacement of bound labeled urinary FSH by urinary FSH (FSH$_u$) and pituitary FSH (FSH$_p$) using an antiserum to urinary FSH. At equal doses a flatter curve was obtained with FSH$_p$ than with FSH$_u$, and at doses equal to or greater than 2 mIU the percentage bound was stabilized at a markedly higher level with FSH$_p$ (33). Reproduced by permission of J. P. Lippincott Company.

THE DIOXANE TECHNIQUE

This is very attractive because of its ease, but in our hands it has proved difficult to apply to the assay of FSH and LH in biologic fluids.

Dioxane does not yield an accurate spearation of free FSH* or LH* from the corresponding antigen-antibody complexes. Thomas et al. (43) have already noted the inadequate separation obtained from LH* and the LH*-anti-HCG complex with dioxane, in contrast to the satisfactory separation of free HCG*-anti-HCG complex.

Regardless of its concentration, dioxane gives rise to a precipitation of free LH* and FSH* in the absence of antibody. The precipitation is even more pronounced when 50 μl of bovine, ovine, or horse serum is added. In the presence of antibody, the influence of protein serums is demonstrated by the finding that the percentage of radioactivity precipitated with dioxane rises when serum is present. The addition of unlabeled hormone produces a slow decrease in antibody-bound radioactivity, which makes both precision and sensitivity poor.

THE IMMUNOSORBENT METHOD

This is based on the use of insoluble polymer-coupled antibodies known as immunosorbents (41, 44). We used cyanogen bromide-activated monocrystalline cellulose (Merk) prepared by the method of Axen et al. (45) as the solid phase material.

The following were incubated for 24 hr at room temperature, using 0.05M phosphate buffer pH 7.5 containing 0.5% bovine albumin for all solutions: (1) 0.5 ml immunosorbent suspended in phosphate buffer; (2) 0.1 ml buffer containing 50 pg of LH*, 0.1 ml unlabeled hormone in increasing doses (0, 1, 5, 10, 50, 100, 250, and 500 pg, 1, 2, 5, and 10 ng) or the biologic fluid to be assayed, and 0.1 ml buffer. Throughout the incubation period the tubes were rotated slowly. The amount of immunosorbent to be added to each tube was calculated by determining the quantity which bound 20 to 40% of 50 pg of LH* in the absence of unlabeled hormone.

At the end of the incubation period, the immunosorbent was separated by centrifugation and washed twice in 2.5 ml 0.05M phosphate buffer, pH 7.5. The radioactivity bound to the solid phase material was measured; this represented the amount of LH* bound by the solid-phase antibodies.

FEATURES OF THE IMMUNOSORBENT

High Stability. After being prepared the immunosorbent is diluted so as to produce a 1 : 1000 dilution of the antiserum initially used for binding. It is then divided into 0.5-ml volumes and frozen at -20 C. For each assay, a tube is thawed and utilized at the appropriate dilution (1 : 45,000). For over 6 months we made use of the same batch of immunosorbent. During this period the percentage of undamaged LH* bound by the diluted immunosorbent remained remarkably stable. It should be noted that the bound antiserum diluted 1 : 250,000 binds 40 to 50% of 50 pg of LH* when separation is performed by the double antibody system, which indicates that a considerable amount of antiserum immunoreactivity is lost during the immunosorbent coupling manipulations. This loss has also been noted by Arends (46).

No Tendency to Nonspecific Adsorption. The immunosorbent obtained with anti-HCG antibodies does not bind HCG* or HTSH* and binds less than 3% of 50 pg of FSH*. However, it does adsorb nonspecifically hormones of lower molecular weight, such as ACTH* and vasopressin*.

LH* is not bound by an immunosorbent prepared with microcrystalline cellulose and nonimmunized rabbit γ-globulins.

EFFECTS OF SERUM PROTEINS

With the immunosorbent separation method, the influence of serum proteins is considerable. If 0.1 ml of undiltued serum (final serum concentration 12.5%) or serum diluted 1 : 1 (final serum concentration 6.25%) from rabbit, ox, guinea pig, sheep, or a hypophysectomized subject is added to the incubation mixture, the percentage of LH* bound by the immunosorbent drops by about one-half. This decrease in the binding affinity of LH* for solid phase coupled antibody in the presence of serum appears to be due, in part, to the greater tendency of the immunosorbent to aggregate in the presence of serum than in its absence. Aggregation is particularly marked with weak dilutions of immunosorbent. The effects of serum proteins are not modified by the addition of Tween at a concentration of 0.5 to 1%. However, if, when the immunsorbent is prepared, it is homogenized with an ultrasound disintegrator, the influence of the serum is reduced.

The serum does not appear to act by damaging the labeled hormone since the radioactivity of the supernatant liquid adsorbs normally to kaolin. Routine use of the method is possible provided the standard curve is performed in the presence of horse serum or serum from a hypophysectomized subject. Results are obtained within 24 hr.

SENSITIVITY OF THE ASSAY

The sensitivity of the immunosorbent technique within 95% confidence limits is 50 pg/tube (preparation of Dr. Hartree containing 7500 IU/mg) or 375 μU of LH. This is lower than that obtained in our hands with the double antibody system.

Labeled Antibodies. These were used to assay LH according to the immunoradiometric method of Miles and Hales (47). The application of this method to LH has been described elsewhere (48).

Incubation was performed in 0.3 ml of 0.05M phosphate buffer containing 0.5% bovine albumin, pH 7.5. The diluted labeled antibodies were incubated with increasing quantities of unlabeled hormone. Incubation was allowed to progress for 48 hr at 4 C for 24 hr at room temperature. To this mixture was added 0.1 ml of a suspension containing a constant amount (250 μg) of LH immunosorbent. The mixture was then shaken for 90 min, the shortest time permitting maximum binding of the free labeled antibodies to the immunosorbent. The mixture was centrifuged and 200 μl of supernatant was drawn off and counted.

Fig. 5 shows the standard curve in an immunoradiometric assay of HLH. The percentage of radioactivity increase in the supernatant (corresponding to the labeled antibody-antigen complexes) is plotted against the amount of HLH added per tube.

In Fig. 6 one of the curves corresponds to an assay performed in buffer alone and the other to an assay performed in buffer containing 20% bovine serum. In the presence of bovine serum, the increase in radioactivity is less marked. The sensitivity is of the order of 10 pg in both cases.

The serum proteins appear to exert their influence on the reaction between the free labeled antibodies and the LH immunosorbent. In the absence of unlabeled LH, the addition of bovine serum causes more radioactivity to appear in the supernatant; conversely, more radioactivity is bound to the LH immunosorbent in the absence of bovine serum (Fig. 6). If the free antibodies which failed to be bound by the immunosorbent are again incubated with it at the same dose, the same percentage of radioactivity will again be bound. This seems to indicate that the serum does not damage the labeled antibodies. Rather, we seem to be dealing with a tendency for the immunosorbent to aggregate in

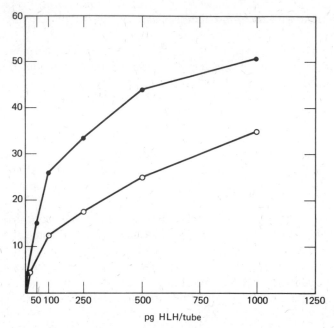

FIG. 5. Immunoradiometric assay of HLH, showing the percentage increase of radioactivity in the supernatant as a function of the HLH dose per tube. The filled circles represent the assay performed in buffer alone; the empty circles represent the assay performed in 20% bovine serum.

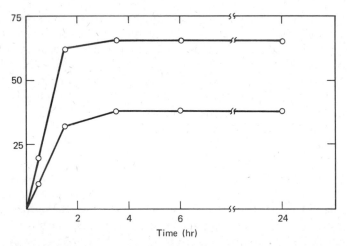

FIG. 6. Immunoradiometric assay of HLH, showing the percentage of radioactivity bound to LH-immunosorbent as a function of time. The filled circles represent the assay performed in buffer alone; the empty circles represent the assay performed in 20% bovine serum.

the presence of serum. Studies are now underway on possible methods of avoiding this phenomen.

The preparation of the labeled antibodies is obviously critical in this technique. In order for the method to be specific, the antibodies must be directed solely against the hormone being assayed, in other words, LH. It is thus essential that they be isolated with a pure hormone preparation bound chemically to the solid phase by an antiserum which does not react with other glycoprotein hormones. Together with Miles and Hales (47), we have verified that labeled antibodies eluted at pH 2.3 have a greater affinity for antigen than those eluted at pH 4.

The immunoradiometric technique is easy to perform since it requires only one centrifugation at the end of a 24-hr incubation period. Under our present experimental conditions, however, it does not heighten the sensitivity of the LH radioimmunoassay.

PHYSIOLOGIC EVIDENCE OF SPECIFICITY

The secretion of gonadotropins in humans can be modified by many factors and under various physiologic and pathologic conditions (50, 51). The finding that certain factors alter the blood levels of one of the gonadotropins without modifying the other offers indirect evidence of the specificity of the FSH and LH radioimmunoassays.

Effects of Estrogen

In postmenopausal women, the administration of small doses of estrogen, 20 μg ethinyl estradiol by mouth, results in a decline in FSH but merely slight changes in LH (Fig. 7). However, when estrogen is withdrawn, undoubtedly as serum levels of the steroid fall, there is a marked rise in LH (42, 49, 50). A true depression of LH is only obtained with higher estrogen doses, such as 50 μg ethinyl estradiol by mouth. The response is slower after methylation of the 3-hydroxy group as in mestranol.

The inhibitory action of estrogen on FSH and LH concentrations disappears when the 17β-hydroxy group is substituted, despite the fact that its peripheral estrogenic properties are preserved.

In our experience, estrogen has never had a stimulatory effect on LH secretion except when treatment is stopped and serum estrogen levels decline.

Effects of Progestogens

The oral administration of low doses (0.3 mg/day) of norethisterone acetate, a progestogen derived from 19-nortestosterone, depresses serum LH although it exerts no effect on FSH (Fig. 8). Norethisterone enanthate (200 mg) when injected intramuscularly reduces both FSH and LH but its effect on LH is more marked and more sustained. The inhibitory action of this particular progestogen

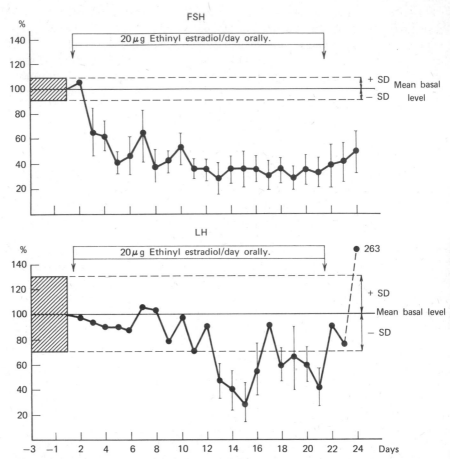

FIG. 7. Changes in serum FSH and LH levels in response to ethinyl estradiol (20 μg/day) administered orally for 19 days to 6 postmenopausal women. The results are expressed as percentage changes relative to mean pretreatment values (= 100%) and each point is shown with its standard deviation.

is exerted preferentially on LH secretion (51).

Effects of Testosterone

Following the intramuscular injection of 50 mg of testosterone propionate in male subjects, LH shows a very marked and prolonged drop. In contrast, FSH levels are unaffected by plasma testosterone, except when large doses of the androgen (100 mg or more) are injected (5). This inhibition of LH and lack of effect on FSH have also been reported by Peterson et al. (52), who injected 25

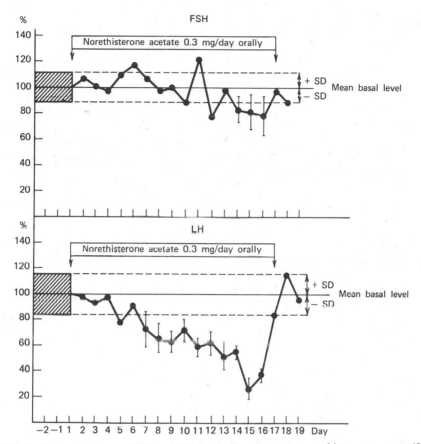

FIG. 8. Changes in serum FSH and LH levels in response to norethisterone acetate (0.3 mg/day) administered orally for 16 days to 4 postmenopausal women. The results are expressed as percentage changes relative to mean pretreatment values (= 100%) and each point is shown with its standard deviation (51). Reproduced by permission of Harper and Row Publisher.

mg of testosterone daily for 3 days in 3 normal subjects. Odell and Swerdloff (53) obtained the same results by administering 50 mg of fluoromesterolone.

In 16 cases of Klinefelter's syndrome verified by biopsy and karyotype, we found consistently high FSH levels accompanied by variable LH concentration, ranging from normal to decidedly elevated values.

In our opinion, the variable levels of LH seem to be related to the degree of Leydig cell insufficiency. We have found an inverse linear relationship between LH levels and plasma testosterone concentrations. Similarly, an inversely proportional relationship between LH and plasma testosterone has been reported during the first few hours after testosterone injection in patients with Klinefelter's syndrome (39).

FSH is independent of plasma testosterone, and the invariably high FSH levels in Klinefelter's syndrome must be considered as resulting from the deficient germinal function in these patients (5, 8, 54).

Consistently elevated FSH levels and variable LH levels ranging from normal to high are also seen in other types of hypogonadism of testicular origin, such as the sequelae of viral orchitis, testicular irradiation, and Steinert's disease (50). The high levels of FSH may be explained by the extensive or even total destruction of the germ cells in such cases, whereas the LH concentrations depend on the functioning of the Leydig cells, which are far more resistant. In addition, androgens are secreted by the adrenals and thus compensate somewhat for the inadequate endocrine secretion of the testis.

REFERENCES

1. Margoulies, M. (Ed.), Protein and Polypeptide Hormones, Excerpta Medica Foundation, Amsterdam, 1968.

2. Diczfalusy, E. (Ed.), Immunoassay of Gonadotrophins, 1st Karolinska Symposium on Research Methods in Reproductive Endocrinology, Stockholm, 1969.

3. Kirkham, K. E., and W. M. Hunter (Eds.), Radioimmunoassay Methods, Churchill Livingstone, Edinburgh and London, 1971.

4. Ferguson, K., and A. Wallace, Nature (London) 190:629, 1961.

5. Franchimont, P., Le Dosage des Hormones Hypophysaires Somatotrope et Gonadotropes et son Application en Clinique, Arscia, Brussels, 1966.

6. Saxena, B. B., H. Demura, H. M. Gandy, and R. E. Peterson, J Clin Endocrinol 28:519, 1968.

7. Franchimont, P., J Labelled Comp 2:303, 1966..

8. Franchimont, P., in M. Margoulies (Ed.), Protein and Polypeptide Hormones, Excerpta Medica Foundation, Amsterdam, 1968, p. 99.

9. Rosselin, G., and J. Dolais, Presse Med 75:2027, 1967.

10. Midgley, A. R., Jr., Fed Proc 26:533, 1967.

11. Midgley, A. R., Jr., J Clin Endocrinol 27:295, 1967.

12. Schlaff, S., S. Rosen, and J. Roth, J Clin Invest 47:1722, 1968.

13. Jeffcoate, S. L., in K. E. Kirkham and W. M. Hunter (Eds.), Radioimmunoassay Methods, Churchill Livingstone, Edinburgh and London, 1971, p. 190.

14. Leyendecker, G., D. M. Saunders, B. B. Saxena, Klin Wschr 49:658, 1971.

15. Hunter, W. M., in E. Diczfalusy (Ed.), Immunoassay of Gonadotrophins, 1st Karolinska Symposium on Research Methods in Reproductive Endocrinology, Stockholm, 1969, p. 134.

16. Franchimont, P., J. J. Legros, B. Deconinck, and A. Brunetti, Hormone Metab Res 1:218, 1969.

17. Franchimont, P., Europ J Clin Invest 1:65, 1970.

18. Odell, W., G. Ross, and D. Rayford, Metabolism 15:287, 1966.

19. Odell, W., G. Ross, and D. Rayford, J Clin Invest 46:248, 1967.

20. Odell, W. D., L. E. Reichert, and R. W. Bates, in M. Margoulies (Ed.), Protein and Polypeptide Hormones, Excerpta Medica Foundation, Amsterdam, 1968, p. 124.

21. Faiman, C., and R. Ryan, J Clin Endocrinol 27:444, 1967.

22. Faiman, C., and R. Ryan, J Clin Endocrinol 27:1711, 1967.

23. Schalch, D. S., A. F. Parlow, R. C. Boon, and S. Reichlin, J Clin Invest 47:665, 1968.

24. Midgley, A. R., Jr., Endocrinology 79:10, 1966.

25. Neill, J. D., E. D. B. Johansson, J. K. Datta, and E. Knobil, J Clin Endocrinol 27:1167, 1967.

26. Aono, T., D. P. Goldstein, M. L. Taymor, and K. Dolch, Amer J Obst Gyn 98:996, 1967.

27. Catt, K. J., H. D. Niall, G. W. Tregear, and H. G. Burger, J Clin Endocrinol 28:121, 1968.

28. Dolais, J., P. Freychet, and G. Rosselin, Compt Rend Acad Sci (Paris) 267:1105, 1968.

29. Thomas, K., and J. Ferin, J Clin Endocrinol 28:1667, 1968.

30. Franchimont, P., in E. Diczfalusy (Ed.), Immunoassay of Gonadotrophins, 1st Karolinska Symposium on Research Methods in Reproductive Endocrinology, Stockholm, 1969, p. 70.

31. Paul, W. E., and G. T. Ross, Endocrinology 75:352, 1964.

32. Goss, D., and J. Lewis, Endocrinology 74:83, 1964.

33. Franchimont, P., and P. Donini, J Clin Endocrinol 31:18, 1970.

34. Ryan, R. J., and C. Faiman, in M. Margoulies (Ed.), Protein and Polypeptide Hormones, Excerpta Medica Foundation, Amsterdam, 1968, p. 129.

35. Stevens, V., in E. Rosemberg (Ed.), Gonadotropins 1968, Geron-X, Inc., Los Altos, 1968, p. 413.

36. Albert, A., E. Rosemberg, G. T. Ross, C. A. Paulsen, and R. J. Ryan, J Clin Endocrinol 28:1214, 1968.

37. Ryan, R. J., and A. Albert, J Clin Endocrinol 28:1076, 1968.

38. Saxena, B. B., G. Leyendecker, W. Chen, H. M. Gandy, and R. E. Peterson, in E. Diczfalusy (Ed.), Immunoassay of Gonadotrophins, 1st Karolinska Symposium on Research Methods in Reproductive Endocrinology, Stockholm, 1969, p. 185.

39. Burger, H. G., in M. Margoulies (Ed.), Protein and Polypeptide Hormones, Part 3, Excerpta Medica Foundation, Amsterdam, 1969, p. 719.

40. Donini, S., and P. Donini, in E. Diczfalusy (Ed.), Immunoassay of Gonadotrophins, 1st Karolinska Symposium on Research Methods in Reproductive Endocrinology, Stockholm, 1969, p. 257.

41. Wide, L., in E. Diczfalusy (Ed.), Immunoassay of Gonadotrophins, 1st Karolinska Symposium on Research Methods in Reproductive Endocrinology, Stockholm, 1969, p. 207.

42. Franchimont, P., and J. C. Hendrick, Hormone Metab Res, in press, 1971.

43. Thomas, K., D. Nash, and J. Ferin, in E. Diczfalusy (Ed.), Immunoassay of Gonadotrophins, 1st Karolinska Symposium on Research Methods in Reproductive Endocrinology, Stockholm, 1969, p. 279.

44. Wide, L., and J. Porath, Biochim Biophys Acta 130:257, 1966.

45. Axen, R., J. Porath, and S. Ernbach, Nature (London) 214:1302,1967.

46. Arends, J., in K. E. Kirkham, and W. M. Hunter (Eds.), Radioimmunoassay Methods, Churchill Livingstone, Edinburgh and London, 1971, p. 426.

47. Miles, L. E. M., and C. N. Hales, Nature (London) 219:186, 1968.

48. Hendrick, J. C., and P. Franchimont, Ann Biol Clin, in press, 1971.

49. Franchimont, P., in L. Martini and W. F. Ganong (Eds.), Frontiers in Neuroendocrinology, 1971, Oxford University Press, New York, 1971.

50. Franchimont, P., La Sécrétion Normale et Pathologique de la Somatotrophine et des Gonadotrophines Humaines, Masson, Paris, 1971.

51. Franchimont, P., J. J. Legros, D. Ayalon, and A. Mutsers, Obst Gyn 36:93, 1970.

52. Peterson, N. T., Jr., A. R. Midgley, Jr., and R. B. Jaffe, J Clin Endocrinol 28:1473, 1968.

53. Odell, W. D., and R. S. Swerdloff, Proc Natl Acad Sci USA 61:529, 1968.

54. Franchimont, P., in W. J. Irvine and J. A. Loraine (Eds.), Reproductive Endocrinology, Livingstone, Edinburgh, 1970, p. 1.

30. Antigen-Antibody Complex Precipitation by Chemical Procedure in Radioimmunoassays

K. Thomas, C. Beckers, and J. Ferin

Among the numerous techniques described for separating unbound from anti-body-bound hormone in radioimmunoassay procedure, selective precipitation of the antigen-antibody complexes with salts, organic solvents, or mixtures thereof, has not been widely employed. It may be, as suggested by Yalow (1), because of separation is seldom as complete as with specific adsorbents and because the specific methods for separation of hormones with different chemical properties have little in common.

Nevertheless, several authors have described salt or organic solvent precipitation methods for the radioimmunological assay of protein, polypeptide, and steroid hormones. These techniques are summarized in Table I.

The purpose of the present communication is to review briefly the data of the literature involving salt or organic solvent fractionation in radioimmunoassay procedures. Special emphasis will be given to an experimental design to obtain a selective precipitation of antibody-bound HCG, LH, HGH, TSH, FSH, and human chorionic somatomammotropin (HCS) by using the following water-soluble organic solvents as precipitating agents: dioxane, propanol-2, methanol, and ethanol. The feasibility of radioimmunologic quantitating HCG (LH) and HCS (HPL) will be briefly described.

Many methods of fractionation of protein mixtures exploit differences in solubility which under suitable circumstances may exist between individual protein species. This solubility is largely a function of the ratio between the

TABLE I. Survey of chemical precipitation methods in radioimmunoassay

Authors and references	Hormone	Biological fluid	Salt and/or organic solvent
Grodsky and Forsham (6)	Insulin	Serum	Sodium sulfite (17%), urea (15%)
Heding (7)	Insulin	Plasma	Ethanol (80%)
Hollemans et al. (17)	Angiotensin	Plasma	Ammonium sulfate (saturated)
Furuyama et al. (18)	Testosterone	Plasma	Ammonium sulfate (saturated)
Heding (8)	Glucagon	Plasma	Ethanol (80%)
Odell et al. (9, 10)	HTSH	Serum	Ethanol (55%), NaCl (5%)
Tomoda and Hreshchyshyn (13)	HCG	Urine	Ethanol, ammonium sulfate (10%)
Arends (15)	HCG	Urine	Ammonium sulfate
Thomas et al. (19, 20)	HCG, HLH	Plasma	Dioxane (52.8%)
Wilson and Hunter (11)	HLH	Urine	Ethanol (55%), NaCl (4.8%)
Stevenson and Spalding (12)	HLH	Urine	Ethanol (55%), NaCl (4.8%)
Kazeto et al. (14)	HLH, HFSH	Urine	Ethanol, ammonium sulfate (10%)
Czygan (24)	HLH, HFSH	Plasma	Dioxane
Leyendecker, Saunders and Saxena (25)	FSH	Plasma	Dioxane
Letchworth et al. (34)	HCS (HPL)	Plasma	Ethanol (66%)
Haour (26)	HCS (HPL)	Plasma	Dioxane (60%)
Thomas and Ferin	HCS (HPL)	Plasma	Propanol-2 (62%) or dioxane (62%)

378

polar, hydrophilic, and the nonpolar, hydrophobic, groups of the molecule. Precipitating agents like salts or water-soluble organic solvents operate essentially by decreasing the activity of the water in the protein mixture, thereby dehydrating the hydrophilic groups of the protein molecules (2), and consequently they influence the solubility of the proteins present in the mixture.

The combination of immunoglobulins (specific antibodies) with hormone molecules will have a tendency to influence the precipitability of the latter and, to some extent, the complex may exhibit solubility characteristics which are essentially those of the immunoglobulins alone. Of prime importance here is the ability of the antigen (hormone)-antibody complex to precipitate in the presence of added salt or organic solvents under conditions that would not affect the unbound antigen. The following survey of the literature reveals that the immunologic binding of hormones to specific antibodies makes it possible to separate the bound antigen from the unbound antigen by taking advantage of the precipitating properties of the immunoglobulins and/or the resulting complex.

Selective removal of antigen-antibody complexes by precipitation with salt and/or organic solvents, but not involving radioimmunologic procedures, was first reported by Berson et al. (3) and later by Gordis (4) and Moloney and Aprile (5) for insulin anti-insulin complexes.

The first mention of a radioimmunologic assay, as such, was reported by Grodsky and Forsham (6) using a technique of preferential salt precipitation of the antibody-bound labeled hormone. The insulin bound to antibody was precipitated by addition of two volumes of water containing sufficient sodium sulfite to attain a final concentration of 17% in the mixture. In order to obtain the same concentration of proteins in the standard assay curves as found in the analytical samples, "insulin-free plasma" or gelatin was used as a carrier. A final concentration of 15% urea was also added to each incubation mixture in order to eliminate coprecipitation of free insulin.

Heding (7) discussed the effect of organic solvents on the precipitation of insulin anti-insulin complexes. She was able to demonstrate that the solvents methanol, propanol, dioxane, and acetone, as used by her, were not adequate for separation of bound from unbound insulin. On the other hand, such separation could be achieved with 80% ethanol. This author also noted that any of the ions Cl^-, NO_3^-, $HCOO^-$, CH_3COO^-, and I^- increase the insulin-antibody reaction rate and, at the same time, increase the total amount of antibody bound insulin. Other ions including Na^+, K^+, NH_4^+, SO_4^{--}, HPO_4^{--}, BO_3^{---}, citrate and oxalate were found to be inactive. It was concluded that a minimum concentration of certain ions is necessary in the assay system. It is important to note that Heding found no dissociation of the antigen-antibody complex within 2 hr after addition of the ethanol to the assay mixture. It was also noted that anticoagulants such as heparin, citrate, oxalate, and EDTA, at 5 times the concentrations normally used, did not affect the results. In a more recent paper (8) the same author reported a similar technique for radioimmunological determination of pancreatic and gut glucagon in plasma. The influence of ethanol, NaCl, and albumin on the assay system is discussed.

For the separation of antibody-bound human thyroid stimulating hormone (HTSH) and free HTSH, Odell et al. (9, 10) developed a chemical procedure based on the solubility of TSH in 55% ethanol-5% NaCl and the insolubility of the TSH-antibody complexes under the same conditions. Using this technique, nonspecific precipitation of free hormone in the presence of serum and in the absence of anti-TSH, amounted to 5 to 15% of the total counts. Washing of the precipitate was omitted since precision was not increased.

Employing the same chemical procedure, Wilson and Hunter (11) described a separation technique for the radioimmunoassay of human LH. With a concentration of 55% ethanol in 4.8% NaCl the antibody-LH complex could be precipitated while free LH remained in solution. Under these conditions, the procedure is only applicable for the assay of LH in human urine and not in serum due to coprecipitation for the assay of ^{131}I-LH with serum proteins. Stevenson and Spalding (12) have successfully employed this method for the assay of LH in concentrated urine samples taken at various stages of the menstrual cycle.

The assay of HCG has been successfully achieved by Tomoda and Hreshchyshyn (13) using ethanol and 10% ammonium acetate. The technique, when applied to urine, proved to be less sensitive than other precipitation methods. An important finding in this paper was the nonspecific inhibition of precipitation of hormone-antibody complexes by unknown factors present in urine. Recently the same group (14) published the applicability of the same technique to the radioimmunologic quantitation of HLH and HFSH in morning urine specimens. Good correlation was found between the values obtained by the alcohol precipitation techniques and those obtained by the double-antibody method.

A radioimmunoassay of urinary HCG was also described recently by Arends (15) using ammonium sulfate at concentrations of 1.9mole/1 as precipitating agent. Particular emphasis was given to the addition of carrier protein (horse serum).

A pretesting of the carrier protein seemed imperative since an increased precipitation of free HCG has been seen with occasional batches of horse serum. The technique was limited to the quantitation of HCG in pregnancy urine.

Hunter (16) attempted to obtain a selective precipitation of antibody-bound HGH using ammonium sulfate. He noted that an important part of the unbound antigen coprecipitated with the bound hormone making this method an unlikely substitute for previously described techniques not involving chemical precipitation.

Hollemans et al. (17) were successful in quantitating angiotensin using techniques in which the bound hormone was precipitated with a saturated ammonium sulfate solution at pH 8.0 and 4 C. Saturated ammonium sulfate was also used by Furuyama et al. (18) to achieve separation of unbound from antibody-bound testosterone in plasma extracts.

From the above mentioned techniques it can be noted that, for the most part, the separation of antibody-bound hormone from the unbound proteins in radioimmunoassay procedures is accomplished by means of precipitation methods using a mixture of salts and organic solvents. The methods described have been designed mainly for assay of hormones in urine and an application to hormones in serum or plasma is often complicated by coprecipitation of free hormone making them inadequate for use in high protein concentration mixtures.

Nevertheless, we were able to report in a preliminary communication (19) that, even in presence of high protein concentrations (25% horse serum or undiluted plasma sample), an excellent separation of free HCG from antibody-bound HCG was obtained by using the organic solvent dioxane at a final concentration of 52.8%. Since then a detailed description of the dioxane technique has been given (20) and also its applicability for radioimmunologic quantitation of HCG and LH in plasma (21, 22) and urine (23). This dioxane technique has been used successfully by Czygan (24) to quantitate plasma LH and FSH levels, and by Leyendecker, et al (25) for the FSH quantitation. Recently, Haour (26) reported a rapid radioimmunoassay of HCG (HPL) also using dioxane as the precipitating agent. It will be shown in the present paper that the organic solvent propanol-2 is also an excellent precipitating agent for the HCS-anti-HCS complex.

MATERIALS

Hormone Preparations

Human Chorionic Gonadotropin. A highly purified sample of HCG (batch A_3R_5) was supplied by Organon, Oss, the Netherlands, and has a biological potency of 14,000 (with 95% confidence limits at 12,200 to 16,100) IU/mg in terms of the Second International Standard of HCG. The purification procedure as well as some of the physicochemical characteristics of this preparation have been described (27). This particular sample was used in the production of specific antisera, preparation of tracer, and as a laboratory standard.

Human LH. This protein (LER-822-2) was obtained through the courtesy of the Endocrinology Study Section, NIH, Bethesda, Maryland. The sample has been reported to have an LH activity of 2.99 x NIH-LH- S_1/mg or 4598 IU 2nd IRP-HMG/mg.

Human FSH. Human urinary FSH "immunochemical grade" (batch E174ter-4) was obtained through the courtesy of Dr. Donini, Serono, Rome. The FSH potency of this preparation was 1108 IU/mg (2nd IRP-HMG).

Human Growth Hormone. HGH HG 1147 DC (Dr. Wilhelmi) was obtained from the Endocrinology Study Section, NIH, Bethesda, Maryland.

Human TSH. Human TSH for iodination was obtained from the Endocrinology Study Section, NIH, Bethesda, Maryland.

Human Chorionic Somatomammotropin. Purified placental protein (human), lot 4508 C 75, was obtained through the courtesy of Lederle Laboratories Division, Pearl River, New York.

Antisera

Anti-Human Chorionic Gonadotropin. Anti-HCG was prepared in rabbits by repeated subcutaneous injections of the highly purified HCG (14,000 IU/mg). Details on the preparation and on the specificity of this antiserum have been described previously (20).

Anti-Human Follicle Stimulating Hormone. Anti-HFSH serum (batch 316) was obtained from Dr. Donini, Serono, Rome. Antibodies directed against contaminating antigens were absorbed with serum and urine extracts from hypophysectomized patients and by addition of purified HCG.

Anti-Human Growth Hormone. Guinea pig anti-HGH (batch no. 2-5-19) was prepared by Drs. R.S. Yalow and S.A. Berson and obtained from the Endocrinology Study Section, NIH, Bethesda, Maryland.

Anti-Human Thyroid Stimulating Hormone. Anti-HTSH was obtained from the Endocrinology Study Section, NIH, Bethesda, Maryland.

Anti-Human Chorionic Somatomammotropin. Anti-HCS serum was prepared in rabbits by repeated injections of the PPP, Lederle, lot 4508 C 75.

Organic Solvents

Dioxane. 1,4-Dioxane, diethylene dioxide, molecular wt, 88.11, technical-grade and analytical-grade dioxane was obtained from Union Chimique Belge (U.C.B.), Brussels, Belgium and Merck, Darmstadt, Germany. Physicochemical properties of this organic solvent have been described previously (20).

Propanol-2. Isopropyl alcohol, molecular wt 60.10; methanol and ethanol were also obtained from the same sources.

Tracer Hormones (^{131}I-HCG, ^{131}I-HLH, ^{131}I-HFSH, ^{125}I-HGH, ^{131}I- HTSH, and ^{125}I-HCS)

The purified hormones were labeled to specific activities of 100 to 450 μCi/μg with ^{131}I according to the method of Greenwood et al. (28). The ^{131}I used for this labeling was freshly prepared by CEN, Mol, Belgium.

Labeled HGH was obtained from Dr. M. de Gasparo, Louvain, and labeled HTSH from Dr. C. Beckers, Louvain. Labeled HCS was obtained from Sclavo-Sorin, Italy. For the iodination of HCG, HLH, and HFSH, 2 to 3.5 mCi ^{131}I was used. These iodinated hormones were separated from inorganic ^{131}I by passage through a Sephadex G-50 column and further purified by filtration on a Sephadex G-200 column.

The buffer used in all test preparations was 0.07M phosphate, pH 7.4 according to Sørensen, and contained 0.0243% Merthiolate. No preservative was added to buffers used in the labeling procedure. Tracer hormones were diluted in phosphate buffer containing 1% bovine albumin.

METHODS AND RESULTS

Experimental Procedure for the Separation of Antibody-Bound from Unbound Hormones

The following experimental procedure has been applied, with variable results, to the separation of bound from unbound HCG, HLH, HGH, HTSH, HFSH, and HCS. A detailed description is given only for the ^{131}I-HCG- ^{131}I and ^{131}I-HCG-anti-HCG complex system since the procedure is essentially the same for the others.

SEPARATION OF ANTI-HCG FROM FREE LABELED HCG

Four groups of 28 tubes (2 ml) were prepared for incubation. Each tube of the first group contained 150 μl of 1% bovine serum albumin in phosphate buffer and 50 μl ^{131}I-HCG (0.25 to 0.050 ng). Each tube in the second group contained 100 μl of 1% bovine serum albumin in phosphate buffer, 50 μl ^{131}I-HCG and 50 μl anti-HCG diluted 1 : 200,000. The third and fourth groups were similar to the second except that they contained antiserum dilutions of 1 : 20,000 and 1 : 400,000 respectively. Each tube was tightly stoppered with a rubber bung in order to prevent evaporation. All operations were carried out at 4 C.

After three days of incubation, 800 μl of aqueous dioxane, in increasing concentrations were added to the four groups. A white flocculent precipitate formed. The contents of each tube were gently mixed and immediately centrifuged at 3000 rpm for 30 min. The supernatant was removed and the precipitate counted in a Packard Autogamma Spectrometer without prior washing. At a concentration of 56% dioxane, free ^{131}I- HCG begins to precipitate and a maximal precipitation is attained at a concentration of 65.6% (Fig. 1, solid lines). Precipitation of the antigen-antibody complex, however, starts at 46.4% dioxane. The majority of the HCG-anti-HCG complex (90%) is precipitated with a concentration of 52.8% dioxane (Fig. 1, dashed lines). The dioxane concentrations mentioned above refer to those present in the final mixture.

In order to assimilate more closely the protein concentration as found in serum, the same experiment was repeated replacing the 50 μl of phosphate buffer with 50 μl horse serum. As can be seen in Fig. 1, the results were essentially the same.

The results obtained from the series of tubes having received antibodies at dilutions of 1 : 20,000 and 1 : 400,000 are also illustrated in Fig. 1. It can be seen that the maximal precipitation levels obtained are a function of the antibody concentration. It will also be noted that the plateau representing

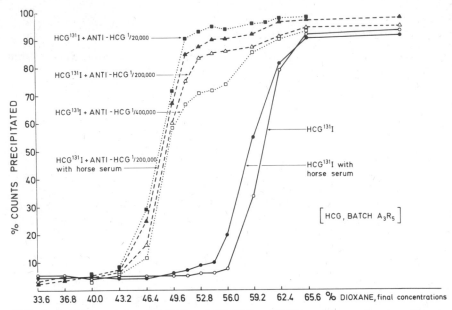

FIG. 1. Solubility of free ^{131}I-HCG and ^{131}I-HCG-anti-HCG complexes at various dioxane concentrations. The abscissa represents total dioxane concentrations of the final mixture.

maximal precipitation of hormone-antibody complexes demonstrated a slight increase in slope with increasing dioxane concentrations. This could mean that the hormone-antibody complex is not completely precipitated at low dioxane concentrations and requires concentrations similar to those precipitating the free hormone. That this is not the case is also illustrated in Fig. 1. The curves representing free hormone precipitates show progressive increases in precipitation at low dioxane concentrations. This observation indicates that some free antigen (labeled hormone) will be precipitated at concentrations lower than expected but higher than necessary for complete removal of complexes from the mixture. The precipitation of free hormone at these lower concentrations becomes manifest as a slight increase in the maximal precipitation slope of the curves representing hormone-antibody precipitates.

That complete removal of the HCG-anti-HCG complex occurs is demonstrated by the fact that by using high antibody concentrations the radioactive complex is precipitated nearly 98%. On the other hand, if the complex is first removed by a second precipitating antibody (double-antibody system) the addition of dioxane to the resulting supernatant precipitates only 1% to 3% of the total counts. This is a proof that dioxane at an adequate concentration precipitates only the HCG-anti-HCG complex and nothing more.

Some factors which may influence the slopes of these precipitation curves were studied in detail.

A comparison of technical grade dioxane with analytical grade dioxane revealed no substantial differences (Fig. 2), so that later experiments were performed using technical grade dioxane.

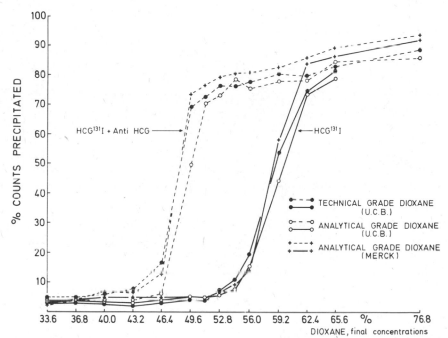

FIG. 2. Influences of different grades of dioxane on the solubility of free ^{131}I-HCG and ^{131}I-HCG-anti-HCG complexes at increasing dioxane concentrations. Abscissa as in Fig. 1.

Variation of pH in the final incubation mixture between 7.0 and 8.0 proved to give identical results (Fig. 3)). Also the presence of EDTA or normal rabbit serum in concentrations usually employed did not influence the outcome of the separation technique (Fig. 4).

Finally the possible dissociation effect of dioxane on the antigen-antibody complexes was investigated by waiting up to 6 hr before centrifugation of the incubated dioxane mixture. The extension of the time between addition of dioxane and centrifugation decreases only slightly the precipitated radioactive complex, which indicates that under the described working conditions dioxane does not significantly dissociate the complex (Fig. 5).

The results of this experiment demonstrate the validity of the dioxane precipitation method for radioimmunoassay of HCG, when dioxane concentrations are used, which will precipitate bound hormone, while at the same time, having little or no effect on the free hormone in solution. Under identical conditions precipitation of HCG-anti-HCG complexes was not adequate using the organic solvents, methanol, ethanol, or isopropyl alcohol.

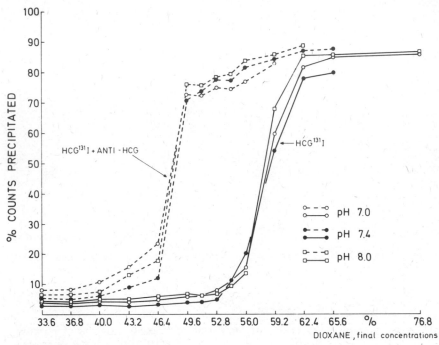

FIG. 3. Influence of pH on the solubility of free ^{131}I-HCG and ^{131}I-HCG-anti-HCG complexes at increasing dioxane concentrations. Abscissa as in Fig. 1.

SEPARATION OF ANTI-HCG BOUND HLH FROM FREE LABELED HLH

The results obtained in this system are represented in Fig. 6. The slopes of the curves representing LH-anti-HCG complexes are identical with those of the HCG-anti-HCG curves found in Fig. 1, if the same antibody dilutions (1 : 200,000) are compared. Nonspecific precipitation of free labeled LH occurs at concentrations of dioxane lower than 56.0% reducing seriously "the zone" where dioxane is assumed to precipitate only the LH-anti-HCG complex. This nonspecific precipitation of free LH is not influenced by high protein concentrations of the assay mixture achieved by the addition of horse serum, since the curves of free HLH with or without horse serum are strictly parallel.

SEPARATION OF ANTI-HGH BOUND FROM THE LABELED HGH

Less than adequate separation of bound HGH from unbound hormone is illustrated in Fig. 7. This series of precipitation curves illustrates that serious

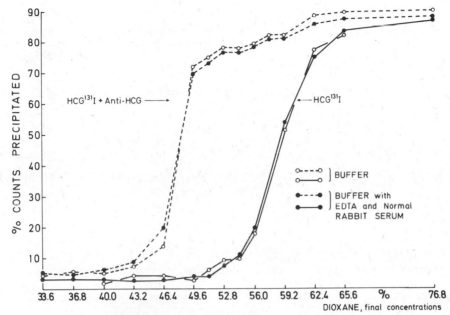

FIG. 4. Influence of EDTA and normal rabbit serum on the solubility of free ^{131}I-HCG and ^{131}I-HCG-anti-HCG complexes at increasing dioxane concentrations. Abscissa as in Fig. 1.

coprecipitation occurs only in the presence of undiluted horse serum. When serum is diluted 1 : 10, as is usual in radioimmunoassay of HGH, the precipitation of free HGH represents only 5 to 12% at dioxane concentrations of 52.8 to 56.0%. Washing the precipitate with corresponding dioxane concentration slightly reduces the apparent precipitation of free hormone.

SEPARATION OF ANTI-HTSH BOUND HTSH FROM FREE LABELED HTSH

Excellent separation is obtained at dioxane concentrations of 49.6 to 56.0% when the procedure is carried out in buffer milieu containing as protein only 1% of albumin (Fig. 8). If horse serum is added to the incubation mixture an important nonspecific precipitation of free HTSH occurs at the same dioxane concentrations. The slope of the HTSH-anti-HTSH complex precipitation curve seems also to be affected.

SEPARATION OF ANTI-HFSH BOUND HFSH FROM FREE LABELED HFSH

In absence of horse serum the vertical distance between the curves is optimal at a dioxane concentration of 56.0% (Fig. 9). This distance is reduced in

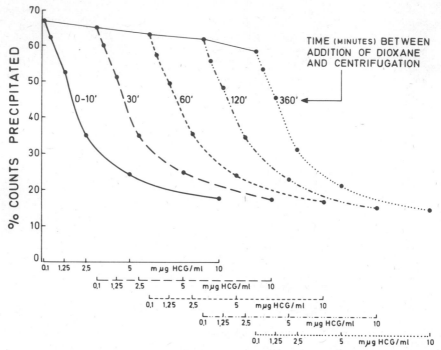

FIG. 5. Stability of the ^{131}I-HCG-anti-HCG complexes in presence of dioxane. The extension of the time between addition of dioxane to the incubation mixture and centrifugation produces an insignificant decrease of the precipitated radioactive complex as is shown by the standard assay curves.

presence of horse serum owing principally to the coprecipitation of free HFSH. In contrast with the separation procedure for the other hormones, difficulties occur with the precipitation of the HFSH-anti-HFSH complexes. Even at final anti-HFSH concentrations of 1 : 200 it was impossible to precipitate more than 70 to 80% of the antigen-antibody complexes at high dioxane concentrations.

SEPARATION OF ANTI-HCS BOUND HCS FROM FREE LABELED HCS

As Fig. 10 illustrates, an excellent separation is observed in this experimental design using either dioxane or isopropyl alcohol (propanol-2). The optimal vertical distance between the curves of antibody-bound hormone and free HCS is around 62% of dioxane or propanol-2. While at this concentration dioxane gives about 10% nonspecific precipitation of free HCS, propanol-2 gives only an insignificant free hormone precipitate. For this reason propanol-2 may be preferred to achieve the separation. Since in radioimmunoassay HCS is usually determined in diluted plasma or serum the experiment was not performed using high protein concentrations (25% horse serum) in the incubation milieu.

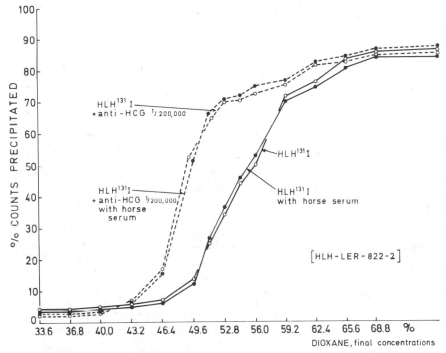

FIG. 6. Solubility of free ^{131}I-HLH and ^{131}I-HLH-anti-HLH complexes at various dioxane concentrations. HLH-LER-822-2 was used as tracer hormone. The anti-HLH antibody is the same as in Fig. 1. The abscissa represents the total dioxane concentrations of the final mixture.

Radioimmunoassay Procedure Using Organic Solvents For the Selective Precipitation of the Antigen-Antibody Complex

The experiments described above clearly indicate that dioxane is an excellent solvent to achieve separation of antibody-bound HCG (LH) from free HCG (LH) and of antibody-bound HCS (HPL) from free HCS (HPL). For the latter system propanol-2 may be preferred, because of the lower nonspecific precipitation of free HCS. Fig. 11 represents a general schedule of the proposed radioimmuno-assay system.

HCG (LH) RADIOIMMUNOASSAY

A detailed description of the procedure for this hormone has been given previously (19, 20) and will not be repeated here. Nevertheless, it may be mentioned, in addition to the previous reported data, that the tracer hormone is added to the incubation mixture 4 hr after the other reactants. The volume of all reactants was doubled (final incubation volume 400 μl instead of 200 μl) and consequently the volume of the dioxane solution was also doubled (1.6 ml)

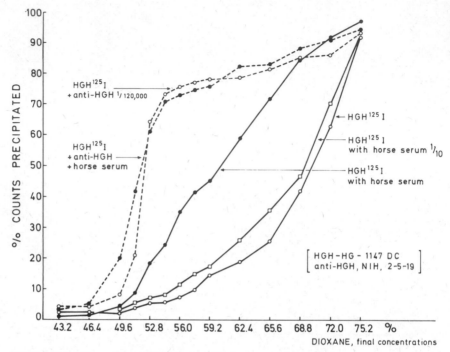

FIG. 7. Solubility of free ^{125}I-HGH and ^{125}I-HGH-anti-HGH complexes at various dioxane concentrations. Tracer protein is HGH-HG-1147 DC; anti-HGH is NIH 2-5-19. Abscissa as in Fig. 1.

giving in the final mixture a concentration of 52.8%. Precision and specificity of this system have already been reported (20, 21) and also its usefulness for radioimmunologic quantitation of LH in plasma (21, 22) and in urine (23).

An example of the plasma LH concentration found every 6 hr during the midcycle LH discharge is given in Fig. 12. The LH levels were quantitated by three different techniques. The dioxane method was compared with the double-antibody technique. In addition, two different labeled hormones, HCG and HLH, were compared using the same anti-HCG. Good correlations were found between the three techniques for the relative fluctuations of LH. The dioxane method, using HCG as tracer and the 2nd IRP-HMG as standard, demonstrated absolute values, which were slightly higher than those obtained with the same tracer and standard, but using the double-antibody technique. Using HLH as tracer and standard, combined with the double-antibody technique, even lower absolute values were observed.

Fig. 13 compares the fluctuations of LH concentrations in plasma and urine during the same periovulatory period. The biphasic pattern of the midcycle LH surge found in plasma is also evident in urine but several hours later (23). This

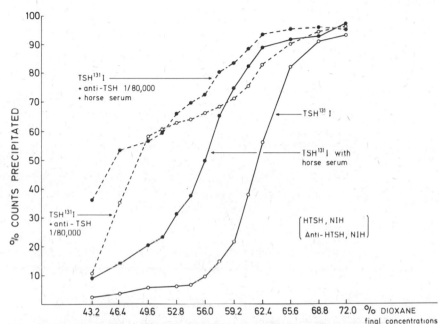

FIG. 8. Solubility of free ^{131}I-TSH and ^{131}I-TSH-anti-TSH complexes at various dioxane concentrations. Tracer hormone is HTSH, NIH; antibody is anti-TSH, NIH. Abscissa as in Fig. 1.

figure demonstrates also urinary LH concentrations found by the hemagglutination inhibition test (29).

HCS (HPL) RADIOIMMUNOASSAY

For this hormone the same procedure was followed as for the HCG radioimmunoassay. However, in determining standard assay curves no horse serum was added, since the analytical samples for HCS determinations are usually diluted. In order to obtain the results more rapidly the total incubation time was reduced to 16 hr. The organic solvent dioxane or propanol-2 was used as precipitating agent. A comparison of the HCS concentrations found by the organic solvent technique with those found by the double-antibody procedure is shown in Fig. 14. A good correlation was observed between the values found by the different assay systems. The HCS kit of Sclava-Sorin, Italy, was employed in the double-antibody technique.

DISCUSSION AND CONCLUSIONS

In comparison with other methods for the separation of antigen-antibody complexes from free antigen the chemical precipitation with salts and/or organic

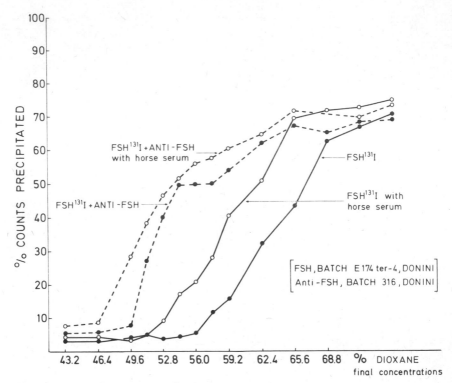

FIG. 9. Solubility of free ^{131}I-FSH and ^{131}I-FSH-anti-FSH complexes at various dioxane concentrations. Tracer hormone is urinary FSH, Batch E 174 ter-4, Donini; anti-FSH is Batch 316, Donini. Abscissa as in Fig. 1.

solvents has the advantage of simplicity and applicability to demands of mass and routine assay. However, the above survey of the literature and the described results indicate that a proper control of protein concentration, temperature, ionic strength, and pH is required.

Among the antigen-antibody systems submitted to our experimental procedure an excellent separation of free from bound tracer was obtained for the HCG-anti-HCG system and the applicability of this system for radioimmunologic quantitation of HCG and LH in plasma and urine demonstrated. Different grades of dioxane and slight variations of pH did not significantly influence the outcome of the technique. Since it has been reported by Grant (30) that dioxane inhibits the antigen-antibody precipitation particular attention was given to this point. The experimental conditions of this author were completely different from ours. He added dioxane (20%) to antiserum dilutions before adding the antigen. We found no significant dissociation within the 6 hr after addition of the dioxane to the assay mixture. Heding (7) obtained similar results in her alcohol system for insulin.

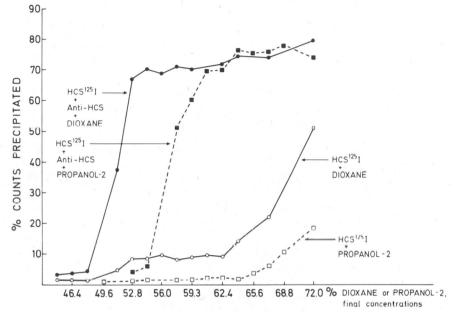

FIG. 10. Solubility of ^{125}I-HCS and ^{125}I-HCS-antibody complexes at various dioxane or propanol-2 concentrations. Tracer hormone is HCS, from the Sclavo-Sorin kit; antibody is obtained in rabbits with PPP Lederle, lot 4508 C 75. The abscissa represents the total dioxane or propanol-2 concentrations of the final mixture.

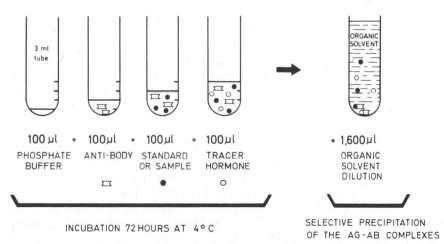

FIG. 11. Schematic representation of the radioimmunoassay procedure using organic solvents.

393

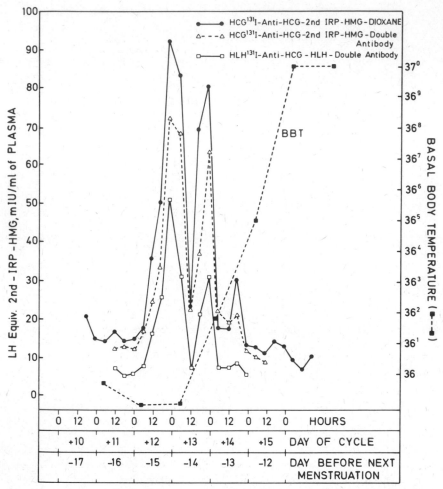

FIG. 12. Comparison of the midcycle LH levels found using three different radioimmuno-assay systems. Plasma was collected every 6 hr for a period of seven consecutive days. Note the biphasic nature of the midcycle LH surge.

For the HLH-anti-HCG system the zone where dioxane was assumed to precipitate only the bound LH was seriously reduced owing to the earlier nonspecific precipitation of the free tracer. Similarly, as in the HCG-anti-HCG system, high protein concentrations (25% horse serum) did not affect the slope of the free tracer curves. It would appear that the nonspecific precipitation of the free LH was probably due to physicochemical characteristics of the labeled antigen (solubility, purity).

In the HGH-anti-HGH system and HTSH-anti-HTSH system the slopes of the

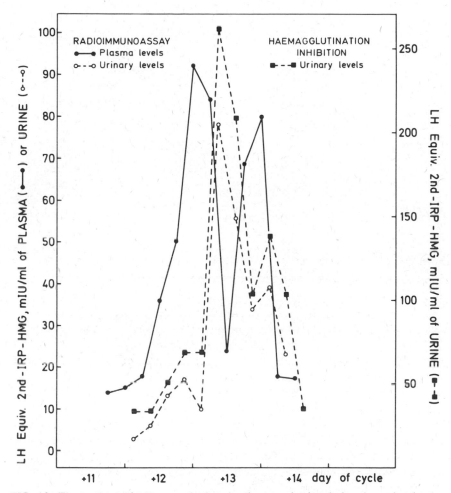

FIG. 13. Fluctuations of LH concentrations in plasma and urine during the periovulatory period, obtained by the dioxane technique and by the hemagglutination inhibition test. The biphasic pattern of the midcycle LH discharge in plasma is also apparent in urine. Same volunteer as Fig. 12. Note the two different ordinate scales.

free hormone curves were greatly influenced by high protein concentrations. For the HGH-anti-HGH system this difficulty may be avoided since radioimmunologic qunatitation of this hormone occurs usually in diluted plasma. In the HTSH radioimmunoassay, working with undiluted plasma, this problem of coprecipitation remains. For this reason Odell (31) stopped using the alcohol saline precipitation technique for this hormone.

In the HFSH-anti-HFSH system difficulties occur with the precipitation of

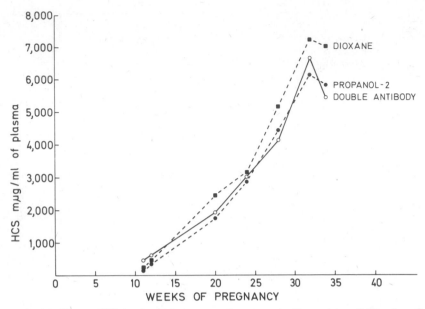

FIG. 14. Plasma HCS levels during a normal pregnancy. Comparison of the values found using three different techniques for the separation of free HCS from antibody-bound HCS.

the antigen-antibody complexes. Hunter (32) made the same observation and found that the bound form of ^{125}I-FSH was much more soluble in his NaCl-ethanol system than the bound form of ^{125}I-LH. This indicates that during the development of a chemical separative system the bound form of a hormone must be examined alongside. Despite these difficulties, Czygan (24) and Leyendecker, et al. (25) were able to develop successfully a dioxane technique for the radioimmunologic quantitation of HFSH in plasma. These discrepancies may be explained by differences in the degree of specificity and strength of the antisera or the purity of the tracer antigen.

Butt (33) compared several solid-phase methods, the polymerized antiserum method, and the dioxane system using the same antibody and the same labeled FSH. He found that the dioxane method was more sensitive than any of the other methods. However, the dioxane method reacted more favorably to HCG.

The most successful separation of free from bound tracer was obtained in the HCS (HPL)-anti-HCS (HPL) system by using propanol-2 as precipitating solvent. In contrast with the data of Haour (26), dioxane usually gives more than 10% nonspecific precipitation of free HCS, but it must be mentioned that working conditions were not strictly the same. Using diluted plasma for the radioimmunoassay of HCS, the problem of high protein concentrations is not encountered. Organic solvent techniques, especially the propanol-2 technique may be recommended for a rapid radioimmunologic quantitation of this hormone. That radioimmunologic measurement of HCS is also possible in undiluted plasma using organic solvent precipitation (ethanol) has been demonstrated recently by Letchworth et al. (34).

This contribution demonstrates that the organic solvent technique is applicable to radioimmunoassay procedures (HCG, LH, HCS), which may encourage further research to find optimal conditions of protein concentration, temperature, ionic strength, and pH for the quantitation of other hormones. It would also be worthwhile to investigate solvents other than those tested here, perhaps more specific for one or the other hormone. Furthermore, the chemical precipitation procedures offer many advantages. First, the chemical precipitation agents are stable, readily available, and inexpensive. Secondly, the technique is rapid, simple, able to process a large number of samples, and consequently particularly suitable for automation.

ACKNOWLEDGMENT

This work was supported by a grant from the Ford Foundation and the Fonds de la Recherche Scientifique Médicale, Belgium.

The authors wish to express their appreciation for the excellent technical assistance of Miss M. Cardon, Miss M. Callewaert, and Miss C. Brulet, and for the secretarial help of Miss E. Jochmans.

REFERENCES

1. Yalow, R. S., in M. Margoulies (Ed.), Protein and Polypeptide Hormones, Excerpta Medica, Amsterdam, 1969, p. 630.
2. Schultze, H. E. and J. F. Heremans (Eds.), in Molecular Biology of Human Proteins, Elsevier, Amsterdam, 1966, p. 236.
3. Berson, S. A., R. S. Yalow, A. Bauman, M. A. Ruthschild, and K. Newerby, J Clin Invest 35:170, 1956.
4. Gordis, E., Proc Soc Exp Biol 103:542, 1960.
5. Moloney, P. J. and M. A. Aprile, Canad J. Biochem 38:1216, 1960.
6. Grodsky, G. M., and P. H. Forsham, J Clin Invest 39:1070, 1960.
7. Heding, L. G., in L. Donato, G. Milhaud, and J. Sirchis (Eds.), Labeled Proteins in Tracer Studies, Euratom, Brussels, 1966, p. 345.
8. Heding, L. G., Diabetologia 7:10, 1971.
9. Odell, W. D., J. F. Wilber, and W. E. Paul, Metabolism 14:465, 1965.
10. Odell, W. D., J. F. Wilber, and W. E. Paul, J Clin Endocrinol 25:1179, 1965.
11. Wilson, P. M., and W. M. Hunter, J Endocrinol 35:i, 1966.
12. Stevenson, P. M., and A. C. Spalding, in M. Margoulies (Ed.), Protein and Polypeptide Hormones, Excerpta Medica, Amsterdam, 1969, p. 401.
13. Tomoda, Y., and M. M. Hreshchyshyn, Amer J Obs Gyn 100:118, 1968.
14. Kazeto, S., A. Sansone, and M. M. Hreshchyshyn, Amer J Obst Gyn 109:952, 1971.

15. Arends, J., Acta Endocrinol (Kbh) 66:611, 1971.

16. Hunter, W. M., in D. M. Weir (Ed.), Handbook of Experimental Immunology, Blackwell, Oxford, 1967, p. 626.

17. Hollemans, H. J. C., R van der Meer, and J. L. Touber, Nature (London) 217:277, 1968.

18. Furuyama, S., D. M. Darrel, and C. A. Nugent, Steroids 16:415, 1970.

19. Thomas, K., and J. Ferin, J Clin Endocrinol 28:1167, 1968.

20. Thomas, K., D. Nash, and J. Ferin, Acta Endocrinol, (Kbh), 142:279, 1969.

21. Thomas, K., R. Walckiers, and J. Ferin, J Clin Endocrinol 30:269, 1970.

22. Ferin, J., and K. Thomas, Bull Schweiz Akad Med Wiss 25:285, 1970.

23. Thomas, K., and J. Ferin, Acta Endocrinol, (Kbh), Suppl 141:75, 1970.

24. Czygan, P. J., Acta Endocrinol, (Kbh), Suppl 152:2, 1971.

25. Leyendecker, G., D. M. Saunders, and B. B. Saxena, Klin Wschr 49:658, 1971.

26. Haour, F., Hormone Metab Res 3:131, 1971.

27. van Hell, H., R. Matthijsen, and J. D. H. Homan, Acta Endocrinol (Kbh), 59:89, 1968.

28. Greenwood, F. C., W. H. Hunter, and J. S. Glover, Biochem J 89:114, 1963.

29. Schuurs, A. H. W. M., Acta Endocrinol, (Kbh), Suppl 142:95, 1969.

30. Grant, R. A., Brit J Exp Pathol 40:551, 1959.

31. Odell, W. D., Acta Endocrinol, (Kbh), Suppl 142:378, 1969.

32. Hunter, W. M., Acta Endocrinol (Kbh), Suppl 142:297, 1969.

33. Butt, W. R., Acta Endocrinol, (Kbh), Suppl 142:381, 1969.

34. Letchworth, A. T., C. N. Hudson, and T. Chard, J Endocrinol 49:V, 1971.

31. Further Characterization of the Radioimmunoassay of Human Pituitary FSH

Brij B. Saxena,[1] Ruby Malva, Gerhard Leyendecker,[2] and Hortense M. Gandy

Radioimmunoassay of human gonadotropins has been used in physiological and clinical studies. Lack of pure antigens uniform standards and suitable antisera has thus far limited the use of this technique as a routine diagnostic procedure. Incomplete knowledge of the structure-function relationship as well as kinetics of the antibody-antigen reaction has resulted in interlaboratory variations in the radioimmunoassay of gonadotropins. In view of recent progress made in the chemistry of gonadotropins, a reassessment of the radioimmunoassay is necessary. This paper describes the purification of tracer by adsorption chromatography on cellulose and the use of dioxane for the separation of free and bound labeled FSH. Standards, aantisera, and tracers has been evaluated by the dioxane method and with chromatoelectrophoresis. Precision, sensitivity, specificity, and statistical manipulations commonly employed in interpretation of assay results are discussed.

MATERIALS AND METHODS

Physicochemically and immunologically homogeneous FSH was isolated from human pituitary glands provided by the National Pituitary Agency, Baltimore,

[1]Career Scientist Awardee, Health Research Council, City of New York, Contract No. I-621.

[2]Present Address, University of Bonn, West Germany.

399

Maryland. The FSH contained 153 NIH-FSH-S3 U/mg and was stable in the lyophilized state (1, 2). Aliquots of 2.5 μg of FSH in 0.05M phosphate buffer containing 0.1M NaCl (solvent) were stored at −60 C until used for labeling with radioactive iodine. Stock solutions for the standard containing 0.01 and 0.001 ng/μl in 0.05M phosphate buffer containing 0.1% human serum albumin (diluent) were also stored at −60 C and thawed prior to the assay. Similarly, suitable aliquots of human pituitary LH containing 8.9 NIH-LH-S1 U/mg (3), the α and β subunits of FSH and LH (4, 5) and 2nd IRP-HMG obtained by the courtesy of Dr. R. Bangham, Medical Research Council, Mill Hill, London were also prepared. Each ampule of 2nd IRP-HMG has been assigned a potency of 40 IU of FSH and 40 IU of LH activity. A pituitary standard, LER-907, containing 20. IU FSH and 48 IU LH/mg was supplied by Dr. Leo E. Reichert. Antisera to FSH were raised in rabbits. These antisera were purified by immunoabsorption and gel filtration on a column of Sephadex G-25 coupled with human pituitary LH (6, 7). Hundred-microliter aliquots of purified antisera at a dilution of 1 : 100 in the diluent were stored at −60 C. Prior to assay, each aliquot was diluted with diluent to yield the initial dilution of the antisera used in the assay.

Morning samples of heparinized blood were obtained from children and thirty adults; daily samples were obtained from 3 women with cyclical menses. Blood specimens were also collected from men and women every 4 hr for a period of 24 hr for determination of FSH, androgens, estrogens, and cortisol. Plasma was separated from cells by centrifugation at 4 C and stored at −20 C until analyzed. The plasma from the 30 normal subjects was divided into two aliquots; one was frozen immediately and the other left at room temperature for 6 hr.

Human pituitary FSH was labeled with carrier-free ^{131}I and ^{125}I (Iso-Serve, Inc., Cambridge, Mass.) by the method of Hunter and Greenwood with minor modifications (8, 9). Labeled hormones were purified by adsorption chromatography on cellulose as shown in Fig. 1 (10). The specific activities of ^{131}I and ^{125}I-FSH ranged from 100 to 150 and 250 to 300 μCi/μg, respectively. The purified tracer was virtually free of 'damage' (Fig. 2).

A protocol for the assay using dioxane is presented in Table I. Chromatoelectrophoretic assay was performed as described earlier (11). In both systems, the same reagents and plasma samples were used. Blanks, standards with human pituitary FSH, LER-907 and 2nd IRP-HMG, and plasma samples were assayed in duplicate in 10.8 × 76.6 mm dioxane-resistant polypropylene tubes (Cat. No. 250 Ivan Sorvall, Inc., Norwalk, Conn.). Prior to the addition of 8000 to 10,000 cpm equivalent to approximately 0.05 ng of the tracer, reagents were allowed to preincubate for 72 hr at 4 C. Incubation was continued for an additional period of 16 to 24 hr. The total cpm in each tube were determined in a well-type autogamma counter (Packard Instrument Co., Downers Grove, Ill.). For the separation of the bound and free tracer, 800 μl of 66% dioxane was added to each tuber (Fig. 3). The tubes were allowed to stand at 4 C for 15 min and then centrifuged at 5000 cpm for 30 min at 4 C in a type RC 2-B Sorvall centrifuge equipped with four modified cups with a capacity for twenty-four 10 × 74 mm

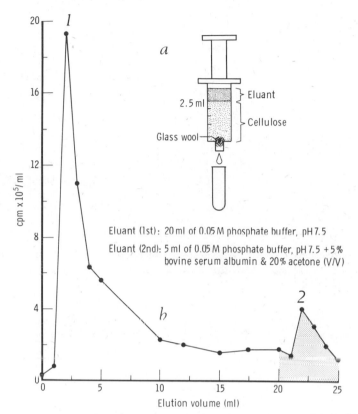

FIG. 1. (a)Purification of ^{131}I-FSH by adsorption chromatography on cellulose, (b) elution profile representing damaged hormone and unreacted ^{131}I in fraction 1 and ^{131}I-FSH in fraction 2. Reproduced by permission of Springer Verlag.

tubes each. The supernate containing free hormone was aspirated. The tubes were then inverted on disposable paper towels to drain since residual dioxane gave spurious counts. The tubes containing precipitate representing bound hormone were then counted. The cpm remaining in the 'blank' were regarded as nonspecific and were substracted from the bound. The standard curve was plotted as the ratio of bound to free (B/F). The linearization of the standard was obtained as shown in Fig. 5b. The FSH levels in the unknown samples were determined from their respective B/F and B_0/B_n ratios using computer programs. The results were expressed in mIU of FSH in terms of 2nd IRP-HMG/ml of plasma. A conversion factor (1 mg FSH equivalent to 5.6 mIU) was determined by assaying 2nd IRP-HMG at six dose levels (Fig. 4).

Testosterone was determined by the double isotope derivative dilution technique (12), cortisol by a modification of Porter-Silber method (13), and estrogens by a modification of the radioimmunoassay procedure (14).

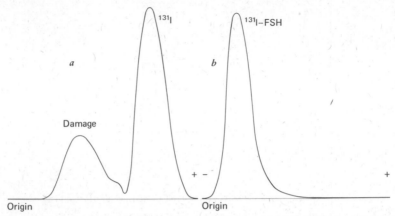

FIG. 2. Radioactivity scans of chromatoelectropherogram of (a) fraction 1 with damaged hormone and unreacted ^{131}I and (b) of fraction 2 containing ^{131}I-FSH. Reproduced by permission of Springer Verlag.

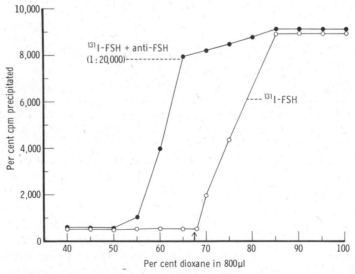

FIG. 3. Precipitation of antibody bound ^{131}I-FSH and free ^{131}I-FSH at various concentrations of dioxane. As indicated by the arrow, 66% dioxane precipitated 85% of the bound ^{131}I-FSH without precipitation of the free ^{131}I-FSH. Reproduced by permission of Springer Verlag.

TABLE I. Quantity of reagents (μl) added to reaction vials

	Diluent[a]	Antisera 1 : 100,000 final dilution	Standard FSH	^{131}I-FSH 10,000 cpm	Control plasma[b]
Blank	130			50	20
Zero	80	50		50	20
Standard (ng)					
0.01	70	50	10 (0.001 ng/μl) Stock I	50	20
0.025	55	50	25	50	20
0.05	30	50	50	50	20
0.075	5	50	75	50	20
0.1	70	50	10 (0.01 ng/μl) Stock II	50	20
Plasma samples (20μl)	80	50		50	

[a] 0.05M phosphate buffer of pH 7.5, containing 0.1% human serum albumin, 1 : 10,000 merthiolate and 0.01M disodium EDTA.

[b] Obtained from hypophysectomized subjects.

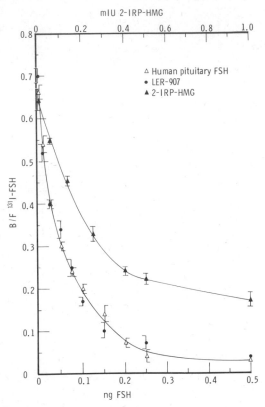

FIG. 4. Pituitary FSH, LER-907 and 2nd IRP-HMG standard curves obtained with anti-FSH serum at final dilution of 1:100,000.

RESULTS AND DISCUSSION

The adsorption chromatography technique used for purification of labeled FSH was convenient and rapid as well as provided a disposable system. It is of interest that this technique is also applicable for purification of labeled LH, HCG, and GH. The tracer was of greater purity than that obtained by gel filtration on Sephadex G-100 columns used previously (15). During chromatoelectrophoretic separation the damage in the tracer migrated with plasma proteins and therefore a tracer with greater damage resulted in lesser adsorption at the origin. The tracer purified by adsorption chromatography on cellulose, however, did not migrate from the origin in the presence of up to 50 μl of plasma from hypophysectomized subjects. Neither significant damage nor loss of immunoreactivity was apparent in the tracer stored at −60 C up to a period of 4 weeks as shown in Fig. 6.

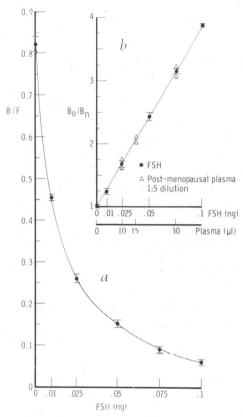

FIG. 5. (a) FSH standard, (b) linear relationship obtained when the ratio of cpm bound at "zero" hormone concentration (B_0) to the cpm found at corresponding concentrations of the unlabeled FSH (B_n) was plotted against various concentrations of the standard. Reproduced by permission of Springer Verlag.

Absolutely specific antisera to gonadotropins have been difficult to obtain. A survey of antisera from approximately 500 bleeds from rabbits and guinea pigs immunized with FSH has invariably shown 25 to 100% cross-reaction with LH and HCG. Immunizations with highly purified FSH have yielded antisera with lesser cross-reaction but failed to generate absolutely specific antisera. The antisera purified either by immunoabsorption or chemically by gel filtration have also shown 5 to 15% residual cross-reaction with LH and HCG (6, 7). Attempts to eliminate residual cross-reaction by absorption with excess HCG resulted in significant losses of the titer to FSH suggesting allosteric effect. On the basis of these observations, Saxena et al. (6) suggested that FSH, LH, and HCG share common antigenic sites. Recently the discovery of an α, the hormone

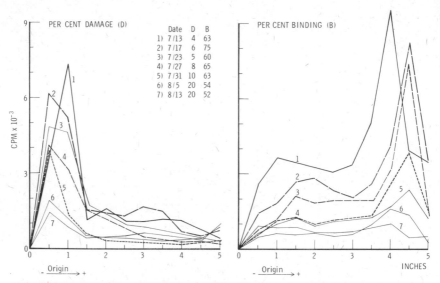

FIG. 6. Percent damage and binding of ^{125}I-FSH determined by chromatoelectrophoresis anti-FSH serum at final dilution of 1:100,000.

nonspecific, and a β, the hormone-specific, subunit of FSH, LH, and HCG and homology of the α subunits of these hormones (16, 17) have confirmed the above suggestion. The subunits of FSH and LH were tested in specific radioimmunoassays. The β subunits exhibited hormone specificity, whereas α subunits were hormone nonspecific (Fig. 7).

The use of excess LH or HCG to render the radioimmunoassay specific to FSH could have two effects. First, excess antigen may inhibit precipitation of HCG bound to cross-reacting antibodies, thus exhibiting a false specificity of the antisera. Second, due to allosteric effects, excess HCG may to some extent also inhibit the precipitation of FSH bound to its antibody resulting in the loss of sensitivity of the assay. The specificity of the assay therefore depends primarily on the use of pure tracer and an antisera of suitable purity. As shown in Fig. 8 the degree of cross-reaction of an antiserum to FSH with LH was greater at lower than at higher concentrations. In view of these findings, it is necessary to examine the specificity of an antiserum at lower concentrations of the cross-reacting antigens. The cross-reactivity of an FSH antiserum should be tested with LH rather than HCG, since the latter is only present in women during pregnancy and has been shown to contain FSH-like activity (16).

The standard curves of human pituitary FSH and 2nd IRP-HMG obtained by the dioxane method are illustrated in Fig. 4. A nonidentity of 2nd IRP-HMG

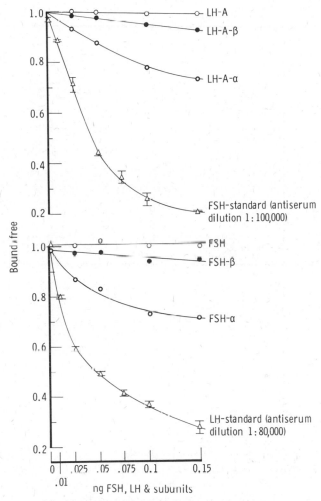

FIG. 7. Cross-reaction of LH and its subunits in a radioimmunoassay specific for FSH (top); cross-reaction of FSH and its subunits in a radioimmunoassay specific for LH (bottom).

with human pituitary FSH and LER-907 was evident. Few antisera revealed complete cross-reactivity with FSH, LER-907, and 2nd IRP-HMG suggesting that these antisera possess antibodies to sites common to both urinary and pituitary FSH (17). Ryan et al. (19) previously suggested the use of standards of pituitary origin in the measurement of plasma FSH by radioimmunoassay.

The sensitivity of dioxane and chromatoelectrophoretic methods was not significantly different. The precision of the dioxane method was approximately

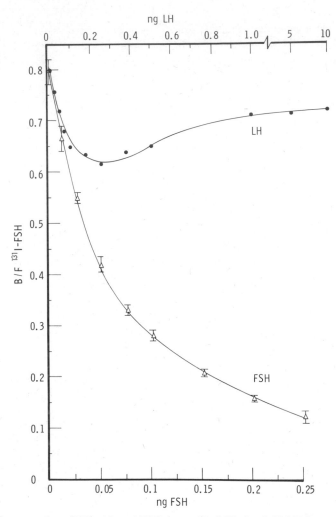

FIG. 8. Cross-reaction of LH with anti-FSH serum, final dilution 1:100,000.

± 5% as compared to ± 10% for chromatoelectrophoresis. The greater purity of the tracer and higher efficiency of a well-type counter may account for improved precision by dioxane method. As shown in Fig. 9, plasma FSH levels at 8:00 AM were significantly higher than at 8:00 PM. Testosterone, estrogen, and cortisol levels showed similar patterns of diurnal variation. The presence of a diurnal rhythm in plasma levels of FSH in men has been described previously (20, 21). However, some investigators have failed to demonstrate diurnal variation of FSH in men (22, 23). A diurnal variation of plasma levels of

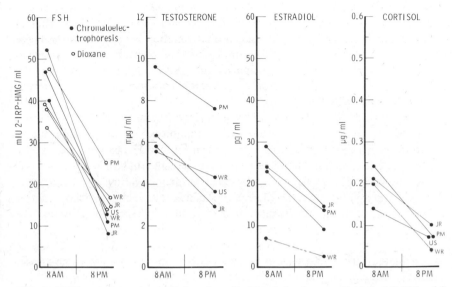

FIG. 9. FSH, testosterone, estradiol, and cortisol levels in plasma collected at 8 AM and 8 PM from men.

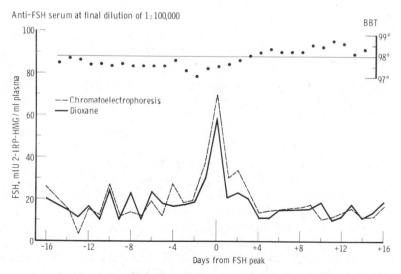

FIG. 10. Composite of daily plasma FSH levels during menstrual cycle from 3 women.

testosterone has been well-documented in humans (6, 11, 26-28). Diurnal changes in the levels of pituitary gonadotropins and in the nucleus volume of Leydig cells have been described in the rat and mouse (24, 25). There is considerable evidence to suggest that diurnal variation is inherent in the higher brain centers which control the hypothalamus. The pineal indoles are known to modify the secretion of gonadotropins. Light inhibits hydroxyindole-o-methyl transferase and thus the formation of melatonin from serotonin, the latter being a gonadotropin inhibitor (29, 30).

Composite of daily plasma FSH levels during menstrual cycle from 3 women, obtained by dioxane and chromatoelectrophoresis methods using human pituitary FSH as the standard are presented in Fig. 10. The patterns were similar and validate that both methods are measuring the same substance.

As shown in Fig. 11 the FSH patterns in children of various ages obtained by dioxane method was similar to those obtained by double-antibody method (31-39). No significant differences in FSH levels were demonstrable in ether boys or girls until approximately 10 and 8 years of age respectively. A progressive rise in FSH levels occurred at these ages and continued until puberty was achieved. These observations further substantiate the validity of the dioxane method.

As calculated from the standard curves in Fig. 4, 1 ng of FSH was equivalent to 5.6 mIU of 2nd IRP-HMG, which was identical with the similar value obtained earlier (6). However, on the basis of bioassay, 1 ng of FSH was equivalent to 3.7 mIU 2nd IRP-HMG (40, 41). As illustrated in Fig. 12, the use of these two factors yielded similar patterns but different values. FSH of comparable physicochemical purity with a range of biological activity from 1250 to 14,000 IU FSH/mg has been reported (42). The use of conversion factor based on bioassay may therefore account for significant interlaboratory differences in radioimmunoassay estimates. We, therefore, propose the use of an immunounit for standards and antisera determined in the radioimmunoassay system. The standardization of the antisera and the standard may be obtained by determining the amount of antisera of a known dilution which will yield a B/F ratio of greater than unity with a fixed amount of labeled antigen of known specific activity. The immunological unit of the standard and the antisera may then be defined as the quantities of each required to yield a ratio of unity or any other convenient ratio; in other words,

$$X \text{ ml antiserum} + Y \text{ ng tracer} \qquad B/F = 2$$
$$X \text{ ml antiserum} + Z \text{ ng standard} \qquad B/F = 1$$

where X = one unit antiserum; and Z = one unit standard with reference to Y; and tracer hormone of highest purity available.

Subsequent antisera and standard preparations may then be calibrated in reference to the first antisera and standard.

Plasma FSH levels during the menstrual cycle calculated from standards obtained by using human pituitary FSH and 2nd IRP-HMG are presented in Fig. 13. The estimates from 2nd IRP-HMG standard were higher than those obtained

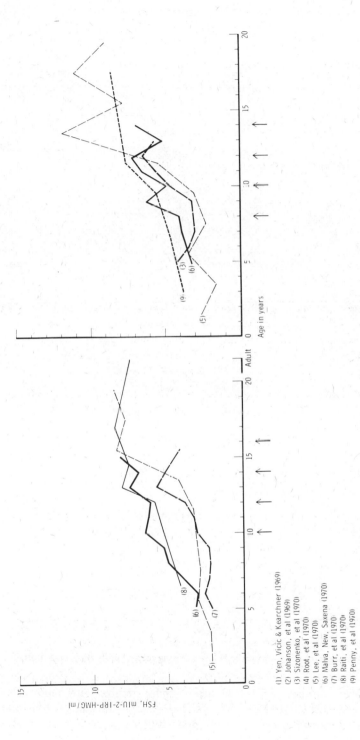

(1) Yen, Vicic & Kearchner (1969)
(2) Johanson, et al (1969)
(3) Sizonenko, et al (1970)
(4) Root, et al (1970)
(5) Lee, et al (1970)
(6) Malva, New, Saxena (1970)
(7) Burr, et al (1970)
(8) Raiti, et al (1970)
(9) Penny, et al (1970)

FIG. 11. Patterns of FSH in children obtained by dioxane and double-antibody methods.

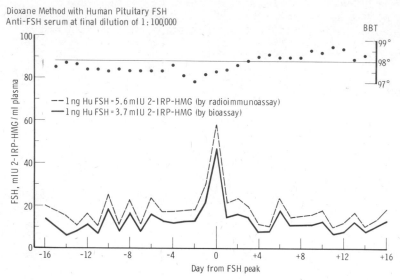

FIG. 12. Composite of daily plasma FSH levels during menstrual cycle from 3 women.

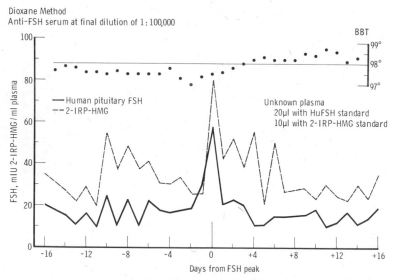

FIG. 13. Composite of daily plasma FSH levels during menstrual cycle from 3 women.

from human pituitary FSH standard. Similar results were reported using
LER-907 and 2nd IRP-HMG in the measurement of FSH and LH in urine by
double antibody and alcohol precipitation methods as shown in Fig. 14 (43).

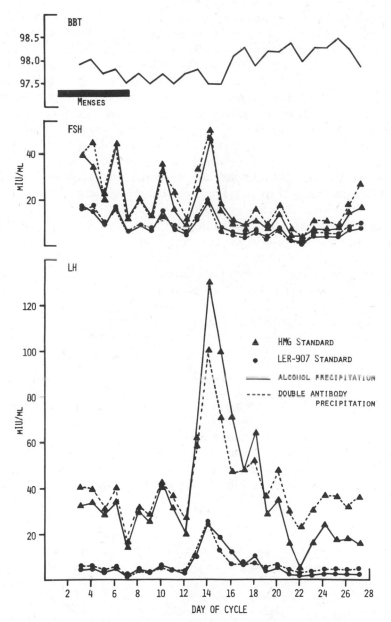

FIG. 14. Basal body temperature and daily FSH and LH values in a subject for the duration of one menstrual cycle (44). Reproduced by permission of C. V. Mosby Co.

The patterns obtained by 2nd IRP-HMG standard were exaggerated. These findings may account for interlaboratory differences in the patterns and introduce bias in the interpretation of plasma FSH levels during menstrual cycle. The FSH activities of purified human FSH, LER-907, and 2nd IRP-HMG are 4921, 20, and 8 IU/mg, respectively. Thus on w/w basis, for each unit of the purified human FSH, 246-fold LER-907 and 615-fold 2nd IRP-MHG are required. These differences in the mass of standard preparations may have little effect in bioassay whereas steric interference on kinetics of the antibody-antigen reaction in the radioimmunoassay could be prohibitive. The use of pure hormones as standards and expression of results in immunounits should therefore result in less interlaboratory differences in the estimates of FSH.

Several methods have been employed empirically in the statistical linearization of the standard (44). It has been pointed out that due to the nonuniformity of the variance around the regression line, the results may be severely biased and invalid. The specificity of an assay fundamentally depends upon the slope of the response. Therefore, a statistical manipulation not consistent with the kinetics of an antibody-antigen reaction may lead to an error of indeterminate degree in the estimates. We have employed a method for the linearization of the standard as shown in Fig. 5 (45, 46). It is assumed in this manipulation, that the tracer contained 'zero damage.' In our experience, the use of tracer purified by cellulose chromatography has permitted a reasonable linearization of the standard as shown in Fig. 5b. The B/F and B_o/B_n ratio of various dilutions of plasma from a postmenopausal subject yielded similar slopes suggesting the validity and similarity of the two standard curves (Fig. 5a and b).

ACKNOWLEDGMENT

This work was supported by grant M 71.26 from the Population Council, Rockefeller University, and AM-11187, R01-HD 04173, and 70-2140 from the National Institutes of Health, Bethesda, Maryland.

We are grateful to Dr. P. Rathnam for the preparation of FSH, LH, and their subunits and to Misses Inessa Epsztein and Rebecca Pascaul for technical assistance. We thank Dr. B. V. Caldwell for a gift of antibody to estradiol-17β.

REFERENCES

1. Saxena, B. B., and P. Rathnam, J Biol Chem 242:3769, 1967.
2. Saxena, B. B., and P. Rathnam, in E. Rosemberg (Ed.), Gonadotropins 1968, Geron-X, Inc., Los Altos, 1968, p. 33.
3. Rathnam, P., and B. B. Saxena, J Biol Chem 245:3725, 1970.
4. Saxena, B. B., and P. Rathnam, J Biol Chem 246:3549, 1971.
5. Saxena, B. B., and P. Rathnam, Fed Proc 30:473, 1971.
6. Saxena, B. B., H. Demura, H. M. Gandy, and R. E. Peterson, J Clin Endocrinol 28:519, 1968.
7. Lehmann, F., and B. B. Saxena, in Proc Congress German Society of Gynecology, Hamburg, in press, 1970.

8. Greenwood, F. C., and W. M. Hunter, Nature (London) 194:496, 1962.

9. Saxena, B. B., G. Leyendecker, W. Chen, H. M. Gandy, and R. E. Peterson, Acta Endocrinol (Kbh) Suppl 142:185, 1969.

10. Leyendecker, G., D. M. Saunders, and BB. Saxena, Klin Wochschr 49:659, 1971.

11. Saxena, B. B., and H. M. Gandy, In Vitro Procedures with Radioisotopes in Medicine, International Atomic Energy Agency, Vienna, 1970, p. 613.

12. Gandy, H. M., and R. E. Peterson, J Clin Endocrinol 28:949, 1968.

13. Peterson, R. E., in D. Seligson (Ed.), Standard Methods of Clinical Chemistry, Academic, New York, 3:160, 1961.

14. Abraham, G. E., J Clin Endocrinol 29:866, 1969.

15. Saxena, B. B., H. M. Gandy, and R. E. Peterson, in E. Rosemberg (Ed.), Gonadotropins 1968, Geron-X, Inc., Los Altos, 1968, p. 339.

16. Saxena, B. B., and P. Rathnam, J Biol Chem 246:3549, 1971.

17. Liao, T. H., and J. G. Pierce, J Biol Chem 245:3275, 1970.

18. Franchimont, P., and P. Donini, J Clin Endocrinol 31:18, 1970.

19. Ryan, R. J., Acta Endocrinol (Kbh) Suppl 142:300, 1969.

20. Faiman, C., and R. J. Ryan, Nature (London) 215:857, 1967.

21. Dolais, J., A. J. Valleron, A. M. Grapin, and G. Rosselin, C R Acad Sci (Paris) 270:3123, 1970.

22. Peterson, N. T., A. R. Midgley, Jr., and R. B. Jaffe, J Clin Endocrinol 28:1473, 1968.

23. Burger, H. G. in M. Margoulies (Ed.), Protein and Polypeptide Hormones, Excerpta Medica, Liege, 1968, p. 412.

24. Fraschini, F., and M. Motta, Program of the 49th Endocrine Society Meeting, Miami, 1967, p. 128.

25. Kovacs, J., Acta Biol Acad Sci Hung 10:69, 1959.

26. Southren, A. L., S. Tochimoto, N. S. Carmody, and K. Isurugi, J Clin Endocrinol 25.1441, 1965.

27. Dray, F., A. Reinberg, and J. Sebaoun, C R Acad Sci (Paris) 261:573, 1965.

28. Rasko, J. A., and K. B. Eik-Nes, J Clin Endocrinol 26:573, 1966.

29. Wurtman, R. J., J. Axelrod, and L. Phillips, Science 141:277, 1963.

30. Quay, W. B., Proc Soc Exp Biol Med (NY) 121:946, 1966.

31. Yen, S. S. C., W. J. Vicic, and D. V. Kearchner, J Clin Endocrinol 29:382, 1969.

32. Johanson, A. J., H. Guyda, C. Light, C. J. Migeon, and R. M. Blizzard, J Pediat 74:416, 1969.

33. Sizonenko, P. C., I. M. Burr, S. L. Kaplan, and M. M. Grumbach, Ped Res 4:36, 1970.

34. Root, A. W., T. Moshang, Jr., A. M. Bongiovanni, and W. R. Eberlein, Ped Res 4:175, 1970.

35. Lee, P. A., A. R. Midgley, Jr., and R. B. Jaffe, J Clin Endocrinol 31:248, 1970.

36. Saxena, B. B., in S. Marcus, and C. Marcus (Eds.), Advances in Obstetrics and Gynecology, Vol II, Williams & Wilkins, Baltimore, in press, 1971.

37. Burr, I. M., P. C. Sizonenko, S. L. Kaplan, and M. M. Grumbach, Pediat Res 4:31, 1970.

38. Raiti, S., A. J. Johanson, C. Light, C. J. Migeon, and R. M. Blizzard, Metabolism 18:234, 1969.

39. Penny, R., J. H. Guyda, A. Baghdassarian, and R. M. Blizzard, J Clin Invest 49:1847, 1970.

40. Steelman, S. L., and F. M. Pohley, Endocrinology 53:604, 1953.

41. Rosemberg, E., in E. Rosemberg (Ed.), Gonadotropins 1968, Geron-X, Inc., Los Altos, 1968, p. 387.

42. Barker, S. A., C. J. Gray, J. F. Kennedy, and W. R. Butt, J Endocrinol 45:777, 1969.

43. Kazeto, S., A. Sansome, and M. M. Hreshchyschn, Amer J Obst Gyn 109:952, 1971.

44. Rodbard, D., P. L. Rayford, J. A. Cooper, and G. T. Ross, J Clin Endocrinol 28:1412, 1968.

45. Hales, C. N., and P. J. Randle, Biochem J 88:137, 1963.

46. Herbert, V., K. Law, C. W. Gottlieb, and S. J. Bleicher, J Clin Endocrinol 25:1375, 1965.

32.   Sialic Acid and the
Immunologic and Biologic
Activity of Gonadotropins

Griff T. Ross, E. V. van Hall,[1] Judith L. Vaitukaitis, G. D. Braunstein, and P. L. Rayford

We have determined immunologic and biologic activities of human chorionic gonadotropin (HCG), human luteinizing hormone (HLH), and human follicle stimulating hormone (HFSH) before and after either complete or partial (graded) enzymatic removal of sialic acid (desialylation) (1-3). We now summarize results of these studies and report some additional observations on the biologic and immunologic properties of HCG in which the sialic acid moiety had been labeled with tritium following successive oxidation with periodate and reduction with tritiated borohydride (4).

MATERIALS AND METHODS

Hormone Preparations

HLH (LER 1486), a purified extract of human pituitary tissue was prepared by Leo E. Reichert (2) and had biologic activity of 1910 IU/mg (Bioassay, 2nd IRP-HMG). D-RA, an extract of urine from eunuchs containing HFSH, had an initial potency of 26 IU/mg (bioassay, 2nd IRP-HMG) and was the generous gift of A. Albert. HCG, a purified extract from the urine of pregnant women was prepared by J. W. Hickman and G. G. Ashwell (1) and had a biologic potency of 11,110 IU/mg (bioassay, 2nd International Standard HCG).

[1]Present Address: Department of Obstetrics and Gynecology, University of Nijmegen, Nijmegen, The Netherlands.

Desialylation and Measurements of Sialic Acid (N-Acetylneuraminic Acid, NANA)

Enzymatic desialylation was carried out using commercial preparations of Clostridium perfringens neuraminidase (Worthington, Sigma) in acetate buffer, pH 5.6 to 6.3, at 37 C (1, 2). In experiments where progressive desialylation was performed, enzyme was separated from hormone by passing the incubation mixture over a sepharose column to which antibodies made against neuraminidase had been covalently linked (1). Chemical desialylation, to determine total NANA content of the various hormones, was achieved by digestion with 0.1N H_2SO_4 at 80 C for 1 hr. NANA was measured chemically in aliquots of the incubation mixture by the method of Warren (5).

Bioassays and Immunoassays

The Second International Standard HCG (2nd International Standard) and the Second International Reference Preparation for Human Menopausal Gonadotropin (2nd IRP-HMG) were used for dose interpolation in biologic and immunologic assays for HCG, and for HFSH or HLH respectively. Details of the ventral prostate weight assay (VPW) and ovarian ascorbic acid depletion assay (OAAD) used to determine biologic potencies of both HCG and HLH as well as the Steelman-Pohley assay (OAR) used for HFSH have been described (1, 3). All assays were parallel-line, graded-dose response assays. Relative potencies and confidence limits of these were calculated after suitable tests for parallelism and homogeneity of variance in responses to unknown and reference preparation.

Radioimmunoassays for HCG, HLH, and HFSH were done using methods described elsewhere (6). The reference preparations used for dose interpolation were the same as those used for biologic assays. The methods of Rodbard and Lewald were used to determine the confidence limits of estimates of immunopotency (7).

Determination of Plasma Disappearance Rates

Disappearance rates for variably desialylated preparations of HCG were followed by immunoassays of plasma samples taken at intervals following single intravenous injections of hormones via tail vein into immature female rats made pseudopregnant in preparation for OAAD assays (8). Initial rates of disappearance were calculated graphically without correction for possible multiexponential rates of disappearance.

Labeling with Tritium

The method used to label HCG with tritium, following successive oxidation with periodate and reduction with tritium labeled borohydride, has been described in detail (4).

RESULTS

Complete desialylation of HLH, HCG, and HFSH resulted in dramatic reductions in biologic activity (Table I). Limited quantities available made an exact determination of the residual activity of HFSH impractical but such determinations were made for both HLH and HCG. Residual biologic activity following complete desialylation was greater for HLH (ca. 15%) than for HCG (less than 1%).

TABLE I. Biologic activity before and after complete desialylation

Hormone	Source	Assay	Activity	
			Before	After
HLH	Pituitary extract	VPW	1910[a]	238[a]
HCG	Urinary extract	VPW	11110[b]	1.2[b]
FSH	Urinary extract	OAR	26[a]	< 3[a]

[a]IU/mg, bioassay, 2nd IRP-HMG.
[b]IU/mg, bioassay, 2nd International Standard HCG.

In contrast to the consistent decrease in biologic activity for all preparations, immunologic activity was variably affected following desialylation (Table II). The apparent small increase in immunologic activity of HCG was not found to be statistically significant while increments for HLH and HFSH were significant ($p < 0.05$).

TABLE II. Immunologic activity before and after complete desialylation

Hormone	Source	Activity	
		Before	After
HLH	Pituitary extract	46[a]	66[a]
HCG	Urine extract	4430[b]	4830[b]
FSH	Urine extract	16[c]	40[c]

[a]mg/mg, immunoassay, LER 907 reference preparation.
[b]IU/mg, immunoassay, 2nd International Standard HCG, reference preparation.
[c]IU/mg, immunoassay, 2nd IRP-HMG, reference preparation.

Having established that complete desialylation significantly reduced biologic and variably altered immunologic activity of gonadotropins, it was of interest to evaluate effects of partial but progressive desialylation on these properties of HCG, the only hormone available in sufficient quantities for such studies. Desialylation ranging from 0 to 100% was achieved and results of biologic and immunologic assays of these preparations are summarized in Table III.

TABLE III. Biologic and immunologic activities following variable desialylation
             of purified HCG

Percent desialylation	Biologic activity[a]		Immunologic activity[b]
	OAAD	VPW	
0	13,500 (11,370-16,170)	11,110 (9,930-13,220)	5,820 (5,650-6,000)
7	7,210 (5,770-9,150)	7,390 (5,570-9,880)	5,520 (5,270-5,770)
13	5,510 (4,290-7,320)	5,070 (3,260-7,760)	5,270 (5,030-5,510)
25	2,990 (2,240-4,160)	2,800 (1,940-3,990)	6,160 (5,870-6,480)
47	1,250 (830-2,070)	220 (150-300)	6,020 (5,730-6,320)
62	60 (44-83)	1.3 (0.9-1.8)	4,140 (3,900-4,400)
70	86 (67-111)	0.7 (0.4-1.1)	4,110 (3,850-4,380)
100	56 (42-73)	1.2 (0.9-1.6)	4,830 (4,600-5,070)

[a]IU/mg, bioassay, 2nd International Standard HCG, reference preparation.
[b]IU/mg, immunoassay, 2nd International Standard HCG, reference preparation.

No clear trend in alteration of immunologic activity was observed and, as
before, we concluded that the variations were not significant. Biologic activities
were similar, irrespective of the method of biologic assay, over the range of 0 to
25% desialylation. In contrast, above 25% desialylation, residual activity was
consistently and significantly lower when potencies determined by VPW were
compared to those measured by OAAD. After 62% desialylation, no further
reduction in biologic activity was observed by either method of assay and the
previously noted differences were maintained.

In an attempt to understand the basis for these discrepant alterations in
activity, we recalled the observations of Parlow (8), who correlated relative
potencies in these two assay systems with plasma half-life of a series of
preparations with LH activity. Parlow's observations led us to hypothesize that
increased metabolic clearance of desialylated HCG could account for the changes
we had observed (9). Credibility of this hypothesis was enhanced further by the

observations that desialylation of a series of glycoproteins, including HCG, exposed galactosyl residues resulting in avid hepatic uptake and rapid disappearance of some of these substances from plasma of rats (10, 11).

Evidence consistent with validity of this hypothesis for HCG is shown in Fig. 1 where changes in the half-time for disappearance from plasma are plotted on simultaneous coordinates with reduction in biologic activity measured by VPW. As biologic activity decreased, plasma halflife decreased at a similar rate, suggesting a cause-effect relationship between the two events.

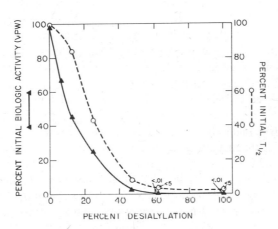

FIG. 1. Percent initial biological activity (biologic assay, 2nd International Standard HCG) of a series of variably desialylated preparations of HCG, ▲—▲; and percent of plasma half-life of the same preparations measured by radioimmuno-assay ○ – ○.

To understand the relevance of these observations to metabolism of HCG in physiologic and pathophysiologic states required that the sialic acid moiety of HCG be labeled without complete loss of biologic or immunologic activity (4). For this purpose, we have produced a tritium-labeled preparation retaining 50% of both biologic and immunologic activity of the hormone prior to labeling. Biologic activities were equal in VPW and OAAD assays, and more than 67% of the isotope introduced into the hormone remained susceptible to removal by hydrolysis with neuraminidase. The tritium removed by neuraminidase was in a compound which cochromatographed with N-acetyl heptulosaminic acid, a seven-carbon analog of NANA. Isoelectric focusing in polyacrylamide gels followed by biologic assay, immunoassay, and assay of tritium eluted from gel slices showed coincidence of peak immunologic, biologic, and physical activities. In preliminary physiologic studies, labeled hormone was concentrated in ovaries of pseudopregnant rats given the preparation intravenously (4).

These observations were interpreted to indicate that exocyclic carbon atoms 8 and 9 of sialic acid residues in HCG could be removed by successive oxidation with periodate and reduction with borohydride labeled with tritium leaving the gonadotropin biologically and immunologically active and labeled with ^{3}H.

DISCUSSION

Complete desialylation of HLH, HCG, and HFSH resulted in a substantial reduction in biologic activity of these gonadotropins. Using HCG as a model, it was shown that progressive desialylation was accompanied by both progressive decrease in biologic activity and progressive decrease in plasma half-life of the hormone. These observations led us to postulate that sialic acid extended the effective plasma half-life of the hormone and thereby enhanced the biologic activity of HCG, and by inference, HLH and HFSH as well.

In contrast to the reduction in biologic activity measured in vivo, immunologic activity measured in vitro was either unaffected (HCG) or enhanced (HLH and HFSH) by complete desialylation.

In the absence of evidence for alterations in primary amino acid sequence (which would be expected to result in reduction rather than enhancement of antigenic activity) alterations in tertiary structure seem to be the most plausible explanation for the changes in immunopotency observed following desialylation of the HLH and HFSH. We would ascribe to sialic acid a role in the maintenance of tertiary structure of these molecules, and thus, indirectly, a role in determining antigenic behavior of these glycoprotein hormones with the antisera used in these studies. It seems reasonable to suppose that antisera produced in response to desialylated immunogens would react more avidly with desialylated than with fully sialylated antigens.

Further elucidation of the role of sialic acid in determining biologic and immunologic behavior of the gonadotropins requires a variety of additional studies. These include the following: (1) Studies of the relative potencies of desialylated and fully sialylated hormones using in vitro systems such as radio-receptor assays. Catt and others have shown that desialylated HCG and HLH compete as effectively as fully sialylated preparations of these hormones for binding with Leydig cells from rat testis (12, 13). (2) Studies of relative potencies in stimulating such in vitro processes as biosynthesis of progesterone by granulosa cells in tissue culture (14) should be relevant to elucidating the role of sialic acid at target organ level. (3) Studies of the tertiary structure of the molecules in solution using physical methods. Finally, degradation of hormone preparations with radioactively labeled sialic acid residues should be followed in vivo to determine whether desialylation is an important mechanism of hormonal degradation.

ACKNOWLEDGMENT

The expert technical assistance of Messrs. Robert Wright, Adrian Coleman, James Brice, and Rudolph Reid is gratefully acknowledged.

REFERENCES

1. Van Hall, E. V., J. L. Vaitukaitis, G. T. Ross, J. W. Hickman, and G. Ashwell, Endocrinology 88:456, 1971.
2. Braunstein, G. D., L. E. Reichert, Jr., E. V. Van Hall, J. L. Vaitukaitis, and G. T. Ross, Biochem Biophys Res Commun 42:962, 1971.
3. Vaitukaitis, J. L., and G. T. Ross, J Clin Endocrinol 33:308, 1971.
4. Vaitukaitis, J. L., J. Hammond, G. Ross, J. Hickman, and G. Ashwell, J Clin Endocrinol 32:290, 1971.
5. Warren, L., J Biol Chem 234:1971, 1959.
6. Odell, W. D., P. L. Rayford, and G. T. Ross, J Lab Clin Med 70:973, 1967.
7. Rodbard, D., and J. E. Lewald, Acta Endocrinol (Kbh) 64:79, 1970.
8. Parlow, A. F., in E. Rosemberg (Ed.), Gonadotropins 1968, Geron-X, Inc., Los Altos, 1968, p. 59.
9. Van Hall, E. V., J. L. Vaitukaitis, G. T. Ross, J. W. Hickman, and G. Ashwell, Endocrinology 89:11, 1971.
10. Morel, A. G., R. A. Irvine, I. Sternlieb, I. H. Scheinberg, and G. G. Ashwell, J Biol Chem 243:155, 1968.
11. Morel, A. G., G. Gregoriadis, I. H. Scheinberg, J. Hickman, and G. G. Ashwell, J Biol Chem 246:1461, 1971.
12. Catt, K. J., M. Dufau, and T. Tsurahara, J Clin Endocrinol 32:860, 1971.
13. Catt, K. J., M. Dufau, and T. Tsurahara, Abstracts of papers presented at meetings of ASCI, Atlantic City, N.J., May 1971.
14. Van Thiel, D. H., W. F. Bridson, and P. O. Kohler, Endocrinology 89:622, 1971.

33.　　　Correlation Between Bioassay and Radioimmunoassay of FSH and LH

Eugenia Rosemberg, Si G. Lee, George Bulat, Griff T. Ross, and Philip S. Butler

---

Published comparisons of biologic and immunologic potency estimates of human pituitary and urinary FSH and LH indicate that potency estimates using biologic methods do not always agree with those obtained by immunoassay. One of the major sources of confusion in the literature concerning both biologic and immunologic potency estimates of gonadotropic hormones has been the use of several standards. In the bioassay field, at least six reference preparations or standards were used to report values of gonadotropin activity in pituitary tissue and body fluids (1). In the radioimmunoassay field, there are now two materials widely used in the United States for the same purpose: a human pituitary extract LER 907 prepared and distributed by the National Institute of Arthritis and Metabolic Diseases and the Second International Reference Preparation for Human Menopausal Gonadotropin (2nd IRP-HMG) distributed in behalf of the World Health Organization by the Division of Biological Standards, National Institute for Medical Research, Mill Hill, London.

If valid comparisons are to be made between the biologic and immunologic potency estimates of human gonadotropins, the physiologic characteristics of the bioassay systems should be understood and the specific characteristics of the immunoassay system should be known. As an example, in the bioassay field, a disparity of some 12-fold in the assay of urinary LH was found when the assays were conducted by the ventral prostate weight method (VPW) and by the

424

ovarian ascorbic acid depletion method (OAAD) (2). The discrepancy was understandable on the basis that it was attributable to the physical and chemical differences and possibly also to metabolic differences in the standard used (NIH-LH-S1, an ovine pituitary LH) and the material (urinary LH) tested (2, 3). The discrepancy disappeared when a urinary standard was used for the assay of urinary LH. A similar observation was made testing a pituitary LH preparation, in both the VPW and OAAD methods using ovine NIH-LH-S1 as standard (4).

As shown in Table I, another example of this discrepancy is illustrated in the assay of ovine NIH-FSH-S1 and NIH-LH-S1 and the 2nd IRP-HMG, a gonadotropic preparation obtained from human urine.

TABLE I. Specific activity of NIH-FSH-S1 and NIH-LH-S1, IU 2nd IRP-HMG/ mg[a]

Assay system	No. of assays	No. of animals	Assay characteristics		Weighted mean potency ratio (95% CI)	
			bc	λ	NIH-FSH-S1 (IU/mg)	NIH-LH-S1 (IU/mg)
AR	10	245	239	0.14	26.5 (24.3-28.8)	
VPW	6	167	18.6	0.21		51.3 (43.9-59.9)
OAAD	21	417	−26	0.30		588 (500-714)

[a]Index of discrimination OAAD/VPW = 11.5.

In the radioimmunoassay field, many reports now available in the literature emanating from various laboratories indicate differences in potency estimates of FSH and LH. These quantitative differences are ascribed not only to the standard used to relate potency estimates of unknown samples (pituitary extracts, serum or urinary gonadotropins) but to differences in the characteristics of the specific radioimmunoassay system used (5, 6).

Moreover, a collaborative study conducted by the National Pituitary Agency (NPA) (7) established that a tissue pituitary extract (LER-907) is satisfactory as a radioimmunoassay reference preparation for FSH and LH in pituitary tissue extracts. The study also showed that the use of the 2nd IRP-HMG (urinary) as a radioimmunoassay standard is associated with an overestimation of FSH and LH content of human pituitary tissue extracts. These discrepancies have been also pointed out by Ryan in an extensive review on the comparison of biologic and immunologic potency estimates of human FSH and LH (8).

The purpose of the present report is to further extend the observations recorded in the literature relative to the biologic and immunologic potency estimates of human gonadotropins.

MATERIALS AND METHODS

Highly purified human pituitary FSH and LH preparations were obtained through the courtesy of the National Pituitary Agency. The purified LH preparations used were: LER 856-1; LER 1371; LER 960; and DEAE 2-II. The purified FSH preparations were: LER 862-A; LER 869-2; and LER 1366.

The details of bioassay methods used as performed in our laboratories (Worcester and Bethesda) have been described (2-9). The LH and FSH radioimmunoassay used were performed as described by Odell et al. (10) and Midgley et al. (11).

All preparations were tested at several dose levels. The concomitant standard and reference preparation used in all assays were the 2nd IRP-HMG and LER 907, respectively. All assays were calculated by appropriate computer programs for parallel-line assays. Results are given in terms of specific activity (SA) by weight of the preparations in terms of weight of LER 907, and by SA in IU of the 2nd IRP-HMG/mg.

RESULTS

Comparison of Relative Potencies

Table II shows the biologic and radioimmunological potency estimation of highly purified human pituitary LH preparations in terms of the 2nd IRP-HMG standard (urinary).

Table III shows the biologic (BIO) and radioimmunologic (IMM) potency estimation of the preparations shown in Table II in terms of LER 907 standard (pituitary extract).

Two points should be emphasized: The potency estimation of LER 907 in terms of 2nd IRP-HMG does not agree with the unitage assigned to this reference preparation [20 IU FSH and 48 IU LH activity/vial = 1 mg (7)]. Moreover, the VPW estimation is higher than that obtained with the OAAD method. The reason for this discrepancy is unknown. As all preparations were assayed concomitantly with the standard, potency estimates obtained by the VPW method are higher than those obtained with the OAAD assay.

The biologic and immunologic potency estimates of pituitary LH preparations using a pituitary standard are in agreement. However, the immunologic potency estimates using a urinary standard are higher than those obtained by bioassay.

Table IV shows the biologic and immunologic potency estimation of highly purified human pituitary FSH preparations in terms of the two standards (urinary and pituitary extract). One LH preparation, LER 856-1, is also shown in this Table.

TABLE II. Bio- and radioimmunoassay of human pituitary gonadotropin preparations

| Preparation | IU 2nd IRP-HMG/mg | | | |
| | Bioassay | | | Radioimmunoassay |
	AR[a]	OAAD[b]	VPW[c]	LH
LER 907	23 (17-30)[e]	54 (32-99)	70 (44-109)	310 (320-340)
LER 856-1	2.5 (2.0-3.1)	510 (320-830)	516 (216-1,396)	1,633 (1,500-1,700)
LER 1371	1.7 (1.2-2.5)	1,320 (760-2,290)	2,032 (930-4,545)	6,235 (6,000-6,560)
LER 960	1.1 (0.8-1.7)	1,465 (630-3,460)	2,514 (962-8,802)	8,526 (8,230-8,800)
DEAE 2-II[a]	2.5 (2.1-3.0)	1,350 (560-3,250)	3,309 (1,536-7,296)	9,349 (8,960-9,720)

[a]Augmentation reaction assay.
[b]Ovarian ascorbic acid depletion assay.
[c]Ventral prostate weight assay.
[d]Prepared by Dr. Parlow for the NPA.
[e]Confidence limits.

TABLE III. Bio- and radioimmunoassay of human pituitary gonadotropin preparations

| Preparation | mg LER 907/mg | | | |
| | Bioassay | | | Radioimmunoassay |
	AR	OAAD	VPW	LH
LER 856-1	0.13 (0.10-0.16)	9 (6-15.4)	6 (3-20)	6 (5.8-6.3)
LER 1371	0.09 (0.06-0.13)	23 (14-42)	26 (13-65)	26 (25-26.6)
LER 960	0.06 (0.04-0.09)	30 (12-64)	31 (14-125)	28 (27.2-29.1)
DEAE 2-II	0.13 (0.11-0.15)	28 (10-60)	39 (22-104)	30 (28-31.4)

TABLE IV. Bio- and radioimmunoassay of human pituitary gonadotrop in preparations

Preparations	2nd IRP-HMG (IU/mg)			LER 907 (mg/mg)		
	AR	OAAD	FSH	AR	OAAD	FSH
LER 907	23 (17-30)	54.0 (32-99)	54 (43-62)			
LER 862-A[a]	800 (690-1,050)	3.7 (2.5-4.7)	794 (690-867)	40 (35-53)	0.08 (0.05-0.09)	16 (13-18)
LER 869-2	2,782 (2,317-3,341)	92.0 (81-110)	2,136 (1,950-2,358)	139 (116-167)	1.9 (1.5-2.0)	43 (36-46)
LER 1366	2,570 (2,230-2,750)	50.0 (43-76)	2,350 (2,135-2,540)	129 (112-138)	1.0 (0.79-1.4)	47 (40-49)
LER 856-1[a]	2.5 (2.0-3.1)	510.0 (320-830)	34.3 (29-40.5)	0.13 (0.10-0.16)	9.0 (6.0-15.4)	0.69 (0.53-0.75)

[a]Distributed by the NPA for clinical investigation.

TABLE V. Purified pituitary LH fractions: comparison of FSH/LH ratios (BIO) using two standards

| Preparation | FSH/LH ratios (BIO) | | | | ID FSH/LH |
| | 2nd IRP-HMG (IU/mg) | | LER 907 (mg/mg) | | LER 907/2nd IRP-HMG |
	AR/OAAD	AR/VPW	AR/OAAD	AR/VPW	
LER 907	0.37	0.33			
LER 856-1	0.005	0.005	0.015	0.023	3
LER 1371	0.0013	0.0008	0.004	0.003	3
LER 960	0.0008	0.0004	0.002	0.002	2.5
DEAE-2-II	0.0019	0.0008	0.005	0.003	2.6

The biologic and immunologic potency estimates of pituitary FSH preparations using a urinary standard are in agreement. However, the immunologic
potency estimates using a pituitary extract are lower than those obtained by
bioassay.

Comparison of FSH/LH (BIO) Ratios

The comparison of the FSH/LH (biologic) ratios using two standards is
presented in Tables V and VI.

TABLE VI. Comparison of FSH/LH ratios (BIO) using two standards

Preparations	2nd IRP-HMG (IU/mg)	LER 907 (mg/mg)	ID FSH/LH LER 907/2nd IRP-HMG
LER 907	0.43		
LER 862-A[a]	216.0	500	2.3
LER 869-2	30.0	73	2.4
LER 1366	51.0	129	2.5
LER 856-1[a]	0.005	0.01	2.0

[a]Distributed by the NPA for clinical investigation.

The index of discrimination, I/D, (LER 907/2nd IRP-HMG) indicate that
when a pituitary extract is used as reference material, the FSH/LH ratios of
highly purified LH and FSH preparations are two to three times higher than
those estimated using a urinary standard.

Comparison of IMM/BIO Ratios

The comparison of the immunoassay/bioassay (IMM/BIO) LH and FSH ratios
using two standards are presented in Tables VII and VIII.

Comparison of the LH IMM/BIO ratios shows that immunoassay overestimates the LH potency of pituitary preparations when a urinary standard is
used; the IMM/BIO ratio, however, was close to unity when a pituitary
preparation was used as the reference material. Comparison of the FSH/BIO
ratios shows that the immunoassay underestimates the FSH potency of pituitary
preparations when a pituitary standard is used; the IMM/BIO ratio, however, was
close to unity when a urinary preparation was used as the standard reference
material.

TABLE VII. Comparison of IMM/BIO LH ratio using two standards

Preparations	2nd IRP-HMG (IU/mg)		LER 907 (mg/mg)	
	RIA-LH OAAD	RIA-LH VPW	RIA-LH OAAD	RIA-LH VPW
LER 907	5.7	4.4		
LER 856-1	3.2	3.2	0.63	1
LER 1371	4.7	3.1	1.1	1
LER 960	5.8	3.4	0.93	0.90
DEAE-2-II	6.9	2.8	1.1	0.77

TABLE VIII. Comparison of IMM/BIO FSH ratios using two standards

Preparations	RIA-FSH/AR	
	2nd IRP-HMG (IU/mg)	LER 907 (mg/mg)
LER 907	2.3	
LER 862-A[a]	0.99	0.40
LER 869-2	0.77	0.31
LER 1366	0.91	0.36
LER 856-1[a]	14.0	5.3

[a]Distributed by the NPA for clinical investigation.

Table IX shows the comparison of FSH/LH biologic ratios and the corresponding FSH and LH IMM/BIO ratios of an LH-rich fraction, LER 856-1, and of an FSH rich fraction, LER 869-2.

TABLE IX. Comparison of purified pituitary fractions

Preparations	FSH/LH ratios (BIO)		IMM/BIO FSH		IMM/BIO LH	
	2nd IRP-HMG	LER 907	2nd IRP-HMG	LER 907	2nd IRP-HMG	LER 907
LH-rich fraction LER 856-1	0.005	0.01	14	5.3	3.2	1
FSH-rich fraction LER 869-2	30	73	0.77	0.31	6.0	1

In LH-rich fractions, the immunoassay detects more FSH than is measured by the bioassay using the two standards. In FSH rich fractions, the immunoassay detects more LH than is measured by bioassay using a urinary standard and is in good agreement with the bioassay when a pituitary standard is used.

COMMENTS

The data presented above confirm the observations recorded in the literature (7-13) in that bioassay and radioimmunoassay potency estimates of LH obtained for pituitary preparations are in agreement when a pituitary standard is used, and that bioassay potency estimates obtained for pituitary preparations are lower than radioimmunoassay potency estimates when a urinary reference preparation is used. These observations also apply when the LH content of purified pituitary FSH fractions was estimated by bio- and immunoassays.

Several factors might be responsible for the radioimmunoassay overestimation of LH content of the pituitary preparations when the 2nd IRP-HMG is used as the standard. One is the possibility that a urinary preparation such as the 2nd IRP-HMG, could have lost immunoreactive sites in the LH molecule as a result of metabolism attendant to its passage from pituitary to blood to urine, or from the extraction procedure used in the preparation of this standard. Another explanation has been introduced by Ryan (8) based on the hypothesis of the formation of hybrid molecules which could account for the immunologic deficiency of urinary LH. This hypothesis implies that a dissociated biologically inactive but immunologically recognizable form of LH, as well as the biologically active associated species of LH, is excreted in urine.

The radioimmunoassay for FSH grossly overestimates the amount found by bioassay when LH-rich fractions are analyzed using two standards although the degree of discrepancy is much less when a pituitary extract is used. This observation also applies when the FSH content of FSH-rich fractions were estimated by bio- and immunoassays using two standards. However, when a pituitary reference material was used, the immunoassay detected less FSH than was measured by bioassay. Although immunologic distinction between urinary and pituitary FSH has been noted (8), the cause of this discrepancy is unknown.

ACKNOWLEDGMENT

This work was supported by USPHS grant AM-07564, National Institutes of Health, Bethesda, Maryland.

We are indebted to the National Institute of Arthritis and Metabolic Diseases, NIH, and to the National Pituitary Agency, Baltimore, Maryland for the supply of immunologic reagents and the supply of hormones used in this study. We wish to thank Dr. D. R. Bangham, Department of Biological Standards, Medical Research Council, Mill Hill, London for the gift of the 2nd IRP-HMG.

REFERENCES

1. Rosemberg, in E. Rosemberg (Ed.), Gonadotropins 1968, Geron-X, Inc., Los Altos, 1968, p. 384.

2. Rosemberg, E., E. A. Solod, and A. Albert, J Clin Endocrinol 24:714, 1964.

3. Albert, A., I. Derner, E. Rosemberg, and W. B. Lewis, Endocrinol 76:139, 1965.

4. Albert, A., C. Hanten, E. Rosemberg, and G. Bulat, Endocrinol 77:588, 1965.

5. Taymor, M. L., and J. Miyata, in E. Diczfalusy (Ed.), Immunoassay of Gonadotropins, Bogtrykkeriet Forum, Copenhagen, Denmark, 1970, p. 324.

6. Stevens, V. C., in E. Diczfalusy (Ed.), Immunoassay of Gonadotropins, Bogtrykkeriet Forum, Copenhagen, Denmark, 1970, p. 338.

7. Albert, A., E. Rosemberg, G. T. Ross, C. A. Paulsen, and R. J. Ryan, J Clin Endocrinol 28:1214, 1968.

8. Ryan, R. J., in E. Diczfalusy (Ed.), Immunoassay of Gonadotropins, Bogtrykkeriet Forum, Copenhagen, Denmark, 1969, p. 300.

9. Rosemberg, E., and I. Engel, J Clin Endocrinol 21:1063, 1961.

10. Odell, W. D., G. T. Ross, and P. L. Rayford, J Clin Invest 46:248, 1967.

11. Midgley, A. R., Jr., Endocrinology 79:10, 1966.

12. Albert, A., in E. Rosemberg (Ed.), Gonadotropins 1968, Geron-X, Inc., Los Altos, 1968, p. 393.

13. Odell, W. D., L. E. Reichert, and R. S. Swerdloff, in E. Rosemberg (Ed.), Gonadotropins 1968, Geron-X, Inc., Los Altos, 1968, p. 393.

34.   Antigenic Similarities Among the Human Glycoprotein Hormones and their Subunits

Judith L. Vaitukaitis and Griff T. Ross

Common antigenic determinants among HCG, LH, FSH, and TSH have made the production of specific antisera for radioimmunoassay difficult (1-4). However, complete cross-reaction between LH and HCG has been used to advantage in developing radioimmunoassays for LH using antisera raised against HCG (2, 5-8,). It has been difficult to determine whether the cross-reaction reflected contamination of hormonal preparations used for immunogen or, alternatively, common antigenic determinants in small portions or entire subunits of the hormone. The recent isolation and separation of subunits of FSH (9), LH (10), and HCG (11, 12) have provided unique materials with which these questions could be explored. We have generated specific antisera to the subunits of HCG and using those antisera, have examined the cross-reactivity among the human glycoprotein hormones and their subunits.

MATERIALS AND METHODS

Purification, preparation, and biologic activity of the subunits of HCG, designated CR 100α and CR 100β have been described previously (11). The α and β subunits of human FSH were generously provided by Dr. Brij Saxena and the LH subunits, LH 89CI and LH 89CII, by Dr. Leo Reichert.

ANTISERA

Female 3-month-old New Zealand white rabbits were immunized with 20 μg CR 100α or β in a vehicle containing complete Freund's adjuvant (Difco) in an equal volume of 0.15M NaC1 and 2 mg dried tubercle bacilli (Difco) in a total vol of 2 ml. The injections were administered intradermally in 30 to 50 sites over the dorsum of the animal and into 2 toe pads of each hind limb. In a separate site, 0.5 ml of crude pertussis vaccine was given subcutaneously. The animals were bled by either cardiac puncture or puncture of the central ear artery 17 days later, then every 7 to 10 days thereafter. When no significant antibody titer was evident in the animals initially immunized with CR 100β, they were reimmunized with 20 μg CR 100β in an emulsion containing saline:marcol: arlacel (2 : 3 : 1 v/v) at multiple sites 39 days after the primary immunization. Animals rechallenged with CR 100β were bled 7 days later and one of those sera used for studies with CR 100β antisera in a final serum dilution of 1 : 5000 or 1 : 10,000. Serum obtained from an animal 46 days after the primary immunization with CR 100α was used for all studies antiserum in a final dilution of 1 : 50,000.

RADIOIMMUNOASSAY

CR 100α and β were labeled with ^{125}I according to the method of Greenwood et al. (13). The double-antibody technique was used for all assays which were initially incubated at 37 C for 2 hr, then 17 to 30 hr at 4 C, second antibody added and incubation continued for 6 to 20 hr at 4 C.

Highly purified human glycoprotein hormones, TSH (Pierce Fraction 4), HFSH (LER 1366), HCG (CR 100 HCG), and LH (LER 960), were provided by the National Pituitary Agency. These hormones were assayed along with the subunits of HCG in either the homologous α system consisting of ^{125}I-CR 100α and CR 100α antiserum, or the homologous β system comprised of ^{125}I-CR 100 β and CR 100β antiserum. The subunits of HCG, FSH, and LH were radioimmuno-assayed in both the homologous α and β systems.

All results are shown as logit transform of the response variable versus log dose of antigen (14). A high-speed digital computer with programs designed by Rodbard et al. (15) was used for all calculations.

RESULTS

Intact Hormones

HOMOLOGOUS α SYSTEM

Figure 1 shows that the dose-response lines of TSH, LH, FSH, and HCG were parallel to CR 100 α. Doses of intact hormones were clustered about a common area of the graph, requiring 10 to 100 times more mass for percent inhibition comparable to the homologous antigen, CR 100 α.

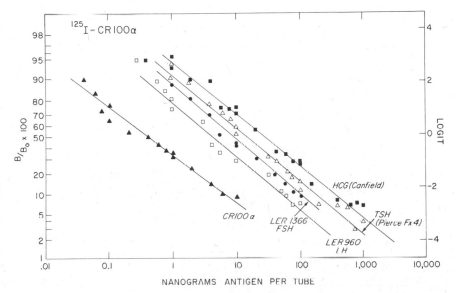

FIG. 1. Dose-response lines for CR100α (▲), LER 960 LH (⊔), LER 1366, FSH (●), TSII, Pierce Fx 4 (△) and HCG, Canfield (■). B_0 = maximum counts bound with labeled ligand alone; B = counts bound in presence of labeled and unlabeled ligand. CR100α antisera used in final dilution of 1:50,000.

HOMOLOGOUS β SYSTEM

Although the dose-response lines of LH, HCG, and CR 100β occurred in the same portion of the dose-response graph, their configuration, slopes, or both were different (Fig. 2). LH failed to effectively inhibit ^{125}I-Cr 100β since the direction of the dose-response line changed sharply when 10 ng or more of LH was added per assay tube.

Figure 3 shows a similar cross-reacting pattern for TSH but the entire dose-response line started at a much higher dose of antigen than that for LH. The dose-response line of FSH was parallel to that for HCG but like TSH, the dose-response line started at a higher dose of antigen.

Subunits

HOMOLOGOUS α SYSTEM

Figure 4 shows the dose-response lines of CR 100α FSHα and HLH 89CI. The slopes were equal. The dose-response line of FSHα, was closer to the dose-response line of the homologous antigen, CR 100α, than was HLH 89CI. Table I shows the slopes of the regression line generated for each subunit studied in the homologous α system and the p value resulting from comparing the slope of each weighted regression with that of the homologous antigen, CR 100α.

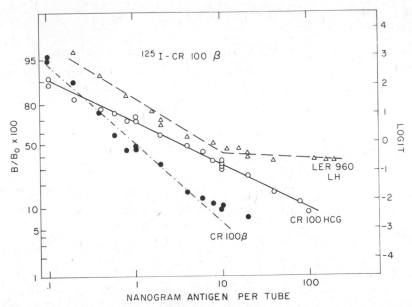

FIG. 2. Dose-response lines for CR100β, CR100 HCG, and LER 960 (LH). B_0 = maximum counts bound with labeled ligand alone; B = counts bound in presence of labeled and unlabeled ligand. CR100β antiserum used in final dilution of 1:5000.

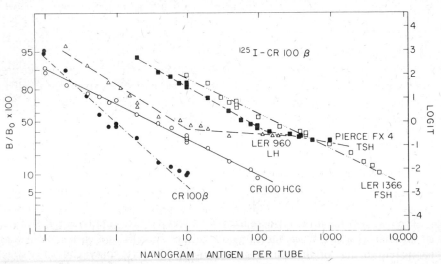

FIG. 3. Dose-response lines for CR100β (●), CR100 HCG (○), LH (△), TSH (■), and FSH (□).

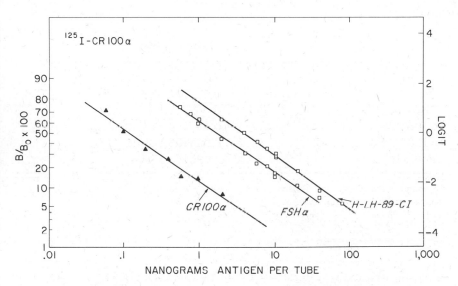

FIG. 4. Inhibition lines for CR100α (▲), FSHα (□), and HLH 89CI (□) generated with ^{125}I-CR100α and CR10 antiserum.

TABLE I.

Antigen	N	Slope ± SE	p[a]
CR 100 α	17	−0.974582 ± 0.059	
CR 100 β	23	−0.778702 ± 0.037	< 0.05
FSH	17	−0.930044 ± 0.049	> 0.05
FSH	14	−0.895882 ± 0.079	> 0.05
HLH 89CI	20	−1.09956 ± 0.043	> 0.05
HLH 89CII	20	−1.06012 ± 0.042	> 0.05

[a]p value computed for parallelism between regression line of CR 100 α and each subunit assayed in the homologous system.

HOMOLOGOUS β SYSTEM

The slopes of the dose-response lines of CR 100β, FSHβ, and HLH 89CII were all different (Fig. 5). When the slope of the regression line for each subunit was compared to that of the homologous antigen, CR 100β, only CR 100α was parallel (Table II). The slopes of the dose-response lines of HLH 89CI and CII were different (p <.05) from each other whereas the slopes of the dose-response lines of FSH α and β were equal. The CI subunit of HLH was parallel to FSH α. In the β-assay system both LH subunits required less mass than the FSH subunits for comparable percent inhibition.

TABLE II.

Antigen	N	Slope ± SE	p[a]
CR 100 β	20	−1.09098 ± 0.027	
FSH	21	−0.529192 ± 0.036	< 0.05
FSH	23	−0.565544 ± 0.022	< 0.05
HLH 89 CI	23	−0.447414 ± 0.018	< 0.05
HLH 89 CII	23	−0.348898 ± 0.012	< 0.05
CR 100 α	19	−1.19033 ± 0.044	> 0.05

[a]p value computed for parallelism between regression line of CR 100β and each subunit assayed in the homologous system.

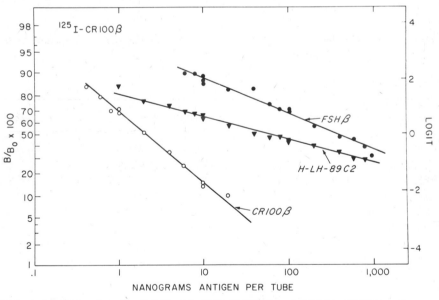

FIG. 5. Inhibition lines for CR100β (o), HLH 89C2 (▲), and FSH (●). CR100β antiserum used in final dilution of 1:5000.

DISCUSSION

Liao and Pierce (15) studied the subunits of bovine TSH and LH. The α subunit of TSH and CI subunit of LH were found to have similar primary amino acid structures (16, 17). Furthermore, those subunits recombined equally well with either the β subunit of TSH or CII subunit of LH. Biologic assays showed that the β or CII subunit contained the intrinsic biologic determinants of the intact hormone whereas the α or CI subunit served as a "carrier" for a complementary subunit. The isolated subunit of LH, FSH, HCG, and TSH have little or no detectable biologic activity but on recombination with the complementary subunit, considerable biologic activity may be restored (9-11, 16).

If the human glycoproteins were to share a common subunit, then cross-reactivity of antisera made with the intact hormone should reflect common antigenic sites on that subunit whereas specific antisera should reflect antibody directed to antigenic sites on the unique subunit of a particular hormone. When antiserum raised to the α subunit of HCG was reacted in a system containing ^{125}I-CR 100α and FSH, HLH, TSH, HCG, CR 100α, all dose-response lines were parallel (Fig. 1). The homologous antigen, CR 100α, had the highest apparent affinity since the dose-response line of that antigen required less mass for equivalent inhibition. FSH, LH, TSH, and HCG shared common antigenic determinants in the homologous α system since their dose-response lines all clustered about the same portion of the graph and all dose-response lines were parallel.

When antiserum generated against CR 100β was introduced into a system with ^{125}I-CR 100β and either CR 100β, LH, HCG, FSH, TSH, or CR 100 α, then the intact hormones displayed different slopes, affinities, or both (Figs. 2 and 3), indicating incomplete cross-reactivity with CR 100β and different antigenic determinants from the homologous antigen and from each other. The configuration of the dose-response lines of TSH and LH were similar with the upper portion of their lines appearing parallel. Both hormones had a sharp break in their dose-response lines indicating interaction with a subset of lower affinity antibodies which were readily saturated with relatively small amounts of antigen. The dose-response lines of HCG and FSH were parallel but the relative affinities of the two hormones quite different since 100 times more mass was required for FSH to attain comparable inhibition in the β assay system. The dose-response lines of TSH and FSH were closer to the α subunit of HCG than were the dose-response lines of HCG and LH which were closer to CR 100β, probably reflecting closer immunologic similarity among HCG, LH, and CR 100β in the homologous β system. That the intact hormones reacted similarly in the homologous system but quite differently in the homologous β system is consistent with there being more common antigenic determinants on the α subunit of HCG and intact glycoprotein hormones than with the β subunit of HCG and the various hormones studied.

When the subunits of HCG, LH, and FSH were assayed in the homologous α system, the dose-response lines of all the α or CI subunits were parallel (Fig. 4), reflecting common antigenic determinants among those subunits. The β subunit of FSH and CII of LH required three to five times more mass, relative to their complementary subunit, for equivalent percent inhibition in the homologous α

system. The latter may reflect either contamination of the β or CII subunit with 20 to 30% intact hormone or α subunit or that common antigenic sites appear on both the α and β subunits of each antigen tested.

When the intact glycoprotein hormones and the β subunits of LH, FSH, and HCG were assayed in the homologous β system, antigenic dissimilarity became apparent. Furthermore, the dose-response lines of intact HCG and LH were different from the dose-response lines of their respective β subunits. The latter observation suggests that on recombination of two complementary subunits, expression of antigenic determinants of the β or CII subunits was altered.

On the other hand, when the intact glycoprotein hormones and the α or CI subunits of HCG, FSH, or HLH were assayed in the homologous α system, all dose-response lines were parallel to the homologous antigen, CR 100α, and to each other. It would appear that recombination of the complementary subunits of a particular hormone did not appreciably affect the antigenic behavior of the α subunit since the same qualitative dose-response line was generated in the homologous α system whether the α subunit or intact hormone were studied. An absolute quantitative analysis cannot be considered here since the subunit preparations were not derived from the specific intact glycoprotein studied in the foregoing radioimmunoassay systems.

The ability of CR 100β antisera to distinguish between intact LH and HCG probably reflected the antigenic dissimilarity between HLH 89CII and CR 100β, as well as between intact LH and HCG. Franchimont (18) has characterized an antiserum raised to intact HCG and demonstrated incomplete cross-reactivity between LH and HCG. In view of the results, it would appear that the HCG-specific antibody was directed to antigenic sites of the β subunit of HCG.

We conclude that the cross-reactivity among the human glycoprotein hormones reflects antigenic determinants on either a common subunit or large segments of the α or CI subunit and that those common antigenic determinants result in the nonspecificity of antisera raised to the intact glycoprotein hormones. The absolute chemical purity of a particular glycoprotein hormone used as an immunogen would appear to be of secondary importance. The β or CII subunit confers the unique immunoreactivity of the intact hormone. Furthermore, generation of specific antisera could be facilitated if the β or CII subunit were used in the immunologic procedure and only those antisera exhibiting complete cross-reactivity with the intact hormone be used in specific radioimmunoassays.

REFERENCES

1. Wide, L. P. Roos, and C. A. Gemzel, Acta Endocrinol (Kbh) 37:445, 1961.
2. Wilde, C. E., A. H. Orr, and K. D. Bagshawe, J Endocrinol 37:23, 1967.
3. Odell, W. A., G. Abraham, H. R. Raud, R. S. Swerdloff, and D. Fisher, in Diczfalusy, (ED.), Karolinska Symposia on Research Methods in Reproductive Endocrinology, Bogtrykkeriet Forum, Copenhagen, Denmark, 1969, p. 54.

4. Schlaff, S., S. W. Rosen, and J. Roth, J Clin Invest 47:1722, 1968.

5. Odell, W. D., G. T. Ross, and P. L. Rayford, Metabolism 15:187, 1966.

6. Odell, W. D., G. T. Ross, and P. L. Rayford, J Clin Invest 46:248, 1967.

7. Midgley, A. R., Endocrinology 79:10, 1966.

8. Rizkallah, T., M. L. Taymor, M. Park, and R. Batt, J Clin Endocrinol 25:943, 1965.

9 Reichert, L. E., and A. R. Midgley, in E. Rosemberg (Ed.), Gonadotropins 1968, Geron - X, Inc., Los Altos, 1968, p. 25.

10. Reichert, L. E., A. R. Midgley, G. D. Niswender, and D. N. Ward, Endocrinology 87:534, 1970.

11. Morgan, F. J., and R. E. Canfield, Endocrinology 88:1045, 1971.

12. Swaminathanan, N., and P. O. Bahl, Biochem Biophys Res Commun 40:422, 1970.

13. Greenwood, F. C., W. M. Hunter, and J. S. Glover, Biochem J 89:114, 1963.

14. Rodbard, D., W. Bridson, and and P. L. Rayford, J Lab Clin Med 74:770, 1969.

15. Rodbard, D., and J. E. Lewald, in E. Diczfalusy, (Ed.), Karolinska Symposia on Research Methods in Reproductive Endocrinology, 2nd symposium: Steroid assay by protein binding, Bogtrykkeriet Forum, Copenhagen, Denmark, 1970, p. 79.

16. Liao, T. H., and J. G. Pierce, J Biol Chem 245:3275, 1970.

17. Liu, W. K., C. M. Sweeney, II. S. H. Nahm, G. N. Holcomb, and D. N. Ward, Res Commun Chem Pathol Pharmacol 2:168, 1971.

18. Franchimont, P., Europ J Clin. Invest 1:65, 1970.

DISCUSSION

S. A. BERSON: Not being a gonadotropinologist, I can be sympathetic with those who are in the field without being frustrated myself at the many years of difficulties in standardizing the various gonadotropin preparations. I think the evidence we have heard today indicates that as far as in vivo biological assays are concerned, the significance of these with respect to gonadotropic activity and the comparison of gonadotropic activity with immunoreactivity, we should simply stop doing bioassays. It is obviously very important for the treatment of a patient that we know the biologic activity. However, if we are interested in the effect of gonadotropins on the gonads or in comparing biologic gonadotropic activity with immunoactivity, we simply cannot rely on in vivo bioassays. We have heard today that removal of sialic acid and subsequent changes in the half-life of the hormone markedly alter the biologic response. Therefore, in vivo bioassay determines not only the gonadotropic activity of the gonadotropin, but also something which is related to its rate of removal. Many years ago, Dr. Yalow and I showed that one of the most sensitive biologic mechanisms for detecting mild alterations in a serum protein such as albumin, that could not be detected by a variety of physical or chemical tests, was the rate at which the liver would recognize this alteration and remove it from the body (J Clin Invest 36:44, 1957). The same thing is true of the desialylated proteins, as shown by studies which began originally with ceruloplasm and transferin and now have been applied to the glycopeptides of the anterior pituitary. Here we stand. We know that desialylation produces a marked increase in the rate of removal and therefore a diminution in the biologic potency, but what about other more occult and minor changes in the peptide portion. We are not as yet able to characterize these very readily, but in the various extraction and purification procedures some minor alteration that makes the liver recognize the abnormality and quickly remove the hormone might so affect its gonadotropic potency that the in vivo biologic assays are useless for the purposes under consideration. What does removal of galactose or the entire carbohydrate fraction do to the biologic activity and the circulatory half-life of these glycopeptides?

G. T. ROSS: If one removes galactose from these desialylated preparations, our preliminary experiments indicate that one, in fact, restores some of the biological activity which has been lost following the removal of sialic acid alone. We would hope to study effects of progressive removal of all of the carbohydrates from the molecules.

M. SAIRAM. I have a comment in relation to the paper by Dr. Ross. Drs. Papkoff and Li have repeatedly found that removal of sialic acid from human LH does not, in any way, affect the biological activity. Using the same enzyme preparation, it has been found that ovine FSH is completely inactivated. I believe Dr. Mori has reported similar findings in one of his papers on the antigenic determinants of human pituitary LH. In the case of human TSH, Dr. Pierce et al. have also found that removal of sialic acid does not affect biological activity. This is in keeping with the fact that removal of sialic acid from ovine LH does not, in any way, affect biological activity. I would like to emphasize that one should make sure of proteolytic contamination before making conclusive statements with respect to the requirement of sialic acid for biological activity of human LH.

G. T. ROSS. I hope I made it clear in my presentation that our material had been tested for proteolytic activity and none had been found. There are two very important factors that lead us to the conclusions that we have made, recognizing that our results are not entirely compatible with those that others have obtained. Firstly, as far as I am aware, changing the primary structure of a molecule by proteolysis rarely, if ever, enhances its antigenic activity. It has been suggested that chymotryptic digestion of LH will enhance its immunologic activity, but even this effect has not been observed consistently. Secondly, Drs. Ashwell and Hickman treated HCG with the same neurominidase which we have used in these studies and showed a decrement in the biological activity of the hormone. The desialylated preparation was then treated with sialotransferase and isotopically labeled sialic acid; labeled sialic acid was found to be reinserted into the molecule with recovery of some biologic activity. It seems unlikely that restoration of sialic acid would have restored biologic activity if proteolysis had been responsible for the loss of biologic activity.

G. E. ROSSELIN: As a comment on Dr. Saxena's finding of the FSH α subunits and on Dr. Vaitukaitis' presentation, I wish to sum up some of the arguments which led us to conclude that there is a common antigenic determinant in human FSH and the other glycopeptide hormones. Using ^{131}I-HFSH and antisera obtained with crude or partially purified HFSH preparations, a complete inhibition of binding could be demonstrated with unlabeled HFSH, but as much as 10,000 times higher molar concentrations of HCG was only partly inhibitory. The relative inhibitory potency of HCG and FSH varied significantly in different antisera indicating the presence of a cross-reacting substance other than FSH in the HCG preparation. Quantitative studies of these antisera with four ^{131}I-glycopeptide hormones and different FSH, LH, TSH, and HCG preparations show a clear-cut difference between pure cross-reactions and the effect of contaminating impurities.

HCG antiserum was found to bind both ^{131}I-HCG and ^{131}I-HLH but not to ^{131}I-FSH at a dilution of 10^6. ^{131}I-FSH is bound at a dilution of 10^3 to 10^4. Under the latter conditions, purified HFSH, HCG, and HLH are equally potent in inhibiting the binding of ^{131}I-FSH and a less pure preparation of HTSH was found to be half as potent. Since it is not likely that all these hormones contain identical amounts of HFSH, the cross-reaction was probably caused by a common antigen in all the glycopeptides.

J. L. VAITUKAITIS. The only explanation I can offer is that the purity of the preparations differs.

R. N. MOUDGAL. Dr. Samy and Mr. Muralidhar in my laboratory have some interesting results on the use of polymerized antisera to prepare hormones in small quantities from pituitary extracts of various species. These hormone preparations were used in radioimmunoassay, both for iodination and as standards. Antisera were polymerized with the use of ethyl chloroformate. With polymerized simian LH antiserum and NIH and Li-LH preparations, it was possible to show that 75 to 80% of the bound LH could be dissociated by treating with either 5.5M KI or 4M guanidine HCl as shown in this slide (Table I). The free LH in the supernatant after dialysis showed both immunological and

TABLE I. Reversible association-dissociation of LH with its antibody polymer.

Experiment number	Amount loaded (μg)	Amount bound (μg)	Dissociating agent	Amount recovered (μg)	Yield (%)
I	2000 NIH-LH-S8	200[a]	5.5 M KI[a] in 0.1M tris buffer pH 8.5	160	76
II	300 Li-LH	190[a]	4M Guanidine HCl[b]	145	76
III	350 Li-LH	200[b]	5.5 M KI[b] in 0.1M tris buffer pH 8.5	160	80

Note: Polymer from 0.5 ml of LH A/S was used in each experiment.

[a]At 22 C.
[b]At 3 to 4 C.

biological activity. Table II shows the application of this technique for the isolation of biologically and immunologically active LH and FSH from rat pituitary extracts and LH from monkey pituitary extracts. Polymerized simian LH, simian FSH and HCG antisera were used in these studies.

H. VAN HELL. I have a slide showing starch-gel electrophoresis of 2 HCG-subunit preparations. The highly purified HCG preparation contained only one band which was prepared by isoelectric focusing. After treatment with 10M urea at 37C for 1 hr the reaction mixture clearly showed the presence of at least 5 bands. Starch-gel immunoelectrophoresis showed that these bands all reacted with an antiserum to highly purified HCG. The five different components could be the subunits of HCG, the desialylated subunits of HCG and desialylated HCG. Partial recombination may also have taken place.

TABLE II. Summary of attempts to isolate hormones using polymerized antisera

Hormone and source	Biological activity[a]	Immunological activity[b]
LH from rat pituitary	+	+
LH from fraction B[c]	+	+[d]
LH from monkey pituitary[e]	+	+
FSH from rat[f]	+	−

[a]LH preparations were assayed for biological activity by the OAAD test. FSH activity was assayed by the Steelman-Pohley test.

[b]The immunological activity was assayed in all cases except that of FSH by precipitin test.

[c]A side fraction obtained during the fractionation of rat pituitary extracts for prolactin, growth hormone etc. (Ellis et al., Endocrinology 83:1029, 1969).

[d]Homogeneous by polyacrylamide disc electrophoresis at pH 4.3.

[e]Anti-HCG polymer used.

[f]Rat pituitary extract treated with LH polymer to remove rat LH was used in this experiment to prepare rat FSH.

Human Prolactin

35.   Studies on Human Prolactin

Andrew G. Frantz, David L. Kleinberg, and Gordon L. Noel

One of the main obstacles which has delayed the recognition of human prolactin as a separate hormone has been a lack of an adequately sensitive and specific bioassay, capable of measuring the hormone in human blood. In the hope of overcoming some of the limitations of the standard pigeon crop sac assay of Riddle and Bates, we began several years ago to experiment with a system employing a mammalian end organ, that of midpregnant mouse breast tissue maintained in organ culture. This system had previously been studied by a number of investigators (1, 2) in terms of its hormonal requirements, but it had not previously been utilized for assay purposes. Two years ago we reported (3) that this system was indeed capable of serving as an assay, with a sensitivity for prolactin considerably below what had previously been observed, and last year we reported on its use for the measurement of prolactin in unextracted human plasma in a variety of conditions (4). Immunologic as well as physiologic studies clearly indicated that the hormone was separate from human growth hormone and that its release was governed by different mechanisms. In this report we extend these observations, and present additional physiologic and immunologic data.

The system we use employs breast tissue from 8- to 9-day pregnant white Swiss mice of a local strain, bred in our own laboratory. The tissue is cut into small fragments and incubated for 4 days and under 95% oxygen and 5% carbon dioxide. The incubation medium is 199, supplemented by 30% pooled normal human male plasma. An important factor in the development of this assay was the discovery that not only is the organ culture system tolerant of human plasma, but that the presence of plasma both enhances the viability of the tissue and increases its sensitivity to prolactin. Ovine prolactin standards are run in every assay at 7 dose levels ranging from 0 to 50 ng/ml. The end point of the assay is histologic. A negative response, seen in the absence of prolactin, is characterized by tubules whose lumina are empty and which lack evidence of secretory activity. A strongly positive response, seen in the presence of prolactin at the 50 ng/ml dose level, shows abundant red staining secretory material present in all or virtually all of the lumina. The response is scored on an arbitrary scale of 0 to 4+, depending upon the amount of secretory material present. In practice scoring is not difficult and the results of different observers have been in good agreement. Further details of the assay have been reported elsewhere (5). When results are plotted for the combined experience of a number of assays, a standard curve of the form shown in Fig. 1 is obtained. The sensitivity of the

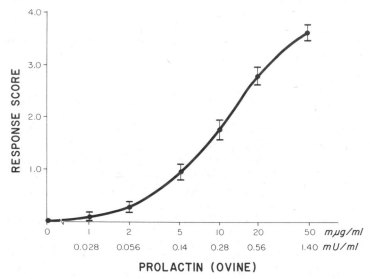

FIG. 1. Standard curve representing combined experience of 44 assays for prolactin. Vertical bars denote SEM.

assay is 5 ng/ml for ovine prolactin in most assays, occasionally as low as 2 ng/ml. When human plasma samples are run in the assay they are generally done in 2 or 4 more dilutions, ranging from 10% or below to 30%; the pooled normal male plasma is correspondingly reduced or completely replaced by the plasma under test. Thus the sensitivity for the plasma unknowns at 30% concentration is approximately 15 ng/ml ovine equivalents or 0.42 mU/ml. Specificity is very high; no substance not known to be a prolactin has given positive results in this assay, including a wide variety of pituitary and nonpituitary hormones. Human placental lactogen, as might be expected, gives a positive response, with preliminary potency estimates indicating slightly less than half the activity by weight of ovine prolactin. Human growth hormone is also strongly lactogenic. The purest preparations we have tested have had potencies ranging from 50 to

70% that of the ovine standard. The precision of the assay depends upon the number of times each sample is assayed and the dilutions used. We consider it important to assay every specimen in at least 2 assays and at 2 dilutions, and many of these specimens reported have been assayed on 3 or more occasions. Under these conditions, for levels not at the threshold of sensitivity of the assay, the standard error of the determination is approximately 25 to 30% that of mean value.

Our experience with prolactin measurement in human plasma is summarized in part in Fig. 2. In normal men and women, of whom we have studied over 50 to date, prolactin is generally undetectable, with levels below 0.42 mU/ml. In an occasional individual, we have noticed detectable levels at or below this limit with unusual assays, but the number of such cases is small and I think their significance is still uncertain.

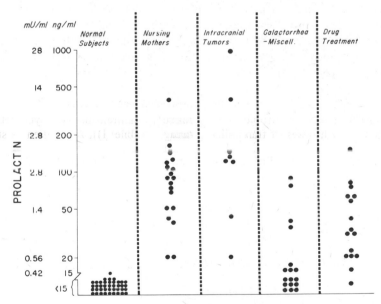

FIG. 2. Results of prolactin measurements on human plasma specimens. Values are expressed in terms of the NIH ovine standard S-8, with a potency of 28 U/mg.

Prolactin has been detectable, often at high levels, in a variety of states associated with lactation. All post-partum nursing mothers in whom we have measured prolactin have had detectable levels, ranging from 0.56 to 10.8 mU/ml. In several nursing mothers, three- to fourfold elevations in prolactin have occurred within half an hour after the beginning of a period of suckling. Plasma growth hormone, as measured by radioimmunoassay (6), was low in all these nursing subjects, ranging from 0.3 to 3.6 ng/ml. These levels are far too low to account for the bioassayable prolactin activity observed. We have observed high prolactin in a number of patients with intracranial lesions, including chromo-phobe adenomas, craniopharyngiomas, and other lesions affecting the hypo-thalamic-pituitary axis. We have found elevated prolactin in a number of patients following pituitary stalk section performed for diabetic retinopathy. In some patients with intracranial lesions, of whom we have studied many more than are shown in Fig. 2, galactorrhea was present and prolactin was measured for this reason. As we have looked, however, we have found an increasing number of patients with high prolactin without galactorrhea. Among these some of the highest levels have been encountered in patients with chromophobe adenomas. In patients with galactorrhea without known intracranial lesions, the highest prolactin levels have been found chiefly in those taking tranquilizing drugs. In limited numbers of patients we have seen prolactin elevations during estrogen administration, in association with alpha-methyldopa, and following withdrawal of birth control medications. We have also studied a number of patients with galactorrhea in whom no cause for the condition could be ascertained. In most of these patients plasma prolactin has been unmeasurably low, in other words, less than 0.42 mU/ml. The majority of these patients, unlike those whose galactorrhea was associated with an identifiable cause, have had regular menses. The lower prolactin levels have thus confirmed the clinical impression of a lesser degree of hypothalamic-pituitary disturbance in these patients.

Because of the known effects of chlorpromazine and related drugs in inducing galactorrhea in some subjects, we examined a number of psychiatric patients on chronic high doses of tranquilizing drugs (Table I). All patients studied, except

TABLE I. Prolactin during chronic tranquilizing drug therapy

Patient	Sex	Drug (time in weeks)	Dose (mg/day)	HGH (ng/ml)	Prolactin (mU/ml)
C.G.	F	Fluphenazine (2)	6	0.3	0.42
A.E.	F	Perphenazine (78)	12	0.3	3.1
M.S.	M	Perphenazine (1)	24	3.3	0.42
A.M.	F	Perphenazine (12) + Amitriptyline (12)	12 100	0.3	2.1
D.V.	M	Chlorpromazine (4)	2000	0.5	1.7
M.M.	M	Chlorpromazine (4)	1500	3.7	0.56
T.B.	M	Chlorpromazine (8)	2000	0.4	0.84
A.J.	F	Imipramine (4)	150	1.1	0.56
M.S.	M	Haloperidol (1)	4.5	0.3	1.7

one, had elevated prolactin levels, with growth hormones generally at the low end of the normal range. Only two of these patients had galactorrhea.

We next examined the effect of acute injection of chlorpromazine on a number of normal individuals. Dosages ranged from 12.5 to 50 mg given intramuscularly. Figure 3 shows the results of 12 tests in 10 normal subjects, 7

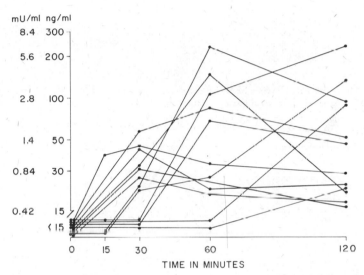

FIG. 3. Plasma prolactin levels following intramuscular chlorpromazine, given at 0 time, in normal individuals. Twelve tests were carried out on 10 subjects, 7 males and 3 females.

men and 3 women, over the first 2 hr. Prolactin, initially undetectable in all subjects, rose within one-half to 2 hr to measurable levels, as high as 6.7 mU/ml, in all subjects. Figure 4 shows the time course of prolactin levels over a more prolonged period of time. Peak levels are achieved at 1 to 2 hrs and remain elevated with little change over the next few hours. By 24 hr, prolactin was detectable in only one of four subjects who were studied at this interval. Growth hormone levels remained in the normal range throughout the duration of the test.

Because chlorpromazine acts in many ways as an antiadrenergic agent, depleting cerebral catecholamine levels, we examined the effect of L-dopa on the response to chlorpromazine stimulation. Two subjects were given 500 mg of levodopa (L-dopa) by mouth prior to the administration of 25 mg of chlorpromazine intramuscularly. The results of this study are shown in Figure 5, in which the responses of the same subjects to prior testing with L-dopa pretreatment are also shown. It can be seen that marked suppression of the normal prolactin rise following chlorpromazine was induced by L-dopa (7). The

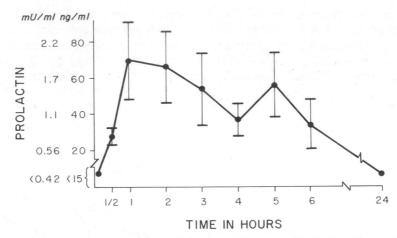

FIG. 4. Mean prolactin levels ± SEM, of the same subjects as in Fig. 3 after chlorpromazine stimulation, showing the response over a longer time period.

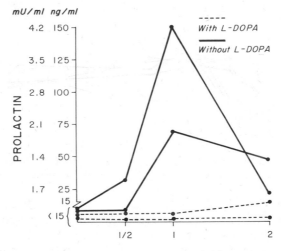

FIG. 5. Prolactin response to 25 mg of chlorpromazine in two normal males. The dashed lines depict the response after pretreatment with L-dopa.

effect of L-dopa on prolactin levels in various pathological conditions is currently under investigation. These studies indicate that despite the paucity of cells thought to be associated with prolactin secretion in the normal pituitary, normal individuals, both men and women, have the capacity to release and perhaps synthesize prolactin within a short time after appropriate stimulation. The secretion so initiated can be maintained indefinitely with continued stimulation.

In all of the individuals so far discussed with high plasma prolactin, growth hormone levels have not been elevated. As we have previously reported (4), high levels of immunoassayable growth hormone in blood are also associated with lactogenic activity. In 14 normal individuals who underwent insulin tolerance tests, prolactin activity in plasma rose from undetectable levels at the start of the test to elevated levels ranging from 0.42 to 1.4 mU/ml coincident with the rise in plasma growth hormone. The lactogenic activity in these patients' plasma, however, could be largely or completely neutralized by exposure to anti-human growth hormone antiserum. Such antiserum had no effect on the elevated prolactin levels of nursing mothers, as discussed below. Similarly, in 16 acromegalic subjects with elevated growth hormone levels, ranging from 13 to 180 ng/ml, prolactin activity was detectable in all at levels from 0.42 to 11 mU/ml. Here, as in the patients studied during insulin tolerance tests, much of the bioassayable activity appeared to be due to growth hormone itself, but in some patients neutralization studies with anti-human growth hormone antiserum indicated that prolactin was being hypersecreted together with growth hormone. These results have indicated that growth hormone in blood resembled the material extracted from human pituitary glands in possessing intrinsic lactogenic activity (4).

Neutralization studies with anti-human growth hormone antiserum have been reported previously (4, 5) and will be only summarized here. We have found that antiserum prepared against a highly purified Wilhelmi growth hormone (HS612A), when preincubated at 1:10 concentrations with normal male plasma in which growth hormone has been dissolved, completely neutralizes the prolactin effect of very large amounts of human growth hormone, up to 2000 ng/ml, when the plasma is subsequently bioassayed at 30% concentration in the usual manner. Under identical conditions of preincubation, the same anti-growth hormone antiserum failed to neutralize the prolactin activity in the plasma of any of the patients we have tested with galactorrhea or postpartum lactation who had high prolactin activity but low growth hormone. The effect on acromegalic plasmas has been variable, with some showing partial and others complete neutralization of prolactin activity following incubation with anti-growth hormone antiserum.

We have also studied the effect of anti-ovine prolactin on the plasma of patients with galactorrhea and postpartum lactation, as shown in Table II. Incubation of the plasma with an antiserum prepared in a rabbit against the NIH ovine standard S-8, under conditions similar to those employed for anti-growth hormone, completely neutralized the prolactin effect in all the samples studied. These studies emphasize, like those of Herbert and Hayashida (8) who used fluorescent techniques, the immunochemical similarity of primate and ovine prolactin.

Preliminary radioimmunoassays for human prolactin have been set up using antisera prepared against baboon prolactin. This material was obtained from organ cultures of baboon pituitaries, obtained from post-partum animals who had been treated with large doses of chlorpromazine for two weeks prior to sacrifice. Under such circumstances large amounts of prolactin, of the order of

TABLE II. Neutralization of prolactin activity in human plasma with anti-ovine prolactin

Patient and sex	Diagnosis	Prolactin (mU/ml)	Growth Hormone (ng/ml)	Prolactin after incubation with anti-ovine prolactin
B.J. (f)	galactorrhea: chromophobe adenoma	3.9 ± 1.0[a]	0.3	undetectable[b]
E.F. (f)	galactorrhea: hypothalamic glioma	3.6 ± 0.7	0.8	undetectable
M.O. (f)	galactorrhea: chromophobe adenoma	3.5 ± 1.0	0.3	undetectable
L.J. (m)	galactorrhea: possible estrogen withdrawal	2.2 ± 0.9	1.3	undetectable
A.C. (f)	galactorrhea: idiopathic	2.1 ± 0.4	0.6	undetectable
J.W. (f)	galactorrhea: idiopathic	0.5	1.2	undetectable
H.L. (f)	post-partum 3 days	10.8 ± 3.1	1.0	undetectable
E.R. (f)	post-partum 2 days	4.6 ± 1.3	0.8	undetectable
L.F. (f)	post-partum 3 days	4.0 ± 0.5	0.6	undetectable
G.W. (f)	post-partum 2 days	3.4 ± 0.8	0.3	undetectable
C.P. (f)	post-partum 4 days	2.8 ± 1.2	0.5	undetectable
M.S. (f)	post-partum 3 days	1.1 ± 0.3	1.6	undetectable

[a]SEM.

[b]Less than 0.4 mU/ml.

several hundred mg/ml, with growth hormone less than 1/10 this amount, have been found in the incubation media. This material has been iodinated and then purified by starch gel electrophoresis. Such assay systems show varying degrees of sensitivity for baboon, human and ovine prolactin. We have been able to measure prolactin by this technique in a number of human plasma samples, but wish to defer presentation of these data until we have had a better opportunity to compare the results of our bioassay and immunoassay measurements.

In summary, the study we have done so far indicates that human prolactin exists as a separate molecule in human plasma and can be measured without preliminary extraction by a sensitive bioassay. The mechanisms governing its release appear to be quite different from those controlling growth hormone. The use of chlorpromazine stimulation and L-dopa suppression afford valuable methods for testing pituitary function.

REFERENCES

1. Elias, J. J., Science 126:842, 1957.
2. Topper, Y. J., Trans N Y Acad Sci 30:869, 1968.
3. Kleinberg, D. L., and A. G. Frantz, Program 51st Meeting Endocrine Society, New York, New York, Abstract No. 32, 1969.
4. Frantz, A. G., and D. L. Kleinberg, Science 170:745, 1970.
5. Kleinberg, D. L., and A. G. Frantz, J Clin Invest 50:1557, 1971.
6. Frantz, A. G., and M. T. Rabkin, New Eng J Med 271:1375, 1964.
7. Kleinberg, D. L., G. L. Noel, and A. G. Frantz, J Clin Endocrinol 33:873, 1971.
8. Herbert, D. L., and T. Hayashida, Science 169:378, 1970.

36. Measurement of Prolactin in Human Serum

William H. Daughaday, Joseph E. Loewenstein, Laurence S. Jacobs, William B. Malarkey, and Ida K. Mariz

Until recently our understanding of physiologic and pathologic secretion of prolactin in man has been rudimentary because of the absence of suitable methods for measurement in biologic fluids. The pigeon crop sac method of assay, which proved so valuable in the study of animal pituitary prolactins, is insufficiently sensitive to detect prolactin in human serum and lacks specificity because it reacts to human growth hormone.

Within the last two years the situation has changed greatly. As you have heard from Dr. Frantz, very satisfactory bioassays for human prolactin are available using explants from mouse mammary glands (1-3). An enzymatic endpoint for this assay which provides improved quantitation is discussed later. These methods are sufficiently sensitive to detect increased levels of prolactin in physiologic and pathologic states.

It is only within the past year that radioimmunoassays for human prolactin have been developed which have great promise for the future. We can certainly anticipate a rapid expansion of our knowledge with the use of these new research tools.

BIOASSAY OF PROLACTIN

The possible use of explants of mammary glands as test objects for the bioassay of prolactin was suggested over a decade ago by Prop (4), but it is only since the painstaking studies of Topper and his group (5) provided the basic understanding of the hormonal induction of lactation in vitro that truly effective in vitro assays have become a reality. Frantz and Kleinberg (1) have used the morphologic

460

appearance of milk as an endpoint, while we have measured the induction of a component of the lactose synthetase enzyme system (2). Turkington (3) has measured ^{32}P incorporation into casein. The incubation conditions which we have adopted are essentially similar to those of Frantz, except that we have stopped our incubations at 48 rather than 96 hr. Explants are homogenized in tricine buffer and N-acetyl lactosamine synthetase activity determined by incubation with N-acetyl glucosamine and UDP-^{3}H-galactose. The enzymatic product is easily separated from the reactants by passage through an anion exchange resin. The radioactivity in the N-acetyl lactosamine is proportional to the time of the enzymatic reaction and the enzyme concentration. Prolactin added to the incubation medium increases N-acetyl lactosamine activity in a dose related fashion. The threshold of the response is between 0.01 and 0.1 mU/ml (Fig. 1).

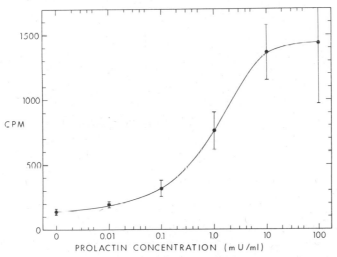

FIG. 1. Standard curve for prolactin bioassay: N-acetyl lactosamine synthetase activity expressed as cpm of the radioactive product vs ovine prolactin concentration of the culture medium (2). Reproduced by permission from J. B. Lippincott Company.

Human growth hormone induces enzymatic activity similar to that produced by prolactin (Fig. 2). Fortunately, this interference can be eliminated by the addition of specific antibodies raised against human growth hormone. The antiserum which we have selected for this purpose does not bind human prolactin or interfere with the measurement of ovine prolactin. We have determined that TSH, LH, FSH, ACTH, vasopressin, glucagon, and thyroxine do not affect the assay. The assay is, of course, responsive to the placental lactogen (HCS).

Prolactin poor plasma produces a nonspecific augmentation of the response

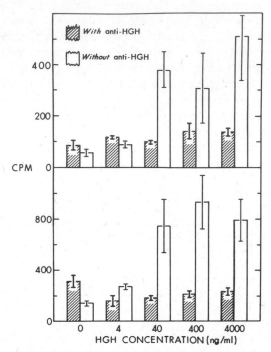

FIG. 2. Effect of different concentrations of HGH on N-acetyl lactosamine synthetase activity in mouse mammary gland explants in two separate experiments. The shaded columns are results obtained with specific anti-HGH added to the medium resulting in neutralization of the prolactin-like effect of HGH (2). Reproduced by permission from J. B. Lippincott Company.

(Fig. 3). For this reason, it is necessary to prepare the ovine prolactin standards in the same concentration of prolactin-free plasma as the specimen which is to be assayed.

The assay is not sufficiently sensitive to detect prolactin in plasma of normal men and nonpregnant women. We can detect prolactin in the expected physiologic condition of lactation. We have also detected increased prolactin in conditions associated with nonpuerperal lactation.

RADIOIMMUNOASSAY OF PROLACTIN

The development of a radioimmunoassay for human prolactin has seemed a hopeless task because the hormone has not yet been isolated from human pituitaries in reasonable purity. Despite these difficulties, workable radio-immunoassays for human prolactin now exist. Bryant et al. (6) have reported preliminary observations on an assay in which tissue culture media from human

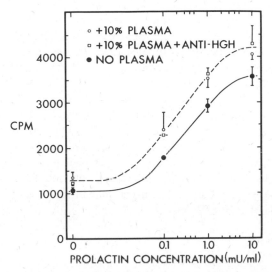

FIG. 3. Effect of plasma from a normal man on ovine prolactin standard curve. The elevation of the curve by the addition of human plasma is significant and reproducible and is not prevented by preincubation of plasma with anti-HGH (2). Reproduced by permission from J. B. Lippincott Company.

pituitary explants were used to induce antibodies and provide the antigen for a crude radioimmunoassay which appeared to detect a peptide associated with lactation which was not growth hormone.

A more successful radioimmunoassay for prolactin has been developed in Friesen's laboratory (7). They also obtained their prolactin from tissue culture medium incubated with primate pituitary tissue. They were able to purify their prolactin by affinity chromatography and eliminate significant growth hormone contamination. This material was used to raise antibodies. Either primate prolactin or ovine prolactin has been used for labeling. The information which has recently been presented is convincing that this radioimmunoassay is measuring human prolactin with little or no interference from growth hormone or other hormonal peptides.

We wished to avoid the difficult task of obtaining prolactin from tissue culture media and we were encouraged by the observation of Herbert and Hayashida (8) that antisera to ovine prolactin cross-reacted with primate lactotrophic cells when examined by immunofluorescent methods. This possibility was further strengthened by the observation of Midgley (9) that serum from post partum women was capable to some extent of displacing ovine prolactin from its antibody. However, when we attempted to repeat this observation with an immunoassay system consisting of ovine prolactin (labeled) and ovine prolactin antibody, displacement was insufficient for assay purposes.

For this reason we have shifted to a mixed heterologous system for assaying human prolactin. Midgley (10) has recently emphasized the principle that if an antiserum raised against a hormone of one species is capable of binding a hormone of a second species, the hormone specific binding site involved may be shared with the hormone of yet another species. With such a mixed heterologous system, he has been able to measure LH in a great variety of animals, an impossibility with any one simple immunoassay. While the concentration of antibody required for a mixed radioimmunoassay is usually higher than for a simple homologous radioimmunoassay, the sensitivity is often very good.

In our human prolactin assay (L. Jacobs, I. Mariz, and W. H. Daughaday, submitted for publication) we have employed labeled porcine prolactin and anti-ovine prolactin antiserum. Because of personal preference, a double-antibody system has been used for separation of free from bound antigen. Displacement curves for four prolactin-rich human sera and for ovine prolactin are given in Fig. 4. All the human sera gave parallel displacement curves which

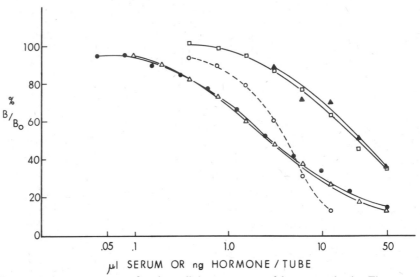

FIG. 4. Displacement curves for the radioimmunoassay of human prolactin. The curves obtained with dilutions of prolactin-rich human sera are shown in solid lines. The solid line connecting the black dots represents the curve of the serum subsequently used for prolactin standardization. The curve described by the dashed line was obtained with different concentrations of ovine prolactin. (Jacobs, Mariz, and Daughaday, unpublished data.)

were somewhat flatter than for ovine prolactin but still very satisfactory for assay purposes. The slope of the curves has actually been an advantage for us because of the extreme range of concentration of prolactin which we encounter in human sera under various circumstances. The differences in slope make it impossible for us to use ovine prolactin for standards in radioimmunoassays and we have resorted to the use of prolactin-rich serum for our standards. Our reference serum (kindly supplied by Drs. Robert Bates and Griff Ross of the National Institutes of Health) was obtained from a lactating man with a pituitary tumor. Dr. Bates has bioassayed this serum and found a potency of about 60 mIU/ml. We have found comparable biological activity in our mouse mammary gland assay. If we assume a biological activity of purified human prolactin of 30 IU/mg, our reference serum contains about 2 ng human prolactin/ml. To avoid later confusion we have reported our results in terms of microliter equivalents (μlEq).

The assay appears to have excellent specificity. No significant cross-reaction was observed with placental lactogen (HCS) or LH (Fig. 5). Very slight cross-reactivity was observed with HCG (potency ratio of 0.000016) and only slightly higher cross-reactivity with human growth hormone (potency ratio of 0.00023). It is impossible for us to determine whether this slight degree of cross-reactivity is specific or due to hormonal contamination with human prolactin.

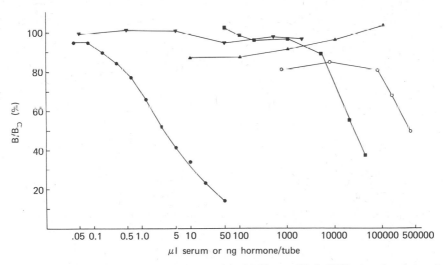

FIG. 5. Displacement curves obtained with highly purified HGH (■–■), placental somatomammotropin (▲–▲) and HLH (▼–▼). Displacement by prolactin-rich serum is shown on the left (●–●). (Jacobs, Mariz, and Daughaday, unpublished data.)

The sensitivity of our assay appears to be sufficient to detect prolactin in some, but not all, sera from normal children and men (Fig. 6). Sera from women obtained at random contained more prolactin. Substantially larger amounts of prolactin were detected in sera from women in late pregnancy and lactation. Patients with nonpuerperal lactation associated with pituitary tumors have high levels of serum prolactin. The concentration of prolactin in the sera of one of these patients was in excess of 1000 μlEq or more than 2000 ng/ml. This is a truly massive amount of prolactin compared to the usual concentration of peptide hormone in serum.

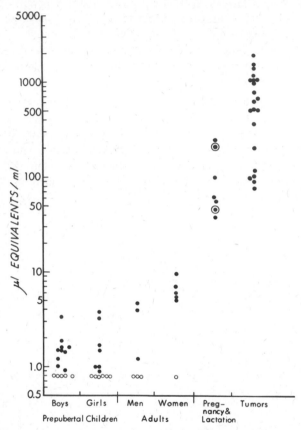

FIG. 6. Levels of prolactin determined by radioimmunoassay in human serum. The sera labeled "tumors" were obtained from 5 patients with pituitary tumors and nonpuerperal lactation without acromegaly. The open circles = less than; encircled dots = third trimester pregnancy. (Jacobs, Mariz, and Daughaday, unpublished data).

Our major interest in the development of assays for prolactin has been to study its secretion by human pituitary tumors. Our experience thus far has established that prolactin hypersecretion is much more common than previously suspected. Certainly the presence or absence of nonpuerperal lactation is not an accurate indication of prolactin secretion.

We have studied sera from 13 patients with active acromegaly and two children with gigantism. Of this group there were four women with nonpuerperal lactation (Fig. 7). All had serum prolactin levels greater than 25 μlEq/ml. Of the nine remaining acromegalics, all had levels less than 20 μlEq/ml and six of the

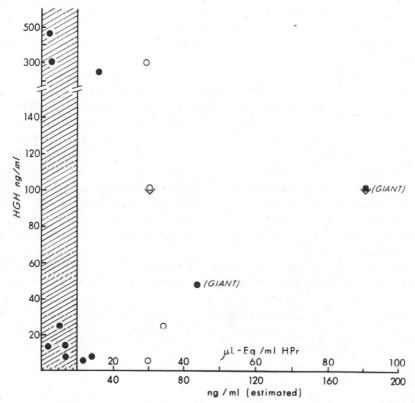

FIG. 7. Correlation between GH and prolactin contrations in the sera of patients with active acromegaly. The open circles represent female acromegalics with nonpuerperal lactation. v = greater than. The shaded area represents our tentative normal range for serum prolactin concentrations (Daughaday, unpublished data).

nine were within the normal range. Both children with gigantism had marked elevation of both hormones. There did not seem to be any correlation between serum growth hormone concentration and prolactin concentration. Two of our most severely affected acromegalic patients had serum prolactin concentrations which were normal. This experience with human growth hormone secreting tumors differs from the experimental pituitary tumors of rats, nearly all of which secrete large amounts of prolactin. These clinical observations are consistent with the well-established morphologic evidence that growth hormone and prolactin are secreted by separate cells. The mammosomatotropic tumors of rats probably arise from a less differentiated precursor cell to both types of secretory cells.

We have studied five patients with nonpuerperal lactation and pituitary tumors unassociated with acromegaly. Of this group all have had elevated serum prolactin. Growth hormone concentrations were usually normal or subnormal. When the 24-hr profile of serum prolactin was monitored by frequent sampling we observed in one case that prolactin levels were highly variable. Glucose administration did not affect prolactin concentrations and arginine administration has caused inconsistent changes.

Of greater interest is the effect of levodopa (L-dopa). This agent is believed to exert its biologic effects by intracellular conversion to dopamine. There is considerable experimental evidence showing that dopamine can affect prolactin secretion in two ways. Dopamine, epinephrine, and norepinephrine are all capable of directly inhibiting the secretion of prolactin by rat pituitary tissue in vitro (11-13). This direct effect may not be predominant in vivo because dopamine also acts on the hypothalamus to increase the secretion of prolactin inhibiting factor. This conclusion is supported most elegantly by observations in Porter's laboratory where dopamine has either been introduced into the third ventricle or into the pituitary by way of the portal vessels (14). The results of such experiments strongly suggest that the critical action of dopamine is on the hypothalamus.

We have given a single oral dose of 0.5 g of L-dopa to five patients with nonpuerperal lactation four of whom had hyperprolactinemia. Three of these patients had pituitary tumors. In each case a profound lowering of serum prolactin occurred; in four patients a rise in serum GH occurred (Fig. 8). The

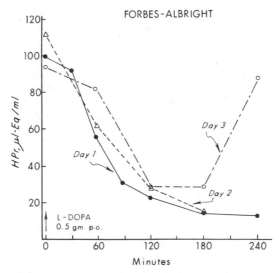

FIG. 8. Changes in serum prolactin in a case of pituitary tumor and lactation before and after the administration of L-dopa on three successive days. (Malarkey, Jacobs, and Daughaday, unpublished data).

nadir was reached after 2 to 4 hr. When the same dose of L-dopa was given four times a day for three days, there was no change in the basal serum prolactin levels in the morning 6 to 8 hr after the last dose of L-dopa and the inhibitory effect following a single dose of 0.5 g remained unimpaired.

We have given L-dopa to five normal women. In three there was measurable prolactin in the basal state and in each case the level of serum prolactin fell markedly or became undetectable.

One patient with pituitary tumor and nonpuerperal lactation received L-dopa in a daily dose of from 0.5 to 3.0 g for 6 weeks. There was no change in the basal level of serum prolactin after this prolonged administration.

In interpreting the responses of serum prolactin to L-dopa, two major possibilities suggest themselves. If we make the assumption that L-dopa acts primarily by increasing hypothalamic dopamine and stimulating release of the prolactin inhibiting factor as suggested by the Dallas group, we must conclude that the patients with pituitary tumors did not react in any way differently from those patients with functional hyperprolactinemia. From this we must conclude that even the tumors do not behave as if they are autonomous and that the pituitary hypersecretory state is dependent on abnormal hypothalamic control. A considerable body of evidence has been presented by us and others that hypothalamic control of GH secretion persists in many patients with acromegaly (15, 16).

The other possible interpretation of our data is that L-dopa might be acting directly on the prolactin secreting cells either directly or by conversion to dopamine. At the present time there is no conclusive way to resolve these two possibilities.

ACKNOWLEDGMENTS

Supported by research grant AM05105, training grant AM05027 and special fellowship grant 5F03 AM48051 from the National Institute of Arthritis and Metabolic Diseases, National Institutes of Health, Bethesda, Maryland. Clinical studies were done on the Clinical Research Center, supported by RR00036, Division of Research Resources, General Clinical Research Centers Branch, National Institutes of Health, Bethesda, Maryland.

REFERENCES

1. Frantz, A. G., and D. L. Kleinberg, Science 170:745, 1970.
2. Loewenstein, J. E., I. K. Mariz, G. T. Peake, and W. H. Daughday, J. Clin Endocrinol, in press, 1971.
3. Turkington, R. W., Program of the 63rd Annual Meeting, Amer Soc Clin Invest, 1971, p. 94a.
4. Prop, F. J. A., Nature 184:379, 1959.

5. Topper, Y. S., Recent Prog in Hormone Res, 26:287, 1970.

6. Bryant, G. D., T. M. Siler, L. L. Morgenstern, B. Webster, and F. C. Greenwood, Excerpta Medica, Internat Cong Sr 236:5, 1971.

7. Guyda, H., P. Hwang, and H. Friesen, Program of the 63rd Annual Meeting, Amer Soc Clin Invest, 1971, p. 41a.

8. Herbert, D. C., and T. Hayshida, Science 169:378, 1970.

9. Midgley, A. R., Presented at the NIH Workshop Conference on Prolactin, Bethesda, Maryland, January 11-12, 1971.

10. Midgley, A. R., G. D. Niswender, V. L. Gay, and L. E. Reichert, Recent Progr in Hormone Res, in press, 1971.

11. MacLeod, R. M., Endocrinology 85:916, 1969.

12. Birge, C. A., L S. Jacobs, C. T. Hammer, and W. H. Daughaday, Endocrinology 86:120, 1970.

13. Koch, Y., K. H. Lu, and J. Meites, Endocrinology 87:673, 1970.

14. Kamberi, I. A., R. S. Mical, and J. C. Porter, Experientia 26:1150, 1970.

15. Cryer, P. E., and W. H. Daughaday, J Clin Endocrinol 29:386, 1969.

16. Lawrence, A. M., I. D. Goldfine, L. Kirsteins, J Clin Endocrinol 31:239, 1970.

37. Homologous Radioimmunoassay for Human Prolactin: Its Development and Results Obtained in Plasma

F. C. Greenwood, T. M. Siler, and G. D. Bryant

We have detailed in a forthcoming paper (1) the use of a human prolactin sample (Pasteel HP) and a rabbit anti-Pasteel HP serum in the development of a radioimmunoassay for the material in plasma. The assay is insensitive to HGH and can measure human prolactin in normal male plasma but precision is less than ideal. Like ovine prolactin the human hormone responds to stress stimuli but rarely to insulin and increases acutely to suckling of the breast and to certain phenothiazines (2). In a patient with galactorrhea both insulin and oral glucose caused marked rises in plasma prolactin. A response to oral glucose was obtained after surgical hypophysectomy. Oral glucose tests in normal subjects, in the absence of stress, did not change prolactin levels. A modest release of prolactin after oxytocin, like a massive release after iv hypertonic saline, in a galactorrhea patient were ascribed to nonspecific stress. A preliminary attempt to correlate an in vitro biological assay with the radioimmunoassay showed an 8/10 agreement on rankings (3).

Sufficient material from tissue culture of human fetal adenohypophyses and from adult pituitary tumors has been accumulated for routine radioiodinations, for the production of better antisera and for preliminary sequence data (4). This work confirmed the pattern of release of human prolactin and other peptide hormones in long term culture shown by Pasteels (5).

REFERENCES

1. Bryant, G. D., T. M. Siler, F. C. Greenwood, J. L. Pasteels, C. Robyn, and P. O. Hubinont, Radioimmunoassay of a Human Pituitary Prolactin in Plasma, Hormones 2:139, 1971.

2. Bryant, G. D., T. M. Siler, L. L. Morgenstern, B. Webster, and F. C. Greenwood, Excerpta Medica Intern Congr Series 236, Abstract 8, 1971.

3. Bryant, G. D., and F. C. Greenwood, in G. E. W. Wolstenholme, and J. Knight (Eds.), Lactogenic Hormones, Ciba Found Coll Endocrn, in press, 1971.

4. Siler, T. M., L. L. Morgenstern, and F. C. Greenwood, in G. E. W. Wolstenholme, and J. Knight (Eds.), Lactogenic Hormones, Ciba Found Coll Endocrn, in press, 1971.

5. Pasteels, J. L., Mémoire de l'Academie Royale de Médicine de Belgique, 11e Series in-8°-Tome VII, 1, 1968.

38.   Problems in the Immunologic Detection of Human Prolactin

John B. Josimovich, Louise Boccella, and Monte J. Levitt

Recent studies in our laboratory (1) demonstrated the presence of a lactogenic antigen in the sera of postpartum and certain galactorrheic patients. The radioimmunoassay (RIA) system used consisted of: trace labeled human chorionic somatomammotropin, ^{131}I-HCS; a standard of fully reduced and alkylated carbamidomethyl-HCS, (CAM)$_4$-HCS; and rabbit anti-serum to the latter, AS/(CAM)$_4$-HCS. The ability of our antiserum to inhibit the pigeon crop sac stimulating activity of postpartum plasma extracts, along with the finding of little or no detectable HCS or growth hormone in the test sera, led us to postulate that the detected antigen was pituitary prolactin. Other investigators have recently presented evidence in support of the existence of this hormone (2-4).

Certain questions remained regarding the character of the prolactin-like antigen measured in our RIA system. Of concern was the possibility that the technique of separation of free from bound trace might introduce an error comparable to that reported by Bryant and Greenwood (5) with goat prolactin. This group, in pursuing this question further (6), claimed that certain radioactive trace separation techniques, such as dextran-coated charcoal, measure aggregates of prolactin. In the studies described here, we have compared the results using dextran charcoal (DC) with double antibody (DA) techniques, and have investigated the extent to which molecular aggregates might influence our RIA.

MATERIALS AND METHODS

ANTIGENS

HCS, 95% electrophoretically pure,[1] was employed as an antigen standard and as starting material for the production of other antigens. Completely reduced and carbamidomethylated HCS,[2] (CAM)$_4$-HCS, was prepared by treatment of HCS with β-mercaptoethanol and iodoacetamide, as described for human growth hormone (7). Half-reduced and carbamidomethylated HCS, (CAM)$_2$-HCS, was prepared by treatment of HCS with dithiothreitol and iodoacetamide (8). A high molecular weight, aggregated form of HCS, [HCS-U]$_{agg}$, was prepared by treatment of HCS with 8M urea for 15 min (7). All antigens were characterized by Sephadex chromatography with ammonium bicarbonate buffer (7) using either absorbancy at 280 mμ for cold antigens or radioactivity for ^{131}I-labeled trace antigens to measure elution volumes.

RADIOIODINATION

Antigens were labeled with ^{131}I by the modified Hunter and Greenwood procedure as described previously (9). Estimation of the amount of intact labeled antigen in the chromatographic fraction used as trace was made by measuring the percent of the radioiodination mixture which remained at the origin after paper electrophoresis (9). For the studies comparing the binding affinity of radiolabeled HCS and a high molecular weight aggregate of (CAM)$_4$-HCS, the previously described fraction eluted with barbital buffer from a cellulose column (9) was used for the former. A void volume fraction eluted from a Sephadex G-100 column with barbital buffer was used in studies of the aggregated (CAM)$_4$-HCS.

ANTISERUM

Rabbit antiserum prepared (9) against (CAM)$_4$-HCS was of a titer which permitted assays with a final incubation dilution of 1 : 10,000 to 1 : 20,000.

IMMUNOASSAYS

For DC assays, incubation of antigen standards, ^{131}I-labeled antigen and rabbit AS/(CAM)$_4$-HCS was carried out as previously described (1, 9). DA assays were performed according to Midgely's technique (10), employing a sheep anti-rabbit gamma globulin serum[3] diluted 1 : 2. The cited technique was modified as follows: trace, unlabeled antigens and first antibody were incubated

---

[1]Kindly provided by Dr. Aaron Glick, Lederle Laboratories, Inc., Div. of American Cyanamid Co., Pearl River, N.Y., Lot no. 717340.

[2]Amino acid analyses of the conversion of half-cystine sulfur to CAM-S were generously provided by Dr. I. R. McManus and Mr. Jean-Paul Vergnes of the Department of Biochemistry, Faculty of Arts and Sciences.

[3]Purchased as anti-rabbit, gamma globulin from Antibodies, Inc., Davis, California.

2 days at 4 C. Additional incubation was carried out for 3 more days after adding the second antibody. The diluting buffer protein concentrations were restricted to those used in our laboratory for DC assays (9). Incubation with both antibodies precipitated 45 to 50% of trace; while omission of the first antibody produced precipitation of only 5 to 6% of the trace.

RESULTS

The presence of two molecular weight species of $(CAM)_2$-HCS, $(CAM)_4$-HCS, and HCS-U are shown by the double peaks of elution from Sephadex in Table I. Radioiodination of the latter two antigens confirmed this finding. The first peaks were eluted near the void volume, signifying high molecular weight aggregates ($_{agg}$). The later peaks exhibited elution behavior similar to that of HCS.

TABLE I. Evidence for low and high molecular weight forms of antigens determined by Sephadex chromatography. For unlabeled antigens, elution volume (V_e) is expressed as a ratio compared to the void volume (V_0) determined with Blue Dextran on 2.5 X 30 cm columns. Labeled materials were chromatographed on 1 X 27 cm columns.

	Sephadex Elution	
Substance	G-75 (V_e/V_0)	G-100 (V_e/V_0)
HCS	1.6	1.8
$(CAM)_2$-HCS	1.0, 1.5	
$(CAM)_4$-HCS		1.1, 1.8
HCS-U, freshly prepared	1.0, 1.6	
		Elution vol (ml)
^{131}I-HCS		13.5
^{131}I-$(CAM)_4$-HCS		10.0, 13.0
^{131}I-HCS-U, freshly prepared		10.5, 14.0
^{131}I-HCS-U, stored O C 1 to 3 wek		12.5
^{131}I		26.0

Table II shows that AS/$(CAM)_4$-HCS apparently bound ^{131}I-[$(CAM)_4$-HCS]$_{agg}$ to a slight extent (5 to 15%). Over one-half of the trace (50 to 70%) was capable of remaining at the origin in paper chromatographs. In contrast, the DA technique revealed 40 to 50% binding of the trace. Using ^{131}I-HCS as trace, there was little disparity between the binding to the antiserum in either DC or DA RIA's.

Investigation of the role that molecular aggregation might make on the

TABLE II. Comparison of apparent binding of radioiodinated HCS and [(CAM)₄-HCS]ₐgg to AS/(CAM)₄-HCS as determined by double anti-body (DA) or dextran charcoal (DC) separation of free from bound trace. The intact fraction was estimated from the material which remained at the origin after paper electrophoresis.

| | | Percent bound | |
Trace	Percent intact	DC	DA
^{131}I-HCS	90-95	50-75	40-50
^{131}I-[(CAM)₄-HCS]ₐgg	50-70	5-15	40-50

immunologic behavior of HCS-related proteins in the DC assay is given in Fig. 1 and Table III. The figure reveals a potent effect of HCS in competing with ^{131}I-HCS for AS/(CAM)₄-HCS; while [(CAM)₄-HCS]ₐgg is much less effective. The partially reduced and substituted protein, (CAM)₂-HCS, was identical in

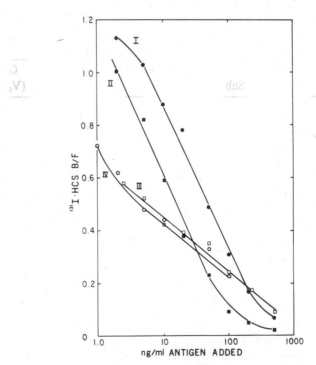

FIG. 1. Comparison of immunoreactivity in ^{131}I-HCS, rabbit AS/(CAM)₄-HCS dextran-charcoal system of HCS and three chemically related antigen standards: I. ●—● [(CAM)₄-HCS]ₐgg; II. ■—■ [(CAM)₄-HCS]ₐgg; III. ■—■ (CAM)₂-HCS; IV. ○—○ HCS.

TABLE III. Immunoreactivity of various antigens in dextran charcoal radio-immunoassay system containing trace ^{131}I-HCS and AS/(CAM)$_4$-HCS.

Antigen	Immunoreactivity parallel to
HCS	HCS
[(CAM)$_4$-HCS]$_{agg}$	[(CAM)$_4$-HCS]$_{agg}$
(CAM)$_2$-HCS	HCS
[(CAM)$_2$-HCS]$_{agg}$	[(CAM)$_4$-HCS]$_{agg}$
[HCS-U]$_{agg}$ (freshly prepared)	[(CAM)$_4$-HCS]$_{agg}$
[HCS-U]$_{agg}$ (after storage)	HCS

effectiveness with HCS in competing for trace; while its aggregate, [(CAM)$_2$-HCS]$_{agg}$, paralleled the activity of the aggregate of the fully reduced molecule, [(CAM)$_4$-HCS]$_{agg}$. Table III summarizes the findings of Fig. 1 and also shows that an aggregate of freshly prepared, urea-treated HCS behaved like [(CAM)$_4$-HCS]$_{agg}$. After storage at 0 C for 1 to 3 weeks, the peak elution volume after radioiodination (12.5 ml, Table I) was nearer that of radioiodinated HCS (13.5 ml) than that expected for the aggregate (10.5 ml). This presumed dissolution of the aggregate was paralleled by a shift in immunoreactivity to one indistinguishable from HCS (Table III).

DISCUSSION

The importance of ascertaining the degree of aggregation of antigen standards and radioiodinated traces in radioimmunoassays for human prolactin is evident from this study. As shown in Fig. 1, the immunologic behavior of an antigen can depend on its state of aggregation as well as on its chemical composition. Moreover, misleading estimates of immunologic potency can occur if an aggregated trace is used in the DC technique. This artifact may result from difficulty of passage of the free trace into dextran coated charcoal. This difficulty does not occur with the double antibody technique.

Our finding that the nonaggregated form of half-reduced and carbamido-methylated HCS, (CAM)$_2$-HCS, behaves immunologically like HCS is in accord with Breuer's results employing complement-fixation immunoassays (11).

Unlike the aggregates of (CAM)$_4$-HCS or (CAM)$_2$-HCS, the aggregates of HCS-U were unstable during storage below 0 C. After 1 to 3 weeks storage, (HCS-U)$_{agg}$ Sephadex elution behavior and immunologic behavior approached that of unmodified HCS.

As reported previously (1), the antigen detected in the sera of post-partum or galactorrheic women has immunological behavior parallel to that of [(CAM)$_4$-

HCS]$_{agg}$. Such behavior may be interpreted to mean that the native antigen is aggregated or that the aggregates in sera result from catabolism of the native, nonaggregated antigen. Further studies will be required to elucidate which of these hypotheses is correct. In either case, however, measurement of the serum antigen levels with AS/(CAM)$_4$-HCS may provide useful data of physiological import.

The importance of the physical state of HCS-like proteins on their activities is illustrated by experiments conducted by C. H. Li and co-workers and confirmed in our laboratory (12). These studies demonstrated that the somatotrophic effects of HCS injected intraperitoneally into hypophysectomized immature rats were significantly greater at pH 3.5 than at pH 8.0 where an entirely different degree of aggregation was found by chemical studies by Dr. Li's group. Whether or not the lactogenic activity of HCS or pituitary prolactin is altered by changes in aggregation is an important question yet to be resolved.

ACKNOWLEDGMENT

Supported by NIH grant HD-05570 and HD-00227.

REFERENCES

1. Josimovich, J. B., L. Boccella, and M. J. Levitt, J Clin Endocrinol 33:77, 1971.
2. Peake, G. T., D. W. McKeel, L. Jarett, and W. H. Daughaday, J Clin Endocrinol 29:1383, 1969.
3. Frantz, A. G., and D. L. Kleinberg, Science 170:745, 1970.
4. Guyda, H., P. Hwang, and H. Friesen, J Clin Endocrinol 32:120, 1971.
5. Bryant, G. D., and F. C. Greenwood, Biochem J 109:831, 1968.
6. Greenwood, F. C., personal communication, presented at NIH Workshop Conference on Prolactin, Bethesda, Md., January 1971.
7. Dixon, J. S., and C. H. Li, Science 154:785, 1966.
8. Bewley, T. A., J. S. Dixon, and C. H. Li, Biochem Biophys Acta 154:420, 1968.
9. Josimovich, J. B., B. Kosor, L. Boccella, D. H. Mintz, and D. L. Hutchinson, Obst Gyn 36:244, 1970.
10. Midgely, A. R., Jr., J Clin Endocrinol 79:10, 1966.
11. Breuer, C. B., Endocrinology 85:989, 1969.
12. Josimovich, J. B., B. Kosor, and L. Boccella, in S. L. Marcus, and C. C. Marcus (Eds.), Advances in Obstetrics and Gynecology, Vol. 2, Williams & Wilkins, Baltimore, in press, 1971.

DISCUSSION

S. A. BERSON. I think I would take a point of minor issue on your estimate of the half-life of prolactin from the initial rate of fall. It seems to me that you do not have a long enough period of observation and that you are measuring distribution of a slug into the circulation at that time rather than metabolic turnover. Would you reply to that?

F. C. GREENWOOD. The human prolactin data reminds me of our sheep data; the half-life of sheep prolactin is 19 min and yet we see much sharper falls in endogenous plasma hormone. I would have thought that with a circulation time of say 2 to 3 min, one should be able to get a not-less-than and a not-greater-than figure from observations over 20 to 30 min.

W. H. DAUGHADAY. I would like to comment on the use of your crude material as a standard. I think this would create a lot of trouble for the correlation of results obtained by different groups of investigators. It might be well, however, if the material is bioassayed until you have completely purified material available to be used as a basis of comparison. Incidentally, Dr. Bates has a fair amount of a serum in his freezer which we have used as a standard. This serum can be provided in sufficient amounts to be used for radioimmunoassay by interest groups.

A. R. MIDGLEY. I would like to comment regarding use of the terms heterogolous and homologous radioimmunoassay. We have found it useful to consider as heterologous a radioimmunoassay system in which the labeled hormone is of different species than that used for the immunization. From the standpoint of specificity, the interaction between antibody and labeled hormone is a critical aspect of an immunoassay. By mixing the species, one has a greater chance of restricting the reaction to something in common between these two hormone molecules. On the other hand, a homologous assay would involve labeled hormone from the same species as that used to generate the antisera. Thus, the assay we have used for measurement of human prolactin is a homologous ovine prolactin assay that uses labeled ovine prolactin and an antiserum against ovine prolactin. This assay happens to show a cross-reaction with human prolactin and, I suspect, with prolactins from many other species. I think it is useful to talk about a cross-reaction in an otherwise homologous assay. Dr. Greenwood commented that his antiserum against ovine prolactin did not work and I am not surprised. Many antisera do not work. I think it is useful, however, to look at mixed systems with the hope that the common regions might be more closely related to the biologically active site of a hormone.

F. C. GREENWOOD. I do not know the homogeneity of our best preparation. Our best preparation has two end groups. We have just assayed our preparation and it gave about 200 ng/ml equivalent of the prolactin standard. What would you call a system with labeled human prolactin and various other antisera for measuring human prolactin? Would that be a homoheteral system?

S. A. BERSON. Both homologous and heterologous immunoassays have been used virtually from the very beginning of the immunoassay era. The important reactions and comparison have nothing to do with the immunizing antigen and the labeled antigen. Irrespective of species one immunizes or species of labeled hormone one uses, it is absolutely essential to use the same standard and in the same form as exists in the unknown biologic sample that one is assaying. With the marked heterogeneity of peptide hormones that has recently been demonstrated for virtually every peptide hormone, I am not sure we will ever actually have the same form, but the important thing is that, since you are comparing the competitive inhibition against the binding of a labeled hormone to an antibody of an unknown versus a standard, they must be identical. The nature of immunizing and labeled hormones are irrelevant for the validity of immunoassay. The second point on which I would take issue with Dr. Midgley is that you never, in any way, actually measure biologically active sites in immunoassay. You are not measuring the hormone qua hormone, that is, its hormonal activity; you measure an immunologic reaction. There is plenty of evidence that the hormonally active site and the immunogenically and immunochemically reactive sites may really be quite distinct. One might have come to this conclusion by a prior reasoning; namely, that when a mutation takes place, it is more likely to survive and be passed on to succeeding generations when that mutation is not in a biologically active site. Since it is the species variation that makes for immunogenecity of a hormone from one species to another species, it is likely that the immunogenecity and the immunochemical reactivity involve biologically inactive sites.

A. R. MIDGLEY. I do not think there is any disagreement. I did not mean to imply that the biologically active sites were going to be identical to immunologically reactive sites. However, the demonstration that a hormone from one species is biologically active in a different species, suggests that hormones from the two species have something in common. The chances of reacting with such a region is enhanced when one goes across species and develops what we term a heterologous assay. We make no claim in being the first to use it. I recognize that you, in particular, have done this for a number of years. Further, I completely agree that the species and the physical chemical characteristics of the standard should be as close as possible to that of the unknown, in other words, they should behave in an identical fashion. The standard and the unknowns must behave in a parallel fashion throughout the entire inhibition curve, and one must be able to measure accurately the amount of standard added to serum "recovery". These considerations are often more important than bioassay to immunoassay ratios.

S. A. BERSON. In comparing hormones of different species and their biological effects, perhaps in some cases, one might get a better immunoreactive system for the closer biologic activity. I am not at all sure of that in any case and I can certainly give evidence for many cases where it is most distinctly not so. For example, many fish insulins have the identical potency (U/mg) as mammalian insulins do and yet in immunoreactive systems developed against the mammalian insulins, many of the antisera will react one thousand- to several thousand-fold weaker with the fish insulins than with the mammalian insulins. (New Engl J Med 270:1171, 1964).

A. R. MIDGLEY. In the case of FSH, it is very clear that antisera against ovine FSH, which are totally worthless for the measurement of ovine FSH, are very suitable when used with labeled FSH of species other than ovine, such as labeled HFSH. This combination, which we term heterologous, will give a specific assay for measuring ovine, rhesus, rat, and other species as well as human FSH. Conversely, antisera against HFSH can be used in combination with ovine FSH. The need for preabsorption with HCG, which is required when using labeled HFSH, is no longer necessary with a heterologous system.

J. L. VAITUKAITIS. In collaboration with Dr. Leo Reichert, we have looked at the cross-reactivity among the subunits of human, bovine, rat, and sheep LH. Using antiserum generated to the α subunit of HCG, we have found no cross-reactivity among the nonhuman LH subunits. On the other hand, the β subunits, which probably carry the biologically active site, do show cross-reactivity in the homologous β system comprised of an antiserum to the β subunits of HCG and ^{125}I-labeled β subunit.

S. A. BERSON. That supports my point that when you get mutations in biologically noncritical regions of the molecule, the mutation is likely to survive. There is a parallel situation in the case of insulin and proinsulin. There are marked differences in the connecting peptides among several mammalian species of insulins that are not reflected in similar quantitative differences in the insulin molecules themselves.

J. WEISZ. How can a hormone exert a precise, regulatory function on its target organ when it fluctuates as wildly as these two hormones do? How does the target organ reject the excess it does not need? How does it discriminate the "signal" from the "noise"? I know that my questions can at this point only be given speculative answers.

S. A. BERSON. We do not know that levels of prolactin achieved even under maximal stimulation are sufficiently high to saturate all receptor sites. Assuming for a moment that prolactin, like other peptide hormones, acts on membrane receptors that eventually stimulate the cyclase system. If you did an in vitro assay and continued to increase your level of peptide hormone, at a certain point you would find a leveling off at maximal activity that might well indicate saturation of all receptor sites. I do not know that it has been proven for any of these concentrations that you are beyond such saturation levels. Even if you were, we might just say that biologic systems are not necessarily absolutely perfect. In this connection, I would like to ask Dr. Frantz if he has looked at the effects of cyclic AMP or dibuturyl AMP on his mammary tissue?

A. G. FRANTZ. No, we have not.

J. B. JOSIMOVICH. It is apparent from the work of all the biologists that circulating steroid levels, particularly estrogen and possibly progesterone, determine whether or not prolactin has galactogenic activity. Thus, high levels of placental lactogen and perhaps pituitary prolactin during pregnancy do not make women lactate. It is circulating levels of steroids which determine whether the lactogenic hormone(s) will be permitted to act on the target organ, the mammary gland.

F. FUCHS. Have any of the four speakers assayed plasma from women during lactation after they have resumed menstruation? One of the problems that concerns us is the question of whether the inhibition of menstruation during lactation is in any way related to prolactin.

A. G. FRANTZ. We have assayed at least a dozen sera from patients with so-called idiopathic galactorrhea who had normal menses. In the majority of these patients lactation had its onset normally, post-partum, and then continued despite the resumption of menses. With very few exceptions, prolactin in these patients was undetectable by our method, that is to say, less than 0.42 mU/ml. This contrasts with the elevated prolactin levels generally found in patients whose galactorrhea was due to tumor or drugs, most of whom have been amenorrheic.

R. B. JAFFE. We have measured serum prolactin in several women following delivery. One patient, who was breast feeding, was studied for 300 days following delivery. During the time that she was breast feeding, levels of prolactin were high. They came down while she was weaning and were low during the post weaning period. Another woman who did not breast feed and did not receive steroids had prolactin levels which came down much more rapidly.

F. FUCHS. Some patients resume menstruation while they are lactating, and I was wondering if prolactin has been measured in such patients?

R. B. JAFFE. No.

J. FURTH. My experience has been with rat prolactin and growth hormone (GH), especially in relation to neoplasia. The situation is not identical with that in man. The following comments are perhaps applicable to studies of human prolactin. The prime role of prolactin is to build up mammary gland tissue in the obese mammary pad. This involves proliferation (DNA synthesis) without milk secretion, which begins late in pregnancy and is much increased during lactation when growth is suppressed. Milk secretion is greatly glucocorticoid-dependent.

Following adrenalectomy in rats bearing prolactin secreting mammary tumors, the mammary gland remains hyperplastic; milk production almost ceases. We have just heard that stress enhances prolactational activity.

The essays of Dr. Frantz and others, just reported, elegantly measure milk production but no growth of the mammary gland. Human mammary tumors very rarely lactate, but some 40% of them are prolactin responsive. A test is needed that determines the specific growth-promoting activity of P. The two hormones are separable in rodents and the body has separate homeostatic mechanisms for their regulation. However, there is some linkage between GH and prolactin. Prolonged administration of estrogen can induce prolactin (mammatropic) secreting tumors in almost 100% of rats and mice. Such tumors invariably produce both GH and prolactin in varying ratios. Biologically, circulating GH activity can be masked (e.g. by high levels of ACTH), and milk secretion can be exaggerated by glucocorticoids. There must be an intimate relation between GH and P secretion. I suppose that there are different molecules for these two hormones with overlapping subunits and that different control mechanisms exist for mammary gland differentiation, growth, and milk secretion.

For us, cancer-oriented workers, the basic problem remains: how to identify in vitro hormone-responsive mammary tumors and predict their responsiveness to supposed antagonists.

W. II. DAUGHADAY. It is interesting that when we give medroxyprogesterone to rats bearing Furth tumors, we increased growth hormone in plasma and in the tumor without similarly affecting prolactin. The pituitary tumor in our acromegalic patients are more differentiated and most secrete growth hormone without excess prolactin.

F. C. GREENWOOD. With regard to the release of prolactin from men and children despite the lack of prolactin cells, Professor Herlant at the recent Ciba meeting, felt there were cells producing prolactin not detected by current staining procedures.

Sexual Maturation

39. Gonadotropins in Relation to Sexual Maturity

Janet W. McArthur

That the immature pituitary is not absolutely quiescent as regards gonadotropic function has long been suggested by the positive bioassays for urinary gonadotropin occasionally obtained in children of prepubertal age with gonadal dysgenesis (1). The patently abnormal genetic milieu of the subjects has led some to reject the physiological implications of these findings. However, the force of the objections is diminished by observations such as those of Hamburger (2). Using the comparatively crude techniques of bioassay available in 1931, he observed an immediate large output of pituitary gonadotropin in a 12-year-old boy castrated for hypersexuality.

These necessarily anecdotal clinical observations are buttressed by a growing body of physiologic knowledge which points to a vibrant, if muted, interaction between the gonads and the hypothalamic-pituitary system. More refined biological assays specific for FSH and LH have yielded information consistent with such an interaction, in that they have enabled the presence of both gonadotropins to be demonstrated in the urine of normal prepubertal children (3, 4). However, the insensitivity of such assays and the difficulty of securing accurate 24-hr urine specimens have combined to impede quantitation. Thus, when the more sensitive method of radioimmunoassay rendered small samples of serum and plasma susceptible to testing for gonadotropin content, the pediatric age group was one of the first to which the new technique was applied. The success of pilot radioimmunoassays in small groups of children was sufficient to encourage the performance of comprehensive surveys, and also to stimulate the application of immunologic methods to the assay of gonadotropins in children's urine.

The present review of the literature on gonadotropins in relation to sexual maturity will be confined to an analysis of recent large-scale immunologic studies in normal children (Table I). Space limitations unfortunately preclude a recapitulation of the important studies (5-8) which demonstrated the feasibility of applying immunologic methods to the body fluids of children. Biological assay data will likewise be omitted, except as they pertain to the interpretation of immunologic findings. For a comprehensive summary of gonadotropin bioassay results in children, the review of Fitschen and Clayton (9) should be consulted.

TABLE I. Recent large-scale studies of gonadotropin levels in the blood and urine of children

Location	Institution	Investigators
Ann Arbor	University of Michigan	Lee et al. (15)
Baltimore	Johns Hopkins University	Johanson et al. (35) Raiti et al. (38) Raiti et al. (37) Baghdassarian et al. (36) Baghdassarian et al. (22) Blizzard et al. (39) Penny et al. (31)
Cleveland	Case Western Reserve University	Yen et al. (34) Yen and Vicic (32)
London	Hospital for Sick Children	Buckler and Clayton (23)
Philadelphia	University of Pennsylvania	Root et al. (40)
Rochester	University of Rochester	Schalch et al. (33)
San Francisco	University of California	Burr et al. (11) Sizonenko et al. (12)
Washington	National Institutes of Health	Kulin et al. (41) Rifkind et al. (21) Rifkind et al. (42)

It is the purpose of this paper to examine the state of our present knowledge with respect to the following questions:

1. At what chronological age and at what stage of sexual maturation are FSH and LH first demonstrable in the body fluids of normal children?

2. At what chronologic age and stage of sexual maturation do FSH and LH begin to rise toward adult levels?

3. What is the subsequent time-course, once the increase in FSH and LH has begun?

4. How do the results of assays of circulating gonadotropins compare with those of excreted gonadotropins?

5. What is the temporal relationship between the changes in the levels of gonadotropins and sex steroids in children, and the increase in the weight of the sex organs?

The chronologic ages and stages of sexual maturation at which the mean levels of circulating FSH and LH are first significantly elevated in groups of children are summarized in Table II. The Tanner schemata (10) for staging the sexual maturation of the subjects, and various modifications thereof, were employed by the majority of investigators. One of the groups also related gonadotropin levels to bone age (11, 12) and to estimates of testicular volume (11). It is important to appreciate that all of the studies from which these data have been drawn are cross-sectional, rather than longitudinal, in character. The potentialities of the longitudinal design are exemplified by the classical bioassay studies of Catchpole and Greulich (13), and of Nathanson and his collaborators (14), to which further reference will be made subsequently. In certain respects, these data are not only unsurpassed but unequaled in the contemporary literature.

It is evident from Table II that the chronologic ages at which FSH and LH were first demonstrable varied widely. However, in the majority of instances assayable levels were detected in the youngest age group with which a given investigator began his series. There is almost universal agreement that immuno-reactive FSH and LH are both demonstrable in the circulation of sexually infantile children.

The chronologic age and the stage of sexual maturation at which the plasma concentrations of FSH and LH first significantly exceed prepubertal levels are shown in Table III. It can be seen that the mean chronologic ages at which FSH and LH begin to rise in girls are 9.8 and 10.9 years, respectively; the corresponding ages in boys are 11.5 and 12.0 years. Thus the rise toward adult levels of both hormones begins one to two years earlier in girls. Appreciable sexual maturation was noted by all investigators to have occurred by the time that the plasma FSH and LH concentrations had begun to increase. However, the degree of maturation varied considerably.

The subsequent time course of the blood FSH and LH levels varies somewhat from one study to another. A representative example, taken from the paper of Lee et al. (15), is depicted in Fig. 1. It can be seen that the concentrations of both FSH and LH tend to rise progressively over a period of approximately four years; thereafter, gradual stabilization occurs within the ranges characteristic of adult reproductive life. Postpubertal values for circulating FSH are approxi-mately twice those of prepubertal values in both sexes; postpubertal concentra-tions of LH are increased three- to fourfold, the increment being somewhat greater in girls than in boys. The pattern of rise in FSH and LH exhibits a striking parallelism in the two sexes. However, because of the earlier maturation of girls, discrepancies necessarily exist between the levels for mean chronologic

TABLE II. The chronologic age and stage of sexual maturation at which gonadotropins are first demonstrable in the circulation of children

Investigator	Total number of normal children studied		Age range studied (yr)		Chronologic age at which circulating gonadotropin first demonstrable (yr)		Developmental stage at which circulating gonadotropin first demonstrable	
	Boys	Girls	Boys	Girls	Boys	Girls	Boys	Girls
FSH								
Raiti et al. (38)	97		5-18		5-8		1	
Penny et al. (32)		89		2-18		2-4		1
Burr et al. (11)	106		5-16		12		1	
Sizonenko et al. (12)		129		5-16		10		2
Lee et al. (15)	111	198	1-20	1-20	1	1	1	1
Yen and Vicic (33)	92	82	8-14	8-14	8	8		
LH								
Schalch et al. (34)	61[a]		<10					
Yen et al. (35)	93	82	8-15	8-15	8	8		
Johanson et al. (36)	100	149	5-18	2-20	5-6	2-5	1	1
Burr et al. (11)	106		5-16		5		3	
Sizonenko et al. (12)		129		5-16		6		1
Lee et al. (15)	115	199	6 mo[b]–20	6 mo–20	1-2	1-2	1	1

[a] Sexes not distinguished.

[b] Children aged 6 mo listed as 1 yr of age.

TABLE III. The chronologic age and stage of sexual maturation at which gonadotropins in the circulation of children first exceed prepubertal
levels

Investigator	First significant FSH rise above prepubertal levels		First significant LH rise above prepubertal levels	
	C.A.[a] (yr)	Stage	C.A. (yr)	Stage
BOYS				
Johanson et al. (36)			9-10	2
Baghdassarian et al. (37)	9-10	2	9-10	2
Burr et al. (11)	10	2	12	3
Lee et al. (15)	13-14	5+	15-16	5
Yen et al. (35)			12	
Yen and Vicic (33)	12			
GIRLS				
Johanson et al. (36)			10-12	2
Penny et al. (32)	5-8	2	9-10	2
Sizonenko et al. (12)	10	2		
Lee et al. (15)	11-12	5	11-12	5
Yen et al. (35)			9	
Yen and Vicic (33)	10			

[a]Chronologic age.

age until both sexes have gained the adult plateau. The changes in FSH and LH
concentration accompanying the transition from late puberty to adulthood are
highly variable and reflect, in part, the limitations of cross-sectional studies.
Such limitations are especially apparent in the case of females. It is difficult to
obtain blood samples at precisely comparable phases of the cycle in groups of
regularly menstruating subjects, and in girls with irregular menses the difficulty
is compounded.

As stated at the outset, one of the attractions of radioimmunoassay to
investigators concerned with pituitary gonadotropin levels in children was the
applicability of this technique to small samples of plasma or serum, and the
deliverance it promised from the labor of securing accurate urine collections.
However, growing experience with plasma gonadotropin assays has prompted
efforts to adapt immunologic and radioimmunologic methods to the urine as the
assay substrate. Among the reasons for this development are: (1) assays of blood
samples yield random estimates not necessarily indicative of mean values over
time, whereas the collection of a 24-hr urine specimen achieves, in effect, an
integration of circulating levels; and (2) no plasma standard has as yet been

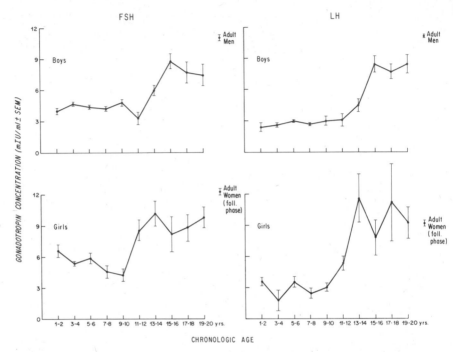

FIG. 1. The serum concentrations of FSH and LH as determined by radioimmunoassay in 198 boys and 111 girls aged 1 through 20 years analyzed at 2-year intervals, 234 adult men aged 29 to 82 years, and 240 adult women during the first 5 days of the menstrual cycle. The brackets indicate SEM. Adapted from Lee et al. (15) and reproduced by permission of the J Clin Endocrinol Metab.

developed, while standards prepared from pituitary tissue do not fulfill the desired condition of similarity. The Second International Reference Preparation (2nd IRP), obtained from human menopausal urine, presumably enjoys a closer immunologic resemblance to excreted than to circulating gonadotropin.

The optimal method for preparing urine for the immunoassay of gonadotropins has not yet been determined. The use of unprocessed urine has been found to yield an undesirably narrow range of variation in subjects known to excrete relatively small amounts of the hormones (16). Presumably, the need to utilize a greater volume of unprocessed urine than of a urine extract in order to achieve a significant response entails a concomitant increase in the concentration of nonspecific interfering substances. The use of dialyzed urine results in an increase in the apparent levels of FSH and LH as measured both by radioimmunoassay and bioassay (17). However, the FSH and LH excretion patterns of urinary dialysates and extracts exhibit as yet unexplained discrepancies (18). The tannic extraction method of Johnsen has been utilized by Sciarra and his collaborators (19) to obtain precipitates for immunoassay by the hemagglutination-inhibition technique of Wide and Gemzell. In normal boys and girls whose ages ranged from 5 to 10 years, LH was detected in every specimen tested. In magnitude, the levels resembled those obtained by workers using radioimmunoassay and increased with age in both sexes.

Ideally, the unknown and standard preparations employed in any given assay should be processed in an identical manner. The present standard, 2nd IRP, is obtained in bulk by the Albert procedure of kaolin-acetone precipitation, plus additional purification steps. When applied to urine samples, the Albert method yields extracts the FSH and LH potency of which exhibit a close immunologic and biologic correspondence (16, 20).

The gain in sensitivity over bioassay achieved by the radioimmunoassay of kaolin-acetone extracts of children's urine has been carefully documented by Rifkind et al. (42). By the use of the Klinefelter mouse uterine weight method, these workers had previously detected "total gonadotropic" activity at the 10 mouse uterine unit (MUU) level in 17% of 459 24-hr urine specimens collected from 44 normal children between the ages of 4 and 10 (21). Subsequently, radioimmunoassays were utilized to measure the FSH and LH content of aliquots taken from 153 of the 459 original extracts. FSH and LH immunoreactivity proved to be measurable in virtually every specimen, whether or not biological activity had originally been demonstrable. Small increases in the excretion of both hormones were observed during childhood. In both sexes, there was doubling of FSH excretion in the 7 to 8 year age group as compared with the 5 to 6 year group, whereas there was only a gradual rise in LH excretion. The LH excretion of children in the 9 to 10 year age group was significantly greater than that of 5 to 6 year old, and in boys it increased to higher levels and at a faster rate than in girls. There was a distinct increase in FSH excretion, but not in LH excretion, prior to and concomitant with the appearance of early signs of puberty.

The addition of organic solvents such as acetone or alcohol to urine without prior extraction with kaolin results in the formation of precipitates which are comparable to kaolin-acetone extracts with respect to FSH immuno and biopotency. However, the LH immunopotency is increased three- to fourfold (22). When immunoreactive LH was added to the urine of hypophysectomized subjects, kaolin extraction recovered less than 20% of the material, whereas direct precipitation achieved virtually 100% recovery. The molecular basis for the enhanced immunoreactivity of the precipitates has not yet been elucidated. It may be that immunologically reactive but biologically inactive LH moieties which are removed by kaolin extraction are conserved, or that organic solvent precipitation dissociates the LH molecule into subunits.

Since the values obtained by the radioimmunoassay of such precipitates

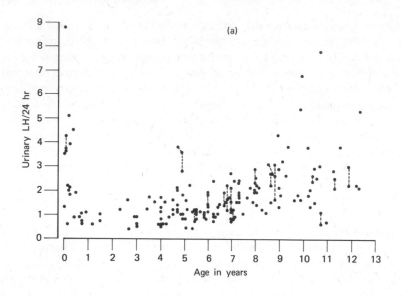

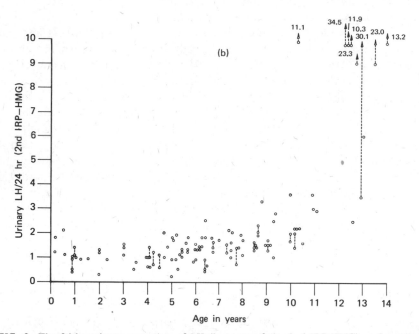

FIG. 2. The 24-hr urinary excretion of LH (in terms of the 2nd IRP-HMG) as determined by the radioimmunoassay of ethanol precipitates in: (a) 152 normal boys aged 3 days to 12½ years, and (b) 104 normal girls aged 3 months to 14 years. Dashed lines connect values for repeat determinations on the same children. Reproduced from Buckler and Clayton (23) by permission of the editor, Arch Dis Child.

appear to vary appropriately in sexually mature, menopausal, and hypophysectomized subjects, the LH immunopotency increment effected by organic solvent precipitation has commended this procedure to pediatric investigators. The majority of the published observations on the radioimmunoassay of direct precipitates of children's urine originate from the Johns Hopkins University group, which developed the technique. Since their findings are to be presented in extenso to this symposium, they will not be recapitulated here. Brief consideration will, instead, be given to the studies of Buckler and Clayton (23), who employed the ethanol precipitation method of Raiti and Blizzard (24) for the preparation of urine samples. High values for LH excretion were found in boys and, less clearly, in girls during the first six months of life (Fig 2a and b). Subsequently, there was a decline to low levels until the age of approximately 6 years. A gradual rise in LH excretion then began in both sexes and continued during the 3 to 4 years which preceded the onset of puberty, when a marked increase occurred. The source of the immunoreactivity observed during early infancy is uncertain. The Leydig cells of newborn males exhibit a hyperplasia attributed to stimulation with chorionic gonadotropin (CG). However, immunoreactive CG is demonstrable in infants for, at most, three weeks postpartum (25)

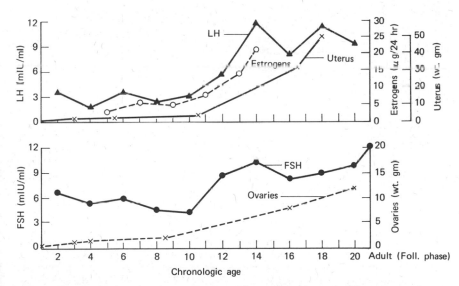

FIG. 3. Changes in the serum concentrations of gonadotropins and of the urinary estrogen excretion in normal girls, compared with the increase in the weight of the uterus and ovaries. The serum FSH and LH concentrations are those of Lee et al. (15). The urinary excretion of total estrogens, as determined by the Brown method, has been obtained by combining the data of Dewhurst (28) with those of Pennington and Dewhurst (29). The weights of the uterus and ovaries are taken from the autopsy findings of Wehefritz and Scammon, and of Roessle and Roulet, as combined by Tanner (10).

and the histologic changes in the testis regress after 4 to 6 weeks. It is conceivable that subunit dissociation is favored by the dilute character of the urine of infants, whose diet is liquid and whose renal concentrating mechanisms are immature.

It now remains to examine the temporal relationship between the changes in the levels of gonadotropins and sex steroids and the increase in weight of the sex organs in maturing adolescents. In Fig. 3 are shown the changes documented in normal girls. A rise in serum FSH can be seen to precede the inflection point marking an increased rate of ovarian growth; a rise in serum LH anticipates a significant trend toward higher levels of urinary estrogen. An increase in estrogen levels, in turn, is well underway before the rate of uterine growth exhibits acceleration.

Parallel changes in boys are depicted in Fig. 4. It is evident that rising FSH levels antedate appreciable increases in testicular weight. Serum LH begins to

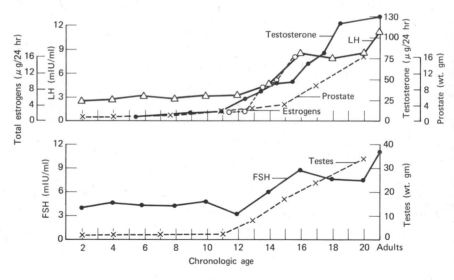

FIG. 4. Changes in the serum concentrations of gonadotropins and of urinary estrogen and testosterone excretion in normal boys, compared with the increase in prostate and testis weight. The serum FSH and LH concentrations are those of Lee et al. (15). The values for the urinary excretion of total estrogens are taken from Steeno et al. (26). The data for the urinary excretion of free testosterone and testosterone glucuronidate are those of Knorr (27). The prostate and testis weights are taken from the autopsy data of Wehefritz and Scammon, and of Roessle and Roulet, as combined by Tanner (10).

increase before urinary testosterone or estrogen levels rise significantly. The prostatic growth pattern exhibits a surprising degree of conformity with the inflection points in the curve for urinary testosterone excretion. Thus despite the paucity of the sex steroid excretion values and the vitiating effect of cross-sectional design upon all of the data, the latter are in fair accord with physiologic expectations.

In the introduction, reference was made to the physiologic interaction between the immature hypothalamic-pituitary system and the gonads, and to the difficulties attending the documentation of this virtually subliminal phenomenon. Clearly, the cross-sectional radioimmunoassay studies performed in recent years have significantly extended our knowledge of the pituitary component of the interaction. However, at least in females, gonadotropin secretion exhibits intermittency, if not periodicity, long before the menarche. Since no overt marker is available as a reference point for sampling during these years, cross-sectional studies cannot but conceal significant trends. The consequences of averaging data cross-sectionally according to chronologic age or stage of maturation can be visualized by considering the urinary gonadotropin results reported by Catchpole and Greulich (13). These workers utilized the mouse

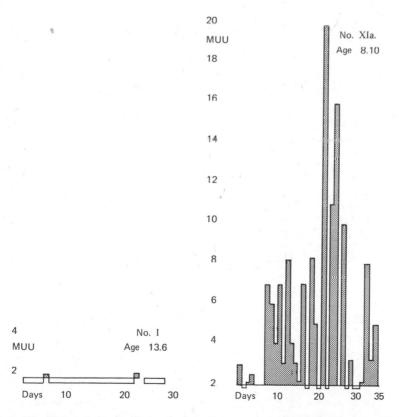

FIG. 5. The 24-hr urinary gonadotropin excretion, expressed in MUU, (a) over a 30-day period in a girl 13 years and 6 months of age, and (b) over a 35-day period in a girl 8 years and 10 months of age. Reproduced from Catchpole and Greulich (13) by permission of the J Clin Invest.

uterine weight method to assay serial 24-hr collections over 30-day periods in 12 subjects. One of these, a girl of 13 years and 6 months, showed little or no excretion over the entire month studied (Fig. 5a). On the other hand, a girl of 8 years and 10 months exhibited a surprisingly active pattern (Fig. 5b), and two months after the collections were completed began to menstruate. Repeat studies in the same subjects often showed a clearcut progression over a twelve months' period (Fig. 6a and b).

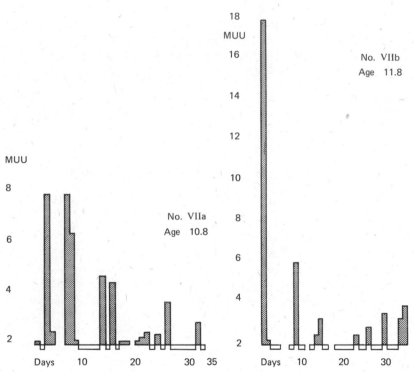

FIG. 6. The 24-hr urinary gonadotropin excretion, expressed in MUU, over a 35-day period in: (a) a girl 10 years and 8 months of age, and (b) the same girl when she was 11 years and 8 months of age. Reproduced from Catchpole and Greulich (13) by permission of the J Clin Invest.

The gonadal aspects of the interaction have been examined with the aid of longitudinal studies by Nathanson et al. (14). They employed the Allen-Doisy bioassay for measurement of urinary estrogens and 17-ketosteroid determinations as an index of urinary androgens in normal boys and girls. For brevity, only the results of the estrogen determinations in girls will be considered. In Fig. 7 is depicted a representative subject in their series. It can be seen that up to the age of 11 years and 4 months this child's estrogen excretion was very low. At 12

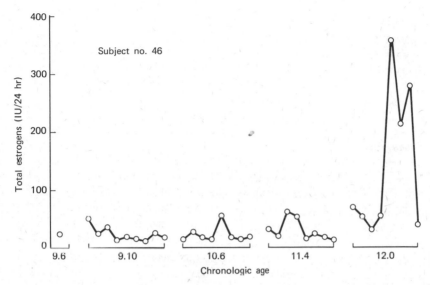

FIG. 7. The urinary excretion of total estrogens during four serial studies in one normal prepubertal girl. The chronologic age at which each series was begun is shown on the abscissa. Adapted from Nathanson et al. (14) and reproduced by permission of Endocrinology.

years of age she was still sexually infantile but exhibited a cyclic excretion which occasionally attained fairly high levels. Eight months later, she developed pubic hair and early breast changes, and at the age of 13 years and 6 months she menstruated for the first time. Cytologic studies by Sonek (31) show an increased proliferation of the vaginal epithelium in girls for approximately three to four years prior to the menarche, and phases of increased and decreased proliferation between the ages of 9 and 12 years. Had vaginal smears been made in Nathanson's subject it is possible that periodic changes in the maturation index might have been noted to accompany the measurements made when she was 10 years and 6 months of age, and perhaps even earlier.

If primitive techniques of biological assay can yield data as descriptive as these, how much more can immunoassays with their capacity to measure several variables in the same specimen be expected to provide! To execute longitudinal studies comprising the simultaneous assay of gonadotropins, sex steroids and, eventually, of hypothalamic releasing factors in individual samples will require strenuous effort. However, from such exertions a precise description of the interaction of the hypothalamic-pituitary system and the gonads of children can be expected ultimately to emerge.

ACKNOWLEDGMENT

This work was supported, in part, by grants from the Ford Foundation and from the Sprague Fund.

REFERENCES

1. Grossman, E. R., Pediatrics 25:298, 1960.
2. Hamburger, C., Ugeskrift f Laeger 93:27, 1931.
3. Brown, P. S., J Endocrinol 17:329, 1958.
4. McArthur, J. W., F. M. Ingersoll, and J. Worcester, J Clin Endocrinol 18:460, 1958.
5. Odell, W. D., G. T. Ross, and P. L. Rayford, J Clin Invest 46:248, 1967.
6. Faiman, C., and R. J. Ryan, J Clin Endocrinol 27:444, 1967.
7. Faiman, C., and R. J. Ryan, Proc Soc Exp Biol Med 125:1130, 1967.
8. Saxena, B. B., H. Demura, H. M. Gandy, and R. E. Peterson, J Clin Endocrinol 28:519, 1968.
9. Fitschen, W., and B. E. Clayton, Arch Dis Child 40:16, 1965.
10. Tanner, J. M., Growth at Adolescence, 2nd ed., Blackwell, Oxford, 1962.
11. Burr, I. M., P. C. Sizonenko, S. L. Kaplan, and M. M. Grumbach, Pediat Res 4:25, 1970.
12. Sizonenko, P. C., I. M. Burr, S. L. Kaplan, and M. M. Grumbach, Pediat Res 4:36, 1970.
13. Catchpole, H. R., and W. W. Greulich, J Clin Invest 22:799, 1943.
14. Nathanson, I. T., L. E. Towne, and J. C. Aub, Endocrinology 28:851, 1941.
15. Lee, P. A., A. R. Midgley, Jr., and R. B. Jaffe, J Clin Endocrinol 31:248, 1970.
16. Kulin, H. E., A. B. Rifkind, and G. T. Ross, J Clin Endocrinol 28:543, 1968.
17. Stevens, V. C., in E. Rosemberg (Ed.), Gonadotropins 1968, Geron-X, Inc., Los Altos, 1968, p. 283.
18. Stevens, V. C., J Clin Endocrinol 29:904, 1969.
19. Sciarra, N., U. Leone, and G. F. Pastorino, J Endocrinol 42:167, 1968.
20. Faiman, C., R. J. Ryan, and A. Albert, J Clin Endocrinol 28:1076, 1968.
21. Rifkind, A. B., H. E. Kulin, and G. T. Ross, J Clin Invest 46:1925, 1967.
22. Baghdassarian, A., S. Fisher, H. Guyda, A. Johanson, T. P. Foley, Jr., R. Penny, and R. M. Blizzard, Amer J Obst Gyn 108:1178, 1970.
23. Buckler, J. M. H., and B. E. Clayton, Arch Dis Child 45:478, 1970.
24. Raiti, S., and R. M. Blizzard, J Clin Endocrinol 28:1719, 1968.
25. Levy, J. M., C. Grunewald, F. Klein, G. Levy, and P. Dellenbach, Arch Franc Pediat 26:73, 1969.
26. Steeno, O., W. Heyns, H. Van Baelen, A. Van Herle, and P. de Moor, European J. Steroids 2:273, 1967.
27. Knorr, D., Acta Endocrinol 54:215, 1967.
28. Dewhurst, C. J., Gynaecological Disorders of Infants and Children, Davis, Philadelphia, 1963, p. 6.
29. Pennington, G. W., and C. J. Dewhurst, Arch Dis Child 44:629, 1969.
30. Sonek, M., Acta Cytol 11:41, 1967.
31. Penny, R., H. J. Guyda, A. Baghdassarian, A. J. Johanson, and R. M. Blizzard, J Clin Invest 49:1847, 1970.
32. Yen, S. S. C., and W. J. Vicic, Amer J Obst Gyn 106:134, 1970.
33. Schalch, D. S., A. F. Parlow, R. C. Boon, and S. Reichlin, J Clin Invest 47:665, 1968.
34. Yen, S. S. C., W. J. Vicic, and D. V. Kearchner, J Clin Endocrinol 29:382, 1969.
35. Johanson, A. J., H. Guyda, C. Light, C. J. Migeon, and R. M. Blizzard, J Pediatrics 74:416, 1969.

36. Baghdassarian, A., H. Guyda, A. Johanson, C. J. Migeon, and R. M. Blizzard, J Clin Endocrinol 31:428, 1970.

37. Raiti, S., A. Johanson, C. Light, C. J. Migeon, and R. M. Blizzard, Metabolism 18:234, 1969.

38. Raiti, S. M. B., C. Light, and R. M. Blizzard, J Clin Endocrinol 29:884, 1969.

39. Blizzard, R. M., A. Johanson, H. Guyda, A. Baghdassarian, S. Raiti, and C. J. Migeon, in R. P. Heald and W. Hung (Eds.), Adolescent Endocrinology, Butterworth's, London, 1970, p. 1.

40. Root, A. W., T. Moshang, Jr., A. M. Bongiovanni, and W. R. Eberlein, Pediat Res 4:175, 1970.

41. Kulin, H. E., A. B. Rifkind, G. T. Ross, and W. D. Odell, J Clin Endocrinol 27:1123, 1967.

42. Rifkind, A. B., H. E. Kulin, P. L. Rayford, C. M. Cargille, and G. T. Ross, J Clin Endocrinol 31:517, 1970.

40. Pituitary-Gonadal Interrelationships in Relation to Puberty

Robert M. Blizzard, Robert Penny, T. P. Foley, Jr., Alice Baghdassarian, A. Johanson, and S. S. C. Yen

In this manuscript our experience in evaluating pituitary gonadal interrelationships, as determined by assaying immunoreactive LH and FSH hormones in serum and urine, in prepubertal and pubertal children, is reviewed.

NORMAL PUBERTAL AND PREPUBERTAL CHILDREN

SERUM GONADOTROPINS IN ORIGINAL REPORTS

We and other investigators (1-8) reported progressively increasing FSH and LH concentrations in serum with progressing age. However, discrepancies exist concerning the ages at which FSH and LH concentrations initially increase, whether the rise occurs in girls before it does in boys, and the comparable levels between boys and girls. When the data of the four major reporting groups are reduced to the same bases and analyzed for similarities (Tables I and II; Figs. 1 and 2) the following becomes apparent.

1. In females a significant increase in mean serum FSH concentration ($p < .05$), as compared to the preceding age groups, was found by all groups at age 11 to 12 years. Three of four groups reported similar findings for LH (Table I).

2. In males the mean serum FSH and LH concentrations increased significantly at ages 11 to 12 years according to two groups (Cleveland and San Francisco). However, our group reported significant increases at 9 to 10 years

TABLE I. Serum gonadotropins in mIU/ml 2nd IRP-HMG follicular stimulating hormone (FSH)

FSH

Age	Ann Arbor (7)[a] Female Mean	SD	Male Mean	SD	Baltimore (1, 3, 8)[a] Female Mean	SD	Male Mean	SD	Cleveland (2, 4)[a] Female Mean	SD	Male Mean	SD	San Francisco (5, 6)[a] Female Mean	SD	Male Mean	SD
5-8	3.1	2.5	2.8	2.2	4.5	0.7	4.2	0.9	4.4	0.9	3.2	0.7	3.1	0.9	2.4	0.5
9-10	3.0	1.9	2.8	1.1	5.4b	1.3	5.4b	1.2	6.3	4.4	4.8b	1.0	3.8b	1.2	2.6	0.7
11-12	5.3b	3.4	3.0	1.4	7.5b	2.2	5.6	1.7	10.1b	6.2	6.9b	2.7	5.9b	2.2	3.5b	1.2
13-14	11.6b	10.2	4.1b	2.7	8.0	3.1	8.1b	2.5	9.5	5.6	9.4b	2.0	5.5		5.4b	1.8
15-16	8.0	4.0	8.0b	3.4	8.2	2.0	8.7	4.2							4.0b	1.4
17-18	11.0	7.0	7.8	1.9	8.6	2.4	9.2	3.8								
Adult													Range			
F[e]	12.3	6.1	11.0	4.6	8.3	0.6	7.4	2.2	12.5	2.1	9.1	1.8	3.1-5.8			
L[f]	6.7	3.4			6.9	0.8							3.6-4.5			

503

TABLE I. Cont'd

<table>
<thead>
<tr><th></th><th colspan="16">LH</th></tr>
</thead>
<tbody>
<tr><td>5-8</td><td>5.2</td><td>2.1</td><td>4.3</td><td>1.0</td><td>2.6</td><td>0.3</td><td>3.4</td><td>0.6</td><td>1.9</td><td>0.3</td><td>1.1</td><td>1.0</td><td>8.7</td><td>2.9</td><td>9.6</td><td>1.7</td></tr>
<tr><td>9-10</td><td>4.3</td><td>2.3</td><td>4.8[b]</td><td>1.1</td><td>4.0[b]</td><td>2.1</td><td>4.8[b]</td><td>1.2</td><td>2.5</td><td>1.3</td><td>0.74</td><td>1.0</td><td>8.1</td><td>2.5</td><td>9.8</td><td>1.8</td></tr>
<tr><td>11-12</td><td>8.6[b]</td><td>4.3</td><td>3.5[c]</td><td>1.4</td><td>8.7[b]</td><td>3.6</td><td>6.8[b]</td><td>1.9</td><td>6.6[b]</td><td>9.1</td><td>1.54[b]</td><td>1.1</td><td>9.1</td><td>3.3</td><td>10.6[b]</td><td>1.5</td></tr>
<tr><td>13-14</td><td>10.0</td><td>3.5</td><td>5.8[d]</td><td>2.7</td><td>8.8</td><td>4.4</td><td>9.4[b]</td><td>2.5</td><td>10.0</td><td>13.1</td><td>4.1[b]</td><td>2.5</td><td>10.7</td><td></td><td>10.9</td><td>1.8</td></tr>
<tr><td>15-16</td><td>8.0</td><td>4.8</td><td>8.4[b]</td><td>3.4</td><td>13.5[b]</td><td>6.8</td><td>9.0</td><td>2.1</td><td></td><td></td><td></td><td></td><td></td><td></td><td>12.5</td><td>1.4</td></tr>
<tr><td>17-18</td><td>8.8</td><td>2.2</td><td>7.6</td><td>2.6</td><td>15.3</td><td>8.5</td><td>14.1[b]</td><td>3.8</td><td></td><td></td><td></td><td></td><td></td><td></td><td></td><td></td></tr>
<tr><td>Adult</td><td></td><td></td><td></td><td></td><td></td><td></td><td></td><td></td><td></td><td></td><td></td><td></td><td colspan="2">Range</td><td></td><td></td></tr>
<tr><td>F[e]</td><td>9.2</td><td>4.7</td><td>11.1</td><td>4.6</td><td>12.8</td><td>2.0</td><td>10.9</td><td>3.8</td><td>13.6</td><td>1.1</td><td>13.1</td><td>1.1</td><td colspan="2">13.8-14.5</td><td></td><td></td></tr>
<tr><td>L[f]</td><td>7.7</td><td>6.7</td><td></td><td></td><td>11.6</td><td>2.6</td><td></td><td></td><td></td><td></td><td></td><td></td><td colspan="2">12.7-17.5</td><td></td><td></td></tr>
</tbody>
</table>

[a]References from which data was taken.

[b]$p < 0.05$ when compared to preceding group.

[c]This value is most likely coincidence since it is lower than the 5-8 or 9-10 age groups.

[d]$p < 0.05$ when compared to 9 to 10 age groups.

[e]F = Follicular phase.

[f]L = Luteal phase.

TABLE II. p values for male vs female mean gonadotropin differences

Age	Ann Arbor		Baltimore		Cleveland		San Francisco		Collaborative study			
									Baltimore		Cleveland	

FSH

Age	Ann Arbor	Baltimore	Cleveland	San Francisco	Collaborative study Baltimore	Collaborative study Cleveland
5-8	0.40 ♀ = ♂	0.10 ♀ = ♂	0.005 ♀ > ♂	0.005 ♀ > ♂	Not done	Not done
9-10	0.40 ♀ = ♂	♀ = ♂	0.10 ♀ > ♂	0.005 ♀ > ♂		
11-12	0.005 ♀ > ♂	0.01 ♀ > ♂	0.01 ♀ > ♂	0.005 ♀ > ♂		
13-14	0.005 ♀ > ♂	0.40 ♀ = ♂	♀ = ♂	♀ = ♂		
15-16	0.40 ♀ = ♂	0.40 ♀ = ♂	no data	no data		
17-18	0.10 ♀ = ♂	0.30 ♀ = ♂	no data	no data		

LH

Age	Ann Arbor	Baltimore	Cleveland	San Francisco	Collaborative study Baltimore	Collaborative study Cleveland
5-8	0.01 ♀ > ♂	0.005 ♂ > ♀	0.025 ♀ > ♂	0.05 ♂ > ♀	— ♀ = ♂	— ♀ = ♂
9-10	0.20 ♀ = ♂	0.01 ♂ > ♀	0.005 ♀ > ♂	0.01 ♂ > ♀	— ♀ = ♂	— ♀ = ♂
11-12	0.005 ♀ > ♂	0.05 ♀ > ♂	0.025 ♀ > ♂	0.05 ♂ > ♀	— ♀ = ♂	0.025 ♀ > ♂
13-14	0.005 ♀ > ♂	0.30 ♀ = ♂	0.025 ♀ > ♂	♀ = ♂	0.05 ♀ > ♂	0.005 ♀ > ♂
15-16	0.40 ♀ = ♂	0.025 ♀ > ♂	no data	no data	— ♀ = ♂	0.05 ♀ > ♂
17-18	0.20 ♀ = ♂	0.30 ♀ = ♂	no data	no data	no data	no data

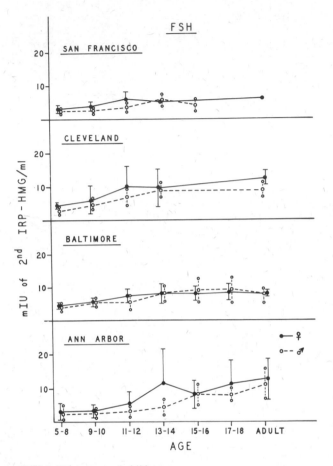

FIG.1 Serum FSH (±SD) in normal children.

and the Ann Arbor investigators reported a significant increase at 13 to 14 years of age (Table I).

3. All four groups reported that mean FSH concentrations, at 11 to 12 years of age, were significantly greater in females than in males. Three of the four groups (San Francisco excluded) also reported significantly higher LH values for females (Table II).

4. The San Francisco group reported markedly less increase in serum LH concentrations from childhood to adulthood than did the other groups. This probably accounts for the discrepant results for serum LH concentrations, when LH results are compared between groups. Although all four groups used the same FSH antiserum, only three groups (excluding San Francisco) used the same LH antiserum. Cargille et al. (9) reported that different antisera can account for discrepant results.

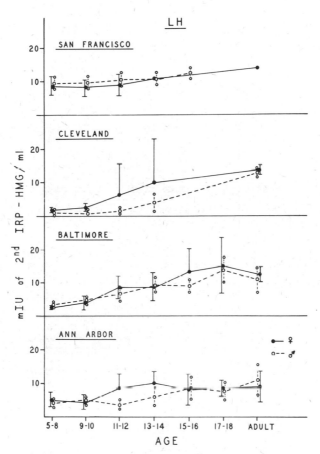

FIG. 2. Serum LH (±SD) in normal children.

SERUM LH IN COLLABORATIVE STUDY

To resolve some of the discrepancies reported, the serums of 153 (80 males and 73 females) randomly selected children were assayed for LH in the Baltimore and Cleveland laboratories (Table III). The role that technique may play in producing discrepant results is suggested by finding in the collaborative study that mean serum LH levels in the males were significantly higher at age 9 to 10 years, as compared to the preceding age group, in the Baltimore laboratory but not in the Cleveland laboratory. Similarly, mean serum LH levels were significantly higher in females than males at 11 to 12 years of age in one laboratory and not the other (Tables II and III). Differences in absolute quantitative values obtained by the two laboratories also are apparent (Table III). However, the influence of population sampling may contribute to the

TABLE III. Serum LH in mIU/ml 2nd IRP-HMG

	Baltimore								Cleveland							
	Collaborative series				Previous series				Collaborative series				Previous series			
Age	No.	Mean	SD	SE	No.	Mean	SD	SE	No.	Mean	SD	SE	No.	Mean	SD	SE
Females																
8	10	3.7	0.9	0.3	6	2.6	0.3	0.1	10	2.0	0.2	0.06	9	1.9	0.3	0.1
9-10	20	4.3	1.4	0.3	18	4.0a	2.1	0.5	20	2.2	0.2	0.04	19	2.5	1.3	0.3
11-12	21	6.9a	2.7	0.6	20	8.7a	3.6	0.8	21	4.9a	0.6	0.1	32	6.6a	9.1	1.6
13-14	13	8.8a	3.9	1.1	19	8.8	4.4	1.0	13	7.0a	0.8	0.2	22	10.0	13.1	2.8
15	9	8.6	3.1	1.0					9	8.4	1.2	0.4				
Males																
8	10	3.8	0.9	0.3	4	3.4	0.6	0.3	10	1.9	0.4	0.1	11	1.1	1.0	0.3
9-10	20	4.5a	0.7	0.2	15	4.8a	1.2	0.3	20	1.9	0.7	0.2	23	0.74	1.0	0.2
11-12	21	6.5a	2.2	0.5	14	6.8a	1.9	0.5	21	3.5a	1.8	0.4	29	1.54a	1.1	0.2
13-14	19	7.0	2.2	0.5	18	9.4a	2.5	0.6	19	4.7a	1.6	0.4	26	4.1a	2.5	0.5
15	10	8.6a	1.9	0.6	9	7.8a	2.0	0.7	10	6.4a	1.1	0.3	4	4.0	0.9	0.5

ap<0.05 when compared to preceding groups.

508

TABLE III. Cont'd

p values for mean LH differences in the two series from each laboratory

	Baltimore	Cleveland
	Females	
Age		
8	0.005	
9-10	0.3	0.2
11-12	0.005	0.2
13-14		0.2
15		
	Males	
8	0.20	0.025
9-10	0.10	0.005
11-12	0.30	0.005
13-14	0.005	0.2
15	0.2	0.005

discrepancies to a greater extent than technical differences. This is suggested when the two series reported from the Cleveland laboratory are compared, and one notes the significant variance between the two male populations which were randomly selected. A similar variance is not observed for the two female populations (Table III). These observations suggest a homogeneity of sexual maturation, as related to age, among maturing females and a heterogeneity of sexual maturation, as related to age, among maturing males; they also are consistent with the clinical finding that there is a disproportionately greater incidence of delayed adolescence among males than females. Therefore, the ages of initial increase in mean serum FSH and LH concentrations reported by the Baltimore and Ann Arbor laboratories may represent the extremes of the variation. The age of initial increase reported for males by the Cleveland and San Francisco laboratories possibly represents the median of the variation. It is of interest to note that the males of the Baltimore initial series were not selected at random but on the basis of their heights being between the 25th and 75th percentile, and this selection may account for the earlier rise of LH in this series than in any other.

The consensus of the data obtained by the 4 groups of investigators on 943 (524 males, 419 females) children, ages 5 to 18 years, is that a progressive increase in mean serum FSH and LH concentration occurs with age. Mean serum FSH and LH concentrations significantly ($p < 0.05$) increase to 11 to 12 years of age in males and females; and mean serum FSH and LH concentrations are significantly (p < 0.05) higher in females than males at 11 to 12 years of age (Table II). In general the data suggest, in a population selected on the basis of age, that mean serum gonadotropin concentrations in maturing females are equal to, or greater than, the mean concentrations of gonadotropins found in maturing males. Mean FSH and LH concentrations comparable to adult levels were attained in females at age 13 to 14 years and in males at age 13 to 14 or 15 to 16 years. The variance between the data of the investigating groups may be related to differences in both technique and population sampling which does not allow for the influence of variation in sexual maturation. It has been demonstrated that a greater correlation exists between gonadotropin concentration and stage of sexual development than gonadotropin concentration and age (8). Complete uniformity of technique and correlation of gonadotropin concentrations with a uniform system for staging sexual maturation should eliminate the discrepancies.

URINARY EXCRETION OF IMMUNOREACTIVE FSH AND LH

Radioimmunoassay and bioassay of kaolin extracts of urine for gonadotropins give comparable values (10-13). Using alcohol or acetone precipitates of raw urine we have found values similar to those obtained on kaolin extracts of urine for immunoreactive FSH, (14, 15) but the values for immunoreactive LH have been 3 to 4 times those obtained on kaolin extracts of urine (16). Parallelism of the dilution curves of 2nd IRP-HMG and of acetone precipitates of raw urine confirmed the validity of the assay (Table IV). Recoveries of 2nd IRP-HMG which was added to the urine of a hypopituitary patient were excellent (95 to 104%). When pools of urine were divided, and one extracted with kaolin before precipitating with acetone and the second precipitated directly with acetone, the

TABLE IV. Recovery and dilutional experiments (mIU/ml)

	Experiment		
	1	2	3
Urine from hypophysectomized patient	1.2	1.4	1.3
+ 16.0 mIU 2nd IRP-HMG	17.8	17.6	17.9
+ 20.0 mIU 2nd IRP-HMG	20.1	21.4	21.8
Urine from normal male adult	26.8	27.0	28.0
1/2 strength	14.0	13.8	14.3
1/4 strength	6.9	6.8	7.1
+ 20 mIU 2nd IRP-HMG	45.0	47.0	47.6
1/2 strength	22.0	23.0	23.2
1/4 strength	12.0	11.8	12.0
Urine from postmenopausal female	64.9	62.0	
1/2 strength	33.0	30.5	
1/4 strength	16.5	15.2	

immunoreactive FSH was essentially identical. However, immunoreactive LH values were 3.7 to 4.3 times higher in direct acetone precipitates than in kaolin extracts, and the discrepancies were comparable for the urines from all age groups (Table V).

TABLE V. Comparison of FSH and LH in kaolin and acetone extracts of urine

Pool	Preadolescent		Male adults		Postmenopausal female	
	Acetone	Kaolin	Acetone	Kaolin	Acetone	Kaolin
FSH						
1	9.6	9.7	13.2	13.2	54.0	53.6
2	7.2	7.4	13.2	13.5	63.5	62.5
3	7.3	7.3	16.5	16.0	lost	
Mean	8.0	8.1	14.3	14.2	58.5	58.0
LH						
1	11.0	3.0	51.0	14.5	192.0	42.8
2	9.3	2.8	62.0	19.5	172.0	47.6
3	12.3	2.8	66.0	16.3	lost	
Mean	10.8	2.9	59.6	16.7	182.0	45.2
Acetone/kaolin	3.7		3.6		4.3	

Measurement of LH daily in serum and direct acetone precipitates of urine during the menstrual cycles of 4 normal women (Fig. 3) demonstrated that the LH measured in acetone precipitates reflected the serum LH concentrations and the physiologic state of an individual. Further confirmation was obtained by suppressing the levels of serum LH and urinary LH in 2 patients with gonadal agenesis with estrogen administration. The mean serum LH concentration of several samples before estrogen treatment was 34.9 ± 12.0 mIU/ml and after treatment 4.3 ± 3.9 mIU/ml. Urinary excretion for the same times was 76.1 ± 11.7 and 7.7 ± 5.0 IU/24 hr. It was not determined whether the LH measured in direct acetone precipitates, but lost in the kaolin extraction, is biologically active. LH aggregates have been described (17), and immunoreactive LH which adheres to kaolin may be aggregates or fragments of LH.

Using the acetone precipitates of aliquots of 24-hr urine specimens, the excretion of immunoreactive FSH and LH by normal boys, ages 5 to 18 years, was determined (15, 18) (Figs. 4-8). Urinary FSH increased 3.2 times from stage I to stage III of sexual development and then plateaued. From stage I to adulthood, on a square meter surface area basis, the increase was 2.3 times. Urinary LH excretion increased progressively throughout each stage of sexual development, did not plateau at stage III as did FSH, increased 12 times from stage I to adulthood, and increased 7.2 times on the basis of surface area, in

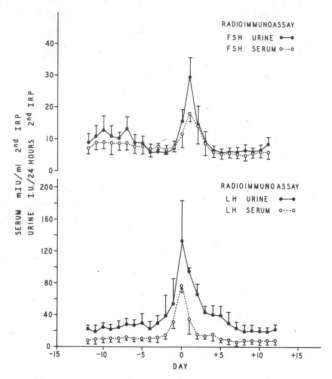

FIG. 3. Gonadotropin patterns during one complete menstrual cycle of 4 normal females (±SD).

other words per square meter. Serum FSH and LH concentrations paralleled urinary FSH and LH excretions. Both serum LH and urinary excretion of LH correlated significantly with urinary 17-ketosteroid values (correlation coefficients, 0.73 and 0.78) while the correlation of serum FSH concentrations and urinary excretion of FSH correlated poorly with the excretion of urinary 17-ketosteroids (correlation coefficients, 0.49 and 0.45).

PREPUBERTAL GONADECTOMIZED SUBJECTS

The significant increase in serum FSH concentrations in 6 of 6 gonadectomized males (XY karyotypes) and serum LH concentrations in 5 of these 6, ages 4 months to 9.8 years, is consistent with a functional prepubertal hypothalamic-pituitary-gonadal axis (Table VI). Severe anomalies of the external genitalia prompted castration and rearing as females. The reason for the disproportionate increase in FSH concentrations, as compared to LH, is unknown. However, the same disproportionate increase is observed in young patients with gonadal dysgenesis (8).

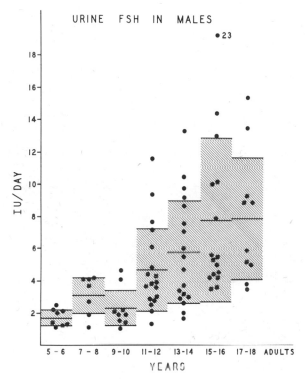

FIG. 4. Twenty-four hour urinary excretion of FSH expressed as IU of 2nd IRP-HMG vs the chronological age in normal males (±SD).

DISORDERS OF SEXUAL DEVELOPMENT (8)

Gonadal Dysgenesis

Thirty-two of 35 gonadal dysgenesis patients (ages 4.8 to 18.9 years) had elevated serum FSH concentrations for age and 19 had serum LH concentrations similarly elevated. No correlation between gonadotropin concentrations and karyotype was found. All patients with elevated serum LH levels were 11 years of age or older. However, 8 of 10 gonadal dysgenesis patients, ages 4.8 to 10.9 years, had serum FSH levels elevated above the normal range (Figs. 9 and 10). These data indicate that serum FSH determinations may be helpful in diagnosing gonadal dysgenesis during childhood.

Idiopathic Isosexual Precocity

Sixteen of 18 girls with idiopathic sexual precocity had serum FSH concentrations elevated above the range of normal for their chronologic age but consistent with their stage of sexual development (Table VII). Eight also had an elevated

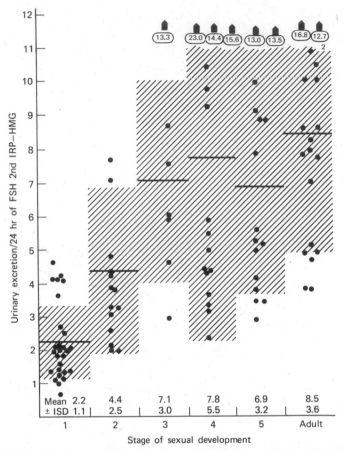

FIG. 5. Twenty-four hour urinary excretion of FSH expressed as IU of 2nd IRP-HMG vs the stage of sexual development in normal males (±SD).

serum LH concentration for age. In contrast 8 patients with premature pubarche (FSH = 4.5 ± 0.2 and LH = 2.7 ± 0.1 mIU/ml), 5 with premature thelarche (FSH = 4.3 ± 0.3 and LH = 2.7 ± 0.3 mIU/ml), and 3 patients with adolescent gynecomastia (FSH 6.3 ± 1.0 and LH 5.5 ± 0.4) had serum gonadotropins within the range of normal for age.

Delayed Adolescence

Serum gonadotropin concentrations in 35 boys (ages 13.1 to 17.8 years) with delayed adolescence correlated with stage of sexual development and, therefore, were often less than those expected for age (Table VIII).

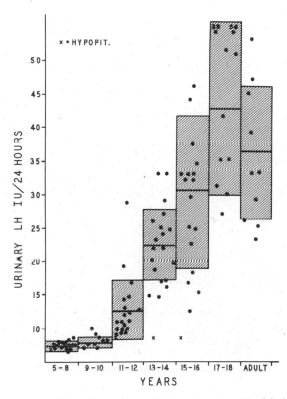

FIG. 6. Twenty-four hour urinary excretion of LH expressed as IU of 2nd IRP-HMG vs the chronological age in normal males (±SD).

SEXUAL DEVELOPMENT IN HYPOPITUITARY SUBJECTS (19)

In a longitudinal study between 1963 and 1970, serum FSH and LH concentrations were correlated with sexual development in 20 males with idiopathic hypopituitarism. Ten of these 20 developed to stage III of sexual development or beyond (Table IX). Six of 10 males with GH, ACTH, and TSH deficiency did not develop beyond stage I. In contrast, 4 of 5 males with GH deficiency without ACTH or TSH deficiency developed to stage III; and 3 of the 4 progressed to stage IV of sexual development. Serum FSH and LH concentrations in these patients were more compatible with stage of sexual development than with age (Table X). The mean serum LH concentration while in stage I (4.5 ± 0.9 mIU/ml) of 7 of the patients who advanced beyond stage I was significantly (p > 0.005) greater than the mean LH concentration (2.4 ± 0.7 mIU/ml) of 7 of the patients who had not advanced beyond this stage. Mean

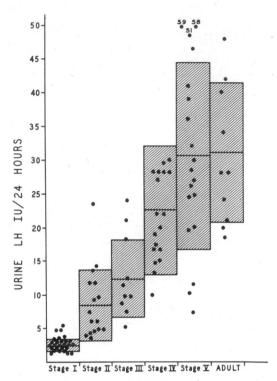

FIG. 7. Twenty-four hour urinary excretion of LH expressed as IU of 2nd IRP-HMG vs the stage of sexual development in normal males (±SD).

serum FSH concentrations were not different. Three of the patients who had not advanced beyond stage I had serum LH concentrations (1.5 to 1.8 mIU/ml) which are less than the normal range of LH (2.5 to 5.8 mIU/ml) in normal males in stage I (Table X).

We suggest that the serum LH concentration is helpful in predicting which patients with growth hormone deficiency will remain sexually infantile as adults.

CONCLUSIONS

1. FSH and LH concentrations increase with age and stage of sexual development. A greater correlation exists between gonadotropin concentrations and stages of sexual development than gonadotropin concentrations with chronological ages.

2. Increase in gonadotropin concentrations following gonadectomy in children, ages 4 months to 9.8 years, is consistent with a functional prepubertal hypothalamic-pituitary-gonadal axis.

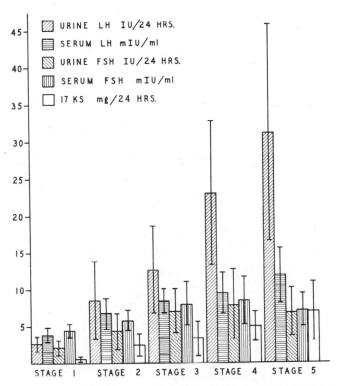

FIG. 8. Urinary LH (IU/24 hr), serum LH (mIU/ml), urinary FSH (IU/24 hr) serum FSH (mIU/ml) and urinary 17-ketosteroids (mg/24 hr) correlated with the stage of sexual development in normal males.

TABLE VI. Preadolescent bilateral gonadectomy

Patient	Chronological age		FSH (mIU/ml)	LH (mIU/ml)
(1) T.R.	4/12 years	Before	2.8	2.4
		7 days after	19.3	7.7
(2) T.D.	5/12 years	Before	2.8	2.2
		6 days after	5.4	3.6
(3) A.B.	2.5 years	2.5 years after	10.5	6.3
(4) G.T.	2.7 years	2.7 years after	178.0	27.8
(5) M.E.	8.3 years	8.3 years after	87.0	9.2
(6) J.E.	9.8 years	9.7 years after	112.0	34.2

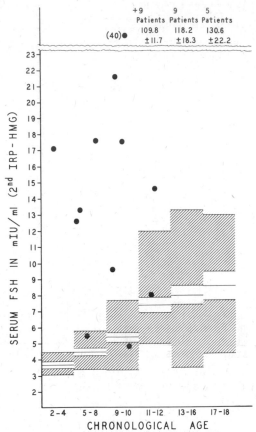

FIG. 9. Serum FSH concentration (mIU/ml, 2nd IRP-HMG) in 35 gonadal dysgenesis patients (black dots) shown with the range (hatch area), mean, and SE (clear area) for normal females of comparable age groups.

3. Patients with gonadal dysgenesis have elevated serum FSH concentrations early in childhood, and, after age 9 to 11 years, elevated serum LH concentrations.

4. Patients with idiopathic isosexual precocity have serum FSH and LH concentrations which are elevated for age but consistent with stage of sexual development.

5. Patients with delayed adolescence have serum gonadotropin concentrations which are consistent with stage of sexual development, and, therefore, are often less than those expected for age.

6. Patients with premature pubarche, premature thelarche, and adolescent gynecomastia have serum gonadotropin concentrations within the range of normal for chronological age.

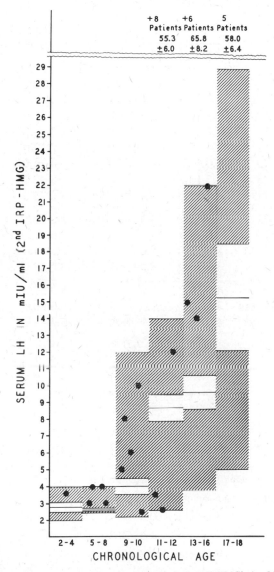

FIG. 10. Serum LH concentrations (mIU/ml, 2nd IRP-HMG) in 35 gonadal dysgenesis patients (black dots) shown with the range (hatched area), mean, and SE (clear area) for normal females of comparable age groups.

7. Data obtained in 20 idiopathic hypopituitary males suggests that serum gonadotropin concentrations, in a prepubertal patient, which are less than the range of normal for stage I of sexual development are consistent with expected sexual infantilism as an adult.

TABLE VII. Normal females and hypopituitary subjects

Stage	Age	No. Pts.	FSH in (mIU/ml)			LH in (mIU/ml)		
			Range	Mean	SE	Range	Mean	SE
	Hypopit							
	All ages	12	2.2- 3.2	2.8	0.1	1.0- 2.0	1.4	0.1
	2- 4	10	3.1- 4.5	3.7[b]	0.2	2.0- 4.0	2.8[b]	0.3
	5- 8	11	3.4- 5.8	4.5[b]	0.2	2.5- 4.0	2.6	0.1
	9-10	18	3.4- 7.7	5.4[b]	0.3	2.2-12.0	4.0[b]	0.5
	11-12	20	5.0-12.0	7.5[b]	0.5	2.4-14.0	8.7[b]	0.8
	13-16	23	3.5-13.3	8.0	0.6	3.8-22.0	9.6	1.0
	17-18	7	4.4-13.0	8.6	0.9	5.0-29.0	15.3[c]	3.2
I	2-12	27	3.1- 5.7	4.2	0.2	2.0- 7.5	2.9	0.4
II	8-12	13	4.6- 7.1	5.5[b]	0.2	2.5-11.5	3.9[b]	0.8
III	9-14	23	5.0-12.0	8.0[b]	0.4	2.5-14.0	8.4[b]	0.6
IV	12-18	26	3.5-13.0	8.0	0.5	3.0-29.0	11.3[c]	1.3
	Adults[a] Follicular		4.0-17.2	8.3	0.3	5.0-57.0	12.8	1.0
	Midcycle peak		13.7-22.5	19.3	2.0	76.0-90.0	83.5	3.7
	Luteal		4.0-15.0	6.9[d]	0.4	3.0-41.0	11.6[d]	1.3
	Idiopathic isosexual precocity							
	2- 4	3	5.5-13.3	9.3[e]	1.9	4.5- 9.5	6.4[e]	1.3
	5- 8	11	3.6-16.0	9.6[e]	1.3	2.5-22.0	6.1[e]	1.6
	9-10	4	9.6-22.6	14.5[e]	2.5	6.0-18.0	11.3[e]	2.2
III	2- 9	11	3.6-14.0	8.4	0.9	2.5-12.0	4.8[e]	0.8
IV	2-10	7	9.0-22.6	14.2[e]	1.8	4.5-22.0	11.4	2.2

[a]Menstrual cycles 4 normal adult females with regular menses.

[b]p of < 0.01 for difference from mean of preceding group.

[c]p of < 0.03 for difference from mean of preceding group.

[d]p of < 0.005 for difference from mean of follicular phase.

[e]p of < 0.01 for difference from mean of normal females.

TABLE VIII. Normal males

Stage	Age	Number of patients	FSH (mIU/ml)			LH (mIU/ml)		
			Range	Mean	SE	Range	Mean	SE
	13-14	18	5.0-14.0	8.1	0.6	5.0-14.0	9.4	0.6
	15-16	18	5.0-13.0	8.7	1.0	4.0-13.0	9.0	0.5
	17-18	10	4.0-14.0	9.2	1.2	7.5-19.0	14.1[a]	1.2
I	5-11	25	2.5- 7.0	4.5	0.2	2.5- 5.8	3.9	0.2
II	10-13	17	3.0- 9.0	5.9[a]	0.3	4.0-12.0	6.8[a]	0.5
III	12-14	11	2.5-14.0	8.1[a]	0.9	6.0-11.0	8.5[b]	0.5
IV	12-17	18	3.5-15.0	8.5	0.8	4.0-15.5	9.5	0.7
Constitutionally delayed adolescent development (males)								
	13-14	23	3.8-16.3	6.6[c]	0.8	2.5- 9.0	4.4[c]	0.4
	15-16	10	2.0- 8.0	4.8[c]	0.5	2.5 6.5	4.1[c]	0.4
	17-18	2	4.7- 4.8	4.8		5.5- 6.0	5.8	
I	14-15	5	3.8- 5.3	4.4	0.2	2.5- 3.5	2.9[d]	0.2
II	13-17	17	3.8- 7.0	4.7[d]	0.3	2.0- 5.5	3.9[c]	0.3
III	14-17	13	2.5-16.3	8.2	1.3	3.0- 7.5	5.5[c]	0.5

[a] p of < 0.01 for difference from mean of preceding group.

[b] p of < 0.03 for difference from mean of preceding group.

[c] p of < 0.01 for difference from mean of normal males.

[d] p of < 0.03 for difference from mean of normal males.

TABLE IX. Hypopituitary subjects

Idiopathic males	No. of Subjects	Stage				
		I	II	III	IV	V
GH; ACTH; TSH deficient	10	6	1	1	1	1
GH deficient only	5		1	1	3	
GH and ACTH deficient	4	1	1	2		
GH and TSH deficient	1			1		
Total	20	7	3	5	4	1

TABLE X. Normal males

Stage	Age	Number of patients	FSH (mIU/ml)			LH (mIU/ml)		
			Range	Mean	SD	Range	Mean	SD
	9-10	9	3.2- 7.1	5.4	1.0	3.5- 7.0	4.8	1.2
	11-12	13	3.0- 9.0	5.6	1.7	4.0-12.0	6.8[c]	2.0
	13-14	18	5.0-14.0	8.1[c]	2.5	5.0-14.0	9.4[c]	2.5
	15-16	18	5.0-13.0	8.7	4.2	4.0-13.0	9.0	2.1
	17-18	10	4.0-14.0	9.1	3.8	2.5- 5.8	14.1[c]	3.8
	Adult	35	4.4-13.2	7.4	1.9	6.0-23.0	10.9	4.0
I	5-11	25	2.5- 7.0	4.5	1.0	2.5- 5.8	3.9	1.0
II	10-13	17	3.0- 9.0	5.9[c]	1.2	4.0-12.0	6.8[c]	2.1
III	12-14	11	2.5-14.0	8.1[c]	3.0	6.0-11.0	8.5[d]	1.7
IV	12-17	18	3.5-15.0	8.5	3.4	4.0-15.5	9.5	3.0
V	15-18	21	4.0-13.0	7.2	2.2	7.0-19.0	11.8	3.7
			Hypopituitary subjects[a,b]					
	9-10	1		3.3			3.0	
	11-12	2	2.9- 2.3	3.1	0.2	3.7- 4.0	3.9	0.2
	13-14	12	2.7- 7.5	4.4	1.5	3.7- 7.6	5.6[c]	1.1
	15-16	10	3.5- 7.6	5.3[f]	1.2	2.7-10.5	5.9	2.3
	17-18	8	3.0- 8.3	5.4	1.8	1.7-10.3	6.0	2.8
	Adult	6	2.6- 8.0	5.0	2.4	1.5-12.5	5.5	4.2
I	9-27	14	2.6- 3.5	3.1	0.3	1.5- 5.4	3.6	1.4
II	13-18	12	4.3- 5.8	5.1	0.4	2.7- 7.6	5.8[c]	1.5
III	14-18	7	5.3- 8.3	6.3[c]	1.2	5.9-10.5	7.3[e]	1.8
IV	15-22	5	5.3- 8.0	6.8	1.1	5.9-12.5	8.6	2.9
V	15- 9	1		7.6			5.5	

[a]p of < .01 for difference from mean of normal males for all ages.

[b]p of < .03 for difference from mean of normal males for stages I and II for FSH.

[c]p of < .01 for difference from mean of preceding group.

[d]p of < .03 for difference from mean of preceding group.

[e]p of < .05 for difference from mean of preceding group.

[f]p of < .03 for difference from mean of 11 to 12 age group.

ACKNOWLEDGMENT

Dr. A. R. Midgley, Jr., supplied the antiserum used in these assays. The immunochemical grade LH and FSH antigens were prepared by Dr. Leo Reichert and provided by The National Pituitary Agency and the National Institutes of

Arthritis and Metabolic Diseases. Dr. Bangham of Mill Hill, England, supplied the 2nd IRP-HMG. This work was supported, in part, by traineeship grant TI AM 5219 from the USPHS, American Cancer Society (T-504), Pardee Foundation of Michigan, and research grants HD 01 852 and 5 Mol-RR-00052 from USPHS.

REFERENCES

1. Johanson, A. J., H. Guyda, C. Light, C. J. Migeon, and R. M. Blizzard, J Pediat 75:416, 1969.
2. Yen, S. S. C., W. J. Vicis, and D. V. Kearcher, J Clin Endocrinol 29:382, 1969.
3. Raiti, S., A. J. Johanson, C. Light, C. J. Migeon, and R. M. Blizzard, Metabolism 18:234, 1969.
4. Yen, S. S. C., and W. J. Vicis, Amer J Obst Gyn 106:134, 1970.
5. Burr, I. M., P. Sizonenko, S. L. Kaplan, and M. M. Grumbach, Pediat Res 4:31, 1970.
6. Sizonenko, P., I. M. Burr, S. L. Kaplan, and M. M. Grumbach, Pediat Res 4:36, 1970.
7. Lee, P. A., A. R. Midgley, Jr., and R. B. Jaffe, J Clin Endocrinol 31:248, 1970.
8. Penny, R., H. J. Guyda, A. Baghdassarian, A. Johanson, and R. M. Blizzard, J Clin Invest 49:1847, 1970.
9. Cargille, C. M., D. Rodbard, and G. T. Ross, J Clin Endocrinol 28:1277, 1968.
10. Albert, A. Rec. Prog Hormone Res 12:227, 1956.
11. Faiman, C., R. J. Ryan, and A. Albert, J Clin Endocrinol 28:1076, 1968.
12. Kulin, H. E., A. B. Rifkind, and G. T. Ross, J Clin Endocrinol 28:543, 1968.
13. Rifkind, A. B., H. E. Kulin, and G. T. Ross, J Clin Invest 46:1925, 1967.
14. Raiti, S., and R. M. Blizzard, J Clin Endocrinol 28:1719, 1968.
15. Raiti, S., C. Light, and R. M. Blizzard, J Clin Endocrinol 29:884, 1969.
16. Baghdassarian, A., S. Fisher, H. Guyda, A. Johanson, T. P. Foley, Jr., R. Penny, and R. M. Blizzard, Amer J Obst Gyn 108:1178, 1970.
17. Ryan, R. J., Biochemistry 8:495, 1969.
18. Baghdassarian, A., H. Guyda, A. Johanson, C. J. Migeon, and R. M. Blizzard, J Clin Endocrinol 31:428, 1970.
19. Penny, R., T. P. Foley, Jr., and R. M. Blizzard, submitted for publication, 1971.

41.   Studies on the
Mechanism of Puberty in Man

Robert P. Kelch, Melvin M. Grumbach, and Selna L. Kaplan[1]

Pubertal development in man is initiated by an acceleration in growth rate and the development of secondary sexual characteristics followed by the attainment of procreative capacity. The age of onset and course of pubertal events is variable (1-4) and is influenced by genetic factors, chronic disease, and altitude but especially by socioeconomic conditions (5). Indeed, the well-established secular trend to earlier pubertal development, for example, the 4 month per decade advancement in   age at menarche since 1830 (6), seems mainly attributable to improved nutritional and health standards and the concomitant earlier attainment of "critical weights".

The concept of "critical weights" for human development, first proposed by Frisch and Revelle (7), is based on the observation that the initiation of the weight growth spurt, the maximum rate of weight gain, and menarche all occur at an "invariant mean weight". (e.g., 47.8 ± 0.51 kg for menarche). It has been suggested that the attainment of a "critical weight" is associated with a change to a "critical" metabolic rate which, in turn, decreases the sensitivity of the hypothalamus to the negative feedback effect of sex steroids.

We shall review the normal progression and correlation of pubertal events with gonadotropin and sex steroid secretion. In the female (Table I), puberty normally begins with breast budding between 8 and 14 years of age. The average duration of female puberty, that is, the time interval between early breast budding (P 2) and the attainment of menses and adult breasts and pubic hair (P 5), is usually 4.5 years. The correlation between breast development and pubic hair growth is high, but there is significant individual variation. For example,

[1]Recipient of a Research Career Development Award, The National Institute of Child Health and Human Development, NIH.

adult-type pubic hair is present in 11% of girls with P 3 breast development, whereas P 4 breast development may occur before pubic hair appears (1). Menarche usually occurs after the peak growth spurt and before full adult breast contours are attained. In our studies, we classify all menstruating females as P 5.

TABLE I. Estimation of female pubertal development

Stage	Physical changes
P 1	Prepubertal. Elevation of papilla only; no pubic hair.
P 2	Breast budding; some labial hair present.
P 3	Further enlargement of breasts with palpable glandular tissue; no separation of breast contours; labial hair spreads over mons pubis.
P 4	Further enlargement of breasts with projection of areola to form a secondary mound; slight lateral spread of pubic hair.
P 5	Single contour of breast and areola; further lateral spread of pubic hair to form an inverse triangle; onset of menstruation.

In the male (Table II), puberty has its onset between 10 and 15 years of age with thinning and reddening of the scrotal skin and testicular enlargement as the first signs and has a mean duration of 4 years. Pubic hair appears shortly after the first genital changes, but subsequent development of the genitalia and pubic hair correlate quite well. The maximum growth rate usually occurs between 14 and 15 years, after midpuberty, and approximately 2 years later than in girls.

TABLE II. Estimation of male pubertal development

Stage	Physical changes
P 1	Prepubertal; infantile genitalia.
P 2	Early testicular enlargement and thinning and reddening of scrotum; minimal straight pubic or scrotal hair.
P 3	Further testicular enlargement; definite phallic enlargement; darker, slightly curled pubic hair and ± early axillary and facial hair.
P 4	Moderate amount of pubic, axillary, and facial hair and acne; voice change; adult body odor.
P 5	Adult-type body habitus, hair distribution, and genitalia.

Although a considerable amount of anthropometric data is available, little is known about the factors governing the initiation and course of human pubertal development. In this report, we discuss the hormonal changes which occur prior to and during puberty and present our concepts of the maturation of the hypothalamo-pituitary-gonadal axis from fetal life to adolescence.

The development of highly sensitive and specific radioimmunoassays for plasma gonadotropins and estradiol and the competitive-protein-binding technique for sex steroids have permitted a correlation of hormonal changes with pubertal development (8-11). Figure 1 illustrates the mean plasma estradiol concentrations of 26 prepubertal children and 76 pubertal females grouped by their stage of sexual development (P 1 to P 5) (11). There was a continuous rise

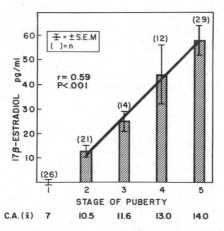

FIG. 1. The concentration of plasma estradiol in 26 prepubertal (22 females and 4 males) and 76 pubertal females grouped by their stage of pubertal development.

in plasma estradiol from the undetectable prepubertal levels (<8 pg/ml) to an average of 58 pg/ml in menstruating adolescents, a significant but equal correlation with bone age (BA) and chronologic age (CA) (r = 0.52 BA, r = 0.54 CA), but a greater correlation with the stage of pubertal development (r = 0.59). In 50 of these girls, plasma gonadotropins were also determined (Table III). Plasma FSH rose sharply in P 2 and then plateaud after midpuberty (P 3 to 4), whereas plasma LH rose slowly throughout puberty. Similar trends in plasma gonadotropins were found by Blizzard et al. (12, 13) in their cross-sectional studies; a significant rise in FSH was observed in 5 to 8-year-old prepubertal girls whereas the LH rise was not significant until 9 to 10 years of age. These studies suggest that a rise in plasma gonadotropins, especially FSH, precedes increased ovarian secretion of estradiol.

Figure 2 illustrates the observed changes in plasma testosterone and

TABLE III. Plasma FSH, LH, and estradiol in females during puberty, P 1 to P 5[a]

Pubertal stage	1	2	3	4	5
FSH(LER-869) ng/ml	0.7 ± 0.1	1.2 ± 0.1	2.3 ± 1.0	2.6 ± 0.4	2.5 ± 0.4
LH(LER-960) ng/ml	0.7 ± 0.1	0.8 ± 0.4	1.4 ± 0.2	1.7 ± 0.2	2.5 ± 0.6
Estradiol pg/ml	< 8	13 ± 2.4	25 ± 4.5	44 ± 12	58 ± 6

[a]$x \pm$ SEM.

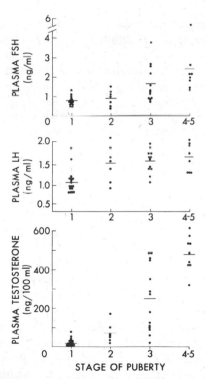

FIG. 2. Correlation between plasma FSH, LH, and testosterone and stage of pubertal development in 51 normal boys.

gonadotropins in 51 normal boys (P 1 to P 4 to 5) (10). The major rise in plasma testosterone was observed between P 2, early puberty 71 ng/100 ml), and P 3, midpuberty (248 ng/100 ml), after plasma LH had risen sharply in P 2. Using a double-isotope derivative technique, Frasier et al. (14) had previously shown a stepwise increase in plasma testosterone throughout puberty with the greatest increment after midpuberty. In our study in boys, plasma FSH concentrations rose progressively from P 1 through P 4 to 5 while plasma LH rose earlier and tended to plateau after midpuberty. Significant increases in the serum concentrations of LH and FSH were noted in 9 to 10-year-old prepubertal males by Blizzard and co-workers (12). They found that serum LH also rose at the onset of puberty but continued to rise slowly throughout puberty. These combined data strongly suggest that the rise in plasma gonadotropins, especially LH, precedes the major increment in testosterone secretion in male puberty. Thus increased gonadotropin secretion, presumably secondary to a decreased sensitivity of the hypothalamic-pituitary negative feedback system is the initial hormonal event of puberty in man.

There is evidence against the proposal that insensitivity or unresponsiveness of the prepubertal gonads to gonadotropins is an important limiting factor in the initiation of human puberty. The prepubertal testis responds to HCG administration, albeit in pharmacologic amounts (14, 15) and this response has been useful in the preoperative detection of functional, abdominal testes before puberty (16, 17). An initial 33-day course of human menopausal gonadotropin combined with HCG treatment for 5 days resulted in ovulation and subsequent menarche in a 15-year-old sexually infantile girl with panhypopituitarism secondary to removal of craniopharyngioma (18).

In our laboratory, Kaplan, Grumbach, and Shepard (19) have studied the synthesis and secretion of pituitary gonadotropins in the human fetus. As early as the end of the first trimester, the presence of immunoreactive FSH and LH has been detected in the pituitaries and FSH and "LH-HCG" in the sera of human fetuses. The fetal pituitary content of FSH peaked at about 200 days with mean values of 5.9 μg for females and 0.5 μg for male fetuses. Serum FSH values ranged from 3.2 to 46.0 ng/ml between 102 and 133 days of gestation, and just as in the pituitary, were generally higher in females than males of comparable gestational ages, and decreased sharply to less than 1 ng/ml in matched umbilical cord and maternal vein specimens. At term, the mean content of pituitary FSH decreased to 0.2 μg. The fetal pituitary LH content rose steadily from a level of 0.06 μg at 90 days gestation to a mean peak of 1.5 μg at 200 days; at term it decreased to 0.9 μg.

These changes in fetal gonadotropins are associated with concurrent histologic changes in the fetal testis and ovary. The high level of HCG in the first trimester correlates well with, and is probably responsible for, the marked hyperplasia of Leydig cells of the fetal testes and secretion of testosterone with its subsequent effects on male sexual differentiation (20). Support for the importance of fetal gonadotropins in the later growth and development of the fetal testis and of the male external genitalia is provided by the higher incidence of cryptorchidism and gonadal hypoplasia in anencephalic and apituitary infants

(21). At the time of the peak rise in LH and FSH of the fetal pituitary, there is sustained Leydig cell activity in the male and active formation of primordial follicles in the female. Marked regression in Leydig cells in the fetal testis and an increased formation of atretic follicles in the fetal ovary is noted when fetal gonadotropins are declining rapidly (22). The absence of a sex difference in testosterone concentrations in umbilical venous plasma at term is further indication that fetal Leydig cell activity parallels fetal gonadotropin secretion (23). From these observations we have suggested that the maturation of the negative feedback mechanism, in the human fetus, gradually occurs during the last trimester after a period of probable unrestrained gonadotropin release in the second trimester.

Recent evidence in man and in the chimpanzee presented by Winter and Faiman (24) and the previous data of Lee et al. (25) suggest that infant females have higher circulating gonadotropins than infant males (0 to 2 years old). These findings are of interest in view of the higher female fetal gonadotropin values and suggest that intrauterine fetal androgens may enhance the negative feedback maturation in the male fetus.

The presence of a prepubertal negative feedback system in the rat was demonstrated in the studies of Kallas in 1929 (26), who showed that prepubertal castration of one of a pair of parabiotic rats resulted in precocious puberty in the other. Recently, Laron and Zilka (27) have reported that highly significant "compensatory hypertrophy" occurs in descended testes of prepubertal males with unilateral cryptorchidism. We interpret this observation as further support for the presence of an operative feedback system in the prepubertal human.

Rifkind et al. (28) demonstrated clearly by bioassay methods that prepubertal children excrete FSH and LH; an increase of approximately 10-fold in LH and 2.7-fold in FSH excretion was found between prepubertal children and adult male subjects. Radioimmunoassay results of plasma and urinary gonadotropins by others (8, 9, 13, 25, 30, 31) and from our laboratory, indicate that normal children have measureable plasma gonadotropins, significantly higher than hypopituitary subjects. Penny et al. (12) detected abnormally elevated serum FSH concentration in 5- to 10-year-old patients with gonadal dysgenesis. The mean serum LH concentration in these patients was significantly higher than controls, but there was a great deal of overlap between the two groups. In a series of 23 patients with XO gonadal dysgenesis, Grumbach and Kaplan (29) observed significantly elevated levels of plasma FSH as early as 2 months of life (Fig. 3), but LH values did not reach castrate or postmenopausal levels until after 11 years of age.

Additional evidence for an operative prepubertal feedback system was obtained by the work of Kulin, Grumbach, and Kaplan (30, 31) when they administered clomiphene citrate, a weakly estrogenic "antiestrogen," to children. The stimulatory effect of clomiphene on gonadotropin secretion and excretion in adult subjects (32-36) is well documented. Clomiphene has been shown to competitively inhibit estradiol binding by "receptors" in various tissues, for

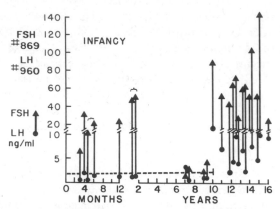

FIG. 3. The concentration of plasma FSH and LH in 23 patients with XO gonadal dysgenesis.

example, uterus, pituitary, and hypothalamus (37, 38). It apparently induces a gonadotropin surge by decreasing or eliminating the negative feedback effect of endogenous sex steroids. However, clomiphene also has intrinsic estrogenic properties (39), which we believe account for our unexpected finding of gonadotropin suppression rather than stimulation in the prepubertal human. Initially, clomiphene was administered in an attempt to stimulate gonadotropin release and to investigate the possibility of an age dependent sensitivity of the negative feedback center(s). Unexpectedly, clomiphene suppressed urinary FSH and LH excretion in prepubertal children. Because of the relative insensitivity of plasma gonadotropin radioimmunoassays in this age group, we could not detect any upward or downward trends. However, by comparing kaolin-acetone urinary concentrates with the urinary gonadotropin reference standard (2nd IRP-HMG), small amounts of gonadotropin excretion were detected and the effects of endocrine manipulations assessed.

Table IV summarizes this experience (30, 31). Prepubertal suppression of urinary FSH was found with doses as low as 0.1 mg/day given for 7 days. Stimulation of gonadotropin excretion was never observed, even when the dose of clomiphene was reduced to 0.01 or 0.001 mg/day. Children in early puberty exhibited suppression of urinary gonadotropins or testosterone on 100 mg/day, but not on 1.0 or 0.1 mg/day. A rise in the excretion of urinary gonadotropins was observed (100 mg/day for 7 days) in 2 midpubertal females who menstruated 17 and 24 days after the initiation of clomiphene. One male adolescent given 100 mg/day for 7 days on three occasions, revealed a change from definite suppression in early puberty to no response at midpuberty.

Since we attributed the suppressive effects of clomiphene to its inherent estrogenic properties, similar studies were performed using very low doses of

TABLE IV. Summary of the effect of clomiphene citrate on urinary FSH, LH, and plasma testosterone in prepubertal and pubertal children (30, 31)

Pubertal stage	No.	Dose (mg/day × 7 d)	Significant suppression
P 1 (prepubertal)	3	100	3/3
	6	10	5/6
	3	1.0	3/3
	5	0.1	2/5
	6	0.01	0/6
	3	0.001	0/3
P 2 (early puberty)	3	100	3/3
	4	10	2/4[a]
	4	1.0	1/4[a]
	4	0.1	0/4

[a]Questionable suppression.

TABLE V. Suppression of urinary FSH with ethinyl estradiol

Pubertal stage	No.	Dose (μg/day × 5 d)	Significant suppression
P 1 (prepubertal)	6	2	3/6
P 1 (prepubertal)	5	5	5/5
P 1 (prepubertal)	3	10	3/3
Total			11/14
P 2 (early puberty)	3	2	1/3
P 3 (mid puberty)	1	10	0/1
P 4 (advanced puberty, premenarche)	2	10	0/2

ethinyl estradiol, a potent estrogen (Table V). Prepubertal children uniformly exhibited a decrease in urinary FSH on only 5 μg of ethinyl estradiol/day, while 2 μg/day elicited definite suppression in 3 of 6 children. Figure 4 shows the pattern observed in A.M., a 11-2/12-year-old prepubertal male, in whom both FSH and LH excretion were suppressed by only 2 μg/day. Males in early puberty could still show the suppressive effects of low dose estrogen administration, but 3 adolescents with more advanced puberty (P 3 to 4) failed to show any detectable change on 10 μg/day.

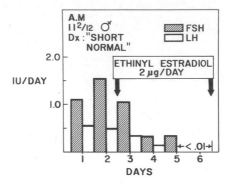

FIG. 4. Ethinyl estradiol suppression of urinary FSH and LH in a short normal 11-2/12-year-old prepubertal male.

The combined data on clomiphene and ethinyl estradiol demonstrate conclusively that the hypothalamo-pituitary-gonadal feedback system is operative prior to the onset of pubertal development and that the sensitivity of the "gonadostat" decreases significantly during puberty. We interpret the lack of suppression in children beyond midpuberty to both clomiphene and low doses of ethinyl estradiol and the positive response to clomiphene in 2 midpubertal females and adults as evidence of the maturation of a positive feedback response in mid- to late puberty. The precise anatomic location, in other words hypothalamic or pituitary, of this "positive feedback center" which is responsive to circulating estrogens and leads to the cyclic release of gonadotropins in the female is unknown. However, recent evidence indicates that: (1) estrogens enhance the gonadotropin-releasing response of the pituitary to exogenous LRF (40); and (2) there may be only a single gonadotropin releasing factor responsible for both FSH and LH release (41), suggesting that the pituitary may participate in the "positive feedback response".

The possible role of "short feedback loops" in the regulation of gonadotropin secretion in man, in other words, pituitary gonadotropins participating in their own neural regulation, as has been demonstrated in the rat (42-46), is yet to be determined.

In summary, we suggest that: (1) maturation of the hypothalamic-pituitary-gonadal axis begins in mid- to late fetal life and may be enhanced in the male by fetal androgen production; (2) an intact negative feedback system is operative in prepubertal children; (3) the initial hormonal event of puberty is an increase in gonadotropin secretion secondary to a marked decrease in the sensitivity of the "gonadostat" to sex steroids; and (4) the development of the positive feedback response to estrogens occurs after midpuberty.

ACKNOWLEDGMENT

This work was supported in part by grants from the National Institute of Child Health and Human Development and the National Institute of Arthritis and Metabolic Disease.

REFERENCES

1. Marshall, W. A., and J. M. Tanner, Arch Dis Child 44:291, 1969.

2. Ibid, Arch Dis Child 45:13, 1970.

3. Donovan, B. T., and J. J. van der Werff Ten Bosch, Physiology of Puberty, Arnold, London, 1965.

4. Zacharias, L., R. J. Wurtman, and M. Schatzoff, Amer J Obst Gyn 108:833, 1970.

5. Zacharias, L., and R. J. Wurtman, New Eng J Med 280:860, 1969.

6. Tanner, J. M., Growth at Adolescence, 2nd ed., Blackwell, Oxford, 1962, p. 152.

7. Frisch, R. E., and R. Revelle, Science 169:397, 1970.

8. Burr, I. M., P. C. Sizonenko, S. L. Kaplan, and M. M. Grumbach, Pediat Res 4:25, 1970.

9. Sizonenko, P. C., I. M. Burr, S. L. Kaplan, and M. M. Grumbach, Pediat Res 4:36, 1970.

10. August, G. P., S. L. Kaplan, and M. M. Grumbach, in preparation.

11. Jenner, M. R., R. P. Kelch, S. L. Kaplan, and M. M. Grumbach, presented to the American Pediatric Society, April, 1971.

12. Blizzard, R. M., A. Johanson, H. Guyda, A. Baghdassarian, S. Raiti, and C. J. Migeon, in F. P. Heald and W. Hung (Eds.), Adolescent Endocrinology, Appleton-Century-Crofts, New York, 1970, p. 1.

13. Penny, R., H. Guyda, A. Baghdassarian, A. Johanson, and R. M. Blizzard, J Clin Invest 49:1847, 1970.

14. Frasier, S. D., F. Gafford, and R. Horton, J Clin Endocrinol 29:1404, 1969.

15. Saez, J. M., and J. Bertrand, Steroids 12:749, 1968.

16. Rivarola, M. A., C. Bergada, and M. Cullen, J Clin Endocrinol 31:526, 1970.

17. Levine, L., and M. I. New, Amer J Dis Child 121:176, 1971.

18. Abrams, C. A. L., M. M. Grumbach, I. Dyrenfurth, and R. L. vande Wiele, J Clin Endocrinol 27:467, 1967.

19. Kaplan, S. L., M. M. Grumbach, and T. H. Shepard, Pediat Res 3:512, 1969.

20. Jirasek, J. E., in G. E. W. Wolstenholme and M. O'Connor (Eds.), Endocrinology of the Testis, Little, Brown, Boston, 1967, p. 3.

21. Bearn, J. G., Acta Paediat Acad Sci Hung 9:159, 1968.

22. van Wagenen, G., and M. E. Simpson (Eds.), Embryology of the Ovary and Testis: Homosapiens and Macaca mulatta, Yale Univ. Press, New Haven, 1965.

23. August, G. P., M. Tkachuk, and M. M. Grumbach, J Clin Endocrinol 29:891, 1969.

24. Winter, J. S., and C. Faiman, Society for Pediatric Research abstract, 1971.

25. Lee, P. A., A. R. Midgley, and R. B. Jaffee, J Clin Endocrinol 31:248, 1970.

26. Kallas, J., C R Soc Biol 100:979, 1929.

27. Laron, Z., and E. Zilka, J Clin Endocrinol 29:1410, 1969.

28. Rifkind, A. B., H. E. Kulin, and G. T. Ross, J Clin Invest 46:1925, 1967.

29. Conte, F., M. M. Grumbach, and S. L. Kaplan, in preparation.

30. Kulin, H. E., M. M. Grumbach, and S. L. Kaplan, Science 166:1912, 1969.

31. Ibid, submitted for publication.

32. Roy, S., R. B. Greenblatt, V. B. Mahesh, and E. C. Jungck, Fertil Steril 14:575, 1963.

33. Thompson, R. J., and R. C. Mellinger, Amer J Obst Gyn 92:412, 1965.

34. Bardin, C. W., G. T. Ross, and M. B. Lipsett, J Clin Endocrinol 27:1558, 1967.

35. Peterson, N. T., A. R. Midgley, and R. B. Jaffee, J Clin Endocrinol 28:1473, 1968.

36. Jacobson, A., J. R. Marshall, G. T. Ross, and C. M. Cargille, Amer J Obst Gyn 102:284, 1968.

37. Wyss, R. H., R. Karsznia, W. L. Heinrichs, and W. L. Herrmann, J Clin Endocrinol 28:1824, 1968.

38. Kahwanago, I., W. L. Heinrichs, and W. L. Herrmann, Endocrinology 86:319, 1970.

39. Wood, J. R., R. T. Wrenn, and J. Bitman, Endocrinology 82:69, 1968.

40. Arimura, A., and A. V. Schally, Prog Soc Exp Biol Med 136:290, 1971.

41. Schally, A. V., A. Arimura, Y. Baba, R. M. G. Nair, H. Matsuo, T. W. Redding, L. Debeljuk, and W. F. White, Endocrine Society abstract, 1971.

42. Ramirez, V. C., in C. Gual and F. J. G. Ebling (Eds.), Progress in Endocrinology, Excerpta Medica Foundation, Amsterdam, 1969, p. 532.

43. Corbin, A., Endocrinology 78:893, 1966.

44. David, A. M., F. Fraschini, and L. Martini, Endocrinology 78:5, 1966.

45. Corbin, A., and J. C. Story, Endocrinology 80:1006, 1967.

46. Martini, L., F. Fraschini, and M. Motta, Recent Progr Hormone Research, 25:439, 1968.

42. Puberty in a Male with 3β-ol-Dehydrogenase Deficiency

Gary A. Parks, Maria I. New, Alfred M. Bongiovanni, Jose A. Bermudez, and Constantine S. Anast

A 13-year-old boy whose male differentiation was incomplete due to 3β-hydroxysteroid dehydrogenase (3β-HSD) deficiency underwent puberty. His puberty was manifested by male secondary sexual characteristics and marked gynecomastia. Bongiovanni (1) reported the first three cases of congenital adrenal hyperplasia due to the deficiency of 3β-HDS in 1961 and subsequently 11 more cases have been reported (2-8). However, none of the cases were of a pubertal age. The case described here (9) gave us an opportunity to investigate the mechanism of puberty and breast development in the presence of an enzyme defect of testosterone synthesis.

CASE REPORT

J. N., a 13-year-old white male student, was the product of an uncomplicated full-term gestation with a birth weight of 2807 g. Hypospadias was not noted at birth and he was considered to be a normal newborn male until one month of age when he was admitted to the hospital in a critically dehydrated condition. Electrolytes revealed: sodium 105 mEq/l and potassium 8.7 mEq/l. He was diagnosed as having 21-hydroxylase deficiency, salt-losing form of congenital adrenal hyperplasia and treated appropriately with saline and cortisone until recovery. His 24-hr urinary 17-ketosteroid excretion was elevated to 3.1 mg.

Subsequently he was treated with oral cortisone,[1] 7.5 mg daily, and 9-α-fluoro-hydrocortisone, 0.05 mg daily. He had twelve subsequent admissions for adrenal insufficiency with electrolyte imbalance and was followed regularly on an out-patient basis.

The family history indicated the parents were not consanguineous and there were two other affected members in the pedigree. The patient had six normal siblings and one male sibling with ambiguous genitalia who died at two days of age with respiratory distress. Electrolytes obtained from that infant at a few hours of age were unremarkable and at autopsy the infant was found to have marked chordee, perineal hypospadias, and a phallus measuring 1.8 cm in length. The testes, scrotum, and vas deferens were normal. The adrenal glands were enlarged (10,11); one weighing 7 and the other 9 g. The patient's paternal first cousin was a female with ambiguous genitalia who died at the age of two months with diarrhea and vomiting. Her electrolytes prior to death were: sodium 95 mEq/l, CO_2 19.4 mEq/l and NPN 41 mg%. At autopsy she was hyperpigmented and had areas of vitiligo. The clitoris and labia majora were enlarged. The uterus and vagina were normal and the ovaries showed follicles at various stages of development. The adrenals were markedly enlarged (10, 11), one weighing 29 and the other 40 g.

The 3β-HSD deficiency is transmitted by an autosomal recessive gene. The presence of congenital adrenal hyperplasia and salt-wasting in first cousins despite the absence of consanguinity in the pedigree is surprising especially in view of the rarity of the 3β-HSD defect. Since the patient's cousin was a female, she could have been suffering from the more common genetic enzyme defect of 21-hydroxylation rather than 3β-HSD defect.

The patient, J. N., had the onset of acne at the age of 11 years. His growth spurt began at the age of 12 years. At the age of 12½ he had pubic and early axillary hair. At a clinic visit at the age of 12½ years his testes were noted to have increased in length from 2.5 cm to 3.5 cm over an 8-month period. It was also at this age that the breast development was first noted and it progressed at a rapid rate in the two months prior to this investigation. The patient was referred to The New York Hospital-Cornell Medical Center for a detailed steroidal work-up as a possible case of the 3β-HSD deficiency.

Physical examination on admission revealed a well-developed, well-nourished, properly proportioned white male. His measurements included: height 145 cm (8th percentile), weight 34.55 kg (8th percentile), span 144 cm, 72 cm upper/73 cm lower, and abdomen 64 cm. His dentition was normal and his thyroid was

[1]The following trivial names and abbreviations are used: 17,21-dihydroxypregn-4-ene-3,20-dione (ll-desoxycortisol; compound S); 5β-pregnane-3α,17α,20α-triol-5β-pregnane (pregnanetriol); 3β-hydroxypregn-5-en-20-one (pregnenolone); preg-5-ene-3β, 17α, 20α-triol (Δ⁵-pregnenetriol); 3β-hydroxy-5β-androstan-17-one (etiocholanolone); 3β,17α-dihydroxypregn-5-ene-20-one (17-OH-pregnenolone); 17α-hydroxypregn-4-ene-3,20-dione (17-OH-progesterone); and 9α-fluoro-16α-methyl-lla, 17α, 21-trihydroxypregn-1,4-diene-3,20-dione (dexamethasone; Decadron).

not enlarged. He had the following signs of puberty: seborrhea; acne on the face, shoulders, and chest; a small amount of axillary hair; a moderate amount of pubic hair (Tanner stage 3) (12); a penis measuring 6.5 cm X 2.5 cm and there was mild hypospadias and chordee; a thin, vascular, rugated scrotum; and testes which were of normal shape and consistency measuring 4.0 X 2.5 cm bilaterally. The over-all size of the external genitalia corresponded to the Tanner stage 3 (12). There was glandular breast tissue which measured 7 cm in diameter on each side. The areolae were enlarged and pigmented corresponding to between the Tanner stage 2 and stage 3 for females (12). His skin was a light golden-brown color and considerably darker than that of his mother, although he had had no recent exposure to sunlight.

METHODS

Secretion rates of cortisol (F), 11-desoxycortisol (S), corticosterone (B), and 11-desoxycorticosterone (DOC) were measured by the method of New et al. (13). Urinary 17-ketosteroids, 17-hydroxysteroids, pregnanetriol, aldosterone and plasma 17-hydroxycorticoids, and plasma renin were measured by previously reported methods (14, 15). Fractionation of urinary 17-ketosteroids was done by two methods (2, 14). Plasma testosterone and dehydroepiandrosterone (DHEA) were determined by a double-isotope dilution derivative technique (16). Plasma values of pregnenolone, 17-hydroxypregnenolone, progesterone, and 17-hydroxyprogesterone were determined by recently reported methods (17-21). Plasma estrogens were determined by the method of Abraham (22). Plasma LH and FSH were determined by a radioimmunoassay (23).

RESULTS

PLASMA HORMONE VALUES

On oral hydrocortisone therapy, plasma 17-hydroxycorticoids were normal (2) (8.2 and 7.2μg/100 ml) but dropped to below normal when the hydrocortisone was discontinued (2.3 μg/100 ml). Plasma 17-hydroxycorticoids (9.8 μg/100 ml) did not significantly rise after ACTH administration (13.6 μg/100 ml). While under dexamethasone suppression, the testosterone level was in the range for a normal male adolescent (0.39 μg/100 ml) and DHEA was greatly elevated (13.5μg/100 ml). While still suppressed with dexamethasone, HCG administration, 5000 U IM daily for three days caused a 9-fold rise (2.86μg/100 ml) to well above the normal adult male range. Plasma gonadotropins were not elevated (FSH = 1.7 and LH = 6.0 to 9.0 mIU/ml) when the patient was treated with hydrocortisone or dexamethasone and when this therapy was discontinued. When hydrocortisone therapy was discontinued and two days after IV ACTH administration, plasma estradiol was normal (30 pg/ml) while the estrone, usually the major estrogen in males, was very low (2 pg/ml).

On the same day, determinations of plasma progesterone (0.73 ng/ml) and 17-hydroxyprogesterone (2.89 ng/ml) were elevated while the pregnenolone (4.6 ng/ml) and 17-hydroxypregnenolone (> 40 ng/ml) were extremely high. Plasma renin was in the low-normal range (2.7 ng of angiotensin/ml/hr) on a day when the patient was on 9α-fluorohydrocortisone, was in positive sodium balance, was on a very high sodium intake, and was hyponatremic. The day following the renin determination, the serum sodium began to approach normal. Karyotype of 12 white blood cells was 46/XY.

URINARY EXCRETION OF STEROIDAL METABOLITES

When maintenance therapy with hydrocortisone was discontinued for 4 days daily urinary excretion of 17-ketosteroids and pregnanetriol was extremely high but did suppress after 4 days of dexamethasone treatment (Table 1). Neither urinary 17-ketosteroid nor pregnanetriol excretion increased after ACTH or HCG administration.

Two 24-hr determinations of pregnenetriol revealed values even higher than pregnanetriol. The 17-ketosteroids were partitioned on 2/1/70 when hydrocortisone treatment was discontinued and on 2/3/70 when ACTH was administered. The markedly elevated values for DHEA, etiocholanolone, and androsterone were much higher than the values seen in the typical 21-hydroxylase or 3β-HSD defect. The ratio of DHEA to androsterone was 4 : 1 in our patient as compared to 1 : 1 in the patient with the 21-hydroxylase defect. Analysis of urinary 17-ketosteroids by means of digitonin precipitation and Oertel reaction (2) reveals most of the 17-ketosteroids to be in the sulfate fraction, to be digitonin precipitable, and to react with the Oertel reagent (Table II). This indicates that the urinary 17-ketosteroid are largely conjugated with sulfate rather than glucuronide and have the $3\beta ol\text{-}\Delta^5$ configuration. These results are consistent with those of Bongiovanni (2). Urinary aldosterone excretion was low irrespective of treatment of sodium balance. The secretion rates of F, S, B, and DOC were low under all conditions of study when compared to normal subjects (13) or to the patient's mother. The ACTH test particularly discriminates between normal secretion rates and those of the patient since none of the patient's secretion rates increased following ACTH stimulation (Table III).

The secretion rates of aldosterone are low despite hyponatremia and no acute response to ACTH administration is evident in the patient. In contrast, the mother did respond to sodium restriction and ACTH with an increased aldosterone secretion. The incapacity to secrete aldosterone was confirmed by an electrolyte balance study.

DISCUSSION

The present report describes a patient who was erroneously diagnosed in infancy as having the 21-hydroxylase deficiency, salt-wasting form of adrenal hyperplasia.

TABLE I. Data after hydrocortisone discontinued for 5 days

Treatment	17-OH (mg/day)	17-KS (mg/day)	Pregnanetriol (mg/day)	Pregnentriol (mg/day)	Aldosterone (μg/d)
9α-fluoro	1.4	153[a]	18	52	0.19
ACTH + 9α-fluoro	1.6	133[b]	14	14	0.65
Dexamethasone + 9α-fluoro	2.2	11	1.5		
Dexamethasone + 9α-fluoro + HCG	2.1	13	0.20		2.8
Normal adult male	4-10	9-22	0.5-1.0		
Typical child with 21-OH hydroxylase		1.1		0	

[a]DHEA = 58, etiocholanolone = 12, and androsterone = 20.
[b]DHEA = 80, etiocholanolone = 22, and androsterone = 28.

TABLE II. Partition of urinary 17-ketosteroids (mg/day)

	Baseline	ACTH	Normal
I. Total 17-ketosteroids	128.0	92.8	
A. Glucuronide fraction			
digitonin precipitable	0	0	
nondigitonin precipitable	24.5	20.1	
Total Oertel	8.5	4.5	
B. Sulfate fraction			
digitonin precipitable	67.5	34.5	
nondigitonin precipitable	36.4	50.0	
Total Oertel	67.5	52.5	
II. Total acetaldehydogenic	127.2	97.0	Maximum 3.5 mg/m^2
A. Glucuronide fraction			
digitonin precipitable	0	6.1	0.2 mg
nondigitonin precipitable	43.0	41.0	3 mg/m^2
B. Sulfate fraction			
digitonin precipitable	65.3	30.3	0.2
nondigitonin precipitable	18.9	20.2	0.2
III. 3α,17α,20α-pregnanetriol	15.4	4.3	

Clinical support for the diagnosis of 3 salt-wasting, (2) hypospadias, and (3) family history of two infants who died with congenital adrenal hyperplasia, ambiguous genitalia, and signs of adrenal insufficiency. Most children reported with the 3β-HSD defect die in early infancy in a salt-losing crisis (2) and probably only those with a partial defect survive into later childhood (2, 4, 6-8). The remarkable aspects of this case are survival to a pubertal age and development of male secondary sexual characteristics and marked gynecomastia at this time. Breast biopsy showed increased periductal stroma and ductal hyperplasia which resembles the juvenile hypertrophied female breast (24, 25). A possible explanation for the gynecomastia at puberty is the proposal by Federman (26) that fetal testosterone deficiency results in failure to inhibit the female breast anlage which results in female breast development at puberty. It is suggested that in the present patient a testosterone deficiency occurred during embryonic development due to the 3β-HSD deficiency. Further support for this concept is seen in animal experiments in which male rats treated in utero with an androgen antagonist (cyproterone acetate), which has no estrogen effects, will show ambiguous

TABLE III. Secretion rate studies in the patient and a family control, the mother

Condition	Date	F	B	DOC (mg/m²/day)	S	Aldosterone	Serum Na (mEq/l)
Patient							
Incomplete treatment with cortisol but on 9α-fluoro	1/29		0.42	0.12	0.52	0.18	132
Three days off treatment, low serum sodium	2/2	1.5	0.33	0.025	0.36	0.22	115
ACTH 40 U IV over 8 hr	2/3	1.5	0.28	0.023	0.31	0.09	118
Dexamethasone 2 mg q.i.d.	2/9	0.17	0.051	0.0054	0.029	0.026	130
Mother							
Baseline	1/29	5.3	0.51	0.028	0.10	0.11	134
Low salt	2/2	8.7	1.06	0.048	0.16	0.28	130
ACTH 40 U IV over 8 hr	2/3	25.1	13.1	0.33	0.83	0.39	138
High salt	2/6	7.5	0.83	0.031	0.23	0.063	134
Dexamethasone 2 mg q.i.d.	2/9	0.50	0.75	0.058	0.05	0.066	131

genitalia and female postnatal breast development (27). When a specific inhibitor of the 3β-HSD enzyme was administered to fetal male rats, they also developed female mammary glands and hypospadias, both of which could be prevented by testosterone administration (28). This latter animal experiment mimics the clinical case presented. Finally, New (29) recently reported that marked gynecomastia occurred in a male pseudohermaphrodite with adrenal hyperplasia due to a 17a-hydroxylase defect which impaired testosterone secretion. The greatly elevated levels of Δ-5-steroids in plasma and urine confirm a 3β-HSD deficiency and exclude a 21 hydroxylase defect. The secretion rate studies confirm the site of enzymatic defect as the 3β-HSD enzyme and, in addition, suggest that the adrenal 3β-HSD enzyme for each pathway—glucocorticoid, mineralocorticoid, and sex-steroids—is the same or under the same genetic control.

Laboratory data which cast doubt on the proposal that the patient suffered from a single enzyme deficiency of 3β-HSD are the elevated urinary levels of total 17-ketosteroids, pregnanetriol, androsterone, and etiocholanolone, and the elevated plasma concentrations of progesterone, 17-OH progesterone, and testosterone. Similar paradoxical data have been observed in other recently reported patients with the 3β-HSD defect (6, 7).

A mechanism which makes these apparently paradoxical laboratory results compatible with a single enzyme deficiency of 3β-hydroxysteroid dehydrogenase is the peripheral conversion of Δ^5 compounds to Δ^4 compounds by a 3β-HSD enzyme in the liver. The liver enzyme would either be different from that of the adrenal or would be the same enzyme but under different genetic control. Thus the liver would be presented with large amounts of Δ^5 precursors from the adrenal such as pregnanetriol, pregnenolone, 17-OH-pregnenolone, and DHEA. Acted upon by liver 3β-ol-enzyme these compounds would be converted to pregnanetriol, progesterone, 17-OH progesterone, and testosterone respectively. There is experimental support for these conversions in the reports of Strott et al. (19) who showed that in man there may be up to 20% peripheral conversion of 17-OH pregnenolone to 17-OH progesterone and of 17-OH pregnenetriol to 17-OH pregnanetriol. Further, Fukushima et al. (30, 31) reported that in patients with adrenal carcinoma and one normal female, 17-OH pregnenolone was converted to pregnanetriol without the intermediate formation of 17-OH progesterone. Bongiovanni (unpublished data) has shown that when slices of calf adrenal were incubated with 17-OH pregnenolone, the 21-hydroxylase enzyme was directly inhibited. Thus the inhibition of 21-hydroxylation by the overproduction of 17-OH pregnenolone from the patient's adrenal coupled with the peripheral conversion of Δ^5-compounds to Δ^4-compounds would suffice to explain the observed increased levels in the urinary 17-ketosteroids, pregnanetriol, and plasma progesterone and 17-OH progesterone. Peripheral conversion of DHEA to testosterone has been described in humans (32) and may account for the patient's normal plasma testosterone. Since HCG may produce a rise in DHEA (33) as well as testosterone, the marked rise in plasma testosterone observed in this patient upon HCG administration may have resulted from an increased DHEA secretion and peripheral conversion to testosterone. The simultaneous administration of dexamethasone with HCG makes the adrenal and therefore DHEA an unlikely source of testosterone. It is more likely that the increase in plasma testosterone with HCG reflects a capacity of the testis to synthesize testosterone at puberty. Kenny (unpublished data) observed a similar response to HCG in two brothers, ages 7 and 9 with the 3β-HSD defect. Rivarola et al. (34) found very low plasma testosterone in a prepubertal 8-year-old boy.

Furthermore in our patient, the normal rather than high castrate levels of FSH and LH are compatible with normal testosterone secretion. This would suggest that the 3β-HSD enzyme was deficient in the fetal adrenal and testis producing hypospadias but was not deficient in the pubertal testis while the adrenal enzymatic deficiency persisted. There is precedence for the development of the 3β-HSD enzyme with age in the normal male infant. Histochemical evidence for 3β-HSD activity is absent in the newborn testis while it is present in the pubertal testis (5). In the human fetal testis, the peak of 3β-HSD activity corresponds to the time of urethral fold fusion and disappears by the time of birth (35).

Other hypotheses have been proposed to explain the presence of pregnanetriol, androsterone, and etiocholanolone in the urine. The dual enzyme defect of 3β-dehydrogenation and 21-hydroxylation has been considered (2, 8). However, it seems unnecessary and genetically improbable to suggest a double enzyme defect when all the data may be explained by a single enzyme defect of the adrenal as proposed here. Lastly, the data may result from a partial enzymatic defect, but a partial deficiency of 3β-HSD would not account for the markedly elevated levels of urinary 17-ketosteroids and pregnanetriol.

In summary, a pubertal boy with the 3β-HSD has manifested clinical and biochemical signs of puberty. The paradoxical laboratory findings can be explained on the basis of a single enzyme deficiency if it is assumed that the liver 3β-HSD enzyme is not deficient. The advent of puberty suggests the acquisition by the testis of 3β-HSD activity.

ACKNOWLEDGMENT

The authors wish to thank Dr. James German for the chromosome studies, Dr. I. Dyrenfurth for the determinations of plasma estrone and estradiol, and Dr. Ralph E. Peterson for the determination of plasma renin. We are also grateful to Dr. F. Kenny for supplying his unpublished data on the plasma testosterone values in his patients with the 3β-HSD defect.

This investigation was supported in part by grants HD 72, HE 12239, and AM 1351 from the National Institutes of Health, USPHS; The American Heart Association Award 69 686, and was also aided by grant RR 47 from the Division of General Medical Sciences, National Institutes of Health, USPHS.

REFERENCES

1. Bongiovanni, A. M., J Clin Endocrinol 21:860, 1961.
2. Bongiovanni, A. M. J Clin Invest 41:2086, 1962.
3. Goldman, A. S., A. M. Bongiovanni, W. C. Jakovac, and A. Prader, J Clin Endocrinol 24:894, 1964.
4. Hamilton, W., and M. G. Brush, Arch Dis Child 39:66, 1964.
5. David, R. R., C. Bergada, and C. J. Migeon, Bull Johns Hopkins Hosp 117:16, 1965.
6. Zachman, M., J. A. Völlmin, G. Mürset, H. -Ch. Curtius, and A. Prader, J Clin Endocrinol 30:719, 1970.
7. Janne, O., J. Perheentuba, and R. Vihko, J Clin Endocrinol 31:162, 1970.
8. Kenny, F. M., J. W. Reynolds, and O. C. Green, Program and Abstracts, 40th Annual Meeting, Society for Pediatric Research, Atlantic City, 1971.
9. Parks, G. A., J. A. Bermudez, C. S. Anast, A. M. Bongiovanni, and M. I. New, J Clin Endocrinol, accepted for publication.
10. Tahka, H., Acta Pediat 40 (suppl 81), 1951.
11. Soffer, L. J., R. I. Dorfman, and J. L. Gabrilove, The Human Adrenal Gland, Lea and Febiger, Philadelphia, 1961.
12. Tanner, J. M., Growth at Adolescence, Blackwell, Oxford, 1962.
13. New, M. I., M. P. Seaman, and R. E. Peterson, J Clin Endocrinol 29:514, 1969.
14. New, M. I., B. Miller, and R. E. Peterson, J Clin Invest 45:412, 1966.
15. Skinner, S. L., Circ Res. 20:391, 1967.
16. Gandy, H., and R. E. Peterson, J Clin Endocrinol 28:949, 1968.
17. Strott, C. A., and M. B. Lipsett, J Clin Endocrinol 28:1426, 1968.
18. Strott, C. A., T. Yoshimi, and M. B. Lipsett, J Clin Invest 48:930, 1969.
19. Strott, C. A., J. A. Bermudez, and M. B. Lipsett, J Clin Invest 49:1999, 1970.
20. Bermudez, J. A., P. Doerr, and M. B. Lipsett, Steroids, in press, 1971.
21. Lipsett, M. B., P. Doerr, J. A. Bermudez, Proc Karolinska Symposia on Research Methods in Reproductive Endocrinology, 2nd Symposium—Geneva, Switzerland, March 1970, p. 155.
22. Abraham, G. E., J Clin Endocrinol 29:866, 1969.
23. Saxena, B. B., H. Demura, H. M. Gandy, and R. E. Peterson, J Clin Endocrinol 28:519, 1968.
24. Stowens, D., Pediatric Pathology, 2nd ed. Williams & Wilkins, Baltimore, 1966, p. 686.
25. Greenblatt, R. B., and B. Perez Ballester, Medical Aspects of Human Sexuality 3:52, 1969.
26. Federman, D. D., Abnormal Sexual Development, Saunders, Philadelphia, 1967, p. 119.
27. Neumann, F., and W. Elger, J Endocrinol 36:347, 1966.
28. Neumann, F., and A. S. Goldman, Endocrinology 86:1169, 1970.
29. New, M. I., J Clin Invest 49:1930, 1970.
30. Fukushima, D. K., H. L. Bradlow, L. Hellman, and T. F. Gallagher, J Clin Endocrinol 22:765, 1962.
31. Fukushima, D. K., H. L. Bradlow, L. Hellman, and T. F. Gallagher, J Clin Endocrinol 23:263, 1963.
32. Mahesh, V. B., and R. B. Greenblatt, Acta Endocrinol (Kbh) 41:400, 1962.

33. Saez, J. M., and J. Bertrand, Steroids 12:749, 1968.
34. Rivarola, M. A., J. M. Saez, and C. J. Migeon, J Clin Endocrinol 27:624, 1967.
35. Goldman, A. S., W. C. Yakovac, and A. M. Bongiovanni, J Clin Endocrinol 26:14, 1966.

43.   Hypothalamic-Pituitary-Gonadal Interrelationships in the Rat During Sexual Maturation

Ronald S. Swerdloff, Howard S. Jacobs, and William D. Odell

Mechanisms initiating the hormonal changes responsible for puberty are not well understood. Previous workers have shown that the immature gonads of rats secrete sex steroids (1) and that the pituitary of immature animals of both sexes secrete gonadotropins (2-4). Hemicastration of immature rats results in compensatory hypertrophy of the other gonad (5), while bilateral castration results in demonstrable increase of gonadotropins in serum (2, 4, 6, 7). These studies indicate the existence in rats before puberty of an intact feedback relationship between the gonad and pituitary gonadotropin secretion.

A number of studies in rats have been reported which suggest that before puberty the hypothalamic control of gonadotropin secretion is more sensitive to feedback inhibition by gonadal steroids than after sexual maturation has occurred (7-10). These observations form the experimental basis of a hypothesis to explain the mechanism of puberty (11). At the onset of puberty, a reduction of the sensitivity for gonadal steroid feedback inhibition of gonadotropin secretion occurs; this alteration causes a greater secretion of gonadotropins, which in turn stimulates secretion of larger quantities of sex steroids. Eventually, a new equilibrium is reached, corresponding to the feedback relationship observed during the period of sexual maturity. This theory implies that serum concentrations of gonadotropins are lower in the immature rat than after sexual maturation. Earlier studies from our laboratory indicated that during sexual maturation in the male rat, serum LH concentrations increased very gradually, while FSH levels fell, rather than rose, as spermatogenesis developed. This observation did not appear to support the theory that a change in the sensitivity of feedback control of gonadotropins was responsible for the initiation of the pubertal process in rats. This has led us to reevaluate several facets of the hypothalamic-pituitary-gonadal interrelationships during sexual maturation in both male and female rats.

MATERIALS AND METHODS

The studies are divided into four categories:

Serum Gonadotropin, Gonadal and Accessory Sex Organ Weight During Sexual Maturation

Serum LH and FSH were measured from weaning (21 days) to sexual maturation in Wister strain male and female rats. Groups of 5 to 8 rats were sacrificed at regular intervals by exsanguination under light ether anesthesia. Gonadal, uterine, and ventral prostate weights were measured.

Castration Effect on Serum LH and FSH in Immature and Mature Rats

Twenty-one and 75-day-old male and female Wister rats were castrated and groups of 5 or 6 rats were bled at 9 hr, 1, 2, 3, 5, and 8 days after operation.

Determination of the Relative Sensitivity for Gonadal Steroid Feedback Inhibition of LH and FSH Secretion in Mature and Immature Male and Female Rats

MALE STUDY

Twenty-one and 75-day-old male Wister rats were castrated; 5 days later a 5-day course of daily injections of testosterone proprionate in sesame oil was begun. Groups of 5 to 6 animals received doses of testosterone ranging from 1 to 1000 μg/100 gm body weight. After 5 days treatment (a total of 10 days after castration), the animals were anesthetized, exsanguinated by aortic puncture, and ventral prostates dissected free and weighed.

FEMALE STUDY

Twenty-one and 75-day-old female Wister rats were castrated and 5 days later treated daily for 3 days with subcutaneous injections of ethinyl estradiol in sesame oil. Groups of 5 to 8 animals received doses of ethinyl estradiol ranging from 0.00012 to 0.4 μg/100 gm body weight/day. After 3 days treatment (a total of 8 days after castration), the animals were anesthetized, exsanguinated by aortic puncture, and the uterus was removed and weighed.

Determination of the Sensitivity of Gonadal Response to Exogenous LH and FSH Stimulation

Immature (21-day-old) and mature (87-day-old) rats of both sexes were hypophysectomized. Five days later LH (NIH-LH-P7) or FSH (NIH-FSH-S4) or a combination of both were injected in varying doses for varying periods of time. Control animals were injected with saline. At the varying time periods, animals were sacrificed using carbon dioxide anesthesia and uterus and ovaries or prostate and testes were removed and weighed.

Serum LH and FSH were determined by radioimmunoassay using reagents supplied by Dr. Albert Parlow through the courtesy of the NIAMD Rat Pituitary Distribution Program. We have previously reported the specificity and sensitivity of these assays as used in our laboratory (3). All samples from each experiment were measured within a single assay. The intraassay coefficient of variation was ±5%, or less, of the value determined.

In the studies requiring gonadotropin injections, the LH used was NIH-LH-P7, the FSH was NIH-FSH-S4. For studies requiring 5 days treatment subcutaneous injections were given twice daily. For the long-term studies, injections were given once daily. In all instances, a volume of 0.5 ml was given in each injection.

All rats were housed in an air conditioned, artificially lit, 12-hr light-12-hr dark environment. The rats in the first three experiments were fed Purina chow. The hypophysectomized rats in the fourth experiment were fed a diet consisting of a ground meat paste mixed with bread and milk.

RESULTS

Serum LH and FSH in Intact Male and Female Immature Rats

There was a progressive, but small, increase in serum LH concentrations between 21 and 91 days of age in male rats (Fig. 1). Serum FSH was strikingly different; FSH concentrations at 21 days of age were 180% of those at 91 days of age. FSH increased further, reaching a peak of 240% of adult levels by 49 days of age, and thereafter fell, reaching adult levels by 63 days of age. Mature sperm first were seen at 49 days of age, and spermatogenesis was complete by 63 days of age.

In the female rats, vaginal opening was noted in 60% of animals at 34 days of age, and in all animals by 36 days of age. This coincided with the time of rapid uterine and ovarian weight increase. Serum LH (Fig. 2) remained unchanged between 21 to 38 days of age, when proestrous values in those rats with vaginal opening were excluded. Serum FSH was highest at 21 days of age (the mean value being 285 ± 26 ng/ml) and fell thereafter as in the male, reaching adult diestrous values by 30 days of age.

Effect of Castration on Serum LH and FSH in Male and Female Rats

Figure 3 represents the effect of orchiectomy on serum LH and FSH in the immature and mature male rat. Blood FSH and LH concentrations increased rapidly in both sexually immature and mature animals. Figures 4 and 5 demonstrate the effect of oophorectomy on serum gonadotropins. FSH increased promptly by 9 hr after castration in both mature and immature females. However, by 3 days post-castration, FSH concentrations were consider-

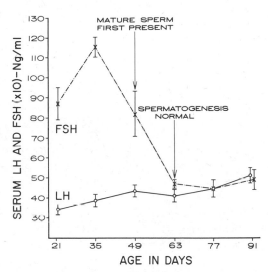

FIG. 1. Serum LH and FSH in male rats from age 21 to 91 days of age. Mature sperm were first noted at age 49 days; spermatogenesis appeared complete by 63 days.

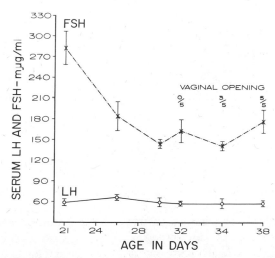

FIG. 2. Serum LH and FSH in female rats from age 21 to 38 days of age. At 34 days of age, vaginal opening had occured in 60% and at 38 days in 100% of animals. After vaginal opening, only serum samples obtained in diestrous were included (19).

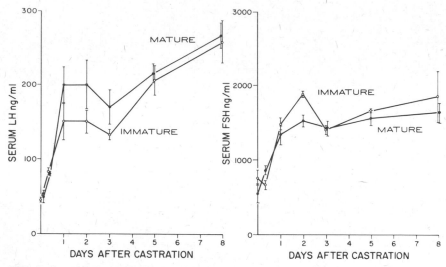

FIG. 3. Serum LH and FSH in immature and mature male rats following orchiectomy (19).

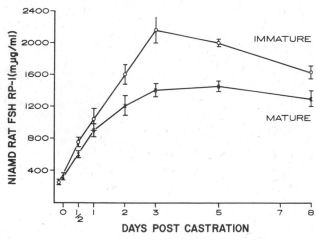

FIG. 4. Serum FSH in immature and mature female rats following oophorectomy (19).

ably greater in immature animals than they were in matures. However, as time progressed the differences were less. The effect of castration on serum LH concentration was considerably different in the mature and immature female rat. Serum LH in the mature rats increased only twofold by 8 days post-castration. In the immature rat, in contrast, LH rose more rapidly, reaching values 3½ times

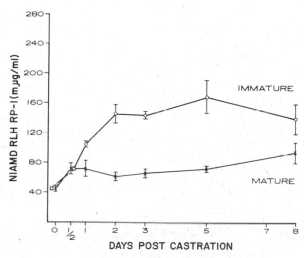

FIG. 5. Serum LH in immature and mature female rats following oophoretomy (19).

greater than those in intact values by only 5 days post-castration. By two weeks after castration, blood LH concentrations were similar in sexually immature and mature animals.

Effect of Gonadal Steroids on Feedback Inhibition of Serum LH and FSH in Mature and Immature Male and Female Rats

The change in serum LH concentration in sexually immature and mature male rats treated with testosterone is shown in Fig. 6. Doses of testosterone which increased the ventral prostate weight in both sexually mature and immature animals failed to effect serum LH (10 μg/100 g body weight). Doses of 30 μg/100 g body weight/day returned serum LH in both groups of animals to a level found in the intact rats. These results indicate that the dose of testosterone required for feedback inhibition of LH secretion was the same in sexually immature and mature animals. Figure 7 shows the changes of serum FSH concentration in both groups treated with testosterone. Doses of 100 μg/100 g body weight/day were required to suppress serum FSH to the levels found in the intact animal. Although this dose was less than that required for maximal stimulation of growth of the ventral prostate, it was greater than that required for feedback inhibition of LH secretion. The dose of testosterone which returned serum FSH concentrations to those observed in intact animals was the same in both immature and mature rats. These results indicate that sexual maturation had no effect on the sensitivity to testosterone in the feedback control of FSH secretion.

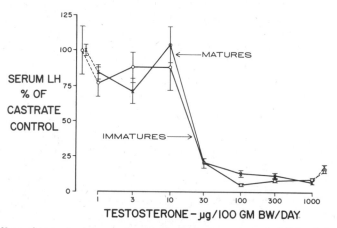

FIG. 6. Effect of testosterone propionate administration on serum LH levels in male rats. Serum LH is expressed as the percent of castrate control levels. Castrate controls are seen on the far left and intact controls on the far right (20).

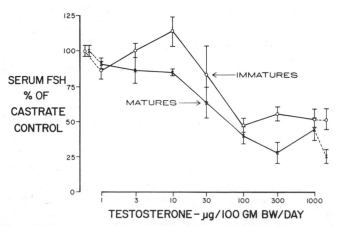

FIG. 7. Effect of testosterone proprionate administration on serum FSH levels in male rats. Serum FSH is expressed as a percent of castrate control levels. Control castrate animals are seen on the far left and control intact levels on the far right (20).

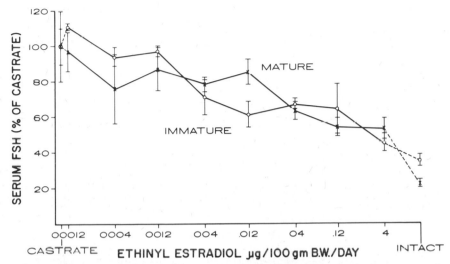

FIG. 8. Effect of ethinyl estradiol administration on serum FSH levels, in mature and immature female rats (19).

Figure 8 represents the effect of ethinyl estradiol on suppression of serum FSH in castrated female rats. As in the male, sexual maturation had no effect on the dose of gonadal steroid required to suppress serum FSH. Figure 9 shows the response of serum LH to ethinyl estradiol administration. The lowest dose of ethinyl estradiol (0.00012 μg/100 g body weight) resulted in an increase of serum LH levels in the immature rat. This increased level was 184% of the control castrate value. The mature rat also responded with an increase in serum LH levels at this lowest dose of ethinyl estradiol administration, but the increase was much smaller. The mean level was only 116% of castrate control values. Further increases in doses of ethinyl estradiol resulted in a fall of serum LH to intact levels at 0.0012 μg/100 g body weight in the mature, and 0.004 μg/100 g body weight in the immature.

Sensitivity to Exogenous LH and FSH Stimulation

STUDIES IN MALE RATS

Figure 10 depicts the prostate weight increment in the 5-day hypophysectomized male rats. Sexually immature males failed to respond to LH in doses up to 2000 μg/100 g body weight given over the 5-day study period. In contrast, the sexually mature male showed a maximal prostate weight response to 100 μg of NIH-LH-P7/100 g body weight.

In contrast to the failure of LH to elicit a response in the immature rats, FSH produced a marked increase in testicular weight (Fig. 11). In fact, the increment in testis weight response was greater in immature than in sexually mature males.

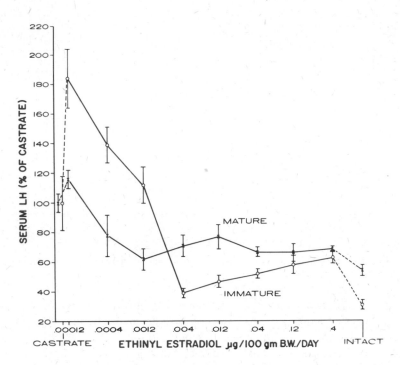

FIG. 9. Effect of ethinyl estradiol administration on serum LH levels in mature and immature female rats (19).

This is probably explained by the fact that the adult testis is nearly maximal in weight and relatively little regression occurs by 5 days after hypophysectomy. Thus further increase is difficult to ascertain. In contrast, the testes in the intact sexually immature animal is only partially developed, and regresses even further after hypophysectomy. FSH administered alone produced little or no increase in prostate weight.

Because the acutely (1 day) hypophysectomized, or intact, immature male is quite sensitive to exogenous LH, but the 5-day post-hypophysectomized immature male was not, we asked whether the difference might be explained by the effects of FSH on the response to LH, for example, might FSH induce sensitivity to LH? Accordingly, studies were performed in the 5-day hypophysectomized rat evaluating the effects of 5-day periods of combined LH and FSH treatment in animals receiving previous treatment with FSH alone.

Table I presents the data for prostate weight response. LH given alone in large doses (100 μg/100 gm body weight) produced a tiny prostate weight increment at 10 days, but no significant effect (over saline injected controls) at 25 and 30

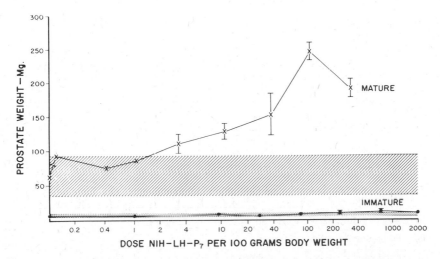

FIG. 10. Effect of 5 days of LH administration on ventral prostate weight in mature and immature male rats. All animals were hypophysectomized at 21 days of age (weaning) and injections were begun 5 days later (26 days of age) and continued for 5 days (31 days of age). The shaded area includes the 95% limits of prostate weight in saline injected control animals. The amount of NIH-LH-P7 administered over the 5-day treatment period is shown on the abscissa (21).

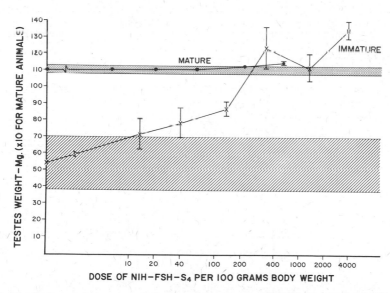

FIG. 11. Testis weight response to 5 days of treatment with FSH. As described in Fig. 10, animals were hypophysectomized at 21 days of age and injections begun at 26 days of age. Shaded areas encompass the 95% limits of testes weight in saline injected control animals (21).

TABLE I. Prostate weight response to LH[a] in rats receiving pretreatment with FSH[b] for varying times[c]

Treatment	Duration of treatment (days)		
	10	25	30
Saline	5.3 ± 0.3	5.2 ± 0.2	4.7 ± 0.4
LH	6.6 ± 0.3	5.6 ± 0.2	4.9 ± 0.3
FSH	6.8 ± 0.4	6.7 ± 0.4	6.2 ± 0.4
FSH and LH	7.2 ± 0.2	8.5 ± 0.6[d]	13.5 ± 2.4[d]

[a]LH−20 μg/day during last 5 days FSH treatment.

[b]FSH−60 μg/day for periods indicated.

[c]The format of this study was to administer FSH for varying periods of time (10, 25, and 30 days), and to combine FSH with LH during the last 5 days of treatment. Prostate weight (± SEM) is given in mg.

[d]At 25 and 30 days, FSH given with LH produced a greater response than either given alone ($p < 0.05$). (From Odell et al. ref. 21.)

days treatment. FSH administered alone also produced a very small increase in prostate weight at 10 days, but no greater response after 25 and 30 days. However, when FSH pretreatment preceded the 5-day LH and FSH treatment, a response to LH became apparent. Most importantly, the prostate weight increased progressively with time of exposure to a constant dose of FSH followed by a constant dose of FSH and LH.

TABLE II. Testes weight response to LH in rats receiving pretreatment with FSH[a] for varying times

Treatment	Duration of treatment (days)		
	10	25	30
Saline	134 ± 6.8	135 ± 5.8	115 ± 3.8
LH	168 ± 6.2	142 ± 7.2	141 ± 2.8
FSH	371 ± 21.2	409 ± 61.3	535 ± 102
FSH and LH	381 ± 10.6	565 ± 92.8	853 ± 145

[a]FSH−60 μg/day for periods indicated. (From Odell et al. ref. 21.)

Table II depicts the testis weight response for the same study depicted in Table I. While FSH alone induced a marked testicular weight increment, a larger response was observed when LH was administered with FSH during the last 5 days of the treatment period.

In separate studies we evaluated the prostate weight response to administered testosterone. This was necessary since any effects of LH on prostate weight are mediated by LH stimulation of testosterone production by the Leydig cells. No significant differences in dose of testosterone required to stimulate prostate growth were observed when sexually immature rats were compared to mature male animals.

These studies then indicate that LH is ineffective in the male in stimulating prostate weight, unless it is preceded by treatment with FSH. Furthermore, the effect of LH administered at constant dose becomes greater with time of pretreatment with FSH; in essence a time-response relationship exists.

STUDIES IN FEMALE RATS

Figure 12 depicts the response of 5-day hypophysectomized female rats to exogenous LH. As in the male, no response of sex accessories (uterine weight or

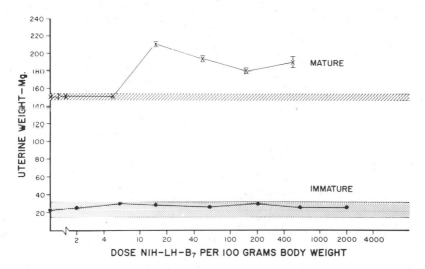

FIG. 12. Effect of 5 days of daily treatment with LH (NIH-LH-P7) to hypophysectomized female mature and immature rats. Experimental protocol as described in Fig. 10 and 11 for male rats. Dose of LH is total dose administered over 5 days (22).

vaginal plate opening) could be elicited in the female immature rat by up to 2,000 μg of LH, administered over 5 days time. This was contrasted with a maximal uterine weight response in adult animals produced by 15 μg LH. FSH response, studied by its effect on ovarian weight, produced large increments in ovarian weight in both sexually immature and mature females; no differences in threshold dose existed (Fig. 13). Thus the female appeared to respond similarly

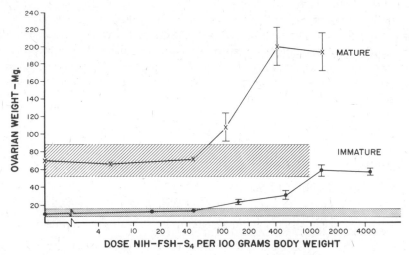

FIG. 13. Effect of 5 days of daily treatment with FSH (NIH-FSH-S4) to hypophysecto-mized female mature and immature rats. Experimental protocol was as described in Fig. 10 and 11. Dose of FSH is total dose administered over 5 days (22).

to the male in these studies. However, in contrast to the studies in males, the 5-day hypophysectomized female rat showed marked sex accessory development in that both uterine weight increase and vaginal plate opening resulted from FSH treatment given alone.

Because of these findings, additional long-term studies were undertaken in the female. The dose of FSH (60 μg) just smaller than the minimal effective dose, judged from the data presented in Fig. 13, was administered each day for 5, 10, 20, and 30 days time. This ineffective FSH dose was accompanied with a maximal dose of LH (judged from data in Fig. 12) during the last 5 days of treatment. In these studies, pretreatment with this low dose of FSH failed to induce any response to the large doses of LH after 10, 20, or 30 days of treatment.

DISCUSSION

We have previously discussed the difficulty of the precise timing of the age of puberty in male rats (3) and have operationally defined the age of sexual maturation as the time at which mature spermatogenesis is fully established. In the strain of rats used in this study, this occurred between 49 and 63 days of age (3). In a similar fashion, we have operationally defined the onset of puberty in female rats as the time of vaginal opening and the onset of growth spurt in uterine and ovarian weight. Accordingly, for the studies reported here, weanling rats of 21 days of age, an age clearly prior to puberty, were selected as representative of immature animals of both sexes. The mature rats (75 days old) were the same age as those used for breeding in the laboratory from which they were obtained.

In the male rat, a slow progressive rise in serum LH levels and a coincident fall in serum FSH levels occurred. In the female rat, serum LH did not change significantly from age 21 through 38 days of age (a period which would appear to encompass puberty). During this same period FSH fell in the female, as it had done in the male rat. Goldman et al. (4) have reported that serum LH and FSH values in male rats during the first 12 days of life were lower than those in adults. In the female rat, serum LH values were quite variable; mean concentrations of LH prior to age 12 days were higher than those of adult diestrous animals; serum FSH was also higher than adult levels and increased progressively throughout the 12-day period. Our data, combined with those of Goldman, would appear to be inconsistent with the hypothesis that serum gonadotropins are low prior to puberty in the rat with an abrupt pubertal increase being responsible for sexual maturation.

Several studies in rats have been reported which suggested that the hypothalamic-pituitary axis was more sensitive to feedback inhibition by gonadal steroids before, as compared to after, sexual maturation (7-10). These studies led to the hypothesis that the puberty process was initiated by an upward set of feedback control mechanisms which resulted in a concomitant increase of gonadotropins and gonadal steroids at the time of puberty.

Because the serum gonadotropin data described above seemed inconsistent with this hypothesis, we undertook studies to test directly the sensitivity of suppression of gonadotropin secretion after administration of testosterone and estrogen. When doses of testosterone and estrogen were given according to body weight, sexual maturation did not influence sensitivity to suppression of serum LH and FSH in male rats and serum FSH in female rats. In the female, the effects of estrogen administration on LH were more complex. Low doses of LH stimulated LH secretion, while higher doses suppressed LH. Despite the difficulties in separating the roles of negative and positive feedback (both might be working simultaneously and in opposite directions) we interpret the data as indicating little difference between age groups with regard to suppression of serum LH levels with increasing doses of estrogen. The observation of a striking increase in serum LH at the very lowest dose of ethinyl estradiol in the immature rat was most interesting. This we feel represents increased sensitivity of the female rat to positive feedback by gonadal steroids. This observation is consistent with those of others in which precocious puberty, including subsequent cyclicity, could be produced by brief estrogen administration to immature animals (9-13) and with the now well-recognized role of estrogen in positive feedback effect on LH secretion in the mature rat (14-16).

The lack of difference in negative feedback between mature and immature animals of both sexes in our study is in direct contrast to those of Ramirez and McCann (7, 9). These workers found that 3 to 4 times larger doses of testosterone or estrogen were required to suppress serum LH in castrated mature than in sexually immature animals. There are a number of differences in the design and execution of the experiments of Ramirez and McCann; they initiated treatment immediately after castration, rather than after a delay of 5 days as in our study. Secondly, the period of treatment was longer in their studies (14 to 23 days) as compared to 3 days in the female rat and 5 days in the male rat in our studies. Lastly, these workers utilized the ovarian ascorbic acid depletion assay to qualify serum LH, an assay which is considerably less sensitive than the radioimmunoassays utilized in our studies.

The studies of Smith and Davidson (10) utilizing hypothalamic implantation of estrogen and androgens also have suggested that the hypothalamus is more steroid-sensitive in prepubertal rats. Interpretation of these results are often complicated because doses of steroids were not adjusted for marked differences in body weight. That the differences in their results and our results could be attributed to different rates of utilization of the hormone in mature and immature rats does not appear to be likely in view of the studies demonstrating that disappearance rate of injected testosterone (17) and metabolic clearance rates of estrogen (18) are similar in mature and immature rats.

Our studies indicate that the pubertal process in male and female rats is not initiated by a change in the sensitivity of the hypothalamic-pituitary unit to negative feedback suppression by testosterone or estrogen.

Our studies of gonadal sensitivity to exogenous LH and FSH may offer an alternative hypothesis to explain sexual maturation in the male rat. The prepubertal male (or female rat) 5 days post-hypophysectomy was totally unresponsive to LH; similarly treated sexually mature animals responded to LH. Presumably this is because the immature gonad "regresses" in 5 days to a near baseline unstimulated state, whereas the mature gonad "regresses," but not to this baseline. Again presumably, in a much longer period post-hypophysectomy, the gonad of the mature animal would also be unresponsive. However, gonads from both mature and immatures responded to FSH. Pretreatment with FSH over 20 to 30 days time returned the testis to a state of responsiveness to LH. Thus in the male, sexual maturation could occur, theoretically in 30 or more days with a constant secretion (or administration) of maximal doses of both LH and FSH. The exact time of sex accessory development in such a theoretical scheme might be altered if lower doses of either LH or FSH were administered. The important point is that a time-response relationship exists.

The studies on the female indicate sexual maturation may be controlled differently in the two sexes. While the 5-day hypophysectomized female rat failed to respond to LH alone, FSH alone did result in increase in uterine weight and vaginal opening. Low dose FSH treatment did not induce sensitivity to LH in 30 days time. At present the mechanism of sexual maturation in the female remains obscure. However, we note that in intact females, LH concentrations did not change during sexual maturation, while FSH fell. Abrupt onset of LH and FSH secretion, changes in feedback sensitivity, or gradually increasing LH and

FSH concentrations do not exist to explain puberty. The mechanisms of maturation in the female remain unknown, and appear to be different than those in the male.

REFERENCES

1. Resko, J. A., H. H. Feder, and R. W. Goy, J Endocrinol 40:485, 1968.
2. Yamamoto, M., N. D. Diebel, and E. M. Bogdanove, Endocrinology 86:1102, 1970.
3. Swerdloff, R. S., P. C. Walsh, H. S. Jacobs, and W. D. Odell, Endocrinology 88:120, 1971.
4. Goldman, B. D., Y. R. Grazia, I. A. Kamberi, and J. C. Porter, Endocrinology 88:771, 1971.
5. Yaginuma, T., A. Matsuda, Y. Murasawa, and T. Kobayashi, Endocrinol Japan 16:5, 1969.
6. Kallas, H., C R Soc Biol 100:979, 1929.
7. Ramirez, V. D., and S. M. McCann, Endocrinology 72:452, 1963.
8. Byrnes, W. W., and R. K. Meyer, Endocrinology 49:449, 1951.
9. Ramirez, V. D., and S. M. McCann, Endocrinology 76:412, 1965.
10. Smith, E. R., and J. M. Davidson, Endocrinology 82:100, 1968.
11. Donovan, B. T., and J. J. Van der Werff ten Bosch, J Physiol 147:78, 1959.
12. Hohlweg, W., Klin Wschr 13:92, 1934.
13. Motta, M., F. Fraschini, G. Guiliani and L. Martini, Endocrinology 83:1101, 1968.
14. Vande Wiele, R. L., J. Bogumil, I. Dyrenfurth, M. Ferin, R. Jewelwicz, M. Warren, T. Rizkallah, and G. Mikhail, Rec Prog Hormone Res 26:63, 1970.
15. Swerdloff, R. S., H. S. Jacobs, and W. D. Odell (Abstract), Program of 52nd Meeting, Endocrine Society, June 10-12, 1970.
16. Wyck, R. F., E. R. Smith, R. Dominguez, A. Chariwal, and J. Davidson, Endocrinology 88:293, 1971.
17. Ulrich, R. S., and J. R. Kent, Proc Soc Exp Biol Med 128:1093, 1968.
18. DeHertogh, R., E. Ekka, I. Vanderheyden, and J. J. Hoet, Endocrinology 87:874, 1970.
19. Swerdloff, R. S., H. S. Jacobs, and W. D. Odell, submitted to Endocrinology, July 1971.
20. Jacobs, H. S., R. S. Swerdloff, and W. D. Odell, submitted to J Clin Invest May 1971.
21. Odell, W. D., R. S. Swerdloff, and H. S. Jacobs, submitted to J Clin Invest, June 1971.
22. Odell, W. D., R. S. Swerdloff, and H. S. Jacobs, submitted to Endocrinology, July 1971.

DISCUSSION

B. LUNENFELD. We have shown on numerous occasions during the last 20 years that single gonadotropic or sex steroid estimates are of little value in elucidating physiological or pathological events in female reproduction. Hormonal patterns yield more information. Moreover, I believe that chronological age has little meaning since it often cannot be directly related to the individual's biological age. Parameters such as "bone age" or "sexual maturation indices" may be more useful. One interesting finding not stressed is the increase of the SD of the LH values. They are small (0.3) in the 8-year-old group of girls and progressively increasing to 13.1 in the 13 to 14 year age group. This increase probably reflects the onset of cyclic activity.

I would like to congratulate Dr. Swerdloff on his most interesting paper. Drs. Eckstein and Hockmann at the Hebrew University in Jerusalem have recently demonstrated that the major steroid metabolite in the rat ovary prior to puberty is 5α-androstane-3α, 17β-diol. They have also shown that FSH can induce an epimerase system which will transform this compound to the 3β-epimer. The 3β-epimer advances vaginal opening and this is followed by normal cyclicity. These findings suggest that the release of FSH occurring prior to puberty leads to the induction of an epimerase system in the ovary, which converts the 5α-androstane-$3\alpha,17\beta$-diol to a biologically active 3β-epimer. This causes, directly or indirectly, vaginal opening, cyclicity, and onset of puberty.

R. S. SWERDLOFF. We are aware of some of the studies of your colleagues. Dr. Grover and I have tried to reproduce this effect of both the α and β epimers in the female immature rat. We have administered 5α-androstane-$3\beta,17\beta$-diol to 21-day-old female rats. We were able to demonstrate precocious vaginal opening in 4 out of 7 animals at 28 days in response to a dose of 5 mg/kg for 7 days. No increase in serum LH or FSH was seen. One mg/kg for 6 days in 21-day-old female rats did not result in precocious vaginal opening. The requirement of such a large dose of this compound for vaginal opening suggested to us that the effect may be due to a metabolite of the compound. We are interested, however, in pursuing this avenue.

R. PENNY. I agree with you that relating FSH and LH levels to age probably is not good We should relate these to stage of sexual maturation. In respect to utilizing a single serum value for evaluation, again, I agree with you. However, I can add that we do have data on 24-hr urines in males which agree with the serum data. At this time we do not have data on females. The single specimen is particularly variable once sexual development is at stage 3 or beyond. This is particularly true for serum LH, and less true for serum FSH, which possibly relates to the difference in half-life.

R. B. JAFFE. Dr. New, there is one possible explanation for your apparently paradoxical finding of increased delta-4,3-ketosteroids in your patient. If, in addition to the relative deficiency of 3β-hydroxysteroid dehydrogenase, your patient also has a relative deficiency of sulfokinase, then there would be increased free delta-5,3β-hydroxysteroids available for conversion to their delta-4,3-keto analogs. Even though there is a relative deficiency of the 3β-hydroxysteroid dehydrogenase enzyme, this might explain your increased concentrations of 17-hydroxyprogesterone.

M. NEW. The patient had a great quantity of sulfates in urine, which I think rules out a sulfokinase deficiency.

R. B. JAFFE. I suppose that plausibility of this thesis and one enzyme being involved rather than two enzymes could be tested if one measured the sulfates.

C. A. PAULSEN. We have all been interested in the concept of the changing sensitivity of the so-called gonadostat. What are your latest data with respect to the ability of clomiphene to inhibit gonadotropin secretion in the adult male or female?

R. KELCH. As you probably remember, Drs. Kulin, Weinstein, Kaplan, and Grumbach reported some preliminary information on gonadotropin suppression in adult males with high doses of clomiphene. These studies, as yet, have not been extended and the data remains as presented. Five hundred mg of clomiphene resulted in a downward trend, but did not suppress the urinary gonadotropins to undetectable levels as in our children.

C. A. PAULSEN. Unfortunately, at the time we evaluated this issue, we utilized the parameter of total urinary gonadotropin excretion titers. However, the administration of as much as 1 g of clomiphene citrate (racemic)/day for 3 months to postmemopausal women did not result in any decrease in urinary gonadotropin excretion titers.

R. M. BLIZZARD. It is important to remember that the clomiphene which was used is a racemic mixture. These studies really ought to be done with pure trans and cis compounds.

R. KELCH. I would like to ask Dr. Swerdloff if he feels that the castrate animal is the appropriate way or perhaps the best way to look at the altered sensitivity of the hypothalamus. I wonder what happens to the hypothalamus after castration before and after the onset of puberty. Our observations on patients with gonadal dysgenesis indicate that although we may achieve sufficient or adequate feminization with physiologic doses of ethinyl estradiol or Premarin, their gonadotropins do not suppress into the normal range. I believe Dr. Penny has other information on it.

R. S. SWERDLOFF. I think Dr. Kelch's point is well taken. There are methodological problems which make it difficult to measure an entire dose response curve of LH in response to graded doses of gonadal steroids in the intact animal.

L. MARTINI. We have approached the problem of changes of sensitivity of the gonadostat at the biochemical level. You know that testosterone must be converted, at tissue level, to dihydrotestosterone (DHT) in order to become fully active.

Confirming data also obtained by Dr. Jaffe, we have been able to show that the amygdala, the hypothalamus, and the anterior pituitary of adult male rats are able to convert testosterone to DHT. The conversion is not as great as that which is found in the prostate and in the seminal vesicles, but it is significant. We wanted to see whether there was a change in the activity of the 5α reductase involved in such a process around the time of sexual maturation. We have found that the conversion of testosterone to DHT in the hypothalamus is more efficient in young animals than in older animals. There are two moments in which a decrease in the converting ability is observed. One occurs between 7 and 14 days of age; the other occurs between 28 and 35 days of age. The pituitary of young animals converts testosterone into DHT to a much greater extent than the pituitary of animals of more advanced age. Again, you find two moments at which 5α reductase activity decreases, the first being again between 7 and 14 days of age and the second between 35 and 60 days of age. It was shown this morning that 60 days is the time at which full maturation of the testis occurs. We feel that our data might provide a biochemical basis for understanding the change in sensitivity of the gonadostat at the time of puberty in male animals.

R. S. SWERDLOFF. I wonder whether anyone here has any idea why the patients with gonadal dysgenesis do not raise their LH levels higher; that is, why the levels of LH often remain in the normal range, while the FSH values are clearly elevated out of the normal range. Are the gonads of these patients producing steroids which are acting as inhibitors on the hypothalamic-pituitary axis?

R. M. BLIZZARD. Possibly, it is not related to the gonadal structure itself. The castrated individuals also have a disproportionate increase of FSH over LH. One finds the same thing in the menopausal women, as you know. We would interpret these data as though there are different feedback mechanisms for these gonadotropins, which is an unsatisfactory answer. Hopefully later on in the morning after some of the other papers are presented, we may be able to come forth with some better ideas.

C. A. PAULSEN. I believe that you have focused on the key issue, that is, there are two different mechanisms for feedback control of the gonadotropins, one for FSH and one for LH. We should remember that an individual who is agonadal by virtue of either a congenital anomaly (e.g., Turner's syndrome) or surgical castration, or in the case of the normal postmenopausal woman, has normal adrenal cortical function. Thus, sex steroids are being secreted which would tend to modulate the delta increase in LH, whereas the negative feedback mechanism for FSH secretion no longer exists.

J. GOLDZIEHER. I want to comment on Dr. Kelch's observation that 2 µg of ethinyl estradiol did not produce an elevation in plasma gonadotropins. This is in contrast to the positive feedback effect that can be seen in the adult and was just demonstrated in the immature rat. I think it is an important observation and its implications are obvious. The things that we heard in the past couple of days on the effect of dose and duration of an estrogen stimulating positive feedback are very relevant to this point. Two µg of ethinyl estradiol is not a small dose in a small child, when 5 µg in a single dose will produce a positive feedback elevation of gonadotropins in the adult. I hope that Dr. Kelch will consider lowering his doses. One might also consider some technical problems that arise when small doses are used. The crystal size and formulation of the medication have a great deal to do with biological effectiveness. Finally, you might consider not just ethinyl estradiol but estradiol benzoate, which was used in some other experiments reported early today. These experiments are so important that I hope they will be expanded to include progressively smaller doses.

W. H. DAUGHADAY. I would like to ask Dr. McArthur or Dr. Blizzard if they could give an adequate explanation of why the urinary gonadotropins, as compared to plasma gonadotropins, show so much difference in pre- and post-puberty. This certainly is true of the biological urinary gonadotropins. I am impressed that plasma gonadotropins at puberty rise, but at the lower limits there is overlap in the pre- and post-pubertal individual. This does not seem to be true in the urinary gonadotropin measurement to the same extent.

R. M. BLIZZARD. As most of you know, we have been interested in extracting urine using acetone or ethanol and then using radioimmunoassay. We have applied this technique to urines collected during various stages of development. The increment of increase in urine LH from prepubertal children to adults is 12 times (2.3 ± 0.8 to 31.3 ± 10.3 IU/24 hr), which is a very significant increase. This is comparable to the increment that has been reported for bioassayable LH utilizing kaolin extracts. The increment of increase for FSH in urine is about 4 times; the increment in serum for LH is approximately 3 times, and for serum FSH, as done in our laboratory, about 2 times. Therefore, the urinary determinations for LH eliminate much of the overlap that one sees when using serum for LH. Part of your question was, "why does one find such high values of immunoreactive material in urine, in contrast to the bioassayable material?" This is related, we believe, to the fact that the kaolin extraction procedure takes out approximately 60 to 75% of the radioimmunoassayable material. This is the same percentage whether it is a prepubertal child's, an adult's or a postmeno-pausal urine that is being tested. We do not know at this point in time whether the material which is removed is biologically active or inactive. There are a lot of difficulties, as you are aware, with using acetone precipitates in the bioassay.

R. B. JAFFE. I would like to ask Dr. Martini a question. In the studies that we did on the conversion of testosterone to dihydrotestosterone in rat hypothalamus and pituitary, we used male rats. In the similar conversion that we showed in the human fetus, we used a female fetus. Was there a significant sex difference in the conversions?

L. MARTINI. We have also studied the brain and the pituitary of the female rat. There is a high 5α reductase activity in the hypothalamus and in the pituitary of the female; the amounts of testosterone converted to DHT are quite similar to those found in adult male rats.

Pituitary-Testicular Axis

44. Gonadotropic and Gonadal Function in the Normal Adult Male

Henry G. Burger, H. W. G. Baker, Bryan Hudson, and H. Pincus Taft

Any review of the factors which control testicular function should take into account not only the relationship between hypothalamus, anterior pituitary, and testis, but also the effects of changes in the internal and external environment on this system. The purpose of this contribution will be to discuss some aspects of the physiology of the gonadotropins in the male, of the control of steroidogenesis and gametogenesis, and of the factors involved in the feedback relationship between testis and pituitary. Finally, some of the external influences (e.g., liver disease) on male reproductive function will be considered. For reference purposes, normal values for plasma gonadotropins and gonadal steroids from the author's laboratory are shown in Table I.

HYPOTHALAMIC CONTROL OF THE PITUITARY

Although a description of current knowledge of the synthesis and secretion of the hypothalamic factors regulating pituitary production of gonadotropins is beyond the scope of this paper, it would seem appropriate to refer briefly to studies in which the presence of LH releasing hormone in hypophyseal portal blood of male rats has been confirmed (5). Figure 1 illustrates the results of injecting saline, and extracts of hypophyseal portal blood into ovariectomized rats pretreated with estrogen and progesterone. Serum levels of LH in the recipient animals, measured by radioimmunoassay (RIA) showed no significant change after the injection of saline: the extract of 1 ml of portal blood caused a

TABLE I. Normal values for gonadotropins and gonadal steroids in adult males

Hormone	Mean	Range	Reference
FSH	3.5 mIU/ml[a]	<1.7-6.6	1
LH	3.6 mIU/ml	0.6-6.6	2
Testosterone	690 ng/100 ml	270-1110	3
Estradiol	3.8 ng/100 ml	0.6-11.0	4

[a]In the authors' laboratory, a crude human pituitary gonadotropin (HPG) has been used as a standard for immunoassay. Immunological potencies of plasma samples have been converted to mIU on the basis of the biological potency (2nd IRP-HMG) of this standard. The potency of the latter in terms of 2nd IRP-HMG, are as follows: 40 IU FSH, 144 IU LH/mg by bioassay and 112 IU FSH, 980 IU LH/mg by immunoassay.

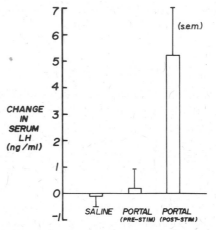

FIG. 1. Mean change (ng/ml ± SEM) in serum LH of ovariectomized, steroid treated rats, after injection of saline, and of the extracts from 1 ml of hypophyseal portal blood from anaesthetized male rats, before and after electrical stimulation of the medial preoptic area of the hypothalamus.

small rise, 0.2 ng/ml ± 0.7 (SEM), but after hypothalamic stimulation in the donor animals, a similar extract caused a rise of 5.2 ± 1.8 ng/ml. Electrical stimulation of the hypothalamus in the donor animals had been shown, in previous experiments, to produce a marked increase in endogenous serum LH.

These observations are consistent with current knowledge of the neuroendocrine control of the pituitary; the details of the mechanism of action of the releasing hormones, and whether these are separate for FSH and LH has been reviewed at another symposium (6). Kastin et al. (7) have recently given material purified from human hypothalamic tissue to 2 normal adult males, and have demonstrated a mean increase of 163% in plasma LH; the material presumably represents human LHRF.

PITUITARY GONADOTROPINS

Pituitary Content and Production Rates

Extensive data on the pituitary content of LH and FSH in normal adult males are not readily available; Ryan (8) reported that the average pituitary content of LH, measured by bioassay, in 10 males ages 19 to 40 who died suddenly was 0.95 mg NIII-LII-S1 (equivalent to 475 IU). Pooled pituitary glands contain approximately 400 IU FSH/gland (9). Estimates of the daily production rates of the two hormones can be derived from measurements of their peripheral plasma levels and metabolic clearance rates (MCR). Kohler et al. (10) found the MCR of LH to be 35 liter/day in premenopausal women and one male subject in their study had a similar MCR. Keller (11) found that the bioassayable LH content of normal male plasma was 14.4 mIU/ml, and Kulin et al. (12) found 6.1 mIU/ml; a daily production rate of 214 to 490 IU can therefore be calculated. For FSH, MCR has been found to be 20 l/day in premenopausal women (13). If a similar figure can be assumed for males, a daily production rate of 176 to 230 IU can be derived from the mean bioassayable FSH content of male plasma, 8.8 mIU/ml (11) and 11.5 mIU/ml (12). These data suggest that there is a daily turnover of between 50 and 100% of the total pituitary content of both gonadotropins.

Peripheral Plasma Concentrations

Table II shows the peripheral plasma concentrations of FSH and LH reported by a number of investigators for the normal adult male both by bioassay and RIA. The standard most commonly used has been of postmenopausal urinary origin (2nd IRP-HMG). A wide range of mean concentrations of both hormones has been reported (4.1 to 16.9 mIU/ml for FSH, 10.9 to 24.2 mIU/ml for LH) even when a single standard has been employed; this may result from the variable properties of different antisera, and other unexplained factors (27).

The question of diurnal variation in plasma gonadotropins has been examined by a number of authors. Faiman and Ryan (28) showed that the concentrations of FSH in the plasma of healthy young adult males were greatest in the early morning, near 5 A.M. and that they decreased between noon and 4 P.M. A diurnal variation in FSH was also reported by Saxena et al. (23), but no such variation could be discerned by Franchimont (14), Peterson et al. (29), and Swerdloff and Odell (30). Evidence regarding LH is also conflicting: no diurnal variation was observed by Odell et al. (18), Peterson et al. (29), and Faiman and Ryan (28), while LH and testosterone appeared to vary concomitantly in the studies of Saxena et al. (23) and Burger et al. (31). A more recent study (32) however, failed to demonstrate significant diurnal change in LH.

In contrast, several studies have confirmed the presence of a diurnal variation

TABLE II. Gonadotropin concentrations in the plasma of adult males

FSH (mIU/ml) Mean (range; SEM)	LH (mIU/ml) Mean (range; SEM)	Standard	Reference
	Bioassay		
8.8[a]	14.4[b]	2nd IRP[d]	Keller (11)
	16.8[c]	2nd IRP	Keller (11)
11.5[a] (10.1-13.3)	6.1[b] (3.8-9.7)	2nd IRP	Kulin et al. (12)
	Immunoassay		
4.1	13.1	2nd IRP	Franchimont (14)
4.9 (2.6-11.8)		HPFSH[e]	Faiman and Ryan (15)
	22.6 (11.7-35.9)	HPLH[f]	Faiman and Ryan (16)
6.0 (3.5-8.6		IRP-2	Midgley (17)
	14.4 (6.4-25.6)	2nd IRP	Odell et al. (18)
5-25		2nd IRP	Odell et al. (19)
1.3-8.2		2nd IRP	Rosselin and Dolais (20)
	22.5 (5-68)	2nd IRP	Burger et al. (21)
	24.2 (15-31)	2nd IRP	Catt et al. (22)
16.9 (3.9-42.0)	14.0 (2.5-31.5)	2nd IRP	Saxena et al. (23)
	10.9 ± 4.0	2nd IRP	Johanson et al. (24)
7.4 ± 1.9		2nd IRP	Raiti et al. (25)
9.1		2nd IRP	Yen and Vicic (26)

[a]Ovarian augmentation assay.

[b]Ventral prostate weight assay.

[c]Ovarian ascorbic acid depletion assay.

[d]Second international reference preparation.

[e]Human pituitary FSH (100 NIH-FSH-SI U/mg).

[f]Human pituitary LH (3.35 NIH-LH-SI U/mg).

in plasma testosterone (31, 33-35). Southren et al. (35) showed that there was no significant diurnal change in MCR of testosterone in the same subjects, and therefore concluded that there is a true diurnal variation in production rate, the cause of which remains obscure. Although Peterson et al. (29) did not waken their subjects, in whom no diurnal variations were seen, a closer study of the concentrations of gonadotropins during sleep is required. Evans et al. (36) recently reported the concentrations of plasma testosterone in normal men during sleep, and showed that peaks occurred in conjunction with or adjacent to periods of rapid eye movement (REM). The presence of diurnal variation was again seen. In view of recent demonstrations that growth hormone (37) and thyroid stimulating hormone (38) rise during sleep, it seems appropriate to examine gonadotropin levels under the carefully controlled conditions of a "sleep laboratory."

Longitudinal studies (29, 31) have shown that the levels of both FSH and LH remain fairly constant from day to day, unlike the cyclical variations in premenopausal females; testosterone concentrations are more variable, but do not show a regular pattern.

The possibility that seasonal fluctuations might occur in gonadotropin and testosterone concentrations has not been widely examined. In the course of two studies (39) on the effects of HCG on plasma gonadotropins and testosterone, however, it was observed that the mean concentrations of LH and testosterone in a group of 5 normal males aged 22 to 27, studied in the Australian spring, were 5.12 ± 0.69 (SEM) mIU/ml and 582 ± 58 ng/ml respectively, compared with values of 3.03 ± 0.23 and 413 ± 20 in 6 males aged 21 to 27 who were studied during winter. These mean values differed significantly at the 2% probability level. FSH concentrations, in contrast, were not significantly different (4.76 to 4.69 mIU/ml). The question of seasonal fluctuation requires further examination.

Several investigators have shown that plasma gonadotropin levels in adult males rise with age. Thus Schalch et al. (40) showed that mean plasma LH in males aged 20 to 40 was 7.0 ± 2 mIU/ml, compared with 17.0 ± 4.0 m IU/ml in males aged 50 to 80. Ryan and Faiman (41) showed that males over 50 years of age may segregate into two populations based on serum concentrations of FSH and LH, with one of the groups showing levels higher than those seen in young men, while the second group had lower values.

TESTICULAR FUNCTION

Steroid Secretion

The subject of steroid secretion by the testes has been extensively reviewed at a recent symposium (6) and by Vermeulen (42). The normal daily production rate of testerone in young adult men is between 5 and 10 mg/day, and fails by about one-third in old age. In excess of 95% is derived from testicular secretion, the remaining 5% from peripheral interconversion from other steroid precursors, notably androstenedione.

The secretion of testosterone is under the control of LH; before puberty, when no mature Leydig cells are identifiable in the testis, levels of plasma and urinary LH are low. Rising levels of testosterone and gonadotropins correlate well with the stages of puberty and with Leydig cell development. Faiman and Winter (43) suggested that the pubertal surge in testicular growth and testosterone production results from the attainment of critical threshold levels of gonadotropins, as plasma testosterone was reported to rise abruptly at age 12, in contrast to the gradual rise in gonadotropins.

In the adult, HCG has been used as an interstitial cell stimulating hormone in the evaluation of testicular function. In the study referred to above (39), plasma testosterone, gonadotropin, and estradiol were measured daily before and during the intramuscular administration of HCG, 1500 IU b.i.d. for 4 days, to 5 young adult males, and the results are shown in Fig. 2. There was a rise in plasma

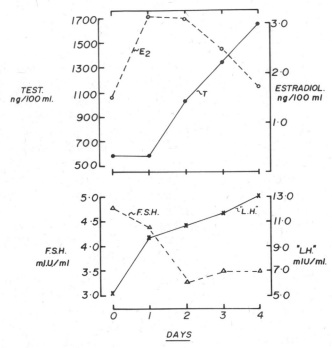

FIG. 2. Mean plasma concentrations (5 subjects, aged 22 to 27) of plasma FSH, LH, testosterone, and estradiol after the daily administration of 3000 IU HCG for 4 days.

testosterone from 582 ± 58 (SEM) to 1648 ± 128 ng/100 ml, elevated levels being seen only on the second day of HCG. Plasma LH-like immunoreactivity rose steadily, from 5.12 ± 0.69 to 13.1 ± 1.3 mIU/ml. There was a transient small rise in estradiol (from 1.52 ± 0.37 to 3.10 ± 0.35 ng/100 ml), and a fall in FSH, from 4.8 ± 0.84 to 3.3 ± 0.45 mIU/ml on day 2, which was statistically significant at the 5% level. No significant change occurred in plasma testosterone-binding capacity (44).

It is of interest that Rosemberg et al. (45) recently reported that the responses of 2 adolescent male subjects with immature testes to the administration of 5,000 IU LH and 5,000 IU HCG daily for 3 days were comparable both in terms of testosterone levels and plasma LH-like immunoreactivity. Other detailed studies of the effects of HCG on plasma testosterone were reported by Lipsett et al. (46).

As would be expected, organic hypopituitarism results in lowered levels of plasma gonadotropin and testosterone. The effects of purified FSH on testicular steroid production in man have not been reported.

Spermatogenesis

Excellent recent reviews of current concepts relating to hormonal control of spermatogenesis are those of Lunenfeld and Shalkovsky-Weissenberg (47) and Steinberger (48). The former authors state that "there is no conclusive evidence that any stage of spermatogenesis in man may be independent of gonadotropic stimulation." The precise roles of FSH and LH in man are not yet clear, although there seems little doubt that LH exerts much of its effect by increasing the local concentration of testosterone in the environment of the seminiferous epithelium. A striking example of the local effects of testosterone is seen in the affected testis of children with Leydig cell tumors, where tubules close to the tumour show evidence of stimulation of spermatogenesis, while more distant tubules, and those in the opposite testis, remain in their normal prepubertal state.

Localization of fluorescein-labeled FSH has been demonstrated in Sertoli cells by Mancini (49); labeled LH was found in the interstitial cells, and this was confirmed by de Kretser et al. (50), using ^{125}I-labeled human LH administered to rats.

INTERRELATIONSHIPS OF PITUITARY AND TESTICULAR FUNCTION

It is generally accepted that a classical endocrine feedback control system operates between the hypothalamus, pituitary, and testis, and some recent evidence for factors influencing the system is reviewed below.

The Effects of Castration

Although little opportunity exists for study of the effects of orchidectomy in the normal male, data has been obtained in patients with prostatic carcinoma (51), and the results in two such patients are illustrated in Figs. 3 and 4.Plasma testosterone fell rapidly in one patient, and there was a slow rise in LH levels to those seen in postmenopausal females; in the second patient, there was a slower fall in plasma testosterone, which was low prior to operation, and there was a slow but steady rise in plasma gonadotropin levels, which had reached a plateau at about 4 weeks postoperatively. Another patient, previously treated with estrogen for 10 years, was studied after orchidectomy which was performed 45 days after cessation of his estrogens. Basal LH and FSH were normal, but failed to rise after removal of the testes. This finding is of interest in the light of the observations of Geller et al. (52), that some patients with prostatic disease may have impairment of both storage and synthesizing capacity for LH.

One normal young male was studied 4 months after suffering a traumatic

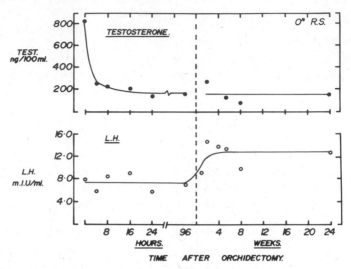

FIG. 3. Plasma testosterone and LH in a male aged 74, after orchidectomy for metastatic prostatic carcinoma. Plasma testosterone fell rapidly and LH rose slowly.

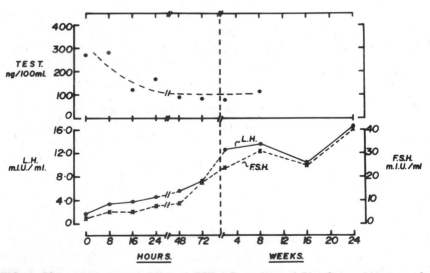

FIG. 4. Plasma testosterone, LH, and FSH in a male aged 71, after orchidectomy for metastatic prostatic carcinoma. Initial levels of plasma testosterone were low and fell slowly. There was a slow simultaneous rise of plasma FSH and LH.

576

haematoma of his only functioning testis (26); plasma testosterone was 340 ng/100 ml, while both gonadotropins were in the postmenopausal range (LH 12.3 mIU/ml, FSH 40 mIU/ml).

From these data, it is clear that castration in the adult male leads to an elevation in the levels of gonadotropins within about 72 hr, an elevation that is somewhat delayed when compared with the prompt fall in plasma testosterone. It may be concluded that orchidectomy removes one or more inhibitors of pituitary gonadotropin release, or that gonadotropins are utilized by testicular tissue, as suggested by Nelson (53) and Heller et al. (54). It is thus appropriate to examine the effects of certain testicular secretions on gonadotropin release.

The Effects of Androgens

Several studies have been reported on the effects of exogenous androgens on pituitary and testicular hormone production and on spermatogenesis. Davis et al. (55) showed that the administration of oral androgens such as 2α-methyl dihydrotestosterone and fluoroxymestrone was followed by a slow, dose-related decline in plasma testosterone over several days. Swerdloff and Odell (30) studied the effects of fluoroxymestrone on plasma LH and FSH in normal males: there was a slight reduction in LH values with a dose of 20 mg daily, but on 50 mg daily, LH became undetectable in 6 of 9 subjects at 4 days. There was no suppression of plasma FSH at either dose. Franchimont (14) also showed a sharp decline in plasma LH following a single intramuscular injection of 50 mg of testosterone propionate, persisting for 18 to 20 hr; again, there was no significant change in FSH reported (although levels had fallen from 6.8 to 4 mIU/ml at 24 hr). Peterson et al. (29) gave 25 mg of testosterone propionate im once a day for 3 days to three normal subjects in all of whom LH levels had fallen significantly after 2 days, whereas FSH fell significantly in one, marginally in another, and rose in the third. Heller et al. (56) gave testosterone propionate, 100 mg daily for 5 days to 2 subjects; LH fell, but again no fall in FSH was detected.

The results of administering a single im injection of 100 mg testosterone propionate to 6 normal males aged 22 to 27 are shown in Figs. 5 and 6 (39). Plasma testosterone rose from 615 ± 69 (SEM) to 2015 ± 126 ng/100 ml on the second day after the injection; plasma LH fell in the first 24 hr in 4 of the 6 subjects, the mean fall being 26.7%, from 4.05 ± 0.99 to 2.96 ± 0.51 mIU/ml; FSH fell in 5 of the 6 subjects, the mean fall being 20.8%, from 4.95 ± 0.62 mIU/ml in the first day, significant at the 2.5% level. By 7 days, FSH was 4.76 ± 0.84 mIU/ml.

These findings are somewhat at variance with those reported by other investigators mentioned above, particularly with regard to an effect of testosterone on plasma FSH, and the differences are not readily explicable; they may reflect differences in numbers of subjects studied, in effective androgen dosage, in period of observation, or in the immunoassay systems.

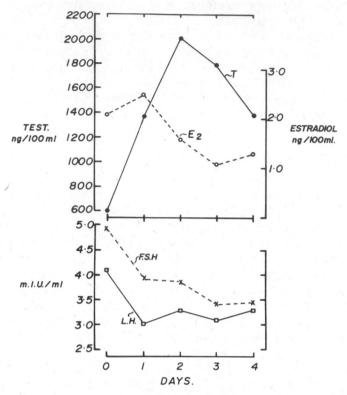

FIG. 5. Mean plasma testosterone, estradiol, LH, and FSH concentrations in 6 normal male subjects aged 22 to 27 after a single IM injection of testosterone propionate, 100 mg.

More speculative conclusions may be drawn from the study described earlier, where plasma FSH was noted to fall following the administration of HCG (Fig. 2); there is again an inverse relationship between plasma testosterone and FSH, although it may be that the FSH-like portion of the HCG molecule is exerting a "short" feedback effect (vide infra), or that the changes are mediated by the rise in plasma estradiol.

To summarize the effects of androgens, it is established that they suppress plasma LH levels, while their influence on plasma FSH is more controversial.

The Effects of Antiandrogens

The availability of antiandrogens, which act by competing with androgens for their receptor sites in target cells (57) has led to a limited number of studies of their effects on gonadotropin secretion in man. Franchimont (58) administered cyproterone acetate, 300 mg by intramuscular injection, or 300 mg daily orally, to two groups of 4 adult males. Plasma FSH and LH fell in both groups. In

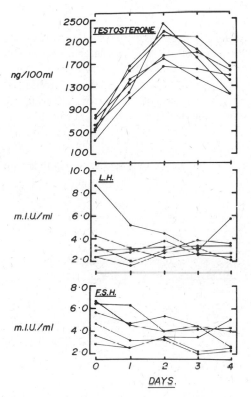

FIG. 6. Individual values for plasma testosterone, LH, and FSH for the 6 subjects shown in Fig. 5.

contrast, Neumann et al. (59) found an increase in urinary LH excretion in healthy men receiving 200 mg daily, which also causes increased testosterone secretion (60, 61). Cyproterone is a pure anti-androgen, while the acetylated compound possesses strong progestational properties (62). The different effects of the two compounds on gonadotropin levels may be due to this fact, as large doses of progestational agents cause a fall in both FSH and LH levels in postmenopausal females (58). The rise in LH and testosterone in response to a pure anti-androgen is in accord with classical feedback concepts.

The Effects of Estrogens

Estrogens, at least in pharmacological amounts, also exert a suppressive effect on gonadotropin and testosterone secretion. Coppage and Cooner (63) showed depression of plasma testosterone to levels seen after orchidectomy in 3 men given diethylstilbestrol, 10 mg daily, for 7 to 10 days. This dose is equivalent to

0.5 mg ethinyl estradiol, which is in turn equivalent to 1.5 mg estradiol. As the average daily production rate of estradiol is 40 ug, these doses clearly lie in the pharmacological range.

Alder et al. (64) further showed that both testosterone and LH levels in plasma fell after the administration of very large doses of stilbestrol (90 mg/day) to men with prostatic carcinoma, and Swerdloff and Odell (30) gave ethinyl estradiol, 0.2 mg daily, to 14 males, in whom both LH and FSH declined significantly by the fourth day of treatment, although the majority of the subjects still had detectable levels at that time. Continued observations in males with prostatic cancer have confirmed that, over the daily dosage range of 15 to 90 mg stilbestrol, there is a significant acute fall in levels of plasma testosterone, LH, and FSH (51). The data are shown in Fig. 7. There is an initial sharp decline

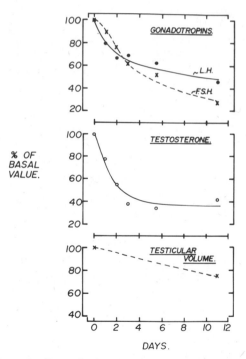

FIG. 7. Acute effects of stilbestrol administration (15 to 90 mg daily) in 21 males with prostatic cancer on plasma gonadotropins and testosterone and testicular volume.

in gonadotropins and testosterone: after 1 day of therapy, the mean FSH level is 89% of the basal value, LH is 79%, and testosterone, 78%. After 3 days, FSH has fallen to 61% of the initial reading, LH to 67%, and testosterone to 38%. The decline in mean testosterone concentration appears to be more rapid than those of the gonadotropins.

The effects of administering stilbestrol, 15 mg daily, to 9 normal young males have also been examined recently (39), and similar results have been observed. After 2 days, FSH was 50% of the basal value, LH was 34.5%, and testosterone 24%, with little further change after 3 days. Similar acute effects of estrogen treatment were reported by Peterson et al. (29).

When the chronic effects of estrogen therapy in prostatic carcinoma are examined (Fig. 8), there is a slow and steady decline in both the pituitary and the testicular hormones, accompanied by a drop in mean testicular volume.

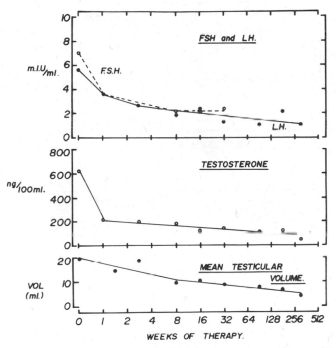

FIG. 8. Chronic effects of stilbestrol administration (15 to 30 mg daily) in 21 males with prostatic cancer. The abscissa is drawn on a logarithmic scale.

Even after months of therapy, testosterone values remain somewhat higher (20 to 200 ng/100 ml) than the normal female range, and gonadotropins are still detectable in the plasma of many subjects, although they lie in the range seen prior to puberty (LH, 0.2 to 2.2 mIU/ml; FSH, < 1 to 5.0 mIU/ml). The pattern of response to large doses of estrogens is therefore a rapid initial fall in gonadotropins and testosterone, with a subsequent prolonged decline. It has been noted, even after some months of treatment, that certain patients, who have ceased to take estrogen for 1 to 2 weeks, show escape from suppression, with a rapid rise of gonadotropins, and a more variable response of plasma testosterone. Thus, a 75-year-old male treated for more than a year with 15 mg stilbestrol was studied after discontinuing treatment for 3 weeks. LH rose from 1.5 to 9.1 mIU/ml, FSH from 3.0 to 8.7 mIU/ml, and testosterone remained low (20 ng/100 ml, previously 90 ng/100 ml). Another example of rebound after estrogen withdrawal is seen in Fig. 9 (vide infra) where the patient temporarily discontinued his treatment for 2 weeks after 7 weeks of stilbestrol. In this instance, testosterone rose from 40 to 430 ng/100 ml.

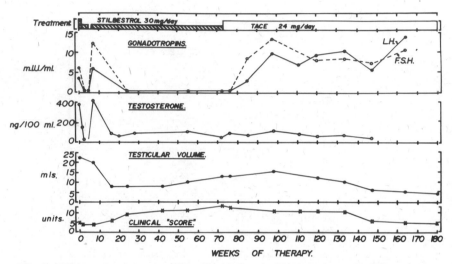

FIG. 9. Effects of treatment with stilbestrol and chlorotrianisene (TACE) on plasma gonadotropins and testosterone, testicular volume and clinical progress in a 73-year-old male with prostatic cancer. For definition of clinical score, see text. A rising score indicates deterioration.

The relationship between pituitary and testis is therefore similar to that of pituitary and adrenal cortex in that, after prolonged corticosteroid suppression, ACTH levels rise to supranormal values before the adrenal cortex responds by increasing secretion of glucocorticoids (65).

The effects described above are those of pharmacological amounts of estrogens. Observations of the responses of plasma gonadotropins in 10 castrated men to physiological and pharmacological doses of ethinyl estradiol (5 to 300 μg/day) were reported by Walsh et al. (66). At a dose of 50 μg daily, a dose which caused gynecomastia and was already pharmacological, FSH and LH were suppressed to normal levels in 50% of the patients while lower doses were largely ineffective. It was concluded that it was "unlikely that estrogen or testosterone acts alone as the primary regulator of FSH secretion in the male," since all the men developed gynecomastia on the lowest dose of ethinyl estradiol which suppressed FSH. It was noteworthy, however, that both gonadotropins were suppressed to normal by a similar dose of estrogen, a dose which is equivalent to about three times the normal daily production rate of estradiol.

The dissociation sometimes seen between plasma LH and testosterone during estrogen treatment, when testosterone values are suppressed while LH is still easily detectable, suggests that estrogen may have a direct effect on testicular steroid synthesis in addition to their effect on the pituitary, and indeed Uchikawa et al. (67) reported a direct influence of estrogen on enzymes of the Leydig cells of male mice and monkeys. Additional evidence for this hypothesis is provided by recent observations (51) on the effects of the orally active estrogen, chlorotrianisene (TACE®). The effects of this substance on plasma levels of gonadotropins and testosterone are shown in Fig. 9. This 73-year old male was originally treated with stilbestrol, 30 mg daily (discontinued temporarily after 7 weeks). After 72 weeks, TACE was substituted for stilbestrol, in a dose of 24 mg daily. Three weeks after commencing TACE, plasma gonadotropins were still undetectable; after 12 weeks, FSH had risen to the upper limit seen in young adult males, and LH lay within the normal range; both gonadotropins were elevated after 25 weeks, and they have remained at high normal or elevated levels. Plasma testosterone stayed within or just above the normal female range throughout this period. Incidentally, testicular volume gradually rose, after an initial fall, during stilbestrol therapy, and fell again with TACE. The patient's clinical progress appeared to be correlated with testicular volume, but not with plasma testosterone. It was assessed by means of a clinical "score," an index consisting of a numerical assessment of the local prostatic lesion, the extent of local and distant spread, and the patient's general condition. Observations have now been made in 5 patients treated with TACE, and in all, plasma testosterone has been suppressed, while gonadotropins have been in or above the normal male range.

The observation that an orally active estrogen suppresses testosterone secretion while gonadotropin levels are normal or elevated is of considerable interest. It suggests that the chemical structure conferring estrogenicity as far as the testis is concerned is not necessarily the same as that recognized as estrogenic by the hypothalamic receptors, although the gonadotropic effect may be interpreted alternatively as an absent or weakly positive feedback response to a weak estrogen (compared with the effects of low doses of estrogens referred to above). It is relevant to note that the chemical structures of clomiphene (vide infra) and chlorotrianisene are closely related, differing only by a triethylamine grouping. Another possible view is that both compounds may act as anti-estrogens at the hypothalamic centers regulating gonadotropin secretion. An orally active androgen, mesterolone, which has a saturated A ring, but closely resembles testosterone in structure, has also been reported not to suppress gonadotropin or testosterone secretion (68), although in high dosage, given by intramuscular injection, it does cause some suppression of plasma FSH, but not LH (58).

The Effects of Anti-estrogen

The administration of clomiphene citrate to normal males has been shown to be followed by an elevation in the levels of gonadotropin and testosterone by several investigators (18, 29, 69-71). Doses of 25 to 200 mg/day were used by these authors. Kulin et al. (72) reported that after the dose was increased to 500 mg daily, suppression of gonadotropin and testosterone occurred. They postulated that the initial stimulatory effects of clomiphene in adults were secondary to positive feedback by this weakly estrogenic compound.

Because of its stimulatory effects, clomiphene has been proposed as a useful agent for the investigation of suspected hypogonadotropic hypogonadism; it has indeed been observed to cause further lowering of plasma LH and testosterone in such patients (73) as well as in prepubertal children (74), suggesting that such individuals lack a functional positive feedback mechanism for estrogens (72). Whether the effects of clomiphene are due to its weakly estrogenic, or to its anti-estrogenic properties, has not been resolved.

The Effects of Gonadotropins on Gonadotropin Production

Evidence has accumulated from studies in experimental animals, that, in addition to the "long" feedback systems, exemplified by the effects of androgens and estrogens, pituitary gonadotropin secretion may be influenced by a "short" feedback system, whereby the gonadotropin may modify its own rate of secretion directly. This concept is discussed by Martini (75) for FSH and by Motta et al. (76) for LH.

A possible example of a "short" feedback mechanism in man was provided by the observation (39) that plasma FSH fell during a period of HCG administration to 5 normal young adult males, from 4.8 ± 0.84 (SEM) to 3.5 ± 0.49 after 4 days ($p < 0.025$). The finding was confirmed in 6 other subjects given a similar course of HCG: FSH fell from 4.7 ± 0.52 to 2.6 ± 0.47 mIU/ml ($p < 0.001$). Several explanations must be considered: it is possible that the effect was through a "long" feedback, through elevation of plasma testosterone or estradiol, but the FSH-like properties of HCG (77) could conceivably have caused a "short" negative feedback inhibition of FSH secretion.

The Effects of Chemical Mediators of Neurotransmission

A CHOLINERGIC MEDIATOR: β-METHYLCHOLINE

Franchimont (58) has examined the effects of β-methylcholine on plasma FSH and LH in 5 normal males. In a dose which causes significant elevations of plasma growth hormone (GH) and cortisol, in addition to an antidiuretic effect, this substance failed to alter gonadotropin levels, and the investigator concluded that the central activation of gonadotropin secretion was not brought about through cholinergic pathways.

A PRECURSOR OF CENTRAL NERVOUS SYSTEM CATECHOL-AMINES: L-DOPA

Several studies in rats, for example, Schneider et al. (78), have provided evidence that the production of LHRH in the hypothalamus may be mediated by dopamine. It was therefore of interest to study the effects of L-dopa, a precursor of dopamine in the central nervous system, on plasma LH and FSH; preliminary observations have been made in 7 males, aged 45 to 61 years, who were chronically receiving 2 to 4 g of the drug daily for the treatment of Parkinson's disease (79). In this acute study, blood samples were taken every 30 min for 2 hr after the oral administration of 1.0 g of L-dopa: there was no significant change in the levels of either FSH or LH, although there was a trend toward a small rise (25%) in LH. Baseline concentrations of both gonadotropins were in the range to be expected in males of that age, and there was thus no clear-cut evidence of an acute or chronic effect of L-dopa on gonadotropin levels in adult males. Recently, Boyd et al. (80) demonstrated that L-dopa caused a significant rise in growth hormone levels following the oral administration of 0.5 g to patients with Parkinsonism, a rise which persisted for 120 min. Franchimont (58) gave dopamine to 4 postmenopausal females, 2 of whom had been pretreated with ethinyl estradiol and 2 with norethisterone. Dopamine produced no effect on plasma gonadotropins in the latter subjects, but caused an elevation of LH in both of the former and of FSH in one. Further experiments are clearly required before definitive conclusions can be drawn.

Other Feedback Mechanisms Concerning FSH

Although much of the data described above indicates that FSH and LH are subject to similar feedback controls, there is evidence that FSH may be controlled by another testicular factor. Thus FSH is not affected by doses of testosterone which cause suppression of LH; following testicular irradiation, when the germinal epithelium is destroyed, but interstitial cells remain intact, plasma LH is normal, but FSH levels rise (58). In Klinefelter's syndrome, FSH levels are invariably elevated, but LH levels may be in the normal range (81) and are inversely related to the levels of plasma testosterone.

Several investigators have proposed mechanisms of FSH control which involve the seminiferous tubules (82-84), but the nature of the hypothetical tubular regulating substance remains obscure. Although FSH levels may be elevated in patients with severe oligospermia and azoospermia, no direct correlation can be made between the sperm count or the germinal cell population, and the concentrations of FSH measured by specific immunological or biological methods (85). Johnsen (86) has recently reviewed his investigations of this feedback mechanism, and believes it to be associated with the last stage of spermatogenesis, and to involve the Sertoli cells. This is an aspect of the relationship between pituitary and testes which certainly merits further study.

OTHER INFLUENCES ON THE PITUITARY-TESTICULAR AXIS

Stimuli of Hypothalamic and Pituitary Function

Several authors have reported that the stimuli frequently used for the evaluation of GH and ACTH secretion are not effective in altering the plasma concentrations of FSH and LH; these stimuli have included insulin-induced hypoglycemia, arginine infusion, and the administration of glucose, pitressin, and pyrogen (30, 31, 41, 58). Ryan et al. (87) showed that convulsive electroshock caused significant rises in gonadotropins in some treated men.

The effects of surgery are of interest. Charters et al. (88) showed that surgery was followed by a transient decline in plasma gonadotropins in otherwise normal subjects, and Matsumoto et al. (89) found corresponding falls in plasma testosterone, decreased levels persisting for at least 6 days following major surgery. The decline in the latter group was from 747 ng/100 ml before surgery to 211 at 2 days, and 243 at 6 days. These effects are in contrast with the elevations found in plasma GH and cortisol under similar circumstances. Ryan and Faiman (41) showed that several polyamines, reported to cause FSH release in rats, were without effect in inducing gonadotropin release in man. Franchimont (81) showed rises in LH and FSH after the administration of posterior pituitary extract to normal male volunteers. Oxytocin caused a rise in FSH, but lysine vasopressin was without effect. The significance of these various observations is not clear, although Franchimont proposed that posterior pituitary extract could be used to stimulate gonadotropin secretion.

Effects of Liver Disease

An intriguing problem, not yet satisfactorily resolved, is the precise nature of the presumed disorder of testicular function which occurs in patients with hepatic cirrhosis. The presence of gynecomastia and of testicular atrophy certainly suggest the possibility that they result from the action of estrogen; it is therefore relevant to review the evidence that exists for the presence of elevated levels of estrogen in such patients, to determine their source, and to examine their effects on levels of gonadotropin and testosterone. Brown et al. (90) showed that patients with cirrhosis, taken as a group, had elevated levels of total urinary estrogen, and Korenman et al. (91) found that plasma levels of estradiol were almost twice those of normal men. These elevations could result from an increased production rate, decreased disposal, an elevated specific binding protein in plasma, or a combination of these factors. Brown et al. (90) gave estradiol to their patients, and found normal rates of metabolism of the steroid except in patients with terminal disease; Shaver et al. (92), on the other hand, showed a diminished capacity of the diseased liver to clear exogenous, isotopically labeled estradiol. Zumoff (93) also demonstrated abnormal estradiol metabolism in cirrhosis. Tarvenetti et al. (94) showed that testosterone binding capacity was increased in the serum of cirrhotic patients. The source of the elevated estrogen levels has thus not been defined, in other words, there may be increased production (90) and decreased disposal, and elevated levels of binding proteins have also been demonstrated.

With regard to consequences of estrogen excess, Coppage and Coorer (63) studied 12 men with alcoholic cirrhosis; all had testicular atrophy and 5 had gynecomastia. Eight of the 12 had testosterone levels below 200 ng/100 ml, in other words, in the range seen after estrogen therapy. Urinary gonadotropins were low or undetectable in the 3 patients in whom measurements were made. There was no apparent correlation with age, nor with specific liver function tests; no mention was made of correlation with gynecomastia. Rosselin and Dolais (20) reported lowered levels of plasma FSH in cirrhosis. The situation in hemochromatosis is less clear-cut. Stocks and Martin (95) studied 15 patients; urinary gonadotropins were normal in 9 and absent or low in 6. Plasma LH was normal in 8 and low in 7, and plasma testosterone was low in 6 of the 13 patients in whom the steroid was measured. Urinary estrogen excretion was normal or low. It was concluded that pituitary failure was not uncommon in hemochromatosis, and was not related to the severity of the liver disease. Gay et al. (96) found normal urinary gonadotropins, and normal or low plasma FSH. In contrast, Franchimont (58) reported on a heterogeneous group of 29 patients with hemochromatosis: 18 had normal plasma FSH, 10 had elevated values (these had diminished spermatogenesis) and in 1 the level was low; LH was normal in 18, increased in 5 and low in 6. In the 5 with elevated LH, urinary 17-oxo-steroid excretion was low, and there was testicular atrophy with evidence of androgen deficiency. He concluded that mean gonadotropin levels were elevated in hemochromatosis, and that there was evidence of pluriglandular insufficiency. The hypogonadism appeared to be due primarily to endocrine and exocrine involvement of the testes; the poor response of the testis to HCG provided confirmatory evidence. However, the pituitary response was less than in healthy subjects, and tended to disappear, resulting ultimately in lowered gonadotropin levels.

In an attempt to define the abnormality in cirrhosis further, a group of 15 patients living in Singapore and suffering from cirrhosis, proven by biopsy, was studied (97). Their endocrine status was investigated fully, but data presented here concern only the levels of gonadotropin, testosterone, and estradiol in plasma, gonadotropin in urine, and in 12 patients, the response of testosterone, estradiol, and FSH to HCG administration. All patients showed marked elevations in plasma estradiol, ranging from 11.5 to 53.5 ng/100 ml, while testosterone ranged from 213 to 702 ng/100 ml (mean 424). There was a strong negative correlation (r = 0.64) between the levels of testosterone, and estradiol. Gonadotropin levels were variable; 3 patients had marked elevations of FSH and LH, together with testicular atrophy and a tendency towards lowered testosterone levels (250 to 365 ng/100 ml). In the remainder, LH was normal, and was not correlated with testosterone; FSH was low in 3, and testosterone was < 300 ng/100 ml in 3 patients. The testosterone response to HCG was impaired in all.

A striking feature was the marked fall in plasma estradiol in response to HCG administration. There were no obvious correlations between the results of the endocrine function tests and the severity, either clinical or biochemical, of the liver disease, nor was there any relationship between clinical evidence suggestive of estrogen excess, and the levels of estradiol. It was concluded that there was evidence of increased levels of estrogen in these patients, that there was no ready interpretation of the effects of the disease on the pituitary and testis, and that the exact mechanisms involved therefore still required elucidation. Comparison of this group of patients with others studied in Australia or in the U.S.A. indicates that the Singapore patients had higher levels of plasma estradiol and testosterone.

Effects of Thyroid Disease

Elevated levels of plasma testosterone in adult males are infrequently encountered. Dray et al. (98) demonstrated that patients with hyperthyroidism had elevated levels of this steroid, accompanied by a lowered MCR, so that the testosterone production rate was within the normal range. Crepy et al. (99) subsequently demonstrated an increase in the serum protein-binding affinity for testosterone in males and females with this disease. The elevation of testosterone has been confirmed (100), and Burger and Hudson (101) found a mean level of 1382 ± 302 (SEM) ng/100 ml in 6 untreated males with the disease, which fell to 737 ± 122 ng/100 ml when they were rendered euthyroid. The basic reason for these findings is obscure, although it is logical to attribute the elevated testosterone to an increase in testosterone-binding globulin in plasma, which emphasizes the importance of binding proteins in adrogen metabolism. It is of interest that Franchimont (58) states that FSH levels in hyperthyroidism are normal, whereas LH levels are generally lower than normal; this observation requires confirmation.

Effects of Sexual Activity

In contrast to the data available in experimental animals, relatively little is known regarding the release of gonadotropins and testosterone at times of sexual activity in the human male. Changes in beard growth, known to be under androgenic control, have been reported after periods of prolonged sexual abstinence. It was noted that with the anticipation of the resumption of sexual activity, there was a significant increase in beard growth (102). In bulls and rams, sharp increases in plasma LH and testosterone occur in anticipation of and at the time of coitus (103), but similar data have not yet been obtained in man.

SUMMARY

In this review, various aspects of the relationship between the hypothalamus, pituitary, and testes of normal adult males have been reviewed, and the effects of certain disease states not primarily affecting the endocrine organs have been discussed. The major area of lack of adequate knowledge is the control of FSH secretion. No attempt has been made to discuss the peripheral effects or the metabolically active form of testosterone.

REFERENCES

1. Burger, H. G., and J. Spinks, in preparation.
2. Reichman, C., M. Fullerton, H. G. Burger, and K. J. Catt, Prog 13th Ann Mtg Endoc Soc, Aust 1970, Abst. 16.
3. Hudson, B., A. Dulmanis, and R. Piper, in preparation.
4. Dufau, M. L., A. Dulmanis, K. J. Catt, and B. Hudson, J Clin Endocrinol 30:351, 1970.
5. Lee, V., G. Fink, and H. G. Burger, submitted for publication.
6. Rosemberg, E. and C. A. Paulsen (Eds.), The Human Testis, Plenum, New York and London, 1970.
7. Kastin, A. J., A. V. Schally, C. Gual, A. R. Midgley, Jr., A. Arimura, M. Clinton Miller, III, and A. Cabeza, J Clin Endocrinol 32:287, 1971.
8. Ryan, R. J., J Clin Endocrinol 22:300, 1962.
9. Roos, P., in C. Gual (Ed.), Progress in Endocrinology, Excerpta Medica, Amsterdam, 1969, p. 377.
10. Kohler, P. O., G. T. Ross, and W. D. Odell, J Clin Invest 47:38, 1968.
11. Keller, P. J., Acta Endocrinol (Kbh) 52:348, 1966.
12. Kulin, H. E., A. B. Rifkind, and G. T. Ross, J Clin Endocrinol 28:100, 1968.
13. Coble, Y. D., P. O. Kohler, C. Cargille, and G. T. Ross, J Clin Invest 48:359, 1969.
14. Franchimont, P., Le Dosage des Hormones Hypophysaires Sometotrope et Gonadotrope et son Application Clinique, Arscia, Bruxelles and Maloine, Paris, 1966.
15. Faiman, C., and R. J. Ryan, J Clin Endocrinol 27:444, 1967.
16. Faiman, C., and R. J. Ryan, Proc Soc Exp Biol Med 125:1130, 1967.
17. Midgley, A. R., J Clin Endocrinol 27:295, 1967.
18. Odell, W. D., G. T. Ross, and P. L. Rayford, J Clin Invest 46:248, 1967.
19. Odell, W. D., A. F. Parlow, C. M. Cargille, and G. T. Ross, J Clin Invest 47:2551, 1968.
20. Rosselin, G., and J. Dolais, Presse Med 75:2027, 1967.
21. Burger, H. G., J. R. Oliver, J. Davis, and K. J. Catt, Aust J Exp Biol Med Sci 46:541, 1968.
22. Catt, K. J., H. D. Niall, G. W. Tregear, and H. G. Burger, J Clin Endocrinol 28:121, 1968.
23. Saxena, B. B., H. Demura, H. M. Gandy, and R. E. Peterson, J Clin Endocrinol 28:519, 1968.
24. Johanson, A. J., H. Guyda, C. Light, C. J. Migeon, and R. M. Blizzard, J Pediat 74:416, 1969.
25. Raiti, S., A. Johnsen, C. Light, C. J. Migeon, and R. M. Blizzard, Metabolism 18:234, 1969.
26. Yen, S. S. C., and W. J. Vicic, Amer J Obst Gyn 106:134, 1970.
27. Albert, A., J Clin Endocrinol 28:1683, 1968.
28. Faiman, C., and R. J. Ryan, Nature 215:857, 1967.
29. Peterson, Jr., N. T., A. R. Midgley, Jr., and R. B. Jaffe, J Clin Endocrinol 28:1473, 1968.

30. Swerdloff, R. S., and W. D. Odell, in E. Rosemberg (Ed.), Gonadotropins 1968, Geron-X, Inc., Los Altos, 1968, p. 155.

31. Burger, H. G., J. B. Brown, K. J. Catt, B. Hudson, and J. R. Stockigt, in M. Margoulies (Ed.), Protein and Polypeptide Hormones, Excerpta Medica Amsterdam, 1968, p. 412.

32. Burger, H. G., D. P. Cameron, and K. J. Catt, unpublished observations, 1968.

33. Dray, F., A. Reinberg, and J. Sebaoun, C R Acad Sci 261:573, 1965.

34. Resko, J. A., and K. B. Eik-nes, J Clin Endocrinol 26:573, 1966.

35. Southren, A. L., G. G. Gordon, S. Tochimoto, G. Pinzon, D. R. Lane, and W. Stypulkowski, J Clin Endocrinol 27:686, 1967.

36. Evans, J. I., A. W. MacLean, A. A. A. Ismail, and D. Love, Nature 229:261, 1971.

37. Takahashi, Y., D. M. Kipnis, and W. H. Daughaday, J Clin Invest 47:2079, 1968.

38. Patel, Y. C., F. P. Alford, and H. G. Burger, unpublished observations, 1971.

39. Baker, H. W. G., H. G. Burger, and B. Hudson, unpublished observations, 1971.

40. Schalch, D. S., A. F. Parlow, R. C. Boon, and S. Reichlin, J Clin Invest 47:665, 1968.

41. Ryan, R. J., and C. Faiman, in E. Rosemberg (Ed.), Gonadotropins 1968, Geron-X, Inc., Los Altos, 1968, p. 333.

42. Vermeulen, A., in C. Gual (Ed.), Progress in Endocrinology, Excerpta Medica, Amsterdam, 1969, p. 863.

43. Faiman, C., and J. S. D. Winter, Prog 52nd Mtg Endoc Soc, 1970, p. 75.

44. Baker, H. W. G., S. O'Connor, and B. Hudson, unpublished observations, 1971.

45. Rosemberg, E., W. F. Jan, S. G. Lee, R. Nakano, and J. F. Crigler, Jr., Progr 52nd Mtg Endoc Soc, 1970, p. 53.

46. Lipsett, M. B., H. Wilson, M. A. Kirschner, S. G. Korenman, L. M. Fishman, G. A. Sarfaty, and C. W. Bardin, Rec Prog Hormone Res 22:245, 1966.

47. Lunenfeld, B., and R. Shalkovsky-Weissenberg, in E. Rosemberg and C. A. Paulsen (Eds.), The Human Testis, Plenum, New York and London, 1970, p. 613.

48. Steinberger, E., Physiol Rev 51:1, 1971.

49. Mancini, R. E., J Histochem Cytochem 15:516, 1967.

50. De Kretser, D. M., K. J. Catt, H. G. Burger, and G. C. Smith, J Endocrinol 43:105, 1969.

51. Burger, H. G., H. W. G. Baker, W. G. Straffon, and B. Hudson, unpublished observations, 1971.

52. Geller, J., A. Baron, and S. Kleinman, J Endocrinol 48:289, 1970.

53. Nelson, W. O., Ciba Found Colloq Endocrinol 4:271, 1952.

54. Heller, C. G., C. A. Paulsen, G. E. Mortimore, E. C. Junck, and W. O. Nelson, Ann N Y Acad Sci 55:685, 1952.

55. Davis, T. E., M. B. Lipsett, and S. G. Korenman, J Clin Endocrinol 25:476, 1965.

56. Heller, C. G., H. C. Morse, M. Su, and M. J. Rowley, in E. Rosemberg, and C. A. Paulsen (Eds.), The Human Testis, Plenum, New York and London, 1970, p. 249.

57. Neumann, F., and R. von Berswordt-Wallrabe, J Endrocrinol 35:363, 1966.

58. Franchimont, P., Secretion Normale et Pathologique de la Somatotrophine et des Gonadotrophines Humaines, Masson & Cie, Paris, 1971.

59. Neumann, F., R. von Berswordt-Wallrabe, W. Elger, H. Steinbeck, J. D. Hahn, and M. Kramer, Rec Prog Hormone Res 26:337, 1970.

60. Voigt, K-D., and H. Klosterhalfen, Ford Found Colloq Conf Phys Human Reprod, Venice, 1966.

61. Rausch-Stroomann, J.-G., R. Petry, V. Hocevar, J. Mauss, and Th. Senge, Acta Endocrinol (Kbh) 63:595, 1970.

62. Wiechert, R., and F. Neumann, Arzneimittel-Forsch 15:244, 1965.

63. Coppage, W. S., Jr., and A. E. Cooner, New Eng J Med 273:902, 1965.

64. Alder, A. B., H. G. Burger, J. Davis, A. Dulmanis, B. Hudson, G. A. Sarfaty, and W. Straffon, Brit Med J 1:28, 1968.

65. Graber, A. L., R. L. Ney, W. E. Nicholson, D. P. Island, and G. W. Liddle, J Clin Endocrinol 25:11, 1965.

66. Walsh, P. C., R. S. Swerdloff, and W. D. Odell, Prog 52nd Mtg Endoc Soc, 1970, p. 40.

67. Uchikawa, T., F. Schick, H. Todd, and L. Samuels, Prog 48th Mtg Endoc Soc 1966, p. 87.

68. Neumann, F., W. Elger, R. von Berswordt-Wallrabe, and M. Kramer, Arch Pharmak Exp Pathol 255:221, 1966.

69. Bardin, C. W., G. T. Ross, and M. B. Lipsett, J Clin Endocrinol 27:1588, 1967.

70. Faiman, C., R. J. Ryan, C. Zwireh, and M. E. Rubin, J Clin Endocrinol 28:1323, 1968.

71. Burger, H. G., J. B. Brown, K. J. Catt, B. Hudson, and J. R. Stockigt, in M. Margoulies (Ed.), Protein and Polypeptide Hormones, Excerpta Medica, Amsterdam, 1968, p. 731.

72. Kulin, H., R. Weinstein, S. Kaplan, and M. Grumbach, Prog 52nd Mtg Endoc Soc, Aust 1970, p. 58.

73. Burger, H. G., B. Hudson, D. M. De Kretser, H. P. Taft, I. Ekkel, and A. Mirovics, Prog 13th Ann Mtg Endoc Soc Aust 1970, Abst. 21.

74. Kulin, H. E., M. M. Grumbach, and S. G. Kaplan, Science 166:1012, 1969.

75. Martini, L., in E. Rosemberg and C. A. Paulsen (Eds.), The Human Testis, Plenum, New York and London, 1970, p. 187.

76. Motta, M., F. Fraschini, and L. Martini, in W. F. Ganong and L. Martini (Eds.), Frontiers in Neuroendocrinology, Oxford Univ. Press, New York, 1969, p. 211.

77. Ashitaka, Y., Y. Tokura, M. Tane, M. Mochizuki, and S. Tojo, Endocrinology 87:233, 1970.

78. Schneider, H. P. G., and S. M. McCann, Endocrinology 85:121, 1969.

79. Burger, H. G., A. C. Schwieger, A. C. Jenkins, and P. M. Dennis, unpublished observations, 1970.

80. Boyd, A. E., III, H. E. Lebovitz, and H. B. Pfeiffer, New Eng J Med 283:1425, 1970.

81. Franchimont, P., in W. J. Irvine (Ed.), Reproductive Endocrinology, Livingstone, Edinburgh and London, 1970, p. 19.

82. McCullagh, D. R., and I. Schneider, Endocrinology 27:899, 1940.

83. Howard, R. P., R. C. Sniffen, F. A. Simmonds, and F. Albright, J Clin Endocrinol 10:121, 1950.

84. Johnsen, S. G., Acta Endocrinol (Kbh) 45:Suppl 90, 99, 1964.

85. Leonard, J. M., R. B. Leach, and C. A. Paulsen, Prog 52nd Mtg Endoc Soc 1970, p. 49.

86. Johnsen, S. G., in E. Rosemberg and C. A. Paulsen, (Eds.), The Human Testis, Plenum, New York and London, 1970, p. 231.

87. Ryan, R. J., D. W. Swanson, C. Faiman, W. E. Mayberry, and A. J. Spadoni, J Clin Endocrinol 30:51, 1970.

88. Charters, A. C., W. D. Odell, and J. C. Thompson, J Clin Endocrinol 29:63, 1969.

89. Matsumoto, K., K. Takeyasu, S. Mizutani, Y. Hamanaka, and T. Uozumi, Acta Endocrinol 65:11, 1970.

90. Brown, J. B., G. P. Crean, and J. Ginsburg, Gut 5:56, 1964.

91. Korenman, S. G., L. E. Perrin, and T. McCallum, Prog 61st Mtg Amer Soc Clin Invest, 1969, Abst. 144.

92. Shaver, J. C., M. S. Roginsky, and N. P. Christy, Lancet 2:335, 1963.

93. Zumoff, B., J. Fishman, T. C. Gallagher, and L. Hellman, J Clin Invest 47:20, 1968.

94. Tarvenetti, R. R., W. Rosenbaum, W. G. Kelly, N. P. Christy, and M. S. Roginsky, J Clin Endocrinol 27:920, 1967.

95. Stocks, A. E., and F. I. R. Martin, Amer J Med 45:839, 1968.

96. Gay, J., G. Tchobroutsky, G. Rosselin, R. Assan, J. Dolais, P. Freychet, and M. Derot, Pathol Biol 16:53, 1968.

97. Taft, H. P., C. S. Seah, H. G. Burger, B. Hudson, in preparation.

98. Dray, F., J. Sebaoun, I. Mowszowicz, G. Delzane, P. Dergez, and G. Dreyfus, C R Acad Sci Paris 264:2578, 1967.

99. Crépy, O., F. Dray, and J. Sebaoun, C R Acad Sci Paris, 264:2651, 1967.

100. Gordon, G. G., A. L. Southren, S. Tochimoti, J. J. Rand, and J. Olivo, J Clin Endocrinol 29:164, 1969.

101. Burger, H. G., and B. Hudson, unpublished observations, 1971.

102. Anonymous, Nature 226:869, 1970.

103. Short, R. V., personal communication.

45. Studies on the Pituitary-Testicular Axis in Male Hypogonadism, Particularly in Infertile Men with "Cryptogenetic" Hypospermatogenesis

Svend G. Johnsen

Recently the author (1, 2) reviewed previous investigations on the relationship between spermatogenesis and gonadotropin level and concluded that the induction of a primary spermatogenetic failure leads, in animals and man, to a great rise in the gonadotropin level and that, accordingly, spermatogenesis must be directly or indirectly accompanied by release of a gonadotropin inhibitor exerting the feedback between spermatogenesis and FSH.

In his own studies the author (1, 2) investigated spermatogenesis and gonadotropin level in a group of 284 patients containing a great variety of primary testicular disorders. In this group, ranging from Klinefelter patients and Sertoli-cell-only cases at one end to cases with fair or good spermatogenesis in the other, a very high negative correlation was found between rate of spermatogenesis and total gonadotropin excretion. A further study showed that the stage of spermatogenesis involved in the testicular-hypophyseal feedback mechanism was the late spermatid stage. An extension of this work in our group by P. Christiansen (chapter 46) employing specific gonadotropin assays showed that the gonadotropin rise in spermatogenetic damage affects primarily FSH.

However, in a study of oligospermic males Paulsen (3) found normal serum

FSH levels and in 12 oligospermic males he was unable to find a correlation between testicular cell count and FSH excretion. To this one might point out that the very large (5- to 10-fold) individual variation in gonadotropin excretion could certainly prevent a correlation from showing up in such a limited number of cases and thus that Paulsen's and our findings are not necessarily in disagreement. On the other hand, it could be argued against our studies that the very high correlation between testicular tubular function and gonadotropin excretion could, to an undisclosed extent, be due to the inclusion of Klinefelter patients, Sertoli-cell-only cases and other patients with an extreme degree of tubular damage.

Therefore, in this study we decided to investigate the relationship between spermatogenesis and gonadotropin excretion in a more narrow group of infertile men with hypospermatogenesis. Attempts are made to perform a further sorting of these selected patients so as to end up with a homogenous group of "cryptogenetic" hypospermatogenesis in which the pituitary-testicular axis could be studied.

METHODS

Urinary hypophyseal gonadotropins (HG) were determined by the method of Johnsen (4, 5). Results are expressed in mouse uterus units (MUU)/24 hr. The MUU was continuously controlled with a HMG standard (1 ampoule of 2nd IRP-HMG = 133 MUU). At FSH/LH ratios found in clinical samples, the MUU expresses FSH + LH (6). However, in our animal strain the MUU is primarily correlated with the FSH content of the urine extracts and less with LH (P. Christiansen, to be published). In analyses of large series of patients and normals the log HG showed no deviation from a normal distribution and log HG is used throughout the study.

Evaluation of spermatogenesis was performed by the testicular biopsy score count method described by the author (7). Full comprehension of this study requires familiarity with this method and with reference to the paper cited, a brief description is given. Each tubular section in one biopsy section is given a score from 10 to 1 according to the following (abridged) criteria: Score 10 = full spermatogenesis, normal germinal epithelium, 9 = many spermatozoa, but disorganized epithelium, 8 = only few spermatozoa present, 7 = no spermatozoa, but many spermatids present, 6 = no spermatozoa and only few spermatids present, 5 = no spermatozoa, no spermatids, but many spermatocytes present, 4 = as 5 but only few spermatocytes, 3 = spermatogonia are the only germ cells present, 2 = no germ cells, but Sertoli cells present, score 1 = no cells in the tubular section. Spermatozoa are defined as cells having achieved the small head form of the spermatozoon.

In order to calculate a mean score (MS) the number of tubuli recorded at each score is multiplied with the score and the sum of all 10 multiplications is divided by the total number of tubuli recorded. The MS is an over-all figure for the quality of the germinal epithelium. The mean number of tubuli scored per biopsy was 113. All testicular biopsy score counts were performed by the author.

The testicular biopsy score count method has permitted a reevaluation of gonadotropin excretion transformed so as to be independent of the rate of spermatogenesis. Values for this transformed log HG in various forms of hypogonadism are being reported (8).

Sperm counts were performed by R. Hammen according to methods previously described (9). The parameter used is the logarithm of the total sperm count per ejaculate in millions (usually the mean of several determinations).

Measurements of testicular and adrenal steroids independent of each other were performed by a combined dexamethasone suppression plus chorionic gonadotropin stimulation test (DXM-HCG test) recently described by us (10). Used in the present study are values for urinary dehydroepiandrosterone (DHA) and androsterone + etiocholanolone (AE) of adrenal origin, and further keto-genic steroids (pregnanetriol) and androsterone + etiocholanolone from the unstimulated testis. All these values were used in log form and normal values for them are given in the paper cited (10).

MATERIAL

From a large series of hypogonadal men seen at the Male Hypogonadism Study Section through the years 1963 to 1968 the following disorders were excluded from the present study: Klinefelter's syndrome, Sertoli-cell only syndrome, eunuchoidism, infantilism, hypopituitarism, adiposo-genital dystrophy, sequelae of previous testicular retention, hypogonadism secondary to other disorders, occlusion of the sperm tract, and varicocele. This left a group of 88 patients with presumably cryptogenetic hypospermatogenesis which was used for this study.

It should be pointed out that this original diagnosing was done according to usual principles and prior to the investigations into the testicular biopsy score count, the evaluation of transformed log HG values and computation of the DXM-HCG test. Since these measures increase the possibilities for diagnosing hypopituitarism and adiposo-genital dystrophy it was anticipated that the group was to some extent contaminated with these and perhaps other disorders and would have to be sorted further (see below). Some of the patients had a high DHA excretion. Since these did not differ in the testicular picture from the rest it was decided to include them in the first round in the total group.

The 88 patients were married men below 40 years of age referred from gynecological departments or from general practitioners for infertility. In some, this was due to oligospermia, in some to poor sperm morphology or poor sperm motility and in many to a combination of these factors. In brief periods, due to heavy patient load, the clinic refused a limited number of men having high sperm count but poor sperm morphology as the only sperm defect. This became known

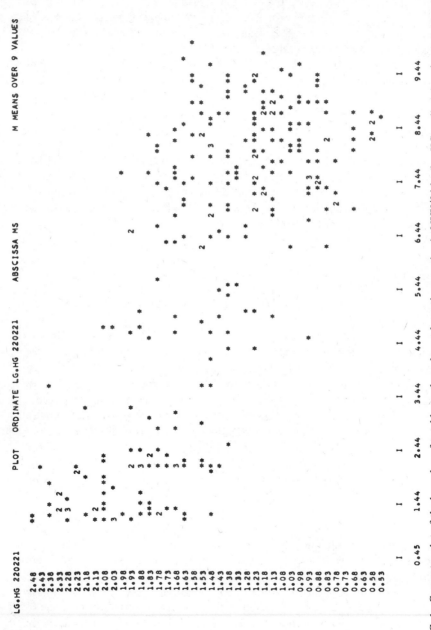

FIG. 1. Computer plot of the log value of total hypophyseal gonadotropin excretion in MUU/24 hr (log HG, ordinate) vs the mean score (MS) of the testicular biopsy score count (abscissa). 284 patients with all kinds of primary testicular disorders (Group 0).

by some of the referring departments and doctors but to what an extent these may have selected patients before referring to us is not known.

After completion of case collection in 1969 all analytical data were punched on cards for computation and the patient names and records no longer consulted.

RESULTS AND DISCUSSIONS

For the sake of clarity and brevity, discussion of the results is included under each successive step.

The Correlation Between Spermatogenesis and Gonadotropins in 284 Patients With All Kinds of Primary Testicular Disorders (Group 0)

This was previously reported (1, 2) but is included for comparison with the following. Figure 1 shows a plot between the mean score (MS) of the testicular biopsy score count (abscissa) and the log value of total gonadotropin excretion (log HG) (ordinate) in 284 patients with a great variety of primary testicular disorders (designated Group 0). The large number of patients with extremely low MS (MS 1 to 2) is due to Klinefelter and Sertoli-cell only cases.

The plot shows a very high negative correlation. The over-all correlation coefficient, r, is 0.732 (p < 0.001). The regression equation, standard deviation of slope, and so on, are stated in Table I. It should be noted that there is a 10-fold rise in gonadotropin level from good spermatogenesis to abolished spermatogenesis (1, 2).

TABLE I. Regression equations and significances against zero in the correlations between the log value of total gonadotropin excretion (log HG) and the mean score (MS) of the testicular biopsy score count[a]

Patient group	Number	Regression equation	SD of slope	t value	p value
O	284	log HG = 2.125 - 0.1130 × MS	0.0062	18.09	<0.001
A	88	log HG = 1.922 - 0.0880 × MS	0.0204	4.31	<0.001
B	75	log HG = 2.089 - 0.1004 × MS	0.0173	5.82	<0.001
C	54	log HG = 2.026 - 0.1005 × MS	0.0170	5.91	<0.001
D	45	log HG = 1.666 - 0.0545 × MS	0.0396	1.38	<0.10 >0.05

[a]Patient Groups O, A, B, C, D: see legends to Figs. 1 to 6.

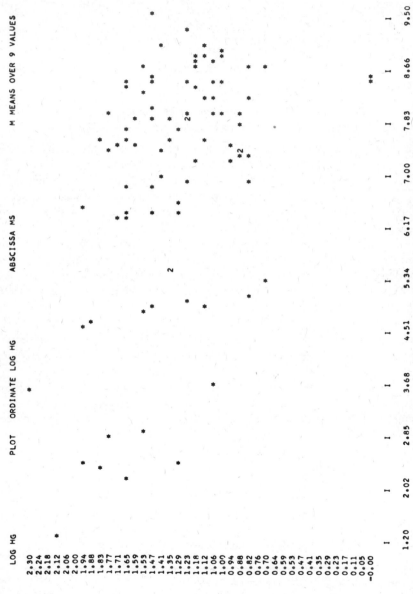

FIG. 2. The total group of 88 infertile men with hypospermatogenesis (Group A). Plot of log HG vs MS (see Fig. 1).

The Correlation in the Total Group of 88 Cases of Hypospermatogenesis (Group A)

For this group consisting of cases originally diagnosed as cases of cryptogenetic hypospermatogenesis but presumably to some extent contaminated with various disorders, the plot between MS and log HG is shown in Fig. 2.

There is, as expected, rather an uneven distribution of values indicating nonhomogeniety of the group. Under these circumstances, correlation analyses must be looked upon with some caution. However, the regression equation and SD of slope (Table I, Group A), indicate a highly significant negative correlation as the first group. The correlation coefficient is 0.421 ($p < 0.001$). This group also shows a significant negative correlation between the log value of the total sperm count and log HG (correlation coefficient 0.459, $p < 0.001$).

Thus, in this infertility group containing no cases of total tubular destruction or total absence of germ cells, the relationship between spermatogenesis and gonadotropin excretion persists.

Exclusion from the Total Group Cases of Hypothalamic and Hypophyseal Disturbances (Group B)

In 1968 the author (11) described that patients with hypothalamic disturbances (organic hypothalamic lesion or functional hypothalamic dysfunction such as adiposo-genital dystrophy and similar conditions) have elevated urinary androsterone/etiocholanolone ratio. Our studies of hypothalamic cases by the DXM-HCG test (to be published) have now shown that besides this defect in androgen metabolism there is a disturbance of adrenal androgen production with a pronounced decrease in urinary DHA and A + E of adrenal origin. The combination of these seems to have high diagnostic specificity and the group of hypospermatogenetic men was searched by these criteria. It was found that 6 patients had data diagnostic for or highly indicative of hypothalamic dysfunction. The findings will be published separately, and in the present study it was decided to take the 6 patients out of the group.

In a separate paper (8) values for the log HG transformed by means of a regression equation to a fixed biopsy mean score of 1.0 found in primary testicular disorders were reported to have a mean of 2.01, ± SD 0.30. It was decided to take out of the hypospermatogenesis group patients with a value below 2.01 to $1.65 \times SD$ = below 1.515. This turned out to be 7 patients which were suspect of hypopituitarism (particularly as the value in most of them was very low) (8). We realized that by such a decision we had to some extent influenced the point of investigation because the patients so removed were patients displaying a particularly low gonadotropin value considered from their spermatogenetic state. However, there is no alternative as long as independent diagnostic criteria for isolated gonadotropin insufficiency do not exist. Fortunately the number of patients is less than 10% of the whole group, and proof

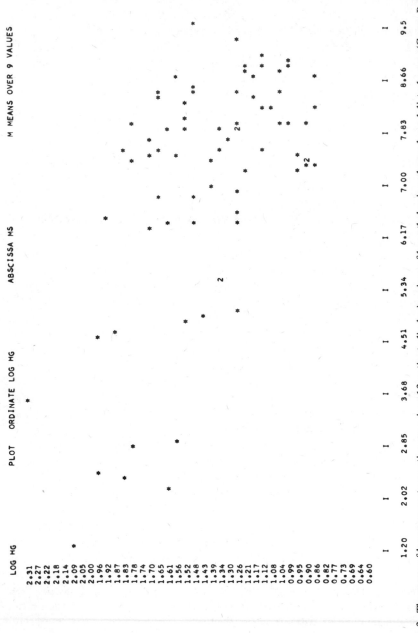

FIG. 3. The group of hypospermatogenetic men minus 13 patients displaying signs of hypothalamic or hypophyseal disturbances (Group B, 75 cases). Plot of log HG vs MS, (see Fig. 1).

that the exclusion of such patients is not the factor which creates the correlation between log HG and MS is evident from the fact that the correlation is present in the total group (Group A) despite the fact that the presence of patients with primary hypopituitarism would tend to blur the correlation.

Exclusion of the 6 hypothalamic cases and the 7 hypopituitarism cases from the total group gives Group B. Figure 3 shows the plot between log HG and MS in this group. It is seen that the distribution of log HG values is less irregular than in group A and the negative correlation more clear. The regression equation is given in Table I. The t value of the slope has increased somewhat from Group A and so has the correlation coefficient which is now in Group B 0.562 (p < 0.001). However, the change in the correlation induced by these patient exclusions is only moderate.

Exclusion of Cases with Presumably Primary Disturbances in Steroid Production of the Adrenals and Leydig Cells (Enzyme Defects): The Purified Group of Idiopathic Hypospermatogenesis (Group C)

In the further screening of the patients it was found by the DXM test that 9 patients in Group B had changes indicating the presence of a borderline adreno-genital syndrome. Eight of these had elevated urinary DHA of adrenal origin, 5 also elevated adrenal A + E, and 7 also somewhat elevated adrenal ketogenic steroids (presumably pregnanetriol). One patient had normal DHA but elevation of both adrenal A + E and ketogenic steroids. The findings indicate that these men suffer from moderate adrenal enzyme deficiencies comparable to the well-known borderline adreno-genital syndrome in women. This condition in men will be described elsewhere. Since, however, increased adrenal steroids could possibly exert an extragonadal influence upon the gonadotropin level it was decided to take these 9 men out of the group.

Primary steroid enzyme deficiencies in Leydig cells have to our knowledge not been described. We tried by mere speculation to find out what changes one would expect to meet if it existed. Logical changes would be: 1) Leydig cell hyperplasia; 2) LH increase which in our study would manifest itself as a high log HG being out of proportion with the spermatogenetic state, in other words, high transformed log HG; and 3) perhaps increase of pregnanetriol of testicular origin (high ketogenic steroids during adrenal suppression in our DXM test).

To our surprise no less than 14 patients in Group B displayed such a combination of changes. Thirteen of these had Leydig cell hyperplasia (which was pronounced in 7 and extremely severe in 1), the transformed log HG was high in 11 and above 2.01 in the remaining 2. Testicular ketogenic steroids was examined in 10, was normal in 4 and high in 6 patients. The patient without Leydig cell hyperplasia had both elevated transformed log HG and elevated testicular ketogenic steroids. Two of the patients turned out to be identical with 2 of the cases of borderline adreno-genital syndrome and these 2 thus displayed signs of steroid enzyme deficiency both in adrenal and Leydig cells. The cases of Leydig cell deficiency will be further described elsewhere. Here it was decided to

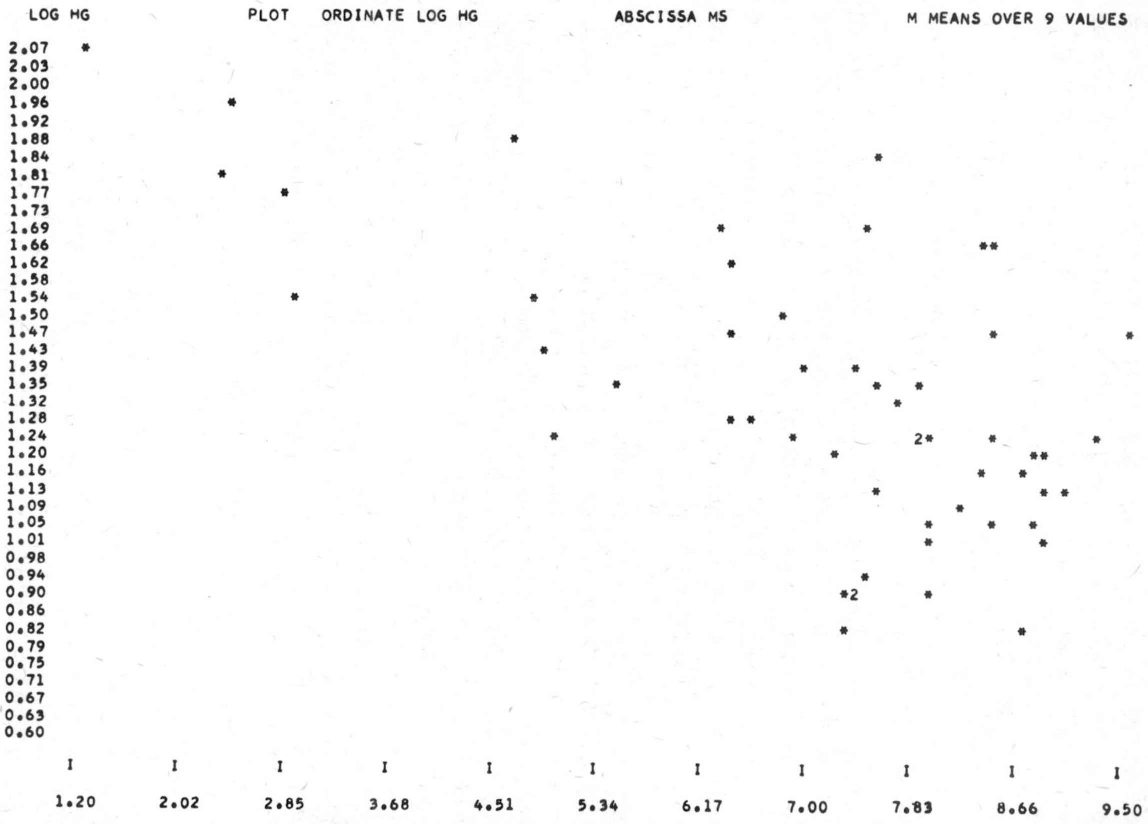

FIG. 4. The group of hypospermatogenetic men minus the 13 cases of hypothalamic/hypophyseal disturbance and minus 21 patients having steroido-genic disturbance in adrenals of Leydig cells. The purified group of hypospermatogenesis (Group C, 54 cases). Plot of log HG vs MS (see Fig. 1).

take them out of the hypospermatogenesis group together with the cases of borderline adreno-genital syndrome, altogether 21 patients.

This step marked the end of our present possibilities for sorting out patients according to diagnostic criteria, and the remaining 54 patients should then constitute a "pure" group of cases of "cryptogenetic" hypospermatogenesis.

Figure 4 shows the plot between log HG and MS in this group of 54 men (Group C). It is seen that the removal of patients with presumably primary disturbances in steroid production has had no effect whatsoever upon the correlation between gonadotropin excretion and spermatogenesis. The regression equation (Table I) shows exactly the same slope as Group B. It has kept its high significance against zero and so has the correlation coefficient which is in Group C, 0.633 (p < 0.001).

As shown in Table I the slope of the regression between gonadotropin excretion and spermatogenesis in this "purified" group of hypospermatogenesis is somewhat lower than the slope originally found when all kinds of primary testicular disorders were included (Group O). Although significant (p < 0.01), the slope difference is, however, only on the order of 10%.

Exclusion of Cases with Severe Tubular Failure from the Purified Group (Group D)

By the original selection of patients and by the subsequent purification of the group by exclusion of cases believed to display extratubular causes of infertility one might perhaps expect to end with a homogenous group of "cryptogenetic" hypospermatogenesis. It appeared, however, that the group was not homogenous. Figure 5 shows the distribution of values for the testicular biopsy mean

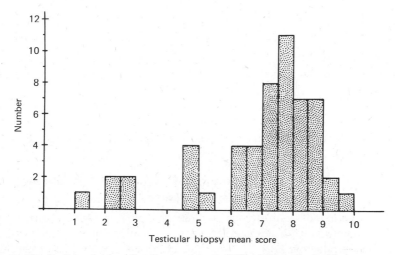

FIG. 5. Distribution of values for the mean score (MS) of the testicular biopsy score count in the purified group of hypospermatogenetic men (Group C), see legend to Fig. 4. In normal men the MS is >8.9.

score. It is seen that the majority of the patients form a homogenous group with MS from 5 to 10. Four patients have, however, MS values between 4 and 5 and these correspond to a much poorer spermatogenesis than that of the majority. Five patients have a MS of only 1.2 to 2.8 and thus suffered from an extensive germinal epithelium damage which is highly different from the condition in all other cases.

From the distribution it appears unlikely that the patients in these two small groups suffered from the same disorder as the rest. What they suffered from is not known at the time of writing but in order to end up with a homogenous group it was tried to take these 4 + 5 patients out.

By doing this the final group of 45 patients (Group D) only contains cases of slight to moderate hypospermatogenesis. The MS in this group shows an even distribution (mean 7.72, SD 0.94) and the log value of the total sperm count has also an approximately normal distribution (with mean 1.68, SD 0.74).

It was clear that a correlation analysis of log HG versus MS in such a group puts the gonadotropin/spermatogenesis relationship to a very hard test because now the rate of spermatogenesis has only a small scale of movement on top of which the very large individual variation of gonadotropin excretion is placed.

Figure 6 shows the outcome in the log HG/MS plot in Group D. There is a wide scattering of the values. However, as shown in Table I, there is still a negative regression between log HG and MS and the slope shows a difference from zero which is close to significance ($p < 0.10 > 0.05$). The mean log HG of the whole Group D is 1.240. Twenty-two patients with a long HG below this mean have a mean MS of 8.071 (SD 0.651); 23 patients with log HG above the mean have a mean MS of 7.452 (SD 1.049). The t value of this difference is 2.37, $p < 0.0125 > 0.01$.

Thus, even in this group with a reduced span of MS there is a negative relationship between spermatogenesis as determined by the testicular biopsy score count method and gonadotropin excretion. This is further substantiated by the fact that this group (as all the preceding groups) shows a negative correlation between log HG and the log value of the total sperm count. In this regression the t value of the slope against zero is 2.61, $p < 0.01 > 0.005$ and thus highly significant.

We have then found that the relationship between spermatogenesis and gonadotropin excretion operates in all groups of hypospermatogenesis, even in a group of moderate hypospermatogenesis where the patients have relatively small differences in the rate of spermatogenesis.

Relationship Between Gonadotropin Excretion and Testicular Androgen Production in Hypospermatogenetic Men

Urinary excretion of androsterone and etiocholanolone (A + E) during total adrenal suppression with dexamethasone is a reliable parameter for testicular testosterone production (10). The log value of testicular A + E [designated XAE

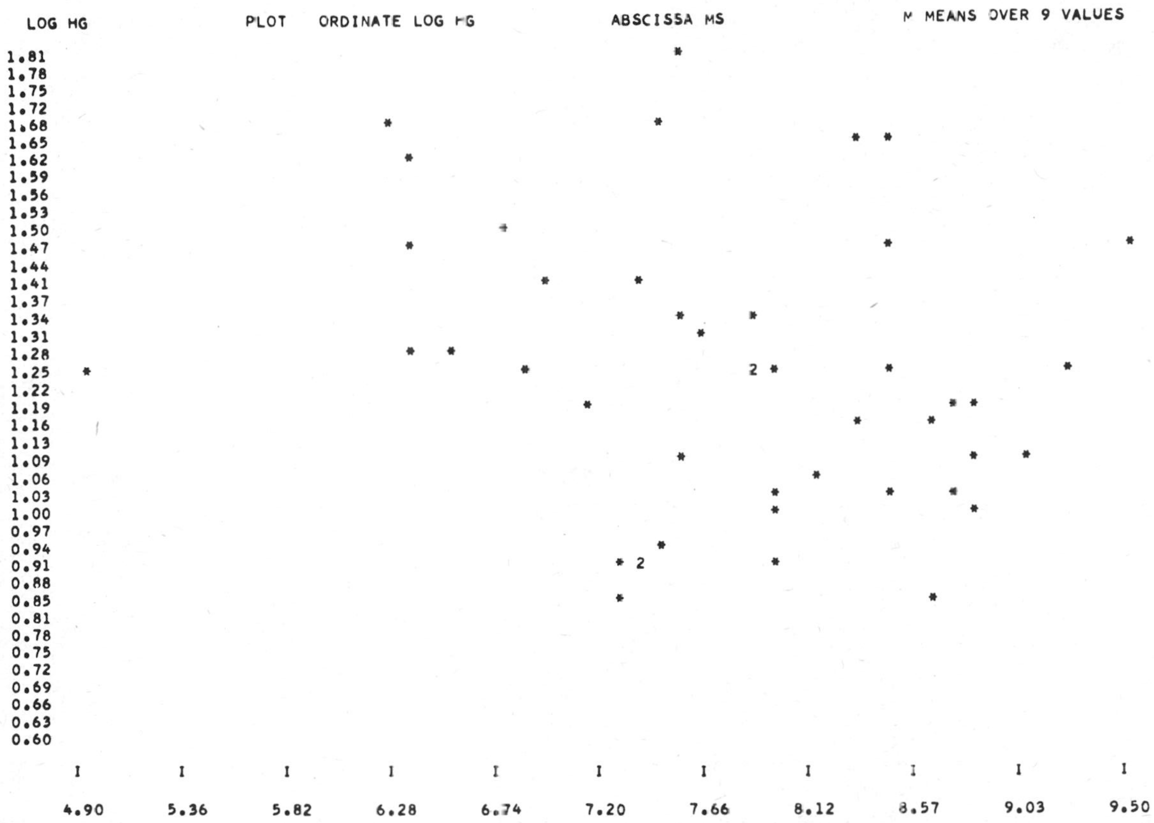

FIG. 6. The purified group of hypospermatogenetic men (Group C, see Fig. 4) minus 9 patients displaying severe tubular failure (Group D, 45 cases). Plot of log HG vs MS (see Fig. 1).

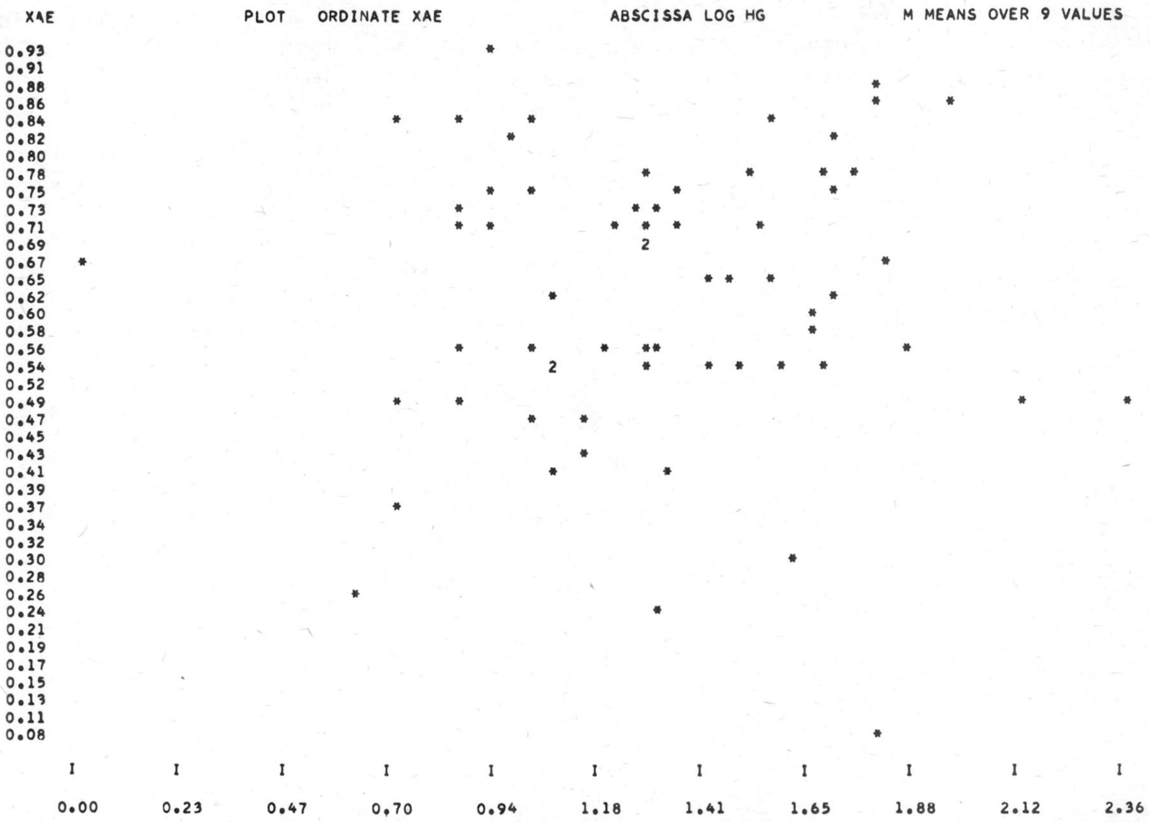

PLOT   ORDINATE XAE   ABSCISSA LOG HG   M MEANS OVER 9 VALUES

XAE

0.93
0.91
0.88
0.86
0.84
0.82
0.80
0.78
0.75
0.73
0.71
0.69
0.67
0.65
0.62
0.60
0.58
0.56
0.54
0.52
0.49
0.47
0.45
0.43
0.41
0.39
0.37
0.34
0.32
0.30
0.28
0.26
0.24
0.21
0.19
0.17
0.15
0.13
0.11
0.08

0.00   0.23   0.47   0.70   0.94   1.18   1.41   1.65   1.88   2.12   2.36

FIG. 7. The total group of hypospermatogenetic men (Group A). Plot of the log value of urinary excretion of androsterone + etiocholanolone during total adrenal suppression with dexamethasone (XAE, ordinate) vs log HG (abscissa). 65 cases.

(10)] was correlated with log HG in all groups. Figure 7 shows the plot between XAE and log HG in the total group of hypospermatogenetic men (Group A). There is no correlation whatsoever, and correlation analyses showed a complete lack of correlation in all groups. The correlation coefficients were: Group A, 0.020; Group B 0.013; Group C, 0.114; and Group D, 0.136. All p values are far above 0.10 and no group shows the slightest tendency of a relationship.

In view of this lack of correlation it should be recalled that the gonadotropin level in severe spermatogenetic failure is considerably elevated. This affects not only FSH. LH is also increased somewhat (12) and our series of hypospermatogenetic males shows a close relationship between gonadotropin elevation and Leydig cell hyperplasia. Nevertheless, as we have also shown previously (13), this gives no increase of testicular androgen production.

The result is that we found no relationship whatsoever between testicular androgen production and excretion of total gonadotropins.

CONCLUSION

The gonadotropin level in the human male with an intact hypothalamic/ hypophyseal system is dependent upon the rate of spermatogenesis. A primary spermatogenetic insufficiency, even in minor degrees, results in gonadotropin increase (primarily FSH) and extensive damage of the germinal epithelium is associated with a 10-fold gonadotropin increase. The close relationship between spermatogenesis and gonadotropin level applies to all kinds of hypospermato-genetic males with intact hypothalamic/hypophyseal system.

As a consequence of this, gonadotropin analyses in men should always be evaluated in relation to the rate of spermatogenesis. As we have described recently (8), one way of doing this is to transform gonadotropin values by means of the general regression equation to a fixed level of spermatogenesis in all patients. Another way is to insert gonadotropin values in a graph showing the relationship between rate of spermatogenesis and gonadotropins in primary testicular disorders. When this is done the scientific and diagnostic value of gonadotropin analyses in hypogonadal men is greatly enhanced.

ACKNOWLEDGMENT

Supported by the Ford Foundation. Testicular biopsies were taken by Professor E. Hasner, Surgical Departmen RE, University Hospital of Copenhagen. Thanks are due for his kind cooperation and interest in these studies without which they could not have been performed.

REFERENCES

1. Johnsen, S. G., Acta Endocrinol (Kbh) 64:193, 1970.
2. Johnsen, S. G., in E. Rosemberg and C. A. Paulsen (Eds.), The Human Testis, Plenum, New York and London, 1970, p. 231.

3. Paulsen, C. A., in E. Rosemberg and C. A. Paulsen (Eds.), The Human Testis, Plenum, New York and London, 1970, p. 246.

4. Johnsen, S. G., Acta Endocrinol (Kbh) 28:69, 1958.

5. Johnsen, S. G., Acta Endocrinol (Kbh) 31:209, 1959.

6. Rosemberg, E. and S. R. Joshi, in E. Rosemberg (Ed.), Gonadotropins 1968, Geron-X, Inc., Los Altos, 1968, p.91.

7. Johnsen, S. G., Hormones 1:1, 1970.

8. Johnsen, S. G., Acta Endocrinol (Kbh) submitted for publication.

9. Hammen, R., Studies on Impaired Fertility in Man with Special Reference to the Male, Munksgaard, Copenhagen, and Oxford Univ. Press, London, 1944.

10. Johnsen, S. G., P. Christiansen, V. Aa. Frandsen, A. Froland, and J. Nielsen, Acta Endocrinol (Kbh) 66:587, 1971.

11. Johnsen, S. G., Acta Endocrinol (Kbh) 57:595, 1968.

12. Wide, L., and B. Kjessler, Acta Endocrinol (Kbh) 62:299, 1969.

13. Johnsen, S. G., Acta Endocrinol (Kbh) Suppl. 124:17, 1967.

46.   The Excretion of FSH and LH in Male Hypogonadism

Peter Christiansen

Recently Johnsen (1), in a large group of patients with all kind of primary testicular disorders, showed a highly significant negative correlation between spermatogenesis and the level of urinary gonadotropins measured by the mouse uterus test. In a "purified" group of 45 men, with "cryptogenic" hyposperma togenesis this relationship was confirmed. Rosen et al. (2), using radioimmuno-assay, found that the plasma level of FSH in 17 normal virile men with "cryptogenic" hypospermatogenesis was significantly higher than in 49 normal men of the same age. No difference in the plasma level of LH was found. Paulsen (3) showed, in investigating men who had undergone acute radiation to the testes, that urinary FSH increased (bioassay) but urinary LH (bioassay) and testorone did not. However, in 12 oligospermic males, using radioimmunoassay, Paulsen (4) found normal plasma levels of FSH and no correlation between testicular cell count and the excretion of FSH.

It is the purpose of this study to compare the excretion pattern of pituitary gonadotropins measured by specific bioassays for FSH and LH in men with severe oligospermia or aspermia to that of normal and castrated men.

MATERIAL AND METHODS

All patients were referred by physicians to the Male Hypogonadism Study Section of the University of Copenhagen for infertility. They underwent standard physical examination, including measurement of the testes volume, analysis of urinary androgens, estrogens, 17-ketosteroids, and gonadotropins;

several sperm counts and testicular biopsy were included. In most of the patients a combined dexamethasone suppression plus chorionic gonadotropin stimulation test (DXM-HCG test) was performed.

All patients collected two to twelve 24-hr urine samples, which were pooled, extracted by the method of Johnsen (5) and divided into three portions for the three bioassays.

Urinary total gonadotropins were measured by the mouse uterus test (6) and expressed in mouse uterus units (MUU)/24 hr (1 ampoule of the 2nd IRP-HMG = 133 MUU).

Urinary FSH was analyzed by the Steelman-Pohley method (7), using 20 IU HCG as total dose per rat for augmentation. The design of the assay was 3 + 3.

Urinary LH was measured by the ventral prostate weight (VPW) method and performed as described earlier (8). The design was 2 + 2. The 2nd IRP-HMG was used as the standard for both FSH and LH assays, and the excretion expressed in IU/24 hr. Statistics were according to a special computer program for bioassays.

Twenty-eight normal virile men, with testes of normal size were used as controls. They had proved their fertility by having at least 2 children. The mean age was 31.2 years, varying from 21 to 44 years. The average excretion of FSH was 6.8 ± 3.1 IU/24 hr and of LH, 6.9 ± 2.7 IU. The FSH/LH ratio was close to 1.0 in all normals.

RESULTS

Table I shows the excretion of FSH, LH, and total gonadotropins in 8 men legally castrated for sexual crimes. The time from castration to collection of urine varied from half a month to 66 months, with an average of 23.6 months. The mean age was 37.4 years. The excretion of FSH ranged from 31 to 190 IU, the mean being 75.5 ± 50.6, which is about 11 times the values in normal men. LH ranged from 15 to 72 IU, with an average of 27.6 ± 18.7, about 4 times the normal level. FSH/LH ratio was 2.7.

Table II indicates urinary FSH, LH, and total gonadotropins in 12 patients with Sertoli-cell-only syndrome. The mean age was 29.8 years. FSH ranged from 5 to 68 IU, in average 27.6, which is 4 times the level in normal men. The difference is statistically significant ($p < 0.05$). The excretion of LH was within normal range, the mean being 9.2 IU. FSH/LH ratio was 3.0.

In Table III is shown FSH, LH, and total gonadotropins in 22 men with "cryptogenis" oligospermia or aspermia. The mean age was 29.8 years. FSH ranged from 11 to 12o IU, the mean being 31.3 IU, about the same level as in Sertoli-cell-only syndrome, and significantly higher than in normal men ($p < 0.05$). LH was within normal range, the mean being 7.4 IU. The FSH/LH ratio was 4.2.

Table IV shows a group of 17 men with severe oligospermia or aspermia combined with hypopituitarism. The average age was 30.5 years. FSH was 3.9 ± 1.2 IU and LH, 5.6 ± 4.4 IU.

TABLE I. Excretion of FSH and LH in 8 castrated men

Identification	Age (years)	Time after castration (months)	FSH (IU/day)[a]	LH (IU/day)[b]	FSH/LH[c]	Total gonadotropins (MUU/day)
O.S.	30	12	190	29	6.5	190
G.L.	44	36	67	15	4.4	160
E.E.	34	60	52	15	3.4	
P.J.	32	12	85	25	3.4	280
V.L.	53	0.5	49	17	2.8	72
P.H.	23	1	40	21	1.9	
U.A.	39	1	90	72	1.2	
J.O.	44	66	31	27	1.1	100

[a]Mean: 75.5 ± 50.6.
[b]Mean: 27.6 ± 18.7.
[c]Mean: 2.7.

TABLE II. Excretion of FSH and LH in men with Sertoli-cell-only syndrome

Identi-fication	Age (years)	FSH (IU/day)[a]	LH (IU/day)[b]	FSH/LH[c]	Total gonado-tropins (MUU/day)
T.E.C.	29	31	5	6.2	64
K.L.	28	50	9	5.6	71
B.J.P.	35	15	3	5.0	12
E.D.C.	26	68	15	4.5	80
P.S.	29	39	10	3.9	41
E.M.	28	42	15	2.8	60
H.E.P.	34	36	18	2.0	33
A.N.	39	13	7	1.9	33
G.K.	26	11	7	1.6	18
W.J.	31	8	5	1.6	28
J.J.	27	14	11	1.3	5
E.J.	25	5	5	1.0	34

[a]Mean: 27.6 ± 19.7.
[b]Mean: 9.2 ± 4.5.
[c]Mean: 3.0.

The 17 patients could be divided into 3 groups: one group of 5 patients with especially low LH (high FSH/LH ratio); a second group of 6 patients with low FSH as well as LH (FSH/LH ratio close to 1.0); and a third group of 6 patients with especially low FSH (low FSH/LH ratio), indicating that the lesion of the pituitary gland may affect FSH and LH separately or both.

DISCUSSION

The data presented here show a monotropic increase of urinary FSH in patients with Sertoli-cell-only syndrome and "cryptogenic" oligospermia and aspermia, using specific bioassays. The level is about 3 times that of normal men, but lower than that of castrated men and of patients with Klinefelters syndrome (9); the FSH/LH ratio is higher. Using the testicular biopsy score count method of Johnsen (10) there is a significant negative correlation between testes morphology and urinary FSH, but no correlation to urinary LH in the 22 patients with severe oligospermia or aspermia. (11).

TABLE III. Monotropic increase of the excretion of FSH in men with severe oligospermia or aspermia

Identi-fication	Age (years)	FSH (IU/day)[a]	LH (IU/day)[b]	FSH/LH[c]	Total gonado-tropins (MUU/day)
K.S.	30	118	15	7.8	70
P.C.	30	120	17	7.0	130
K.C.	38	82	14	5.8	76
K.T.	25	22	4	5.5	21
F.E.	31	25	5	5.0	36
T.P.	30	15	3	5.0	35
K.E.O.	27	15	3	5.0	27
L.S.	29	17	4	4.2	47
P.V.	27	25	6	4.1	66
E.P.	26	21	6	3.5	8
K.M.J.	26	14	4	3.5	35
G.J.	35	27	8	3.3	64
W.M.	31	13	4	3.3	11
P.O.H.	28	15	5	3.0	18
T.K.H.	32	15	5	3.0	19
P.A.	31	37	13	2.8	70
N.J.S.	30	14	5	2.8	60
T.H.	28	11	4	2.7	13
B.P.	32	22	8	2.7	50
F.L.S.	27	35	17	2.0	61
H.L.	31	12	6	2.0	20
P.C.	32	15	8	1.8	25

[a]Mean: 31.3 ± 32.1.
[b]Mean: 7.4 ± 4.5.
[c]Mean: 4.2.

TABLE IV. Excretion of FSH and LH in men with severe oligospermia or aspermia combined with hypopituitarism

Identi-fication	Age (years)	FSH (IU/day)[a]	LH (IU/day)[b]	FSH FSH/LH[c]	Total gonado-tropins (MUU/day)
F.V.	28	6	2	3.0	8
B.R.	27	5	2	2.5	9
K.U.	32	4	2	2.0	18
B.N.	32	4	3	1.3	8
P.T.	30	5	4	1.2	23
H.H.P.	24	5	5	1.0	17
R.B.	33	4	4	1.0	11
P.D.	31	3	3	1.0	8
K.C.	28	3	3	1.0	5
H.S.	28	2	2	1.0	8
B.C.	27	4	5	0.8	9
H.J.	33	4	7	0.5	9
J.S.	31	4	7	0.5	28
B.J.	35	4	8	0.5	11
J.K.H.	44	4	13	0.3	40
B.E.	27	5	19	0.2	24
S.E.H.	28	1	7	0.1	6

[a]Mean: 3.9 ± 1.2.

[b]Mean: 5.6 ± 4.4.

[c]Mean: 0.7.

The study points to the fact that FSH is the regulator of the spermatogenesis, either alone or in combination with other factors and that the germ cells produce a hormone, which is the second link in the feedback mechanism. The role of the androgens (if they have one) is not yet explained, but in our 22 oligospermic men, only 2 had slightly decreased testicular androgens.

ACKNOWLEDGMENT

Supported by the Ford Foundation.

REFERENCES

1. Johnsen, S. G., in E. Rosemberg, and C. A. Paulsen (Eds.), The Human Testis, Plenum, New York and London, 1970, p. 231.
2. Rosen, S. W., and B. D. Weintraub, J Clin Endocrinol 32:410, 1971.
3. Paulsen, C. A., in E. Rosemberg, (Ed.), Gonadotropins 1968, Geron-X, Inc., Los Altos, 1968, p. 163.
4. Paulsen, C. A., in E. Rosemberg, and C. A. Paulsen (Eds.), The Human Testis, Plenum, New York and London, 1970, p. 246.
5. Johnsen, S. G., Acta Endocrinol (Kbh) 28:69, 1958.
6. Johnsen, S. G., Acta Endocr (Kbh) 31:209, 1959.
7. Steelman, S. L., and F. M. Pohley, Endocrinology 53:604, 1953.
8. Christiansen, P., Acta Endocrinol (Kbh) 56:608, 1967.
9. Christiansen, P., Unpublished.
10. Johnsen, S. G., Hormones 1:1, 1970.
11. Christiansen, P., Endocrinol (Kbh) 31:209, 1959.

47. Response of the Human Testes to HLH and HCG

Eugenia Rosemberg, John F. Crigler, Jr., Si G. Lee, Wan F. Jan, and Philip S. Butler

Bioassay [ovarian ascorbic acid depletion (OAAD) and ventral prostate weight (VPW) assays] and radioimmunoassays of HLH ad of HCG indicate differences in biologic activity and immunologic reactivity of these preparations. As information concerning the comparative effect of these hormones in the human testes is meager, it was decided to investigate the acute effect of HLH and HCG following short administration of both hormones in adolescent male subjects with immature testes.

MATERIAL AND METHODS

The preparations used in this study were a commercial preparation of HCG (Follutein, Squibb) with an activity of 10,000 IU HCG/vial (biologic potency) and a purified HLH preparation supplied by the National Pituitary Agency (Lot A1, LER 856-1) with an LH activity of 200 IU 2nd IRP-HMG/vial; the FSH contamination was 2.5 IU 2nd IRP-HMG/vial (biologic potency).

Assays

Plasma testosterone levels were determined by the competitive protein binding assay (1). The LH activity in plasma was determined using the double-antibody radioimmunoassay described by Odell et al. (2). All samples from an individual subject were assayed in the same assay at two dose levels. The reference materials used in all assays were: LER 907 (distributed by the NPA); the Second

616

International Reference Preparation for Human Menopausal Gonadotropin (2nd IRP-HMG); LER 856-1, and HCG Second International Standard (2nd IS). All reference preparations were tested at four dose levels. Radioimmunoassay results were calculated by appropriate computer programs for parallel line assays. In our assay system, the immunoreactivity of 1 mIU of biological activity of 2nd IRP-HMG is equivalent to that of 3.2 ng of LER 907, 0.63 ng of LER 856-1, and 0.28 mIU of biological activity of HCG (2nd IS); 10.6 mIU of biological activity of HCG-2nd IS is equivalent to that of 1 μg of LER 907. In this discussion all concentrations will be expressed in terms of μg LER 907/ml of plasma.

Subjects

Two sexually immature male patients were selected for these studies. The first patient (J. K.) age 18 6/12 years, was referred to the Childrens Hospital Medical Center at 8 years of age because of short stature. On examination, his height age was 4 6/12 years, his bone age 3 2/12 years, his weight 40.2 lb and his genitalia were normal for his age. The usual laboratory procedures revealed deficiencies in GII, TSII, and ACTII, and a diagnosis of idiopathic hypopituitarism was made. The patient was treated with l-thyroxine (T^4), 0.1 to 0.15 mg/day from age 10 3/12 years to age 11 9/12 years. At 13 years of age, the patient was treated with human growth hormone (2 mg q.d.); T^4 was restarted while on growth hormone at age 15 3/12 years. Both medications were given continuously until the time of the present studies. At 18 years of age, the patient showed lack of secondary sexual development. On examination, the testes measured 3.8 x 2 cm, the phallus measured 5.3 x 1.8 cm, and axillary and pubic hair were absent. A testicular biopsy performed at 18 years of age revealed the presence of small tubules without a lumen, arrest of spermatogenesis at the spermatocyte stage, immature Sertoli cells, some thickening of the tubular wall, and a diminished number of Leydig cells. Prior to the present studies, the patient was never treated with gonadotropin preparations.

The second patient (W.S.) age 19 10/12 years, the second born of twins, was referred to the Childrens Hospital Medical Center at age 13 9/12 years for difficulties in school work. His IQ was 115. Remedial training was recommended and he did well. He returned with his twin brother at age 15 2/12 years because of lack of sexual development. Treatment was not recommended at that time. Subsequently, his twin brother developed normally. However, the patient remained sexually immature. On examination at age 19 5/12 years, his height corresponded to a chronological age of 15 6/12 years, and his weight was 192 lb (39% overweight for height). His penis measured 4.0 cm (stretched) and 2 cm in diameter. The right testis measured 4 x 2.1 cm and the left testis measured 3.6 x 1.9 cm. Axillary and pubic hair were present. Buccal smear was negative and chromosome analysis showed a normal male karyotype. The testicular biopsy performed at age 19 revealed the presence of small tubules with arrest of spermatogenesis at the spermatid stage, immature Sertoli cells, and diminished number of Leydig cells. Prior to the present studies, the patient was never treated with gonadotropin preparations. Nine courses of medication were given. The details are given in Table I.

TABLE I. Sequential courses[a] of human gonadotropins administered intramuscularly

Course	HCG (IU/day × 3)	HLH (IU/day × 3)
1	5000	
2		5000 (1800; 1600; 1600)
3		5000 (1800; 1600; 1600)
4	5000	
5[b]		1000 (400; 400; 200)
6[b]	1000	
7[b]		100 (40; 40; 20)
8[b]	100	
9[c]	10	

Note: HCG: Follutein, Squibb - 10,000 IU/vial. HLH: (NPA) LH, 200 IU 2nd IRP - HMG; FSH, 2.5 IU 2nd IRP - HMG/vial.

[a]Separated by 2 to 3 week intervals.

[b]Patient JK and WS only.

[c]Patient JK only.

Both patients received four identical courses of medication separated by an interval of two to three weeks. During the first and fourth course, 5000 IU of HCG was given as a single intramuscular injection given each day at 8:30 A.M. for three consecutive days; during the second and third courses, 5000 IU of HLH was given intramuscularly in three divided doses each day for three consecutive days. In addition, four additional courses of medication were given. During the fifth and sixth course, 1000 IU of HLH and HCG respectively, were given. During the seventh and eighth course 100 IU of HLH and HCG, respectively, were given. A final course (course nine) of 10 IU of HCG was given to patient J.K. The dosage schedules used on courses five to nine were identical to those followed when 5000 IU of HLH and HCG were used. Each course of medication was also given at intervals of 2 to 3 weeks. Blood samples were drawn daily at 8:30 a.m., 2:30 p.m., and 8:30 p.m., the day prior to initiation of medication, during medication days, and for 3 to 6 days after cessation of therapy.

Effect of HLH and HCG

Figure 1 depicts the plasma gonadotropin concentration and testosterone levels during each of the first four courses of medication given to patient J.K.

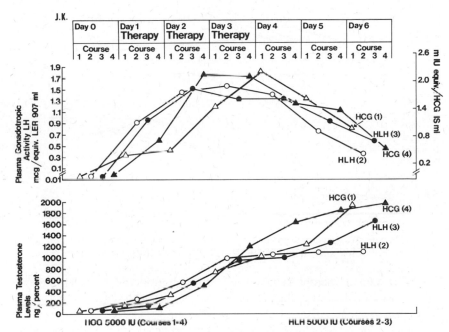

FIG. 1. Patient J.K. Plasma gonadotropic and testosterone concentration during four courses of medication with 5000 IU of HCG, HLH, HLH and HCG, respectively.

During each of the four courses of therapy, plasma gonadotropin concentration increased to 11 to 32 times the control level on the first day of therapy and reached peak values of 32 to 63 times the control level on the third day of therapy. Values 21 to 51 times the control level persisted on the first and second day, and remained above control levels on the third day after cessation of therapy. The response of the testes judged by the testosterone levels was quite striking. During each of the four courses of medication, plasma testosterone concentration increased 2 to 7 times the control level on the first day of therapy, and increased steadily thereafter: 25 to 38% over control levels on the second day of therapy, 28 to 52% and 29 to 63% on the first and second day after cessation of medication. Testosterone levels were still elevated (29 to 99%) on the morning of the third day after withdrawal of medication.

Figure 2 depicts the plasma gonadotropin concentration and testosterone levels during each of the first four courses of medication given to patient W.S.

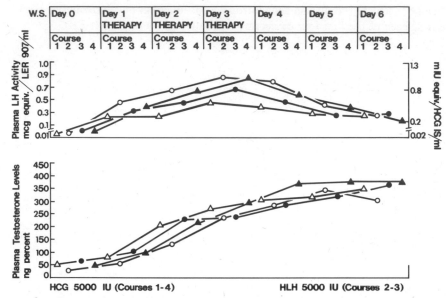

FIG. 2. Patient W. S. Plasma gonadotropic and testosterone concentration during four courses of medication with 5000 IU of HCG, HLH, HLH and HCG, respectively.

The pattern of plasma gonadotropin concentration and testosterone levels was similar to that seen on the first patient, J.K., although the absolute levels of testosterone were lower than those recorded on J.K.

Figure 3 depicts the plasma gonadotropin concentration and testosterone levels during medication courses with 5000,1000, 100, and 10 IU of HCG given to patient J.K.

The pattern of plasma gonadotropin concentration was similar in all courses but, the absolute levels were 2 to 10 times lower when 1000 and 100 IU of HCG were given than those recorded when 5000 IU were administered. With 1000 IU of HCG, plasma testosterone levels were similar to those recorded when 5000 IU were given. However, with 100 IU, testosterone levels were about 2 times lower than those recorded when 1000 IU were given. Moreover, testosterone levels were still elevated on the sixth day after withdrawal of medication with 1000 IU and remained elevated for only four days after withdrawal of medication with 100 IU. There was no increase in plasma testosterone levels when 10 IU of HCG were given.

Figure 4 depicts the plasma gonadotropin concentration and testosterone levels during medication courses with 5000; 1000, and 100 IU of HLH given to patient J.K.

The pattern of plasma gonadotropic concentration was similar in all courses but the absolute levels were 2 to 17 times lower when 1000 and 100 IU,

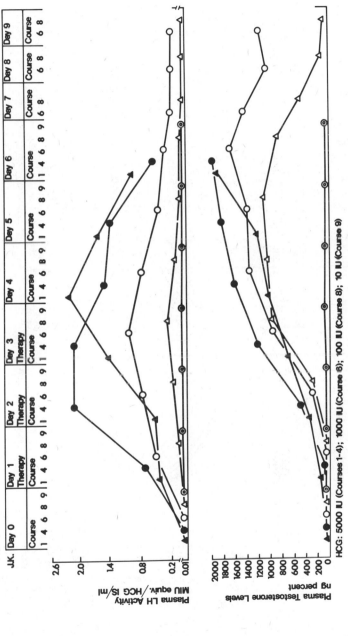

FIG. 3. Patient J.K. Plasma gonadotropic and testosterone concentration during courses of medication with 5000, 1000, 100, and 10 IU of HCG.

HCG: 5000 IU (Courses 1–4); 1000 IU (Course 6); 100 IU (Course 8); 10 IU (Course 9)

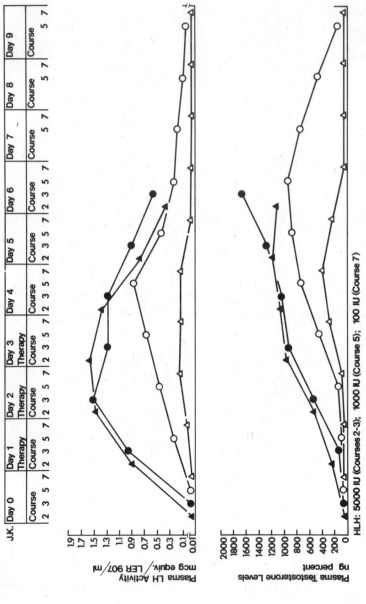

622

FIG. 4. Patient J.K. Plasma gonadotropic and testosterone concentration during courses of medication with 5000, 1000, and 100 IU of HLH.

HLH: 5000 IU (Courses 2-3); 1000 IU (Course 5); 100 IU (Course 7)

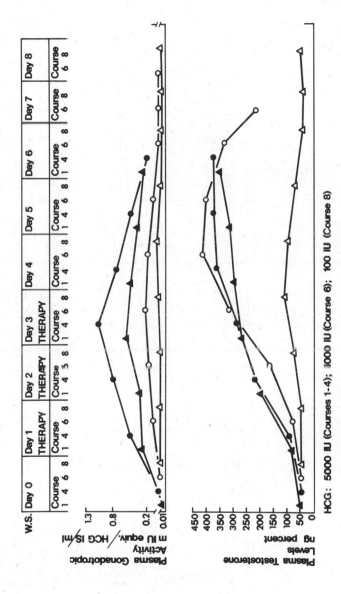

FIG. 5. Patient W.S. Plasma gonadotropic and testosterone concentration during courses of medication with 5000, 1000, and 100 IU of HCG.

HCG: **5000 IU (Courses 1-4); 1000 IU (Course 6); 100 IU (Course 8)**

623

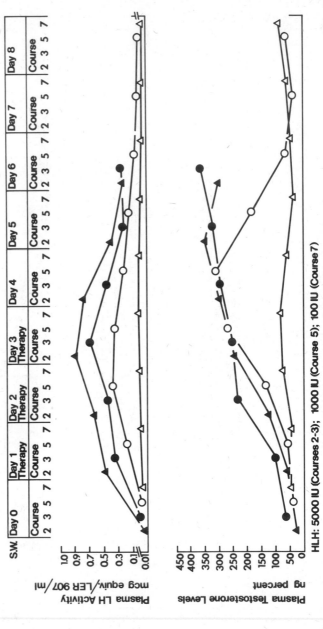

FIG. 6. Patient W.S. Plasma gonadotropic and testosterone concentration during courses of medication with 5000, 1000, and 100 IU of HLH.

HLH: 5000 IU (Courses 2-3); 1000 IU (Course 5); 100 IU (Course 7)

624

respectively, of HLH were given than those recorded when 5000 IU were administered. In contrast to the results observed with HCG, the plasma testosterone values in response to 1000 IU of HLH were 2 times lower than those recorded when 5000 IU were given. When 100 IU of HLH were given the levels of plasma testosterone were about 2 to 3 times lower than those recorded when 1000 IU were administered. Moreover, testosterone levels were still elevated on the fourth day after withdrawal of medication with 1000 IU and for only two days after withdrawal of medication with 100 IU of HLH.

Figures 5 and 6 depict the plasma gonadotropin concentration and testosterone levels during medication courses with 5000; 1000 and 100 IU of HCG and HLH, respectively, given to patient W.S.

Although, the absolute levels of plasma testosterone were lower than those recorded on J. K., the pattern of response was similar to that observed in the first patient.

Figure 7 depicts the response observed in the two patients to the administration of the various dosages of HCG and HLH used in this study.

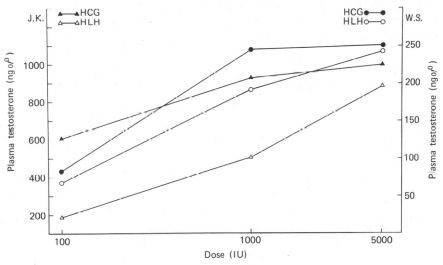

FIG. 7. Plasma Testosterone levels in response to the administration of 100, 1000, and 5000 IU of HCG and HLH, respectively.

DISCUSSION

The data indicate that in terms of dose, both HLH and HCG induced, within the same patient, comparable stimulation of the Leydig cells. Moreover, a dose-response relationship was observed.

The disappearance rate of endogenous and exogenously administered gonadotropins have been studied in the human by several investigators (3-11). The studies utilizing the IV infusion of a tracer dose of hormone indicate that the half-life ($t^{1/2}$) of HLH is approximately 1 hr, that of HFSH is approximately 3 hr, and that the $t^{1/2}$ of HCG shows a fast and slow component of approximately 5 to 23 hr, respectively. The study of the disappearance rate of endogenous gonadotropins indicates that the $t^{1/2}$ of HLH has a fast and slow component of 21 min and 3.9 hr, respectively, and the $t^{1/2}$ of HFSH has a fast and slow component of 3.9 and 70.4 hr, respectively. The $t^{1/2}$ of HCG has a fast and slow component of 8 to 11 hr and 23 to 37.3 hr, respectively. The calculations of metabolic clearance rates (MCR) (5 and 8) of HLH and HCG indicate that the MCR and HCG is approximately 1/10 that of HLH.

In these studies, the pattern of gonadotropin concentration in plasma during all courses of medication was similar in both subjects. The slow disappearance of plasma immunoreactive gonadotropin (HLH and HCG) was coupled with a steady increase in testosterone levels after withdrawal of both hormones. It could be postulated, therefore, that the immunoreactive circulating gonadotropins induced a prolonged biologic effect on the Leydig cells. However, HCG exerted a longer stimulatory effect than that observed with HLH. This effect could be attributed to differences between the two hormones relative to their rate of disappearance from the injection site, differences in peripheral halflife and metabolic clearance rates or, to differences in their halflife at the target cell site.

ACKNOWLEDGMENT

This work was supported by grants AM-07564 and RR 00128, USPHS, National Institutes of Health, Bethesda, Maryland and by a grant from the Theodore Schulze Foundation, New York, New York.

We are indebted to the National Institutes of Arthritis and Metabolic Diseases, NIH, and to the National Pituitary Agency, Baltimore, Maryland for the supply of immunologic reagents and the supply of HLH and HGH used in this study. We wish to thank Dr. E. C. Reifenstein, Jr., Squibb Institute for Medical Research, New Brunswick, New Jersey for the gift of Follutein (human chorionic gonadotropin), and Dr. D. R. Bangham, Department of Biological Standards, Medical Research Council, Mill Hill, London for the gift of HCG 2nd IS and the 2nd IRP-HMG.

REFERENCES

1. Mayes, D., and C. A. Nugent, J Clin Endocrinol 28:1169, 1969.
2. Odell, W. D., G. T. Ross, and P. L. Rayford, J Clin Invest 46:248, 1967.
3. Parlow, A. F., Rec. Prog Hormone Res 21:201, 1965.
4. Schalch, D. S., A. F. Parlow, R. C. Boon, and S. Reichlin, J Clin Invest 47:665, 1968.
5. Kohler, P. O., G. T. Ross, and W. D. Odell, J Clin Invest 47:38, 1968.

6. Yen, S. S. C., O. Llerena, B. Little, and O. H. Pearson, J Clin Endocrinol 28:1763, 1968.

7. Yen, S. S. C., L. A. Llerena, O. H. Pearson, and A. S. Littell, J Clin Endocrinol 30:325, 1970.

8. Rizkallah, T., E. Gurpide, and R. L. Vande Wiele, J Clin Endocrinol 29:92, 1969.

9. Wide, L., E. Johannisson, K.-G. Tillinger, and E. Diczfalusy, Acta Endocrinol (Kbh) 59:579, 1968.

10. Midgley, A. R., and R. B. Jaffe, J Clin Endocrinol 28:1712, 1968.

11. Rosemberg, E., J. F. Crigler, Jr., W. F. Jan, G. Bulat, R. Nakano, and S. G. Lee, in E. Rosemberg, and C. A. Paulsen, (Eds.), The Human Testis, Plenum, New York, 1970, p. 381.

48. Interrelationship Between Spermatogenesis and Follicle-Stimulating-Hormone Levels

C. Alvin Paulsen, John M. Leonard, David M. de Kretser, and Robert B. Leach

Despite an improved understanding of the interaction between the anterior pituitary and testicular interstitial cells, the regulatory mechanisms for FSH secretion by the anterior pituitary remain undefined. Basically, two hypotheses have been formulated to explain the FSH-spermatogenic interrelationship: (1) the utilization theory and (2) the negative feedback theory.

With regard to the first hypothesis, Heller and Nelson (1) and Heller et al. (2) suggested that the germinal epithelium utilized or metabolized FSH in some fashion which controlled FSH levels encountered in the pituitary, serum, and urine. To comply with this theory, an inverse relationship between spermatogenesis and FSH levels should exist, among other requirements.

With the respect to the negative feedback hypothesis, investigators have been concerned with the identity and cellular origin of the hormone presumed to be produced by the seminiferous tubular compartment. Mottram and Cramer (3) followed by McCullagh (4) suggested that the germinal epithelium secreted a substance designated "inhibin" which affected gonadotropin secretion. Later del Castillo et al. (5) proposed that the Sertoli cells secreted an estrogen which controlled "FSH" secretion. Howard et al. (6) in their studies agreed that the Sertoli cells secrete an FSH inhibitor and suggested that this inhibiting agent might be Δ^5-pregnenolone.

Lacy (7) and Johnsen (8, 9) independently have suggested a more elaborate scheme for the control of FSH. Lacy proposed that the residual bodies shed by the mature spermatids and phagocytized by the Sertoli cells are involved in the control of FSH secretion. Although Lacy has not indicated the identity of the inhibiting substance, his in vitro steroidogenic studies demonstrate that isolated seminiferous tubules can produce testosterone and 20α-dihydroprogesterone from appropriate precursors.

Johnsen also has focused on the later phases of spermatogenesis and has suggested that either the phagocytized residual bodies or the mature spermatozoa, by direct contact, alter the secretory function of the Sertoli cell so that estrogens are released into the circulation to inhibit FSH. To comply with Lacy's or Johnsen's proposals, an inverse relationship between spermatogenesis (later phases of maturation) and FSH should also exist.

The availability of more sensitive and specific methods for measuring FSH and LH levels has permitted reassessment of the relationship between FSH and seminiferous tubular function. This communication presents data from our laboratories which are pertinent to this issue. Portions of these studies as well as additional details have been documented elsewhere (10-12).

MATERIAL AND METHODS

Patients

Three groups of oligospermic males were studied. Individuals with obvious pituitary hypothalamic disorders, sex chromosomal abnormalities, or companion interstitial cell disorders were excluded in order to minimize the variables in our investigation.

GROUP I

Sixty-four patients, age 21 to 45 years, with either oligospermia (sperm count $<$ 40 million/ml) or azoospermia were evaluated. Clinically they were androgenically normal and exhibited normal plasma LH levels. Measurement of plasma FSH was performed and correlated with the seminal fluid sperm concentration.

GROUP II

Eleven oligospermic males from another clinic were also studied. In this group quantitative histologic studies were not performed. However, the histologic pattern of the testicular biopsy specimen was correlated with seminal fluid sperm concentration and serum FSH levels. The age range was similar to Groups I and III. In addition to normal serum LH levels, each patient demonstrated normal plasma testosterone levels.

GROUP III

Twelve additional patients of the same age range and clinical characteristics underwent testicular biopsy. The quantitative histologic characteristics of the germinal epithelium were correlated with urinary FSH titers.

GROUP IV

Sixty-two normal males, aged 17 to 45 years with repeated sperm counts over 40 million/ml served as our control subjects.

Serum FSH and LH

Serum FSH was measured by the radioimmunoassay technique of Midgley (13). All reagents for this immunoassay system were generously supplied by the National Pituitary Agency except for the second antibody; this was our own sheep antirabbit gamma globulin. LER 869-2 was utilized as the labeled purified FSH. Human Pituitary Reference Preparation LER 907 served as the standard. In our laboratory 1 mg LER 907 equals 38 IU 2nd IRP-HMG. Sensitivity for the FSH assay is 78 ng/ml. The intraassay and interassay coefficients of variation for a midslope plasma pool are 5 and 13%, respectively. Serum LH was measured by the double-antibody radioimmunoassay method of Morgan et al. (14) as adapted by Midgley for LH (15). The 2nd IRP-HMG served as the LH standard, the precision and sensitivity of the LH assay in our laboratory have previously been reported (16).

Urinary FSH

Urinary FSH titers were determined by the Steelman-Pohley method (17) after kaolin-acetone precipitation (18). Titers are expressed as IU /24 hr; the 2nd IRP-HMG was used as the standard. Relative potency estimates were determined by the parallel line assay computer program of Thorslund and Paulsen (19). The normal adult male range by this method in our laboratory is 3.8 to 25.0 IU /24 hr (16), although occasionally urinary FSH cannot be detected in normal adult males using a 12-hr aliquot, which is the maximum aliquot we inject into each assay rat.

Plasma Testosterone

Plasma testosterone was measured by the double isotope derivative technique (20). In Dr. Hudson's laboratory, the normal adult male range varies between 0.35 and 1.05 $\mu g\%$ (21).

Seminal Fluid Analysis

The seminal fluid sperm concentrations were determined by either the standard hemocytometer (22) or Coulter counter methods (23) in a minimum of three specimens per study subject. The mean number of semen analyses performed in the azoospermic and oligospermic patients was nine. In addition, attention was paid to the sample volume and motility of spermatozoa.

Histologic Studies

Testicular biopsy specimens were obtained and processed as previously described (24) from each patient in Groups II and III. Germinal cell quantitation (Group III) was performed in the following manner: a low-power photomicrograph of an entire testicular biopsy stained section was taken and those seminiferous tubules which had been cut perpendicular to their long axis were identified and numbered consecutively. Tubules cut at oblique angles were disregarded. The numbered tubules were then examined under the light microscope and the individual germinal cells were identified using the cytologic criteria of Clermont (25). The germinal cells were counted in 10 tubules for each biopsy specimen and the resultant counts expressed as the mean cell count per tubule. The cell types scored separately in this manner were: A dark, A pale, and B spermatogonia; resting, leptotene-zygotene, and pachytene primary spermatocytes; spermatids.

For our control values testicular biopsy specimens were obtained from 17 normal adult males, aged 21 to 45 with sperm counts above 40 million/ml, were processed, and quantitated in an identical fashion.

RESULTS

In the adult male control population (Group IV) with normal spermatogenesis, serum FSH titers ranged from 200 to 600 ng/ml. The mean value was 343 ng/ml (Fig. 1). Serum LH levels in each individual were within the normal adult male range for our laboratory, 4 to 19 mIU /ml 2nd IRP-HMG.

The serum FSH titers encountered in the 64 patients with either oligospermia

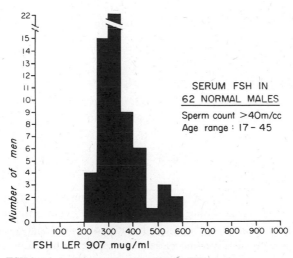

FIG. 1. Serum FSH levels in 62 normal males (Group IV) are shown.

or azoospermia (Group I) are shown in Fig. 2. Fifty-four of these men demonstrated serum FSH titers which were within our normal male range. FSH levels in the remaining 10 patients were elevated, 4 slightly and 6 markedly. There was a definite difference between the serum FSH levels in those men with

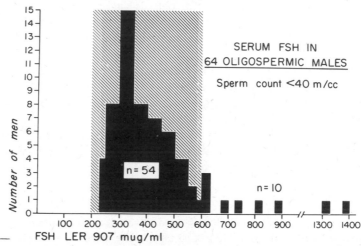

Fig. 2. Serum FSH in 60 males with oligospermia and 4 with azoospermia (Group I). The cross-hatched area represents the range of serum FSH in the normal control population.

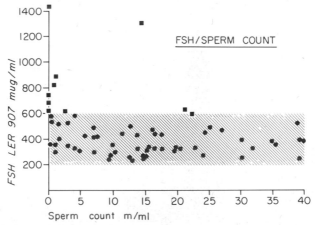

Fig. 3. A comparison of serum FSH and mean sperm count in the patients comprising Group I are shown. The normal range of serum FSH in the control population is indicated by the cross-hatched area.

oligospermia as compared to those with azoospermia, mean titers of 415 and 865 ng/ml, respectively. No direct reciprocal relationship existed between the seminal fluid sperm concentration and the serum FSH titers in the men with oligospermia, $r = -0.18$, $p > 0.05$ (Fig. 3). The mean serum LH level for entire group of oligo-azoospermic patients was 11.0 ± 4.4m IU/ml.

Additionally, the serum FSH titers were compared to the seminal fluid sperm concentration, plasma testosterone levels, serum LH titers, and testicular histologic pattern in an additional 11 oligospermic males. In these patients chromosomal analysis of peripheral blood cultures was performed along with the routine buccal smear analysis. Each patient demonstrated a normal sex chromosomal complement (Table I). The serum FSH titers were entirely normal except in one patient. He demonstrated severe oligospermia (0.1 to 0.3 million/ml) and his testicular histologic picture revealed a pattern compatible with the classification of Sertoli-cell-only syndrome. The degree of oligospermia in the patients with normal FSH titers was variable, mean sperm counts ranging from 0.3 to 22.0 million/ml. Plasma testosterone levels as well as serum LH titers were well within our normal ranges.

In Table II the quantitative analysis of germinal cells in the testicular biopsy specimens from the twelve oligospermic men are tabulated. These men were divided into two groups based on their urinary FSH titers. The patients' ages and the severity of oligospermia in the two groups were comparable. No significant difference could be detected between these two groups of patients with respect to the numbers of specific germinal cell types. Therefore, no relationship between the germinal cell counts and FSH titers emerged.

A summary of germinal cell counts from these two patient groups are presented again in Table III, this time for comparison with mean germinal cell counts from 17 normal adult males who were part of another study (26). Inspection of these data reveal that the major histologic defect present in the oligospermic males was a decrease in the numbers of spermatids.

DISCUSSION

The data derived from our studies failed to demonstrate a significant inverse relationship between serum FSH titers and the degree of oligospermia. Since this finding was unexpected, at least one question was raised. Perhaps our FSH radioimmunoassay system was not accurately estimating the levels of circulating FSH. This seemed unlikely in view of the investigations carried out by the National Pituitary Agency prior to distribution of FSH and LH radioimmunoassay reagents and standard (27). Validation of our serum FSH results was achieved by another dimension. The demonstration that oligospermic patients could be subdivided into two groups with elevated and with normal FSH levels in urine by bioassay further supports the results obtained by radioimmunoassay measurement of serum FSH.

TABLE I[a]

Case No.	Sperm Count (million/ml)		Serum		Testosterone (μg%)	Buccal smear	Karyotype	Testicular biopsy
	Mean	Range	FSH (ng/ml)	LH (mIU/ml)				
16	0.1	0.1- 0.3	620	12.0	.35	-ve	N	Sertoli only
29	3.3	1.3- 5.2	560	13.8	.35	-ve	N	Hyal. Sert.
31	0.3	0.2- 0.4	225	16.0	.43	-ve	N	Hyposperm.
33	0.9	0.5- 1.1	600	15.0	.38	-ve	N	Hyposperm.
34	0.9	0.3- 0.9	452	8.8	.40	-ve	N	Hyposperm.
41	10.0	7.0-13.0	235	15.0	.78	-ve	N	Hyposperm.
44	14.0	6.0-21.0	335	11.5	.61	-ve	N	Hyposperm.
46	14.0	12.0-20.0	345	6.5	.61	-ve	N	Hyposperm.
49	16.0	14.0-18.0	345	7.8	.45	-ve	N	Hyposperm.
50	17.0	10.0-20.0	545	13.0	.45	-ve	N	Hyposperm.
53	22.0	10.0-33.0	375	10.0	.50	-ve	N	Hyposperm.

[a]The details of patients comprising Group II of this study are shown. Case numbers refer to patients also used in a study reported elsewhere (12). Hyal. Sert. = hyalinization of tubules with Sertoli cells. Hyposperm. = hypospermatogenesis.

TABLE II. Histologic data of testicular biopsies in 12 oligospermic subjects[a]

Subject	Age (yr)	FSH (IU/24hr)	Sperm count (million/ml)	Mean germinal cell count/tubule						
				Ad	Ap	B	R	LZ	P	Sp
I. Normal FSH										
T.J.	25	18.2	2.5	25.4	11.8	7.1	0.4	10.0	51.0	66.0
W.C.	29	16.5	8.0	14.8	4.8	2.6	0	6.0	14.3	20.0
J.V.	43	8.0	1.6	15.8	4.7	4.3	0.9	13.2	42.1	70.1
C.A.	21	9.0	24.0	18.8	2.4	3.4	1.2	5.6	32.0	76.2
B.C.	28	3.0	37.0	16.2	3.8	3.1	0.8	4.5	26.0	64.3
H.M.	36	12.0	0.3	14.5	4.4	2.7	1.3	12.9	20.4	0
C.M.	31	10.0	7.0	20.0	2.8	3.9	1.2	7.2	38.3	47.3
Mean		11.0	11.5	17.9	4.9	3.9	0.8	8.5	32.0	49.1
±SD		±5.2	±13.8	±3.9	±3.2	±1.5	±0.5	±3.6	±12.8	±28.7
II. Elevated FSH										
L.R.	27	31.0	7.8	9.6	3.5	4.1	0.6	7.2	21.8	26.1
C.S.	40	26.0	11.6	24.5	5.0	6.6	0	12.5	44.7	54.9
E.R.	33	36.0	13.2	13.6	4.3	3.3	0	6.8	26.7	33.8
R.S.	24	54.0	24.2	10.4	3.7	4.7	0	8.0	27.7	49.8
E.K.	26	26.0	8.3	13.7	2.0	2.8	1.1	4.9	27.3	7.8
Mean		34.6	13.0	14.4	3.7	4.3	0.3	7.9	29.6	34.5
±SD		±11.6	±6.6	±6.0	±1.1	±1.5	±0.5	±2.8	±8.7	±18.9

[a]The quantitative analysis of the testicular histology of the patients comprising Group III is tabulated. Abbreviations: Spermatogonia = Ap (A pale), Ad (A dark), B; primary spermatocytes = resting (R), leptotene-zygotene (LZ), pachytene (P); spermatids (Sp).

TABLE III. Summary of histologic data from the 12 oligospermic patients compared to 17 normal adult males[a]

Subjects (number)	Mean germinal cell count including Sertoli cells per tubule[b]							
	S	Ad	Ap	B	R	LZ	P	Sp
I. Oligospermic, normal FSH (7)	14.6 (4.3)	17.9 (3.9)	4.9 (3.2)	3.9 (1.5)	0.8 (0.5)	8.5 (3.6)	32.0 (12.8)	49.1 (28.7)
II. Oligospermic, elevated FSH (5)	14.7 (2.2)	14.4 (6.0)	3.7 (1.1)	4.3 (1.5)	0.3 (0.5)	7.9 (2.8)	29.6 (8.7)	34.5 (18.9)
III. Normal (17)	15.0 (3.7)	16.8 (4.1)	5.9 (2.8)	3.4 (1.2)	1.4 (0.7)	12.3 (3.1)	33.6 (7.6)	68.5 (22.6)

[a]Quantitative data of the testicular germinal cells from patients in Group III are compared to those from 17 normal men. Abbreviations: Spermatogonia = Ap (A pale), Ad (A dark), B; primary spermatocytes = resting (R), leptotene-zygotene (LZ), pachytene (P); spermatids (Sp); Sertoli cells (S).

groups of patients based on the bioassay of FSH also failed to demonstrate that an inverse relationship between spermatogenesis and FSH titers exists.

The recent report by Rosen and Weintraub (28) appears at first glance to be at variance with our findings. These workers reported an increase in mean serum FSH levels in a group of patients with either oligospermia or azoospermia. Furthermore, they also noted that the majority of oligospermic patients exhibited serum FSH levels which were within their normal adult male range. In contrast, serum FSH titers were elevated in all their patients with azoospermia. These observations are in agreement with our findings. Although serum FSH levels were found by them to be inversely correlated with sperm concentration when both azoospermic and oligospermic subjects were analyzed, if just the oligospermic group is inspected, the inverse correlation becomes less convincing and does not support the inhibin theory.

It had been previously suggested that perhaps our oligospermic patients with normal FSH levels were examples of "occult" pituitary deficiency (10). Therefore we administered clomiphene citrate (racemic) to three oligospermic males (Table IV). Serum FSH and LH levels increased significantly in each patient which makes the presence of pituitary disease highly unlikely.

TABLE IV. Changes in serum FSH and LH titers following clomiphene administration to three oligospermic males

Patient	Seminal fluid sperm count (million/ml)		Serum	
			LH (mIU/ml)	FSH (ng/ml)
M.R.	6-25	Control	13.0	323
		Day 7[a]	31.9	420
H.S.	0-3	Control	9.0	590
		Day 7[a]	16.0	770
M.P.	6-24	Control	11.8	555
		Day 7[a]	26.0	900

[a]Dosage of clomiphene 50 mg twice daily for 7 days.

Our data indicate that the germinal cells do not play a role either directly or indirectly in the feedback regulation of FSH secretion but that this is a function of "an independent testicular station" as yet undefined. The integrity of this "independent testicular station" would not then be directly correlated to the integrity of spermatogenesis but might be disrupted by some of the same underlying factors that cause oligospermia.

Although these conclusions reject the feedback theory as interpreted by Lacy (7), Johnson (8, 9) and by Franchimont et al. (30), they do not exclude the

Sertoli cell as the "independent testicular station." It is possible that this cell may be the site for the secretion of hormonal "signal" which controls FSH secretion. Indeed, with the recent ultrastructural studies which highlight the presence of smooth endoplasmic reticulum as a prominent organelle within its cytoplasm, the mature Sertoli cell appears to be the best candidate.

ACKNOWLEDGMENT

Supported by National Institutes of Health grants AM 05161, AM 05436, and HD 05105. The USPHS International Postdoctoral Fellowship 5F05TWO-1572-02, which supported Dr. de Kretser, aided these studies.

The authors wish to thank Donald J. Moore and Margaret Couture for their able technical assistance.

REFERENCES

1. Heller, C. G., and W. O. Nelson, Rec Prog Hormone Res 3:229, 1948.
2. Heller, C. G., C. A. Paulsen, G. E. Mortimore, E. C. Jungck, and W. O. Nelson, Ann N Y Acad Sci 55:685, 1952.
3. Mottram, J. C., and W. Cramer, Quart J Exp Physiol 13:209, 1923.
4. McCullagh, D. R., Science 76:19, 1923.
5. del Castillo, E. B., A. Trabucco, and F. A. de la Balze, J Clin Endocrinol 7:493, 1947.
6. Howard, R. P., R. C. Sniffen, F. A. Simmons, and F. Albright, J Clin Endocrinol 10:121, 1950.
7. Lacy, D., and A. J. Pettit, Brit Med Bull 26:87, 1970.
8. Johnsen, S. G., Acta Endocrinol (Kbh) Suppl 90:99, 1964.
9. Johnsen, S. G., in E. Rosemberg, and C. A. Paulsen (Eds.), The Human Testis, Plenum, New York, 1970, p. 231.
10. Paulsen, C. A., in E. Rosemberg, and C. A. Paulsen (Eds.), The Human Testis, Plenum, New York, 1970, p. 246.
11. Leonard, J. M., R. B. Leach, and C. A. Paulsen, Clin Res 18:169, 1970 (abstract).
12. de Kretser, D. M., H. G. Burger, D. Fortune, B. Hudson, A. R. Long, C. A. Paulsen, and H. P. Taft, submitted J Clin Endocrinol 1971.
13. Midgley, A. R., Jr., J Clin Endocrinol 27:295, 1967.
14. Morgan, C. R., and A. Lazarow, Diabetes 12:115, 1963.
15. Midgley, A. R., Jr., Endocrinology 79:10, 1966.
16. Paulsen, C. A., D. L. Gordon, R. W. Carpenter, H. M. Gandy, and W. D. Drucker, Rec Prog Hormone Res 23:321, 1968.
17. Steelman, S. L., and F. M. Pohley, Endocrinology 53:604, 1953.
18. Albert, A., Rec Prog Hormone Res 12:227, 1956.
19. Thorslund, T., and C. A. Paulsen, Endocrinology 72:663, 1963.
20. Hudson, B., J. P. Coghlan, A. Dulmanis, M. Wintour, and I. Ekkel, Aust J Exp Biol Med Sci 41:235, 1963.
21. Hudson, B., H. G. Burger, D. M. de Kretser, J. P. Coghlan, and H. P. Taft, in E. Rosemberg, and C. A. Paulsen (Eds.), The Human Testis, Plenum, New York, 1970, p. 423.

22. Hotchkiss, R. S., Fertility in Men, Lippincott, Philadelphia, 1944.

23. Gordon, D. L., J. E. Herrigel, D. J. Moore, and C. A. Paulsen, Amer J Clin Pathol 37:226, 1967.

24. Paulsen, C. A., in R. H. Williams, (Ed.), Textbook of Endocrinology, Saunders, Philadelphia, 1968, p. 417.

25. Clermont, Y., Amer J Anat 112:35, 1963.

26. Paulsen, C. A., AEC Progress Report RLO-1781-10, April, 1969.

27. Albert, A., E. Rosemberg, G. T. Ross, C. A. Paulsen, and R. J. Ryan, J Clin Endocrinol 28:1214, 1968.

28. Rosen, S. W., and B. D. Weintraub, J Clin Endocrinol 32:410, 1971.

29. Franchimont, P., and J. J. Lyros, in L. Martini, M. Motta, and F. Fraschini (Eds.), The Hypothalamus, Academic, New York, 1970, p. 1.

49. Ultrastructural Studies of the Human Sertoli Cell in Normal Men and Males with Hypogonadotropic Hypogonadism before and after Gonadotropic Treatment

David M. de Kretser and Henry G. Burger

The Sertoli cell of the mammalian testis has been implicated as an important factor in many aspects of the spermatogenic process. The results of several studies have suggested that the Sertoli cell transports and provides the nutritive needs of the centrally placed germinal cells (1) and may be involved in the cyclic control of spermatogenesis (2). More recent studies of the steroid biosynthetic activities of the seminiferous tubules have led to the postulate that the Sertoli cell component may elaborate steroid compounds which are necessary for complete spermatogenesis or which may be involved in the feedback control of FSH secretion (3).

Electron microscopic studies of the human Sertoli cell have demonstrated that these cells are individual units and that their cytoplasmic prolongations surround all germinal cells other than spermatogonia (4-6). These investigators also described some of the nuclear and cytoplasmic features of the Sertoli cells in man. This report describes additional ultrastructural features of the Sertoli cells of the normal human testis and compares these findings with the fine structure of the Sertoli cells from the testes of men with hypogonadotropic hypogonadism. These results are compared with the changes in the fine structure of Sertoli cells in testicular biopsies from two men with hypogonadotropic hypogonadism seen after treatment with human pituitary and chorionic gonadotropin.

MATERIAL AND METHODS

Ultrastructure

Testicular biopsy specimens from normal fertile males and from six patients with hypogonadotropic hypogonadism are included in this study. The tissue was immediately fixed in 5% phosphate buffered glutaraldehyde or 2.5% osmium tetroxide buffered with a potassium dichromate-calcium chloride mixture (7), dehydrated in graded concentrations of acetone, and embedded in Araldite. Thin sections stained with uranylacetate (8) and lead citrate (9) were examined in a Siemens Elmiskop IA or Hitachi 11E electron microscopes.

Subjects of Study

1. Normal. Six normal fertile males aged between 23 and 45 years formed the subjects of the normal study.

2. Hypogonadotropic Hypogonadism. The six patients with hypogonadotropic hypogonadism were aged between 17 and 37 years and their general appearance was prepubertal. The diagnosis of hypogonadotropic hypogonadism was established by demonstrating low levels of FSH and LH in serum by radioimmunoassay or in urine by bioassay together with low levels of testosterone in plasma. The histological appearance of the testes by light microscopy was prepubertal. All patients were untreated at the time of the first testicular biopsy.

Two of the above patients with hypogonadotropic hypogonadism were treated with human pituitary and chorionic gonadotropin. The first patient (Case 1) was treated for a total of approximately two years. Initial therapy consisted of human pituitary gonadotropin containing 150 IU FSH and 500 IU LH thrice weekly for five months and subsequently HCG 500 IU thrice weekly was added to the regimen. A second testicular biopsy was performed at the end of the initial five months of treatment before HCG was added. During the initial five months of treatment he remained azoospermic but six months after the addition of HCG to the regimen sperm appeared in his ejaculate reaching a count of 20 million/ml at which time his wife became pregnant. Due to unavoidable circumstances this patient received HCG only for two months during which his sperm count fell from 8 million/ml to azoospermia. Human pituitary gonadotropin was subsequently restored to the therapeutic regimen and his sperm count rose rapidly to the levels at which pregnancy was achieved. The rapid fall in sperm count during this unfortunate interlude suggests that HCG alone was insufficient to maintain spermatogenesis.

The second patient (Case 2) was treated with human pituitary and chorionic

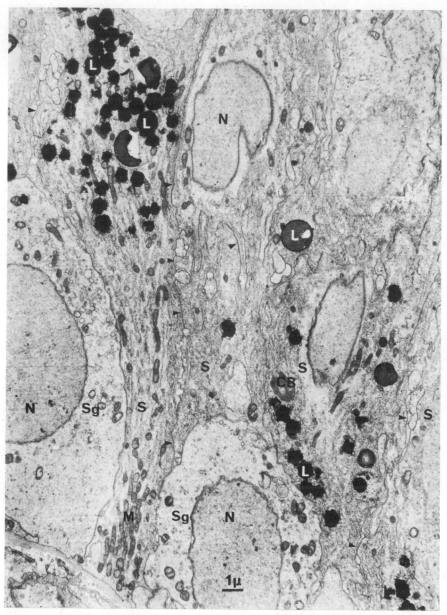

FIG. 1. Several Sertoli cells (S) which contain lipid collections (L), nucleus (N), crystal of Charcot-Böttcher (CB), and basal collections of mitochondria (M) are shown extending between spermatogonia (Sg). Inter-Sertoli cell junctions are shown (arrow heads). X5250.

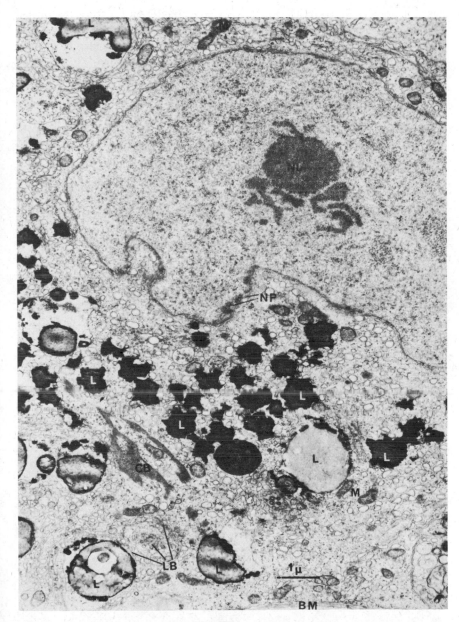

FIG. 2. The nucleus (N), nucleolus (NL), nuclear pores (NP), lipid inclusions (L), mitochondria (M), lamellar body (LB), and vesicles of smooth endoplasmic reticulum in an adult Sertoli cell are shown. BM = basement membrane of tubule. X11,500.

gonadotropin (150 IU FSH, 500 IU LH and 500 IU HCG) from the outset. Despite the development of an adequate ejaculate volume, he did not produce sperm in his ejaculate and after eight months, a second testicular biopsy was performed. Treatment has been continued and results are awaited.

OBSERVATIONS

Normal Adult Sertoli Cells

The Sertoli cells in the normal adult males extended from the basement membrane of the seminiferous epithelium to the luminal aspect of the seminiferous tubule (Fig. 1). The shape and profile of these cells was markedly irregular due to the relationship of adjacent germinal cells which tended to indent the cytoplasm of the Sertoli cell. Many cytoplasmic prolongations of the Sertoli cells extended between all germinal cells other than spermatogonia, thereby surrounding and forming a network in which the germinal cells were placed. At all times the germinal cells were separated from the Sertoli cells by a distinct pericellular space bounded by their cell membranes.

The nucleus of the Sertoli cell was situated basally, exhibited an irregular infolding and contained a prominent nucleolus (Fig. 2). The centrally placed nucleolus was composed of a large spherical granular electron-dense body from

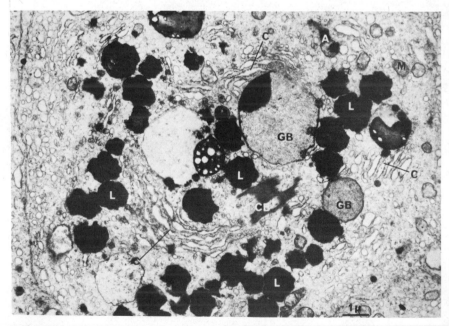

FIG. 3. Part of a lamellar body in the adult Sertoli cell demonstrates the lipid inclusions (L) and lipofuscin deposits (GB) in the cytoplasmic core surrounded by cisternae (C). Crystal of Charcot-Böttcher (CB) and mitochondria (M) are also present. X6750.

which irregular prolongations of similar electron density extended constituting the nucleolonema (Figs. 2 and 8). Amongst the prolongations of the nucleolonema one or two less electron-dense round bodies could be seen frequently.

The cytoplasm of the Sertoli cell was characterized by a well developed smooth endoplasmic reticulum which was present as vesicles of variable diameter (Fig. 2). Prominent localized aggregations of smooth membraned cisternae, of variable size and form, were present in the cytoplasm (Fig. 3). These collections appeared to be cylindrical in shape often with a cytoplasmic core that contained lipid or mitochondrial elements. The cisternae comprising these bodies were interconnected by pores 430 to 460 Å in diameter and in keeping with existing terminology these collections have been termed lamellar bodies (10). Profiles of rough endoplasmic reticulum were seen relatively infrequently in comparison to the smooth endoplasmic reticulum.

The mitochondria of the Sertoli cell were generally rod-shaped with both plate-like and tubular cristae extending across a moderately electron-dense matrix. Prominent collections of mitochondria were present at the bases of Sertoli cells immediately adjacent to the basement membrane (Figs. 1 and 4). The Golgi complex was perinuclear and was composed of vesicles and closely arranged lamellated cisternae. Lipid and lipofuscin inclusions were seen frequently in the perinuclear region of the Sertoli cells. Crystalline inclusions,

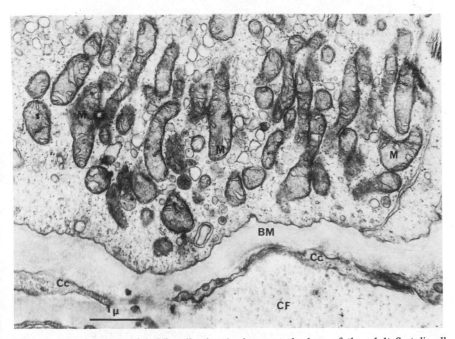

FIG. 4. The mitochondrial (M) collection is shown at the base of the adult Sertoli cell immediately adjacent to the basement membrane (BM) surrounding contractile cells (CC) and collagen fibers (CF). X14,250.

representing the crystals of Charcot-Böttcher, composed of electron-dense filaments and extending up to 4 μ in length were seen frequently in the Sertoli cell cytoplasm (Figs. 1 and 2). These inclusions often were found close to the lamellar bodies. Filaments, 30 to 40 Å in width were seen throughout the cytoplasm but were more numerous in the perinuclear and basal aspects of the cell.

The junctions between adjacent Sertoli cells frequently revealed complex interdigitations and folds of the cell membranes (Figs. 5, 6). The intervening intercellular space was narrow being 60 to 90 Å in width over extensive regions. On both sides of the cell membranes forming the inter-Sertoli cell junction, a narrow band of cytoplasm was demarcated from the rest of the cell by a linear series of smooth-membraned cisternae. In the cytoplasmic band so delineated,

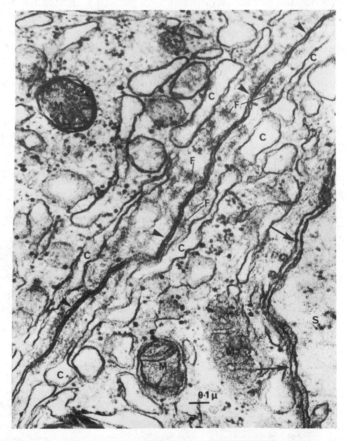

FIG. 5. An inter-Sertoli cell junction shows the narrow intercellular space (arrowheads), adjacent cisternae (C), and bundles of fibrils (F). Mitochondria (M) and a Sertoli-spermatogonial (S) intercellular space (arrows) are indicated. X55,000.

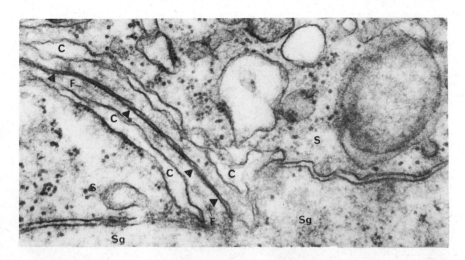

FIG. 6. The inter-Sertoli cell junction (arrowheads) is shown with adjacent cisternae (C) and fibrils (F). It can be seen to intersect with a spermatogonial (Sg) Sertoli cell (S) junction which lacks this organization. X41,250.

filaments 200 to 250 Å in width are found. Over small distances the intercellular space was reduced even further and was obliterated occasionally.

The Immature Sertoli Cells in Hypogonadotropic Hypogonadism

The seminiferous cords were composed of two types of cells, the gonocytes and the immature Sertoli cells. This arrangement could be easily recognized by light microscopic examination (Fig. 10). The gonocytes were large and few in number, being easily recognized by their electron lucid cytoplasm and paucity of organelles. The principal component of the seminiferous cord was the immature Sertoli cells which extended radially towards the center of the cord (Fig. 7). The nuclei were ovoid and were situated basally close to the basement membrane of the seminiferous cord. Many nuclei did not contain nucleoli which if present were small, variable in appearance and peripherally placed (Fig. 8). Their size and simplicity contrasted markedly with the centrally placed elaborate nucleoli found in the adult Sertoli cell (Fig. 8).

The cytoplasm of immature Sertoli cells contained less smooth endoplasmic reticulum than in Sertoli cells of the normal adult testis. Also in contrast to the normal adult Sertoli cells, profiles of rough endoplasmic reticulum were seen frequently especially at the apical regions of these cells (Fig. 9). The mitochondria were pleomorphic and were scattered evenly in the cytoplasm of the immature Sertoli cell. The basal collections of mitochondria found in the normal adult Sertoli cell were not seen in the immature state. Lipid and lipofuscin inclusions were not as prominent in the immature Sertoli cells. Occasionally small crystalline inclusions identical in appearance to the crystals of

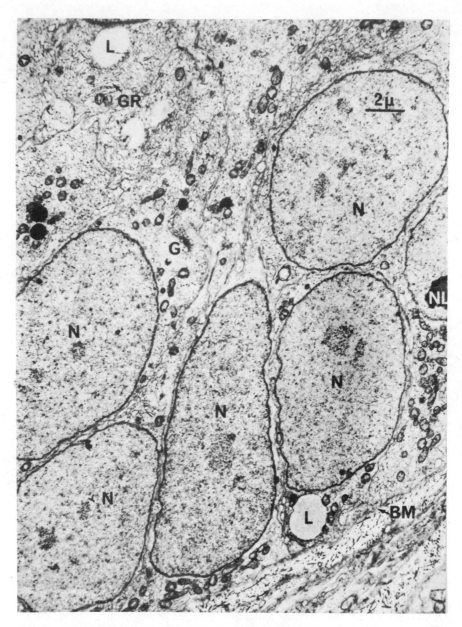

FIG. 7. A group of immature Sertoli cells in hypogonadotropic hypogonadism show nuclei (N), nucleolus (NL), lipid inclusions (L), Golgi complex (G), and granular endoplasmic reticulum (GR). Basement membrane of seminiferous cord = BM. X5000. Reproduced with permission from Virchows Arch Abt B Zellpath 1:283, 1968.

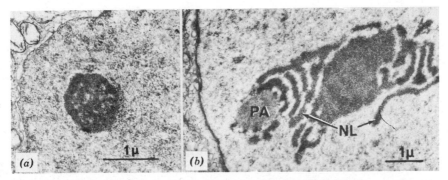

FIG. 8. (a) Nucleolus from immature Sertoli cell. X15,000.(b) Nucleolus from normal adult Sertoli cell. X9,750.

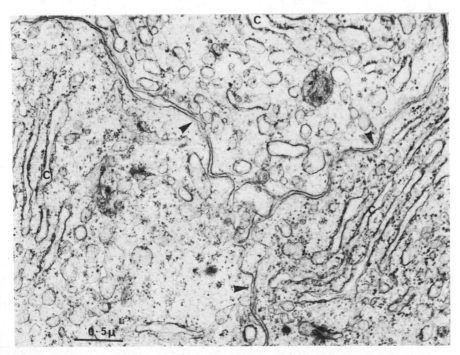

FIG. 9. The apices of adjacent immature Sertoli cells show well-developed cisternae (C) of rough endoplasmic reticulum. The unspecialized wide intercellular space between immature Sertoli cells is indicated (arrows). X25,000. Reproduced with permission from Virchows Arch Abt B Zellpath 1:283, 1968.

Charcot-Böttcher were found. Cytoplasmic filaments, 30 to 50 Å in width were prominent in the basal and perinuclear regions of the immature Sertoli cells.

An intercellular space of approximately 250Å separated adjacent Sertoli cells except toward the apices of the cells where in small areas this space was reduced to about 90Å. In these areas, some increase in the electron density of the surrounding cytoplasm could be seen and ocasionally contained tubular structures 125Å in diameter. No specialized inter-Sertoli cell junctions as seen in the adult testis could be found.

Ultrastructual Observations in Hypogonadotropic Hypogonadism after Treatment with Human Pituitary Gonadotropin

Light microscopic study of biopsies from both patients after treatment showed a marked increase in seminiferous tubule diameter, development of a lumen, and an apparent central movement of the Sertoli cell nuclei (Figs. 10 and 11). In addition, the gonocytes had given rise to a number of germinal cells in Case 1 to the primary spermatocyte stage (Fig. 11) and in Case 2 to the spermatid stage. It should be noted that the ultrastructural changes in the Sertoli cells described below had occurred before the time of biopsy in Case 1 despite the limited maturation of the germinal cells.

After treatment, the Sertoli cells showed striking changes. Their nuclei had been displaced toward the lumen and each contained a prominent, well-developed centrally placed nucleolus (Fig. 12). The amount of smooth

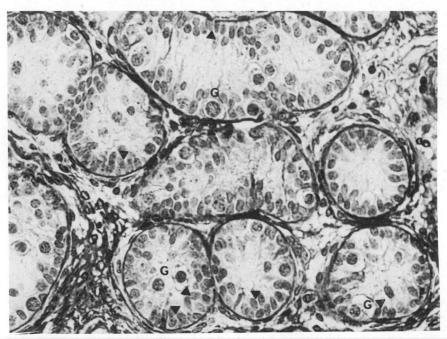

FIG. 10. The seminiferous cords of the testes in hypogonadotropic hypogonadism show gonocytes (G) and immature Sertoli cells (arrowheads). X410.

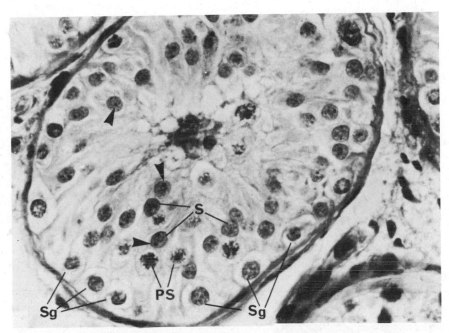

FIG. 11. A seminiferous tubule in Case 1 after treatment with gonadotropin illustrates the tubular lumen, spermatogonia (Sg), primary spermatocytes (PS), and Sertoli cells (S) with nucleoli (arrowheads). X400.

endoplasmic reticulum had markedly increased and completely overshadowed the few cisternal profiles of rough endoplasmic reticulum that were found. It was not possible to assess whether the amount of rough endoplasmic reticulum had decreased after treatment.

The other remarkable change was the development of the specialized inter-Sertoli cell junctions which characterized the adult testis. The width of the intercellular space was reduced to approximately 60 to 90Å and smooth membrane cisternae demarcated a band of cytoplasm on either side of the cell junction (Figs. 12 and 13). Fibers 200 to 250Å in width were present in the cytoplasmic band so delineated.

DISCUSSION

The results of this study demonstrate that a significant difference exists between the electron microscopic features of Sertoli cells from the normal adult testis and from the testis in hypogonadotropic hypogonadism. There were striking differences between the immature and adult Sertoli cells. These consisted of the basal position of the nuclei, the poorly developed nucleoli, the decreased smooth endoplasmic reticulum, and the absence of the characteristic inter-Sertoli cell

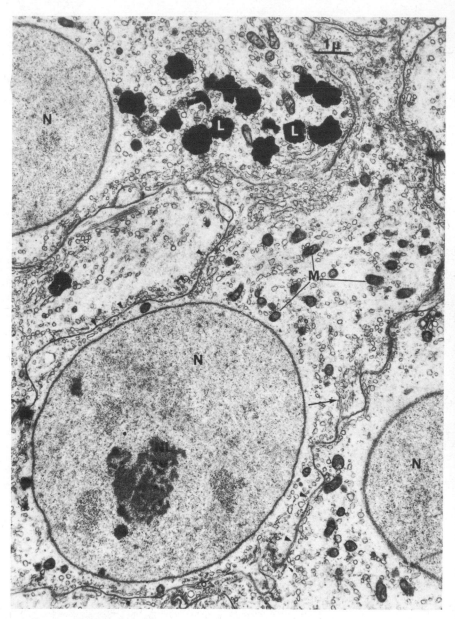

FIG. 12. A number of Sertoli cells after treatment with gonadotropins in Case 1. Nuclei (N), nucleolus (NL), lipid inclusions (L), mitochondria (M), and inter-Sertoli cell junctions (arrowheads) closely associated with fibrils (arrows). Note increased vesicles of smooth endoplasmic reticulum. X9000.

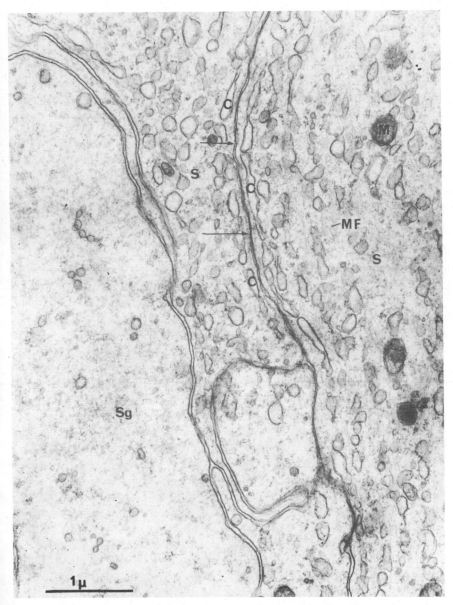

FIG. 13. The specialized inter-Sertoli cell junctions in Case 2 after gonadotropin treatment is characterized by cisternae (C), fibrils (arrows), and narrow intercellular space. A Sertoli cell (S) spermatogonial (Sg) interface is also present. X23,000.

junctions in the immature state. The study has demonstrated that replacement therapy with human pituitary and chorionic gonadotropin can transform the immature Sertoli cell into the adult type. Although patients with hypogonadotropic hypogonadism cannot be entirely equated with the normal prepuberal state, the ultrastructural features of their testes do not differ markedly from those of the normal prepuberal testis as described by Vilar (11). In addition, their testes do retain the ability to respond to gonadotropic therapy (12, 13). Consequently, it is likely that the transformation of immature Sertoli cells to the adult type occurs as part of the normal puberal maturation of the testis.

Studies in other species have shown that nucleolar development in Sertoli cells occurs as part of the normal maturation of the testis (14). The demonstration in the present study that the development of prominent nucleoli and abundant smooth endoplasmic reticulum occurs during treatment suggests that some change occurs in the metabolic processes of these cells. In this regard smooth endoplasmic reticulum has been shown to be present in all steroid secreting tissues (15-17) and it has been established that this organelle contains the majority of enzymes necessary for steroid biosynthesis (17). The presence of well-developed smooth endoplasmic reticulum in adult Sertoli cells has led many investigators to postulate a steroid secretory role for the Sertoli cell (5, 18). Further support for this role is available from the results of studies which indicate that isolated seminiferous tubules are capable of steroid biosynthesis (19, 20). Lacy (3) extended these studies and demonstrated that rat seminiferous tubules have metabolic pathways distinct from those of the intertubular tissue. He postulated that the Sertoli cell may be the source of these steroids which may influence spermatogenesis by local action. The results of the present study suggest that if steroid biosynthesis is a function of these cells, the postpubertal Sertoli cell is more likely to be capable of such action. From the sequence of events in Case 1, it would appear that the increase in smooth endoplasmic reticulum occurs prior to the onset of full spermatogenesis and may well be a necessary preliminary.

The development of prominent nucleoli and smooth endoplasmic reticulum during gonadotropin-induced pubertal maturation of Sertoli cells has an interesting parallel. A similar transformation occurs in the peritubular mesenchymal cells of the immature testis during puberty under the influence of the gonadotropic hormones. During the transformation of mesenchymal cells to interstitial cells, nucleolar development and increases in smooth endoplasmic reticulum are associated with increasing levels of plasma testosterone. The similarity of these changes to those occurring in Sertoli cells lends further support to the concept of a steroid biosynthetic role for the Sertoli cells of the adult testis.

This study demonstrates that the Sertoli cells of the adult human testis exhibit specialized inter-Sertoli cell junctions similar to those described in other mammals (21-24). The recent elegant study by Dym and Fawcett (23) indicates that these specialized inter-Sertoli cell junctions prevent intercellular transport of materials beyond the spermatogonial cells. They propose that the inter-Sertoli cell junctions together with tight junctions found between the peritubular myoid cells constitute the blood-testicular barrier described in earlier studies (25, 26).

It is of interest that these cell junctions are not present between the immature Sertoli cells in males with hypogonadotropic hypogonadism and that they appear to develop during gonadotropin treatment. These findings indicate that the formation of the specialized inter-Sertoli cell junctions may be part of the gonadotropin- controlled pubertal maturation of the testis. The development of these cell juntions virtually isolate all germinal cells other than spermatogonia from the direct influence of external factors other than those transmitted via the Sertoli cell. It is possible that the relative isolation of these cells may provide a highly specialized environment necessary for meiosis and spermiogenesis. The other component of the blood-testicular barrier, namely the peritubular myoid cells, also undergoes changes during the pubertal process (27, 28).

The presence of a blood-testicular barrier in part formed by the inter-Sertoli cell junctions suggests that the isolated germinal cells probably are dependent on the Sertoli cells for their metabolic needs. In this regard the localized collections of mitochondria at the bases of the Sertoli cells may serve as an energy source for transport across the basement membrane.

In conclusion, the remarkable differences between the immature and adult Sertoli cells and the transformation of one to another during puberty suggests that the Sertoli cell plays a central role in the development of spermatogenesis. The unique situation of the Sertoli cell places it in a favorable position to coordinate and influence the spermatogenic process.

ACKNOWLEDGMENTS

This study was supported by grants from the National and Medical Research Council of Australia. Part of the work was performed during the tenure of a USPHS International Postdoctoral Fellowship No. F05TW 1572.

REFERENCES

1. Mancini, R. E., O Vilar, B. Alvarez, and A. C. Seigeur. J Histochem Cytochem 13:376, 1965.
2. Cleland, K. W., Aust J biol Sci Series B 4:344, 1951.
3. Lacy, D., P. Vinson, P. Collins, J. Bell, P. Fyson, J. Pudney, and A. J. Petit, in C. Gual and F. J. G. Ebling (Eds.), Progress in Endocrinology, Excerpta Medica, Amsterdam, 1968, p. 1019.
4. Vilar, O., P. Del Cerro, and R. E. Mancini, Exp Cell Res 27:158, 1962.
5. Nagano, T., Z Zellforsch 73:89, 1966.
6. Vilar, O., C. A. Paulsen, and D. J. Moore, in E. Rosemberg and C. A. Paulsen (Eds.), The Human Testis, Plenum, New York, 1970, p. 63.
7. Richardson, K. C., J Anat (Lond) 96:427, 1962.

8. Watson, M. L., J Biophys Biochem Cytol 4:475, 1958.

9. Reynolds, E. S., J Cell Biol 17:208, 1963.

10. Bawa, S. R., J Ultstruct Res 9:459, 1963.

11. Vilar, O., in E. Rosemberg and C. A. Paulsen (Eds.), The Human Testis, Plenum, New York, 1970, p. 95.

12. Paulsen, C. A., in C. Gual (Ed.), Proc. 6th Pan-American Congr. Endocrinology, Int Cong Series 112, Excerpta Medica, Amsterdam, 1966, p. 398.

13. Johnsen, S. G., Acta Endocrinol (Kbh) 53:315, 1966.

14. Flickinger, C. J., Z Zellforsch 78:92, 1967.

15. Brenner, R. M., Amer J Anat 119:429, 1966.

16. Blanchette, E. J., J Cell Biol 31:501, 1966.

17. Christensen, A. K., J Cell Biol 96:911, 1965.

18. Brökelmann, J., Z Zellforsch 59:820, 1963.

19. Christensen, A. K., and N. R. Mason, Endocrinology 76:646, 1965.

20. Hall, P. F., D. C. Irby, and D. M. de Kretser, Endocrinology 84:488, 1969.

21. Flickinger, C. J., and D. W. Fawcett, Anat Rec 158:207, 1967.

22. Nicander, L., Z Zellforsch 83:375, 1969.

23. Fawcett, D. W., P. M. Heidger, and L. V. Leak, J Reprod Fert 19:109, 1969.

24. Dym, M., and D. W. Fawcett, Biol Reprod 3:308, 1970.

25. Setchell, B. P., J Physiol 189:63P, 1967.

26. Waites, G. M. H., and B. P. Setchell, in K. W. McKerns (Ed.), The Gonads, Appleton-Century-Crofts, New York, 1969, p. 649.

27. Leeson, C. R., and T. S. Leeson, Anat Rec 147:243, 1963.

28. de Kretser, D. M., Virchows Arch Abt B Zellpath 1:283, 1968.

50. The Initiation and Maintenance of Human Spermatogenesis with Urinary Gonadotropins Following Hypophysectomy

John MacLeod[1]

There is strong evidence in support of the view that initation and maintenance of human spermatogenesis is regulated by both FSH and LH but the exact roles of the two hormones is not known. Human FSH from postmenopausal urine (1) in conjunction with HCG from pregnancy urine has been used to treat hypogonadotropic hypogonadism (2-4) and sexual involution after hypophysectomy (5). In terms of stimulation of the secondary sex characteristics, HCG alone has proven eminently successful (6) and several other workers, particularly Heller (3), Paulsen (6), Bartter et al. (7), and Raboch (8), have confirmed the observation originally made by Plum (9) that the long-term administration of HCG to eunuchoidal individuals may result in the initiation of a full cycle of spermatogenesis and the appearance of active spermatozoa in the ejaculate. It should be pointed out, however, that sperm counts after the HCG regimen seldom reach a high level even though ensuing normal pregnancies have been reported. Treatment with a combination of HCG and Human Menopausal Gonadotropin (HMG) which contains substantial amounts of FSH, produces a marked augmentation in spermatogenesis as determined by testicular biopsy (3, 4, 10).

[1]Career Scientist, Health Research Council of the City of New York.

Reports on the effect of gonadotropin therapy in male sexual involution following hypophysectomy are relatively sparse (5, 11, 12). The first known posthypophysectomy case in which spermatogenesis was arrested at the spermatid level was reported by Gemzell and Kjessler (11). They used gonadotropins from human pituitaries to stimulate a complete cycle of spermatogenesis from arrest at the active spermatid level. Spermatozoa appeared in the ejaculate during the third week of the injections and the sperm count level reached 61 million/ml in the 13th week. These authors concluded that the influence of pituitary gonadotropins in human spermatogenesis "is mainly restricted to the maturation process of transforming early spermatids into mature spermatozoa." In the same year, MacLeod et al. (5) reinitiated a full cycle of spermatogenesis with HMG (Pergonal, Serono) containing 103 IU FSH and 75 IU LH/ml within 67 days in a hypophysectomized patient with involution of spermatogenesis to the spermatogonium level 14 weeks after hypophysectomy. It seems that the LH component was not sufficient to restore Leydig cell function and secondary sex characteristics, but a full qualitative cycle of spermatogenesis had been stimulated in the absence of interstitial cell activity. The initial, if not continuing, action of FSH appeared to be exerted at the level of the spermatogonium. By subsequent administration of HCG a full restoration of spermatogenesis and of the secondary sex characteristics, including a complement of active spermatozoa in a normal ejaculate, was obtained.

Mancini et al. (12) reported varying degrees of spermatogenesis in 6 partially hypophysectomized patients after administration of HCG and HMG (Pergonal) over a period of three months. During that latter period HCG alone stimulated spermatogonia to the primary spermatocyte while HMG alone appeared to stimulate all germinal cell phases up to spermatozoa. They confirmed that HMG does not stimulate Leydig cell development and that combined HMG-HCG therapy fully restored spermatogenesis.

Johnsen (10) produced an aspermic ejaculate with 3000 IU of HCG twice weekly for 2 months followed by 60 IU of FSH and 350 IU of HCG three times weekly in a patient with sexual involution 9 years after hypophysectomy. After 9 weeks of treatment, he observed an occasional spermatozoon in the ejaculate and at 17 weeks 16 million sperm/ml with good motility were present. Subsequently, the patient's wife conceived and a normal pregnancy ensued. The acquired level of spermatogenesis was maintained with HCG alone for an unspecified period. The author concluded that a small amount of FSH together with HCG is necessary to restore spermatogenesis and that spermatogenesis can be maintained but not recreated with only HCG.

The following report deals with the effect of long-term administration of HCG and HMG on spermatogenesis in two hypophysectomized patients.

CASE 1

A 28-year-old married man with two children underwent hypophysectomy for infarcted pituitary adenoma in August 1965. Following surgery, he was placed on cortisone and thyroid but no androgen support was given. Eighteen months later he returned to us because of a desire to have another child. In the intervening period he was able to have sporadic intercourse with normal erection and orgasm after much stimulation, but was unable to produce an ejaculate by masturbation. He complained of loss of chest, axillary, facial, and pubic hair. Most of these complaints were verified by physical examination.

The blood testosterone level was extremely low. The gonadotropin bioassay by mouse uterine (MU) weight showed a detectable but low level (3 MU/24 hr). The 17-ketosteroid excretion was 8.0 mg/24 hr. Testicular biopsies showed all stages of spermatogenesis in selected tubules but a marked quantitative depletion. Many of the mature spermatozoa showed bizarre headshapes. Peritubular fibrosis was absent in both testes. The basement membranes and the tubular diameters were normal but the interstitial tissue in both testes was edematous and relatively acellular.

This patient was then treated with a combination of HMG (Perganol) and HCG (APL) on alternate days. Pergonal (Batch 20714) contained 75 IU FSH 2nd IRP-HMG and 75 IU LH 2nd IRP-HMG/ml and APL contained 4000 IU/ml.

RESPONSE TO GONADOTROPIN. Twenty-nine days after the initiation of combined HMG-HCG therapy, an acellular ejaculate of 1.40 ml was obtained (Fig. 1) and at 61 days a 2.2 ml ejaculate contained 4 million sperm, a few of which showed sluggish activity. The morphologic characteristics of these cells (head shape) showed abnormalities similar to those seen in the pretreatment germinal ephithelium. Immature forms such as middle stage spermatids were present in considerable numbers (13% of the total germinal cells). Since no spermatozoa or spermatids were found in the ejaculate 45 days after the beginning of the treatment and a minimum of 14 days must be allowed for transit of the spermatozoa from the lumens of the seminiferous tubules to the ejaculate, the assumption was made that spermatozoa found at 61 days had not been liberated from the germinal epithelium until at least 30 days after initiation of therapy. The importance of this particular point will be considered in more detail later. On day 69, the total sperm count in the ejaculate had doubled (7 million), the spermatozoa showed fully normal motility, and the sperm morphology had improved.

At 90 days, the total sperm count had reached 132 million and the volume was 3.0 ml. The sperm motility was excellent and the sperm morphology continued to improve. Until day 144, the total sperm count varied between 44 and 228 million with continuing excellence of motility and improved morphology. At this point, the patient informed us that his wife had decided against having another child and had used contraception knowing that active spermatozoa were present in the ejaculate. The patient was subsequently informed that the HMG therapy could not be continued and that he would now be treated with 2000 IU of HCG three times weekly. This series of events permitted us to follow both the effect of withdrawal of HMG and the effect of continued maintenance with HCG only.

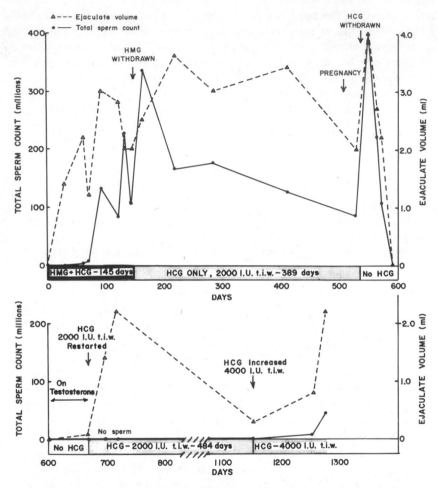

FIG. 1. Case 1. Restoration of spermatogenesis by treatment with HMG and HCG in combination and maintenance of spermatogenesis with HCG only.

Spermatogenesis and otherwise good semen quality was maintained during the HCG treatment as evidenced by a total sperm count ranging from 94 to 336 million. This state continued for a period of 390 days and pregnancy ensued in the 4th cycle of contraception-free intercourse (Fig. 1). At this point, the patient agreed to withdrawal of HCG, being fully aware of the possibility that he might revert again to sexual involution. During the succeeding 28 days without treatment the total sperm count ranged from 221 to 400 million with excellent motility and morphology; the ejaculate volume ranged from 2.7 to 4.0 ml. On the 35th day, the total sperm count fell to 106 million; the volume was 2.2 ml. The low percentage of active cells with no change in sperm morphology suggested that involution had occurred. Seminal fructose was virtually undetectable. Forty-nine days after the withdrawal of HCG, the ejaculate volume fell to a very low level and only occasional spermatozoa were found. Plasma testosterone level was 0.01 μg %. The patient again complained of loss of libido and lethargy. On the 63rd day of HCG withdrawal, only a drop of sperm-free ejaculate was obtainable. An attempt was made to restore the secondary sex characteristics with testosterone enanthate 200 mg im twice weekly. After 70 days, only one perceptible cell-free ejaculate of 0.3 ml containing a low level of fructose (34 mgs %) was elicited.

HCG in a dose of 2000 IU twice weekly was reinitiated. After 28 days, a 1.4 ml cell-free ejaculate was obtained and at day 45 the volume was 2.2 ml. Thereafter, and for a period of 484 days, on this regimen, with the exception of three periods of 37, 14, and 28 days when the self-administered HCG injections were interrupted, the ejaculate volumes remained between 1.0 and 2.2 ml but without spermatozoa. Eight million spermatozoa with good motility and morphology appeared in the ejaculate after 586 days of HCG therapy. The patient had doubled the triweekly dose of HCG over a period of 102 days. He then returned to the original treatment schedule; 22 days later the total sperm count had risen to 46 million and the volume to 2.2 ml. Subsequent total withdrawal of HCG again resulted in disappearance of ejaculate and spermatozoa.

CASE 2

An enlarged sella turcica was discovered at age 23 on a routine skull x-ray following an auto accident. The patient was treated with cobalt irradiation to the sella over a period of 20 weeks with a reduction in size of the pituitary adenoma. He was seen for endocrine evaluation in December, 1968. He had married two months previously but was unable to have intercourse. Facial hair was sparse and axillary hair was normal. Pubic hair was normal but the escutcheon was female. He had noticed a marked failure in libido and potency. Penis and testes were of normal size and consistency. At that time urinary 17-ketosteroids were 2.5 mg/24 hr; the urinary testosterone was low and urinary gonadotropins were less than 6.6 MU/24 hr. The 17-hydroxysteroids were 3.9 mg/24 hr, and did not rise following Metopirone.

A testicular biopsy showed a depleted germinal epithelium and disorganized spermatogonia in a fair number. Middle and late stage spermatids were occasionally found but many were prematurely sloughed into the tubular lumens. Moderate to extensive peritubular fibrosis was present. No Leydig cells were seen and the interstitial tissue was mesenchymal and fibrocytic. The latter finding was consistent with the sexual involution but not with the plasma testosterone value.

He was initially treated with replacement cortisone, thyroid, and depo-testosterone. After six months he was enjoying frequent, normal intercourse.

The ejaculate volume was normal as was the fructose concentration, but was devoid of spermatozoa.

A strong desire to have a child was expressed. Testosterone was withdrawn for 7 weeks. At the end of this period the plasma FSH level was barely detectable. Plasma testosterone was 0.26 mg %. Eighty days after testosterone withdrawal complete sexual involution was apparent; libido and erections were poor. Even though orgasm could be induced, an ejaculate could not be produced. HCG in a dose of 3000 IU three times weekly was given. HMG was withheld until the secondary sex characteristics were restored.

RESPONSE TO GONADOTROPIN. One week after institution of HCG therapy his wife reported a return of sexual activity. At 50 days, a 3.1 ml acellular ejaculate with 165 mg % fructose was obtained (Fig. 2). HMG (75 IU FSH and

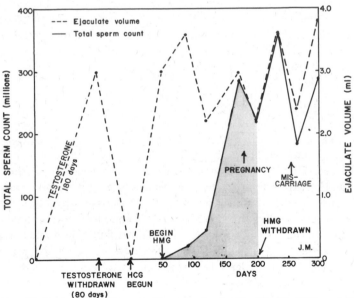

FIG. 2. Case 2. Restoration of spermatogenesis by treatment with HCG and HMG in combination. Shadowed area indicates the HMG treatment period.

75 IU LH) twice weekly was added to the HCG regimen at this point. Forty-two days later the sperm count was 21 million and rather sluggish spermatozoa with abnormal head shapes were found in the ejaculate. On the 84th day of the combined HMG-HCG regimen, the total sperm count had reached 224 million and the motility and morphology were excellent. A pregnancy, confirmed by HCG assay, ensued on the 150th day of treatment. Menstrual data indicated that conception occurred on the 131st day. HMG was withdrawn at this point, but the HCG was continued. A miscarriage occurred in the second month.

A second pregnancy occurred during the next period of 320 days of HCG treatment (Fig. 3) during which time the semen quality was maintained at a high level. After delivery of a normal child, HCG was discontinued and testosterone

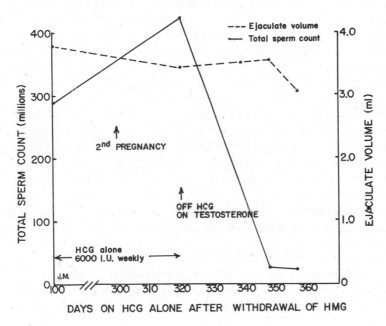

FIG. 3 Maintenance of spermatogenesis with HCG only in Case 2.

was given since it had already been shown that the secondary sex characteristics could be maintained with synthetic testosterone only. After 33 days, during which time two injections of 250 mg cyclopentyl propionate were administered, his sexual activity and ejaculate volume were maintained but the sperm count fell from 430 to 25 million with a normal morphology. The sperm motility index was severely depressed. An HCG regimen of 3000 IU twice weekly was therefore reinstituted.

SUMMARY

In the hypophysectomized patient (Case 1) a combination of HMG-HCG restored an acellular ejaculate within 29 days and a good level of spermatogenesis within 90 days. Subsequent withdrawal of HMG and a continuance of HCG for a period of 398 days did not diminish the cellular quality of the ejaculate. Complete withdrawal of gonadotropin therapy resulted in an involution of the reproductive tract within 56 days. Synthetic testosterone did not restore secondary sex characteristics when administered for 70 days. Subsequent HCG therapy (2000 IU) over a period of 484 days maintained the ejaculate and the secondary sex characteristics, but did not stimulate spermatogenesis to the point of return of spermatozoa in the ejaculate. A doubling of the HCG dose to 4000 IU, however, resulted in the appearance of active spermatozoa in low concentration.

In Case 2, synthetic testosterone restored the secondary sex characteristics, ejaculate and normal sexual activity but did not initiate spermatogenesis. Withdrawal of testosterone was followed by sexual involution as measured by loss of the ejaculate and libido. HCG promptly restored full sexual function and the combination of HMG-HCG resulted in full restoration of spermatogenesis as further confirmed by pregnancy. As in Case 1, subsequent withdrawal of HMG and the continuance of HCG resulted in full maintenance of spermatogenesis for about one year. Withdrawal of HCG and the successful substitution of testosterone, which maintained secondary sex characteristics, resulted in a precipitous fall in the sperm count within 30 days, even though the ejaculate volume was normal. These experiments are still in progress.

In both cases the conclusions are essentially the same. Relatively large amounts of FSH are probably necessary to initiate and develop a full cycle of human spermatogenesis but maintenance of spermatogenesis can be facilitated by much lower FSH levels. The evidence favors the concept that the HCG molecule possesses sufficient FSH-like activity to maintain spermatogenesis once fully established by treatment with HMG.

Our results support the concept originally presented by Albert (13) that the HCG molecule possesses FSH-like activity. It seems that this FSH activity is sufficient to maintain spermatogenesis once fully established by treatment with HMG.

ACKNOWLEDGMENT

This research was performed under grants from the Population Council, Rockefeller University, and the National Institutes of Health grant HD00481.

REFERENCES

1. Donini, P., D. Puzzuoli, and R. Montezemolo, Acta Endocrinol (Kbh) 45:321, 1964.
2. Johnsen, S. G., Acta Endocrinol (Kbh) 53:315, 1966.
3. Heller, C. G., in C. A. Paulsen (Ed.), Estrogen Assays in Clinical Medicine, Univ. Washington Press, Seattle, 1965, p. 275.
4. Paulsen, C. A., Proc. 6th Pan-American Congr Endocrinol International Congress, Excerpta Medica Series No. 122, 1966, p. 398.
5. MacLeod, J., A. Pazianos, and B. R. Ray, Fertil Steril 17:7, 1966.
6. Paulsen, C. A., in C. A. Paulsen (Ed.), Estrogen Assays in Clinical Medicine, Univ. Washington Press, Seattle, 1965, p. 274.
7. Bartter, F. C., R. C. Sniffen, F. A. Simmons, F. Albright, and R. P. Howard, J Clin Endocrinol 12:1532, 1952.

8. Raboch, J., Fertil Steril 11:191, 1960.

9. Plum, P., Acta Med Scand 115:36, 1943.

10. Johnsen, S. G., in E. Rosemberg (Ed.), Gonadotropins 1968, Geron-X Inc., Los Altos, 1968, p. 515.

11. Gemzell, C., and B. Kjessler, Lancet 1:1196, 1964.

12. Mancini, R. E., A. C. Seiguer, and A. Perez Lloret, J Clin Endocrinol 29:465, 1969.

13. Albert, A., J Clin Endocrinol 29:1504, 1969.

DISCUSSION

U. K. BANIK. Dr. Burger, you have shown that after the administration of HCG, the circulating levels of estrogen, testosterone, and LH were elevated, whereas the FSH was decreased. I wonder if this low FSH was due to the negative feedback mechanism of these steroids and whether the elevated LH was due to the positive feedback effect of estrogen. Are you sure that you are not measuring some LH depived from exogenously administered HCG?

H. G. BURGER. I am sorry, if I didn't make it clear that the immunoreactivity marked LH in quotation marks on the slide was meant to indicate the cross-reactivity of HCG in the immunoassay system. We did not attempt to, and I think it would actually have been very difficult to specifically quantitate endogenous pituitary LH after the administration of HCG. With regard to your question on the effects of HCG on FSH, I do not think that we are in any position to give a firm answer. There are a number of possibilities to explain the fall in FSH including, as you have suggested, a rise in testosterone, a rise in estradiol, or possibly the effects of the FSH-like portion of or alternatively the common α subunit which is shared between HCG and FSH. It may be that this is an example of short negative feedback of a gonadotropin on itself or it may be via a long feedback, for which we intend to try to find an answer to that question.

E. ROSEMBERG. Dr. Johnsen, you have defined your "total" gonadotropin assay as an "FSH" assay. I think you recall that we, as well as Dr. Lunenfeld studied the characteristics of the mouse uterine weight assay very thoroughly. Our studies indicated that the mouse uterine weight assay is dependent upon the FSH/LH ratio contained in the preparation being tested. Would you please explain why you called the mouse uterine weight assay an FSH assay?

S. G. JOHNSEN. Dr. Peter Christiansen and I have performed a large number of assays on the same extracts using both the mouse uterus test (HG) and specific FSH and LH bioassay. Correlation analyses showed, throughout the ranges, a much greater correlation between log HG and log FSH than between log HG and log LH. So, in our hands the mouse uterus test measures primarily FSH.

P. FRANCHIMONT. We have recently studied serum FSH levels in cases of azoospermia and oligospermia and correlated them with the results of testicular biopsies. As shown in this slide (Fig. 1) FSH levels were consistently higher than the normal mean value of 4.14 ± 2 SD (SD ± 2.69) mIU/ml in stages 0 through

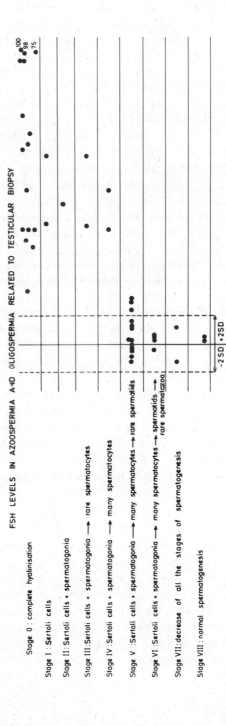

FSH LEVELS IN AZOOSPERMIA AND OLIGOSPERMIA RELATED TO TESTICULAR BIOPSY

Stage 0 : complete hyalinisation

Stage I : Sertoli cells

Stage II : Sertoli cells + spermatogonia

Stage III : Sertoli cells + spermatogonia ⟶ rare spermatocytes

Stage IV : Sertoli cells + spermatogonia ⟶ many spermatocytes

Stage V : Sertoli cells + spermatogonia ⟶ many spermatocytes ⟶ rare spermatids

Stage VI : Sertoli cells + spermatogonia ⟶ many spermatocytes ⟶ spermatids ⟶ rare spermatozoa

Stage VII : decrease of all the stages of spermatogenesis

Stage VIII : normal spermatogenesis

Franchimont, Millet, Vendrely, Netter 1971

FIG. 1.

4. However, in cases of azoospermia or oligospermia, when spermatids were visible on biopsy (stages 5 through 8) the levels of serum FSH were normal. Thus the transformation from the spermatocyte into the spermatid must induce or permit formation of a factor controlling the secretion of FSH.

A substance which depresses FSH was found to be present in the seminal plasma of normal subjects and patients with oligospermia, but not in subjects with azoospermia caused by inhibition of gonadogenesis. The seminal plasma from the three types of subjects was administered to castrated male rats in 4 subcutaneous injections (1 or 0.1 ml) at 18-hr intervals. Seminal plasma from normal subjects and oligospermic patients produced a decrease in rat serum FSH, while the seminal plasma from azoospermic patients failed to reduce serum FSH.

J. S. GOLDZIEHER. I am rather surprised to see people still using dexamethasone as a drug which allegedly suppresses only the adrenal so that one can look at the function of the gonads. It has been known since the days of Thomas McGavack in the early 50's that corticosteroids and more recently, dexamethasone, do lots of things to endogenous gonadotropin production. As a matter of fact, dexamethasone injected intrahypothalamically in the rat does very interesting things to gonadotropin release (Endocrinology 84:308, 1969). I wonder whether the availability of immunological anti-estrogen might not be a very nice way to find out what the role of estrogen is in the feedback control of FSH and the spermatogenic tubules. It seems to me that there are fairly obvious experiments that could be done in rats with anti-estrogen, looking at their plasma FSH and LH under various testicular manipulations. It appears so obvious, that I wonder whether somebody in the Columbia group has done this.

F. C. GREENWOOD. Has anybody measured acute changes in FSH and LH during mating in the human? The present scenarios of the menstrual cycle in the human and the monkey assume that human prolactin does not exist. Presumably one cannot neglect a hormone which, in the sheep and goat rises very acutely during sexual excitement and satisfaction and which surges after the LH peak. I do not think we are that much different from rams.

G. G. GORDON. Dr. Horton has data in the literature showing no changes in LH activity in humans during sexual intercourse.

R. B. JAFFE. I would have to take some issue with Fred about the lack of difference between the sheep and the human, in certain respects at least. In the menstrual cycle, there does not seem to be cyclicity in prolactin.

A. L. SOUTHREN. The studies done on the diurnal rhythm showing that plasma testosterone is higher in the morning or at night seems to argue against a realtionship to sexual behavior. Although this has provoked some humor over the years, I do not think that anyone has established a relationship between the changes in testosterone and sexual behavior.

H. G. BURGER. One of the things that came out in the paper of Evans, who showed the episodic rises in testosterone related to rapid eye movement in sleep, was that the rises in testosterone were also correlated with penile erections.

S. G. JOHNSEN. I am, of course. very much concerned about the difference between C. Alvin Paulsen's results and ours. I am not referring to the small group of 12 men investigated by testicular cell counts, but rather to your big group studied by radioimmunoassay of gonadotropins. I have the feeling that there must be something wrong with the radioimmunoassays and this derives from the very small scale of movement of FSH and LH values when measured immunologically. For example, we have heard today that there is a rise of FSH and LH during puberty by a factor of 2 or perhaps 3 by radioimmunoassays. If you measure urinary gonadotropins by bioassay, you find that adult men have 20 to 30 times more gonadotropin than prepubertal children. By bioassay you find that castration in the human male leads to a 10-fold increase of FSH. The castrate has some 200 to 300 times more gonadotropin than the child. The very small change in radioimmunoassay values do not fit into this and I fear there must be something fundamentally wrong. It would appear that things would fit together if some 80 to 90% of what you measure by radioimmunoassay in low level samples is not gonadotropin.

C. A. PAULSEN. That is precisely why we performed the urinary FSH bioassay studies. Now it is possible that our two laboratories perform this assay differently which might account for the discrepancy in results. However, as I examine Dr. Christiansen's assay results in his patients with Klinefelter's syndrome, the range for urinary FSH is approximately 53 to 100 IU/24 hr. These values are reasonably comparable to our experience (Rec Prog Hormone Res, 24:339, 1968). Thus, our two laboratories appear to perform the Steelman-Pohley FSH assay in a comparable fashion. Therefore, this aspect does not afford an explanation for our differences in FSH values for adult males with idiopathic oligospermia.

E. ROSEMBERG. It will be very important for Drs. Paulsen and Johnsen to arrive at some agreement. Dr. Johnsen bases his conclusions on a bioassay which is not specific for FSH and Dr. Paulsen bases his conclusion on an assay specific for FSH. However, the number of patients studied is small. I would think that more work should be done in order to resolve this problem.

C. A. PAULSEN. I will accept the first point, namely, that we do not have direct proof. Second point, although I appreciate Svend Johnsen's thinking I believe we should continue to work independently so that we might get nearer the "truth."

Pituitary—Ovarian Axis

51.   Some Aspects of CNS-Pituitary-Ovarian Interrelationship

Judith Weisz and Charles W. Lloyd

"In the making of eggs sundry parts are of great use."
Diemberbroeck, 1694

It was during the course of the century in which the great institution, The Society of the New York Hospital, was established that the idea of the ovary as the source of the ovum, the female's contribution to the offspring, was on trial. By the end of the 17th century what had until then been called the female testis or stone acquired a name of its own—the ovary. The name was the result of the suggestion that it contained the mammalian equivalent of the eggs of the ovipara (1). But then along came the sperm, seen for the first time through the newly invented microscope, moving and very much alive. Delanpatius' imaginative eye had even made him see a minute but complete human being, the homunculus, within it (2) (Fig. 1). The mammalian ovum on the other hand had not yet been sighted. The nature of the link between the Graafian follicle, which de Graaf had mistaken for the ovum, and the early embryo was missing. For many, then, the sperm became sufficient to account for human reproduction or generation as it was then called—pitting "spermatists" against "ovulists." By the time this institution was established, the spermatists were definitely losing, and the ovary's role could only become accepted as a reality with the demonstration of the human ovum by von Baer in 1827 (3).

In tracing the recognition and acceptance of the importance of the ovary, one can follow, as if it were in slow motion, the hazards and vicissitudes facing new observations and insights before they could become fully assimilated to serve as a basis for further new observations and insights.

For our presentation, we have selected a few recent observations and concepts derived from studies of the experimental animal as well as of human

673

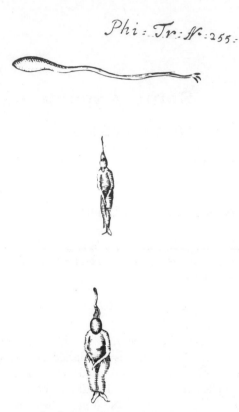

FIG. 1. The sperm as seen by Leeuwenhoek and the homunculus by Delanpatius (21). Reproduced by permission of Proc Royal Soc.

males and females that are relevant to the understanding of the CNS-pituitary-ovarian circuit and how the ovulatory cycle is regulated.

They are ideas and observations that we believe have the credentials to warrant their inclusion in our thinking about the regulation of the circuit. They are, however, still generally considered to be only of specialized or peripheral interest. This seems an appropriate contribution to the bicentennial of this dynamic institution whose life has encompassed the spawning and reevaluation of so many concepts. By our choice of subjects we hope to avoid duplication of material, which is no easy task on the third day of so comprehensive a meeting.

NON STEADY-STATE SECRETION OF PITUITARY TROPIC HORMONES AND STEROIDS

We have recently published the results of a study carried out in collaboration with the Department of Obstetrics and Gynecology of the University of Chile

(4). This project involved measurement of the estrogens, androgens, and gestagens, in the ovarian and peripheral venous blood of 18 normal women with regular menstrual cycles. The samples were collected at the time of elective tubal ligation at known stages of the cycle. The findings were somewhat disconcerting. The results would not fit neatly into the expected pattern of cyclic changes. Since there was, of course, only one set of samples per subject, the cyclic pattern of steroid values could be expected to be less marked than is found when consecutive specimens from the same subject are analyzed. The most unexpected finding, however, was the very wide range of values of the ovarian vein steroids in specimens from patients at corresponding stages of the menstrual cycle. This was particularly evident for estradiol, androstenedione, and progesterone (Figs. 2 and 3).

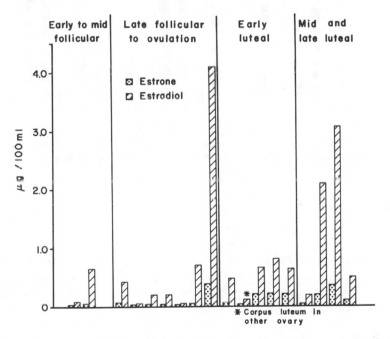

FIG. 2. Concentration of estrone and estradiol in the ovarian venous plasma of 18 women with regular menstrual cycles. The subjects have been grouped according to the stage of the cycle indicated by the endometrial biopsy.

This wide variability of the ovarian vein steroids is evident from the ratios of ovarian to peripheral vein concentrations of estrogens and androgens. The great range of the ratios is essentially due to variations in the concentrations of ovarian vein steroids since the peripheral vein values varied relatively little.

To us, one possible explanation for the findings was that the ovaries may

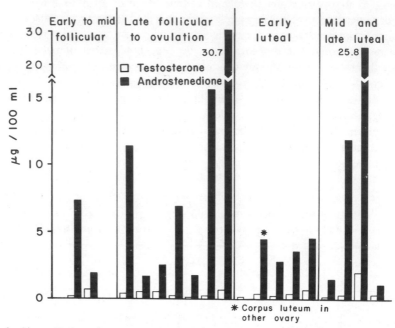

FIG. 3. Concentration of testosterone and androstenedione in the ovarian venous plasma of 18 women with regular menstrual cycles. The subjects have been grouped according to the stage of the cycle indicated by the endometrial biopsy.

secrete at a fluctuating rather than at a steady rate. This idea that the ovaries secrete episodically is not too novel since considerable evidence exists that this type of secretion occurs in other glands.

The adrenal cortex unquestionably secretes corticoids intermittently, presumably because ACTH is discharged in bursts (5-8). Fluctuations in ACTH not related to environmental stress were demonstrated by Berson and Yalow when they first applied their newly developed radioimmunoassay to the serial measurement of ACTH in blood (5). They also reported parallel fluctuations in the levels of 17-hydroxycorticoids. Abrupt changes in corticoid levels in the early morning hours in a sleeping subject were first observed by Weitzman (6). Because the majority of the bursts of corticoid secretion coincided with REM sleep, this investigator suggested that fluctuations in ACTH discharge, which presumably cause the fluctuations in corticoids, may be the result of bursts of neural activity initiated perhaps by the reticular activating system and more evident during sleep.

The intermittent nature of cortisol secretion was clearly demonstrated in a meticulous study by Hellman and associates (7). The bloods for the measurement of cortisol were collected at frequent intervals through a catheter without the subject's knowledge. Whether or not the adrenal was secreting during a particular period of time was determined by monitoring the changes in specific activity of infused labeled steroid. During the day as well as the night, there were discrete secretory episodes and the gland was estimated to be nonsecreting during a large part of the 24 hours.

It is, of course, relatively easy to accept the proposition that the adrenal secretes its hormones intermittently. Its business, after all, is to respond rapidly to varying needs. However, this intermittent secretory activity does not appear to depend on varying stresses and the phenomenon of intermittent secretion does not appear to be a peculiarity of the pituitary-adrenal axis. It may be a more general phenomenon, related perhaps to some characteristic of CNS activity which is transmitted to the hypothalamus and causes the discharge, in bursts, of the releasing factors. Thus there is reason to think that episodic secretion is a basic characteristic also of the pituitary-gonadal axis. The evidence for this, though scanty as yet, is suggestive.

First, in the human male the pattern of secretion of testosterone, at least during sleep, appears to be quite similar to that of cortisol (Fig. 4) (9). The

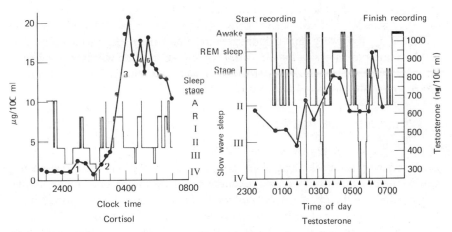

FIG. 4. Fluctuations in cortisol (on left) on testosterone levels (right) during sleep. Electroencephalograms were recorded throughout the period of blood collection.

studies in which this was demonstrated were patterned after those that had been used to study the fluctuations in corticoid levels. Samples of blood were taken at frequent intervals without disturbing the subject and EEG recordings were made at the same time.

Just as with the corticoids there were, towards morning, major fluctuations superimposed on a general upward trend and again there was a suggestion that the bursts of secretion were associated with REM sleep. Unfortunately, the gonadotropin levels were not measured.

In the female, on the other hand, there have been measurements made of LH levels but not of the gonadal steroids in samples of blood collected at frequent intervals. In the oophorectomized monkey, LH appears to be discharged in bursts with a periodicity of about 60 min (10). The short loop feedback apparently can not be implicated in the periodic decreases in LH secretion. In contrast, in the intact monkey, no oscillations in LH were found either during the luteal or the follicular phase. The exact stages of the cycle in which the bloods were collected were not specified. However, there are data from Kapen, Boyar, Hallman, and Weitzman (11), as yet unpublished, indicating that in the intact human female there are major fluctuations in LH at least during certain stages of the cycle. The fluctuations become increasingly evident during the late follicular phase and are damped out after ovulation. Most of the data have been collected from sleeping subjects, at night. Fluctuations were, however, also evident in the few subjects in whom samples were taken throughout the day.

As with the corticoids and testosterone there is a suggestion that at least some of the increases in hormone levels are related to REM sleep. Again, as with the corticoids, the increases in LH do not necessarily coincide with those of growth hormone. We don't yet know exactly how such fluctuations would influence steroid secretion by the ovary or how such variable signals might be integrated by the gonadotropin-responsive cells within the ovary. Should hormone secretion by the ovary prove indeed to be fluctuating, the mechanisms that would damp out the variations in peripheral blood, in other words, extraglandular metabolism and binding of steroids to specific proteins in the circulation, to be discussed later, assume added significance.

STEROIDS SECRETED BY THE OVARY AND THEIR POSSIBLE ROLE

In considering feedback control of gonadotropin secretion, there has been a tendency to concentrate almost exclusively on estradiol and progesterone. Admittedly, the drama of the preovulatory LH surge may depend primarily on these two hormones and at least in the experimental situation they can certainly cause the release of a surge of LH. But the ovary secretes a wide variety of steroids besides estradiol and progesterone and there is, of course, a lot more to the cycle than just the ovulatory surge of gonadotropins. There are some neglected phases of the cycle; for example, the period immediately after the beginning of corpus luteum regression. A rise in circulating FSH levels begins at this time and continues uninterrupted into the next menstrual cycle (Fig. 5) (12). From histological studies of monkey ovaries we may deduce that the growth spurt of the follicles from which the one to ovulate will be selected, begins at this time (13). This period, then, is essentially a part of the next ovulatory cycle and may have an influence on the outcome of the next

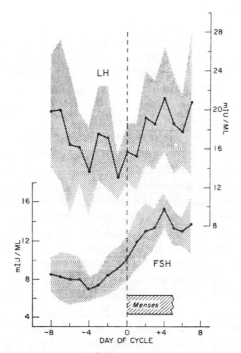

FIG. 5. Plasma gonadotropin levels during the late luteal and early follicular phase showing the steady rise in FSH characteristic for this period of the ovulatory cycle.

ovulation, a point obscured by our convention of thinking in terms of the menstrual rather than the ovulatory cycle.

The range of hormones secreted by the ovary may be deduced from a comparison of the concentrations of several steroids in ovarian and peripheral venous bloods. On this basis, there is evidence that besides estradiol and progesterone the ovary also secretes pregnenolone, 17- and 20α-dihydroprogesterone,[1] testosterone, androstenedione, and estrone and dehydroepiandrosterone (4, 14, 15). We have recently also found the dihydrotestosterone levels to be higher in ovarian than in peripheral venous blood of human subjects and have observed a rise in the concentration of dihydrotestosterone in the ovarian venous blood of anovulatory rats after the administration of an ovulatory dose of LH. Unquestionably, there will be additional steroids that will be found to be secreted by the ovary.

With the newer, simpler methods for steroid measurements, it is feasible to carry out longitudinal studies throughout the ovulatory cycles on individual

[1]The following trivial names are used: 20α-dihydroprogesterone (20α-hydroxypregn-4-en-3-one); 17α-hydroxyprogesterone(17α-hydroxypregn-4-ene-3,20-dione); and dihydrotestosterone (5α-androstan-3-one-17β-ol).

subjects and establish which steroids of ovarian origin vary cyclically in the peripheral blood. The patterns of cyclicity could provide clues as to function.

The levels of at least one until now little considered steroid, 17α-hydroxy-progesterone, have indeed been found to change cyclically (12). It has been proposed that this parallels and reflects estradiol secretion, its source being the same as that of estradiol, presumably the theca interna. Our own data, however, show that actually larger amounts of this steroid may be secreted by the ovary which is less active in terms of estrogen secretion. This is particularly evident when the patterns of steroids are compared in the ovarian venous blood from the two sides in the same subject. In the two cases studied, one in the follicular and one in the luteal phase, the concentrations of 17α-hydroxyprogesterone were higher in the blood from the side in which the estradiol was lower. If 17α-hydroxyprogesterone and estradiol levels are parallel, it is not necessarily because they both originate from the same site, but because they reflect activity proceeding pari passu in different components of the ovaries.

Do the changes in the various steroids have a function or do they simply represent a kind of redundancy in the system, a leakage of intermediates in the metabolic pathway? Our prejudice is that at least some of these steroids will turn out to have a role in feedback control and that the interrelationships, the ratios of different steroids, are of importance in subtler aspects of regulation. Observations such as that of Hilliard that 20α-dihydroprogesterone is needed for the maintenance of the LH surge in the rabbit (16) encourages us to continue measuring systematically a variety of steroids both in the ovarian and peripheral blood. These less popular steroids, which we call "wallflowers" may turn out to be quite sexy once one starts playing around with them.

REGULATORY MECHANISMS INTERPOSED BETWEEN COMPONENTS OF THE CIRCUIT: EXTRAGLANDULAR METABOLISM AND BINDING OF STEROIDS TO SPECIFIC TRANSPORT PROTEINS

The pattern of ovarian hormones which feed back to the CNS and the pituitary, differs radically from the pattern of hormones secreted by the ovary. This is evident from comparison of the concentrations of the different hormones in the peripheral circulation with those in the ovarian venous blood (4, 14, 15). The fate of exogenous steroids also indicates that the pattern of substances that circulate must be very different from their pattern when they are secreted. Steroid hormones released into the circulation are not only catabolized to inert substances, but may also be converted into other steroids with different physiological actions. It is this latter phenomenon that has given rise to the concept of the prehormone (17). We know little about the sites where these metabolic processes take place or about the mechanisms that regulate them, particularly in the human. The liver is without doubt one important site. The way the liver handles steroid hormones is modified by many factors including the steroid hormones themselves (18-24). The liver itself must, therefore, be considered a target organ of steroid hormone action. In experimental animals differences have been shown between the sexes in the way they handle steroids (18, 23). Some of these can be abolished by the administration of the appropriate sex hormones to the mature animals. Others are apparently imprinted permanently by the sex hormones during differentiation (23). For example, if a newborn female rat is given an injection of testosterone propionate her liver, after puberty, will metabolize corticoids, progesterone, and testosterone as that of a male rat. This change may conceivably play a role in the development of polycystic ovaries that follows the administration of testosterone propionate to the newborn female rat.

The observation that testosterone is metabolized to its active form or forms, dihydrotestosterone and the "androstandiols" (5α-androstan-3α,17βol and 5α-androstan-3β,17β-ol), within the secondary sex structures, has added a new dimension to the concept of prehormones (25-27). There are data, including our own, which suggest that the metabolites of testosterone that act on the brain may differ from those that act on the secondary sex structures. We have found that in the rat an injection of 100 μg dihydrotestosterone propionate or of 5α-androstan-3β,17β-diol propionate at 5 days of age masculinizes the external genitalia, but does not induce the syndrome of androgen sterilization. Testosterone propionate at the same dose level, on the other hand, does not affect the external genitalia but causes the development of sterility and polycystic ovaries, abnormalities that are attributed to a change in the gonadotropin regulating centers of the CNS.

Estradiol, in contrast to testosterone, does not seem to be a prehormone. All evidence points to its acting on its target cells as estradiol. Progesterone, however, may turn out to be more akin to testosterone. Like testosterone, it is rapidly metabolized to a variety of other steroids within its target tissues. Recently, Wilson has demonstrated preferential binding of one of its metabolites, dihydroprogesterone, to the nuclei of the hen oviduct, a finding suggesting that this may be the active hormone (28). Thus conversion of a prehormone to an active one by the target organ exemplified by the testosterone-dihydrotestosterone system may turn out to be of great importance in the female also.

There have thus far been few systematic studies to determine what changes in peripheral metabolism of steroids take place throughout the normal cycle. We suspect that there may be such changes. Our studies indicated differences in the metabolic clearance rate of androstenedione in the two phases of the cycle (29). Precise and detailed data for many hormones are needed before the regulatory significance of such changes can be evaluated.

The nature of the metabolic changes the gonadotropins undergo after they are secreted into the circulation is not known. No gross differences have been observed in the half-life of LH in the pre- or the postmenopausal women (30, 31). From various papers presented at this symposium it is quite evident that the biological half-life of LH may be greatly influenced through the carbohydrate and sialic acid content of the hormone. We do not yet know whether structural changes affecting the sialic acid or carbohydrate moiety occur in vitro to alter the rate of utilization or destruction of the gonadotropins in different physiological states. The normal ovary appears to metabolize LH—at least that is the interpretation we have given to our finding of a consistently lower level of LH in the ovarian than in the peripheral venous blood of the women with normal cycles (32). These differences were not found in specimens from patients taking contraceptives. In contrast, the differences in peripheral and ovarian FSH levels were quite variable. The number of pairs of samples at our disposal were too few to determine whether there were systematic differences in the utilization of FSH in different stages of the ovulatory cycle. However, our data suggest that there may be greater difference between peripheral and ovarian FSH values during the late luteal than the fillicular phases.

The specific binding of transport proteins represents a second system that is interposed between the ovary and the other components of the CNS-pituitary-ovarian circuit. The main features of this system are summarized in Table I and II.

Clearly, if binding modifies the physiological effectiveness of steroid hormones (33), a knowledge of only the absolute levels of hormones is not

TABLE I. Circulating steroid-binding "transport" proteins

Types	
Sex hormone binding	2 to 3 mg/l[a]
Corticoid binding	40 mg/l
Characteristics	
High affinity for a relatively few specific steroids	
Small capacity	
Therefore	
Over 90% of the specific steroids are bound at the low concentrations characteristic of circulating hormone levels.	
Binding proteins become saturated when hormone levels rise 2- to 3-fold above normal levels.	
Protein bound steroid is physiologically inactive.	
Presumed Functions	
To protect hormones from catabolism; e.g., by liver.	
Buffer organism from fluctuations in hormone levels.	
Make hormone available at target site.	

[a]Data from E. Baulieu et al. Rec Prog Hormone Res 27:351, 1971.

TABLE II. Circulating steroid-binding "transport" proteins; relative affinity

Sex Steroid Binding Protein[a]

High affinity		Low affinity
Testosterone	100	Estrone
Dihydrotestosterone	300	Estriol
5α-Androstane-3α,17β-diol	160	Stilbesterol
5α-Androstane-3β,17β-diol	160	Androstenedione
Androst-4-en-3β,17β-diol	95	Epitestosterone
Estradiol	60	17α-Estradiol
Androst-5-en-3β,17β-diol	50	

Corticosteroid Binding Protein[b]

High affinity			Low affinity
	4 C	37 C	
Corticosterone	100	33	Testosterone
Progesterone	70	100	Dihydrotestosterone
Cortisol	60	33	"Androstandiols"
			Testosterone Conjugates
			Estradiol

[a]Data from Vermeulen, A., and L. Verdonck, Acta Endocrinol Suppl 147:239, 1970.

[b]Adapted from data of Westphal, U., Acta Endocrinol Suppl 147:122, 1970.

sufficient. Ultimately, we will have to obtain information about the proportion of the hormone that is free and the extent or ease with which the bound portion can be freed and trapped at the different target sites. Because different steroids compete for the same binding site, changes in the level of one may modify the availability of another. The concentration of a metabolite such as dihydrotestosterone may be raised locally in the vicinity of the target organ in which it was formed and displaced bound testosterone to make it available where it is needed—forming a kind of positive feedback system.

Systematic evaluation of steroid binding function in normal and abnormal states has only just begun (34-36). It is too early to say whether alterations in binding play specific roles in the regulation of ovarian cyclicity. No significant changes in total binding capacity have been found in a small number of blood samples obtained during the two stages of the cycle (34). Serial measurements in individual subjects have not yet been made.

The potential importance of these two regulatory mechanisms is demonstrated by the feminizing testis syndrome in which an abnormality in the metabolism of testosterone by the target organ and/or in the plasma steroid binding have both been implicated in the etiology of the abnormality (37-40). A decrease in the activity of 5α reductase in the target tissues, possibly secondary to increased binding of testosterone to the specific proteins, may be the basis of the unresponsiveness of these patients to either their own or to administered testosterone (38).

Thus a number of variables—fluctuations in secretion, interactions of different hormones, variations in metabolism and binding as well as the absolute levels of the hormones—contribute to their physiological actions and must be considered when evaluating them. No matter how precise the methods for their measurement may become, knowledge of the absolute amount of a specific hormone will probably be useful only in recognizing gross abnormalities. Thus the endocrine laboratory does not offer a great deal more diagnostic help with the recent development of the more sensitive methods for measurement of hormones. The concepts we have discussed today are currently of little practical importance to those responsible for the care of patients; nevertheless, it will be through incorporation of these concepts into the study of endocrine diseases that fuller understanding of their pathogenesis will be achieved.

ADENOHYPOPHYSIS AS A SITE FOR FEEDBACK CONTROL BY STEROIDS

In the 18th century the preoccupation with the importance of the sperm delayed the explorations that would lead to recognition of the function of the ovary. In the past two decades, concentration on the hypothalamus has resulted in slighting of the importance of the pituitary as an independent entity which contributes directly, as well as by responding to messages from the CNS, to regulation of ovarian function. During these years there were few lone champions of the pituitary (41). The tide now seems to be turning and new data are being generated on the role of the pituitary as a site for feedback regulation.

The anterior pituitary has the characteristics of a steroid target organ; it concentrates estradiol and contains in the rat, per miliigram tissue, as much specific 8S estradiol receptor protein as does the vagina and per milligram DNA, almost as much as the uterus (42-44).

The effects of gonadal steroids on the adenohypophysis and on its response to releasing factors seem to depend on the circumstances.

In vivo, response to LRF can be increased by prior short term treatment with estrogen and decreased by pretreatment with gestagens (45-48). In the sheep, the response varies with the phase of the cycle (49). In man, the administration of estrogen for a longer time may produce a different response since Reichlin et al. have found increased levels of LRF and decreased levels of LH in plasma of men who have received estrogens (50). In all of these situations, it is difficult to distinguish precisely between direct effects on the pituitary and those that may be secondary to changes in CNS function. This is true even in those experiments in which the releasing factors were administered directly into the pituitary.

For more unequivocal evidence, one has to rely on experiments, however artificial, in which the hormones are placed into and remain confined to the gland itself or to studies of the pituitary in vitro. Estradiol implanted into the pituitary has been shown to advance ovulation in the rat by 24 hr. This effect is obtained only if the estradiol is implanted for a specific time the day before the advanced ovulation (46). In an isolated older study, using bioassay techniques, estradiol has been found to increase the output of LH by pituitaries incubated in vitro for 1 hr with a hypothalamic extract (51). With our colleagues, Drs. Dowd, Chaudhuri, and Barofsky, we have been exploring the dynamics of gonadotropin release by the adenohypophysis in vitro using radioimmunoassay and an adaptation of the superfusion technique developed for the study of adrenocortical secretion (52). In this system, rat pituitaries respond to hypothalamic extract in a reproducible manner for as long as 12 hr. There is a definite dose response. There is remarkably little variation in the response of any given pool of pituitaries to repeated infusions (pulses) of identical amounts of hypothalamic extract (coefficient of variation, 2 to 7% depending on the duration of the pulse). We find that following a brief, 60-min exposure of pituitaries to estradiol at low concentrations (3 X 10^{-9}M) there is a significant decrease in the amount of LH released by a pulse of hypothalmic extract; whether given concurrently or 30 min after the withdrawal of the estradiol (Figs. 6 and 7).

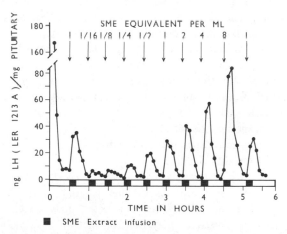

FIG. 6. Changes in the amount of LH released by pituitaries superfused in vitro in response to successive infusions (pulses) of stalk median extract (SME) of different concentrations ranging from 1/16 to 8 SME eq ml. The duration of each pulse was 10 min. The superfusion rate was 12 ml hr. Each point in the graph represents the amount of LH in superfusate collected during a 5-min period and measured by radioimmunoassay. Unpublished data (A. Dowd, N. Chaudhuri, L. Barofsky, J. Weisz, and C. W. Lloyd).

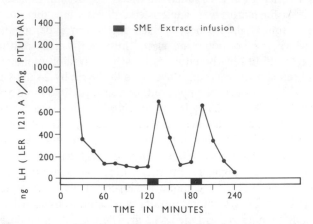

FIG. 7. Amount of LH released by pituitaries superfused in vitro in response to two successive 15-min infusions (pulses) of stalk median eminence extract (SME). The pituitaries were superfused at a rate of 4 ml hr with a concentration of 1.5 SME Eq/ml. Each point represents the amount of LH in the superfusate collected during 15 min and measured by radioimmunoassay. The increase in LH output following exposure of the pituitaries to the two pulses of SME was 758 and 773 ng, respectively. Values were corrected for LH activity in the SME. The initial high concentration of LH in the superfusate is characteristically found during the first 30 min of incubation. The first pulse was given only after base line levels had been reached. Unpublished data (A. Dowd, N. Chaudhuri, L. Barofsky, J. Weisz, and C. W. Lloyd).

It would seem then that the steroid hormones that feedback to the hypothalamus to regulate the production and discharge of the gonadotropin releasing factors may also act on the adenohypophysis to modify its response to the releasing factors. Such a dual mechanism would provide a greater precision and control in the regulatory machinery than could be provided by either alone. However, the difficulties in unraveling the complexity of these controlling mechanisms are suggested by the fragmentary data that not only are there at least two sites of response, the pituitary and the hypothalamus, but that there are differences in response, depending on the duration of the exposure as well as the level of the steroids at both sites.

As in all interacting systems, it will not be easy to differentiate clearly between direct effects of hormones on the pituitary and effects that are mediated via the hypothalamus. The dual site of feedback action, while introducing added complications, may help ultimately to explain some of the puzzling double-threshold and biphasic phenomena which characterize hormone action on gonadotropin release.

These, then, are some additional "sundry parts" to use a phrase from Diemerbroeck's entertaining chapter "Of the secret parts of women serving to the generation of seed and egg." There will undoubtedly be many more "sundry parts" recognized in the future and future generations will no doubt wonder at our not seeing what to them will be so obvious and our interpreting wrongly what to them will be so clear.

ACKNOWLEDGMENT

These studies were supported by grants AM-08184 and HD00282 from the National Institutes of Health, Bethesda, Maryland and the Ford Foundation, New York, New York.

REFERENCES

1. de Graaf, R., Opera Omnia, 2nd ed. Amsterdam, 1705.
2. Delanpatius, quoted in a letter by A. Leeuwenhoek, Philosophical Transactions of the Royal Society, 21:301, 1699.
3. Von Baer, De Ovi Mamalium et Hominis Genesi . . ., Leopold Voss, Leipzig, 1827.
4. Lloyd, C. W., J. Lobotsky, D. T. Baird, J. A. McCracken, J. Weisz, M. Pupkin, J. Zanartu, and J. Puga, J Clin Endocrinol 32:155, 1971.
5. Berson, A. S., and R. S. Yalow, J Clin Invest 47:2725, 1968.
6. Weitzman, E. D., H. Schaumburg, and W. Fishbein, J Clin Endocrinol 26:121, 1966.
7. Hellman, L., F. Nakada, J. Curti, E. D. Weitzman, H. Roffwarg, S. Ellman, D. K. Fukushima, and T. F. Gallagher, J Clin Endocrinol 32:411, 1970.
8. Krieger, D., W. Allen, F. Rizzo, and H. P. Krieger, J Clin Endocrinol 32:266, 1971.
9. Evans, J. I., A. W. MacLean, A. A. A. Ismail, and D. Love, Nature, 229:261, 1971.
10. Diershkee, D. J., A. N. Bhattacharya, L. E. Atkinson, and E. Knobil, Endocrinology 87:850, 1970.
11. Kapen, S., R. Boyar, L. Hellman, and E. D. Weitzman, personal communication.
12. Ross, G. T., C. M. Cargille, M. B. Lipsett, P. L. Rayford, J. R. Marshall, C. A. Strott, and D. Rodbard, Rec Prog Hormone Res 26:1, 1970.
13. Koering, H. J., Amer J Anat 126:73, 1969.
14. Gandy, H. M., and R. E. Peterson, J Clin Endocrinol 28:949, 1968.
15. Mikhail, G., Gyn Invest 1:5, 1970.
16. Hilliard, J., R. Penardi, and C. H. Sawyer, Endocrinology 80:901, 1967.
17. Baird, D. T., R. Horton, C. Longcope, and J. F. Tait, Rec Prog Hormone Res 25:611, 1969.
18. Rubin, B. L., and H. J. Strecker, Endocrinology 69:257, 1961.
19. Barzilai, D., and G. Pincus, Proc Soc Exp Biol Med 117:711, 1964.
20. Jellinck, P. H., and I. Lucieer, J Endocrinol 32:91, 1965.
21. Heinrichs, W. L., H. H. Feder, and A. Colas, Steroids 7:91, 1966.
22. Denef, C., and P. deMoor, Endocrinology 83:791, 1968.
23. Wenzel, M., M. Langold, and P. Hallac, J Biol Chem 244:4523, 1969.
24. Bercovici, J. P., and P. Mauvais-Jarvis, Ann Endocrinol 31:1111, 1970.
25. Wilson, J. D., and R. E. Gloyna, Rec Prog Hormone Res 26:309, 1970.
26. Baulieu, E. E., A. Alberga, I. Jung, M. Lebeau, M. C. Mercier-Bodard, E. Milgrom, J. P. Raynaud, C. Raynaud-Jammet, H. Truong-Richard-Foy, and P. Robel, Rec Prog Hormone Res 27:351, 1971 (in press).

27. Fang, S., and S. Liao, J Biol Chem 246:16, 1971.
28. Morgan, M. D., and J. D. Wilson, J Biol Chem 245:3781, 1970.
29. Abraham, G. E., J. Lobotsky, and C. W. Lloyd, J Clin Invest 48:696, 1969.
30. Kohler, P. O., G. T. Ross, and W. D. Odell, J Clin Invest 47:38, 1968.
31. Coble, Y. D., P. O. Kohler, C. M. Cargill, and G. T. Ross, J Clin Invest 48:359, 1969.
32. Llerena, L. A., A. Guevara, J. Lobotsky, C. W. Lloyd, J. Weisz, M. Pupkin, J. Zanartu, and J. Puga, J. Clin Endocrinol 29:1083, 1969.
33. Kwai, A., and F. E. Yates, Endocrinology 79:1040, 1966.
34. Pearlman, W. H., and O. Crepy, J Biol Chem 242:182, 1967.
35. Crepy, O., H. P. Klotz, D. Jouin-Courzier, M. A. Ducret, and A. Schwob, Ann Endocrinol 31:437, 1970.
36. De Moor, P., Ann Endocrinol 31:437, 1970.
37. Mauvais-Marvis, P., J. P. Bercovici, O. Crepy, and F. Gauthier, J Clin Invest 49:31, 1970.
38. Mauvais-Jarvis, P., O. Crepy, and J. P. Bercovici, J Clin Endocrinol 32:568, 1971.
39. Rosenfield, R. L., A. M. Lawrence, S. Liao, and R. Landau, J Clin Endocrinol 32:625, 1971.
40. Northcutt, R. C., D. P. Island, and G. W. Liddle, J Clin Endocrinol Metab 29:422, 1969.
41. Bogdanove, E. M., Vitamins Hormones 22:205, 1964.
42. Kato, J., and C. A. Villee, Endocrinology 80:1133, 1967.
43. Jensen, E. V., M. Numata, S. Smith, T. Suzuki, P. I. Brecher, and E. R. De Sombre, Dev Biol Supp 3:171, 1969.
44. Notides, A. C., Endocrinology 87:987, 1970.
45. Hilliard, J., A. V. Schally, and C. H. Sawyer, Endocrinology 88:730, 1971.
46. Weick, R. F., E. R. Smith, R. Dominguez, A. P. S. Dhariwal, and J. M. Davidson, Endocrinology 88:293, 1971.
47. Arimura, A., and A. V. Schally, Proc Soc Exp Biol Med 136:290, 1971.
48. Arimura, A., and A. V. Schally, Endocrinology 87:653, 1970.
49. Reeves, J. J., A. Arimura, and A. V. Schally, J Anim Sci 32:123, 1970.
50. Seyler, L. E., and S. Reichlin, personal communication.
51. Piachek, E. B., and J. Meites, Endocrinology 79:432, 1966.
52. Schulster, D., S. A. S. Tait, J. S. Tait, and J. Mrotek, Endocrinology 86:451, 1970.
53. Diemberbroeck, Isbrand de, Anatomy of Human Bodies, W. Whitewood, London, 1694.

52. Induction of Ovulation by Therapeutic Agents

Bruno Lunenfeld, Vaclav Insler, and Mitchell Snyder

An engineer receives specifications and his problem is to design according to them. In biology the design is given and the blueprint must be determined. Interdisciplinary research must strive toward final elucidation of this blueprint. The more complete the blueprint, the more rational the therapy. Thus if one wishes to control reproductive processes, knowledge of normal ovarian functions is essential, key compounds in the regulatory processes have to be characterized, and the failure or failures leading to ovarian dysfunction have to be located and understood. Armed with this knowledge, ideal drugs capable of stimulating or modifying ovarian functions can be developed. Such drugs should act as substitutes of, supplements to, or antagonists to the natural key substances responsible for regulation of reproductive processes. This paper is primarily an attempt to analyze the current state of knowledge on these topics with a view to achieving this aim.

Ovulation is the result of a perfectly balanced and coordinated function of gonadotropin releasing factors, gonadotropic hormones, and ovarian response. Any disruption in this complex system may lead to anovulation. At present ten different types of such disturbances may be postulated. These possible defects are illustrated in Table I.

Class 1 illustrates a theoretical group of patients where the disturbance is due to lack or production of both gonadotropic hormones. In classes 2, 3, and 4 the disturbance is caused by faulty release of gonadotropic hormones (premature, delayed, inadequate, or excessive). In such classes the ovulatory mechanism could be corrected by causing release of gonadotropins in the correct sequence,

TABLE I. Hypothetical defects in gonadotrophic secretion

Class	FSH Production	Release	LH Production	Release	Ovarian response
1	Impaired		Impaired		Normal
2	Normal	Impaired	Normal	Impaired	Normal
3	Normal	Impaired	Normal	Normal	Normal
4	Normal	Normal	Normal	Impaired	Normal
5	Impaired		Normal	Normal	Normal
6	Normal	Normal	Impaired		Normal
7	Normal	Impaired	Impaired		Normal
8	Impaired		Normal	Impaired	Normal
9	Normal	Normal	Normal	Normal	Impaired
10	Normal	Normal	Normal	Normal	None

magnitude and time. In classes 5 and 8 FSH production is impaired, while in classes 6 and 7 LH production is impaired. In patients with such defects only therapy providing the required gonadotropic hormones as a substitute will induce ovarian function. In class 9 the ovarian response is impaired. Such impairment might be the result of a low sensitivity of the ovary to gonadotropic stimulation, and such cases will respond to appropriate supplementary doses of gonadotropins.

Impairment could also be due to interfering steroids which directly or indirectly affect ovarian activity. Such steroids may be secreted by the ovary itself or by the adrenal gland. Inhibition of the interfering steroids might normalize the condition. Inborn errors of steroid metabolism in congenital adrenal hyperplasia may serve as an example to illustrate such a condition. Enzymic impairment along the biosynthetic pathway of cortisol results in cortisol deficiency. Such a deficiency sets up a feedback with the hypothalamic and pituitarytropic tissues and "instructs" them continuously to increase ACTH release (1). This may result in abnormally high levels of androgens (2-5) which, in turn, may affect the pituitary-ovarian feedback mechanism leading to impairment of gonadotropic release. Administration of cortisone or its analogs will inhibit the increased ACTH release, and thus decrease androgen levels. This will result in a decrease of urinary 17-ketosteroids and occurrence of ovulatory cycles (6, 7). Response to corticoid treatment implicates abnormal function of the adrenal as one of the possible causes of anovulation or of the polycystic ovary syndrome and may help to distinguish this group of patients from that in which anovulation or polycystic ovarian syndrome is caused by excessive androgen of ovarian origin.

Theoretically, the impairment of the ovarian response to gonadotropins may be primary, in other words, when the cause is inherent in any of the ovarian compartments, such as an abnormality in the aromatization of Δ^4-androstene-dione or in 3β-hydroxysteroid dehydrogenase activity (8) or secondary, in other words, when ovarian failure is caused by abnormality of the regulating mechanism. It follows logically that any one of the factors operating in classes 1 to 8 could eventually lead to morphological and functional changes in the ovary provided the disturbance persists for sufficient time. The impairment of the ovary may also be the result of a genetic disturbance, even though this may not be detectable by available cytogenetic techniques. Class 10 will in most instances be genetic, for example, Turner's syndrome, although conditions such as precocious menopause must be taken into consideration.

Table I presents only a simplified and hypothetical classification of various conditions that might lead to anovulation and must therefore be regarded as incomplete and arbitrary, primarily because there is only minimal laboratory evidence to prove the existence of these conditions. An additional and serious handicap in attempting such a classification lies in the fact that only the static disturbance is actually classified, whereas the dynamics of ovulation control (time of appearance, magnitude, and sequence of operation of the different factors) is not taken into account. With the advancement in FSH and LH determinations and with the development of dynamic tests of pituitary and ovarian function, it should become possible, in the not too distant future, to verify the existence of such classes. This handicap is even more serious since there is no clear boundary between static and dynamic disturbances. Indeed it is practically impossible in most cases to determine and locate the primary event which caused the over-all defect in the feedback mechanism. Such a situation might be illustrated by the polycystic ovary syndrome originating, for example, from disturbed timing of FSH and LH secretion.

One possible variant of the mechanics leading to polycystic ovary may be the premature release of LH with normal FSH secretion leading to premature luteinization of insufficiently developed follicles, in other words, hyperthecosis, which in turn will result in the premature onset of steroidogenesis. Ill-timed steroidogenesis exerts imperfect feedback action, thus preventing ovulation. The prematurely luteinized follicles, none of which reach the stage of ovulation, undergo disintegration or atresia and become incorporated into the ovarian stroma or become encysted. If this sequence of events continues long enough, this will finally result in a permanent disturbance of the regulatory mechanism and will subsequently lead to morphological changes of the ovary, thus rendering it incapable of normal response to gonadotropins. Even when the proper magnitude, timing, and sequence of appearance of FSH and LH is ensured by appropriate therapy, the response of the diseased target organ might be disturbed to such an extent as to prevent induction of ovulation.

It would seem from the above that in most conditions where the ovary is essentially responsive, gonadotropic hormones applied in the correct amounts in the correct sequence and for the correct duration, should be able to stimulate ovarian function and induce ovulation. Practically, gonadotropic preparations are most effective when used as substitution therapy in patients lacking endogenous gonadotropins and having ovaries capable of a normal response (class 1, and 5 to 8). The presenting symptom in these women is usually primary or secondary amenorrhea. Low or undetectable urinary gonadotropins and lack of endogenous estrogen activity are common characteristic findings in these patients—Group I according to Insler et al. (9). In this group, in a series of 135 patients, a pregnancy rate of 68.5% was obtained. A second group of amenorrheic patients with urinary gonadotropins within the normal range and evidence of estrogenic activity (Group II according to the above classification) also benefits from gonadotropic therapy but to a lesser extent. In our series of 74 cases only 32.9% conceived following therapy.

The discrepancy of the effectiveness of gonadotropic therapy between Groups I and II which according to the X^2 test is significant at a level beyond 0.001, is probably caused by several factors. While the patients in Group I are a-menorrheic and have uniformly low urinary gonadotropins and estrogen, patients of Group II display a wide range of cycle disturbances, urinary gonadotropins, and estrogen levels. Accordingly, the interference of patient's own pituitary gonadotropins during the course of treatment is probably negligible in Group I. In Group II, on the other hand, the patient's hypophysis may release LH in response to ovarian stimulation as evidenced by well-documented cases in which ovulation took place after stimulation with exogenous HMG only, without additional HCG. However, the endogenous LH release, appearing at an improper time, could cause premature luteinization of follicles, thus interfering with ovulation and conception. Clinical data available so far seem to support this theory. It also has to be remembered that Group II represents a selected population. Patients of this group were treated with clomiphene citrate and only those who failed to conceive were subsequently subjected to gonadotropic therapy. At least some of these patients have other disturbances in addition to anovulation. These factors (mechanical, immunological, male) may themselves significantly hinder the reproductive performance of patients. When coupled with anovulation these factors would of course influence the effectiveness of ovulation-inducing therapy.

When comparing our own material with the computer tabulations of pooled data on 1286 patients treated for 3002 cycles (10) it was interesting to note that there were no significant differences in the incidence of hyperstimulation (0.79 and 1.3% respectively) and multiple pregnancy rate (36 and 28%). However, the over-all pregnancy rate reported by the above authors was 25% whereas the pregnancy rate in our series was 53%. This significant discrepancy between the pregnancy rates could be due to four factors: (a) selection of patient; (b) intensity of treatment; (c) dose of gonadotropins used, and (d) treatment scheme.

Data reported by Thompson and Hansen (10) were compared with our own material in an attempt to determine the relative importance of these four factors with regard to the effectiveness of gonadotropic therapy. First the results obtained in a very vaguely defined group of "clomiphene failures" were compared. Thompson and Hansen (10) report on 634 patients treated over 1548 cycles resulting in 169 pregnancies (27%). In our series of 74 patients, 205 treatment courses yielded 27 pregnancies (32.9%). Intensity of treatment and pregnancy rates in both series were similar. However, in this group of patients the basic impairment underlying the ovulatory failure is extremely variable as reflected by the wide range of cycle disturbances and levels of urinary gonadotropins and estrogen. Moreover, these patients represent a population a priori selected on the basis of their failure to respond to clomiphene, and it is possible or even probable, that, at least in part of them, factors other than anovulation are involved. Therefore, in this particular group the influence of unrelated factors is so overwhelming that proper comparison of the results of gonadotropic therapy with regard to the selection of patients, dose of gonadotropins and treatment schemes employed is made practically impossible. Pregnancy rates obtained in this group of patients may just as well be due to a chance element as to intelligently planned therapy.

A meaningful analysis of the results of gonadotropic therapy could be carried out when well-defined groups of patients were used for comparison. Patients with primary amenorrhea of pituitary origin were selected for analysis. In this group differences due to selection should be negligible. Pooled data of Thompson and Hansen (10) report on 54 patients treated over 156 cycles resulting in 12 pregnancies (22%). In our material the pregnancy rate in this group was 67%. (48 pregnancies in 56 patients treated over 175 cycles). The intensity of treatment was similar, 2.9 in their series and 3.1 in ours. The gonadotropic preparations in both series contained approximately 75 IU FSH and 75 IU LH/ampoule. It seems justified therefore to conclude that the differences in the effectiveness of gonadotropic therapy in this well-defined group of patients were due to the differences in the dose of gonadotropins and treatment scheme employed.

A comparison of the efficiency of gonadotropins according to daily dosage irrespective of selection of patients, length of time of administration or scheme of therapy is shown in Table II. From this, the relative importance of the daily dose of gonadotropins becomes apparent.

Clinical experience, showed that ovarian response can be elicited only when a certain dose of HMG, in other words, the effective daily dose (11), has been applied. Application of gonadotropins at levels significantly below the effective daily dose did not cause any measurable effect even when prolonged therapy was used. The effective daily dose of gonadotropins was found to be significantly different in various groups of patients. The mean effective daily dose was 217.5 IU FSH in Group I and 143.2 IU in Group II, respectively. Due to marked individual variations however, the effective dose can not be predetermined and has to be arrived at in every patient during each treatment cycle. When fixed treatment schemes are used the dose of gonadotropins is successively increased

TABLE II. The result of gonadotropin therapy tabulated according to mean daily dose, irrespective of selection of patients, duration or scheme of administration

Parameter	Thompson and Hansen (10)			Our series		
Ampoules	1	2	3	1	2	3 or >3
Courses	217	1923	141	143	434	110
Pregnancies	11	230	25	19	122	23
Pregnancies %	5.0	11.9	17.7	13.3	28.1	21.0

in consecutive treatments until the effective daily dose is reached. This process might take 3 to 5 cycles in patients with lower sensitivity to gonadotropins. In the individually adjusted treatment the dose of gonadotropins and the length of therapy are determined according to the patient's response in each treatment (11). Thus with the same intensity of treatment, the latter scheme will, of course, yield a higher pregnancy rate in comparison to the predetermined schedules. It may be concluded from our data that, if properly selected and monitored, 68.5% of patients of Group I will conceive and 58.5% will take home at least one living child.

In conditions where the pituitary is capable of synthesizing gonadotropins and the lack of ovulation is due to inadequate release, an attempt might be made to use releasing factors. Releasing factors from the median eminence of beef hypothalami (12), ovine hypothalami (13), and porcine hypothalami (14), have been shown to be effective in man. Contrary to earlier reports that the releasing factor of FSH (FSH-RF) is a polypeptide with molecular weight of 1500 to 2000 (15), it seems (16) that FSH-RF appears to be a polyamine derivative with a molecular weight not greater than 300. The releasing factor for LH (LH-RF) was also hitherto believed to be a polypeptide of molecular weight 1200 to 2000. It may be assumed from recent work that the actual molecular weight of LH-RF is much smaller (17).

Although the releasing factors have been found to be effective in humans, further thorough investigation and their wide scale use as therapeutic agents are subject to two main limitations. 1) They seem to be stored in hypothalami in minor amounts and many thousands of brains have to be extracted to obtain a few mg of purified releasing factors. However, when their structure is fully elucidated, it should not take too long before they will be synthesized. 2) From the few clinical investigations carried out so far, it is apparent that following their administration releasing factors very rapidly induce gonadotropic secretion, but only of short duration. This has been demonstrated for the releasing factor of LH by Root et al. (13) who showed that 5 min after the initiation of infusion, LH concentration in blood increased significantly but fell again within

2 hr Kastin et al. (14) showed that following the administration of releasing factors, serum LH and FSH reached a maximum at 23.5 and 24.5 min, respectively. The rapid effect of releasing factors and their short duration of action makes the clinical application of these compounds difficult. The amount, timing, and mode of administration will be crucial for the desired effect.

In view of these considerations, synthetic releasing factors may be of limited value in evoking the desired response. For clinical use it may be necessary to prepare long-acting derivatives. A long-acting releasing factor for FSH may more readily find clinical application since treatment has to be of prolonged duration to allow FSH stimulation for several days in order to evoke adequate follicular development. The time of initiation of treatment is not crucial since the required response is not a continuation of previous development. This is in contrast to the LH-RF or exogenous LH administration where initiation of treatment has to be adjusted to the stage of the development of the follicles, since too early stimulation might provoke luteinization of follicles instead of ovulation. It may also be postulated that in case of a localized FSH-RF deficiency, and hence a lack of LH as a secondary manifestation (i.e., no triggering of the LH release in the absence of follicular development), treatment with FSH releasing factor might initiate the chain of events in the ovary which would subsequently lead to the release of endogenous LH at the proper time. The application of releasing factors for LH for induction of ovulation might be more difficult. Their administration must be accurately coordinated with that particular stage of follicular development in which the follicle will respond to LH stimulation by ovulation. Such synchronization is a formidable task.

The continuous cyclic activity of the hypothalamic-pituitary-ovarian axis is a manifestation of a dynamic and coordinated relationship regulated by feedback stimuli between steroids and gonadotropin releasing factors. Thus administration of gonadal steroids or their analogs will change the normal dynamic equilibrium between sex hormones and their respective hypothalamic receptors. Their effect will depend on the physiological stage of the ovary, hypothalamus, and pituitary. They can be used as inhibitors of ovarian activity, as amply illustrated by the oral contraceptives, or they may stimulate ovarian function when used at the correct time and in the proper dosage. Thus it can be postulated that steroids have a twofold action.

Indeed, numerous investigators have reported during the past twenty years on the application of estrogens or their analogs for inducing ovulation (18-22). A common feature of most of the reports was a significantly lower pregnancy rate than that obtained during the last few years by the use of human gonadotropins. Analysis of the data reveals marked variations in the results obtained by the investigators. The so-called "ovulation" rate obtained by investigators applying the therapy to patients who had manifested estrogenic activity before treatment, was higher. Polishuk et al. (20) for example, obtained 15 "ovulations" and 4 pregnancies in 21 anovulatory patients who had shown evidence of estrogenic activity before treatment, while only 4 in 20 amenorrheic patients with no prior estrogen activity ovulated following the same treatment. This group has found that even out of selected patients only 20% became pregnant, although presumably 74% ovulated.

The above authors claim that ovulation occurs within 24 to 48 hr after intravenous injection of estrogen. It could therefore be speculated that intravenous administration of estrogen promoted a rapid LH secretion. Since the criteria of ovulation of these authors were based on vaginal smears, endometrial biopsy, and basal body temperature the discrepancy between the "ovulation" rate (74%) and the pregnancy rate (20%) could be attributed to the fact that in many cases the LH secretion might have occured at an inappropriate time leading to luteinization of unripe follicles rather than to ovulation.

Indirect evidence both in humans (20) and in animals (23) as well as direct measurements of plasma LH (24) indicate that estrogen administered after appropriate follicular stimulation does evoke release of LH. Assuming that estrogens provoke LH release, the prerequisites for successful treatment would be: 1) a pituitary capable of normal response to releasing factors; 2) a hypothalamus capable of responding to peripheral stimuli; and 3) follicles adequately developed to respond by ovulation following the induced LH stimulation.

Recently Keller et al. (25) and Schmidt-Elmendorff et al. (26) reported on the use of 3-methoxyestra-1,3,5(10)-triene-16α,17α-diol, an estrogen derivative, for inducing ovulation. Further basic and well controlled clinical investigations will be necessary before the effectiveness and suitability of this compound as a "fertility inducing agent" can be evaluated. It might be argued that the clinical application of estrogen analogs may be premature since the precise role of each of the natural estrogens in gonadotropic hormone regulation has not yet been experimentally elucidated. Our knowledge of the steroid and gonadotropic hormone patterns of normal menstrual cycles has made it possible to postulate the regulation of the ovarian cycle. However the precise role of estrogen has yet to be assessed by clinical investigation. Even after this goal is achieved, the interpretation of data concerning events occuring in the normal cycle as compared to the deranged condition of anovulatory cycles might prove difficult.

Harris and Naftolin (27) believe that progesterone seems to have a biphasic feedback effect. For some hours after acute administration of progesterone, ovulation is evoked or hastened, estrous behavior is facilitated. Following this initial and transitory phase, the action of progesterone seems to be reversed and ovulation is inhibited. The first acute effect of progesterone has been used by many veterinary surgeons to synchronize ovulation mainly in sheep. Rust (28) treated 35 patients with anovulatory cycles with 5 mg of progesterone for 4 days, or 30 mg of 17α-hydroxyprogesterone caproate. In 60% of the treatments "ovulation" could be induced and six patients became pregnant. In 1957 Swartz and Seegar-Jones (29) reported on 15 cases with anovulatory bleedings treated with progesterone. In only one of these did it seem at all likely that the treatment might have triggered the ovulatory mechanism. Holmstrom (30) used a single dose of 25 to 50 mg of progesterone in 30 patients with primary amenorrhoea. In 12 "ovulation" occurred in the first four months after the beginning of the treatment. Rothschild and Koh (31) reported that the time of ovulation in the human female could be advanced through the use of progesterone.

Holmstrom (30) found an increase of FSH after the administration of progesterone. Buchholz et al. (32) studied the effect of progesterone on the endocrine activity of the pituitary gland. On the day 5 of the cycle, when 200 mg of progesterone were injected, the urinary excretion of gonadotropins was elevated within the first 24 hr following the injection. The peak was followed by a drop three days later. Administration of progesterone on the fourth day before the shift of basal body temperature was followed by an increase in urinary gonadotropins for three days. Swerdloff and Odell (33) demonstrated that in four out of eight subjects an LH peak occurred in patients under administration of sequential contraceptives immediately after the addition of progesterone. No FSH peak was noted. From these data it cannot be determined whether the rise of LH was due to a cumulative effect of estrogens or to the acute effect of gestagens. Keller (34) found an immediate but slight increase of LH following administration of progesterone from the sixth to the eigth day of the cycle. Motta et al. (35) support the hypothesis, which is based on data obtained both in women and in experimental animals, that progesterone facilitates LH release in the presence of estrogen activity.

Progesterone analogs were also evaluated for their effect on ovarian activity. A number of authors have investigated the capacity of 1,6-bisdehydro 6 chloro-retroprogesterone (Ro 4-8347) to induce ovulation in women. Data from 14 authors on 582 patients suffering from anovulation, secondary amenorrhoea, functional sterility or corpus luteum insufficiency, were available for evaluation (Table III).

The "ovulation" rate, as assessed by clinical means, such as basal body temperature, vaginal smears, and sometimes steroid estimation, varied between 12 and 71%. "Ovulations" did occur during treatment, immediately after treatment, or only in the following cycle, thus implying two different mechanisms of action, namely; (1) a release of gonadotropins (as shown in some experimental work); and (2) indirect stimulation via a rebound effect.

Stamm et al. (36) concluded that the compound provokes LH release. Mancuso and Moneta (37) believe that it has a direct stimulatory effect on release and/or production of both FSH and LH. Haller (38) found that 8 mg of Ro 4-8347/day, or even a smaller dose, apparently stimulated gonadotropic activity. Keller (34) found that in some of the treatment phases there was a slight increase of LH activity, but concluded that it generally provoked no significant alterations in the LH secretion pattern. Ferin and Thomas (39) found

TABLE III. Incidence of ovulation and pregnancy under the treatment with Ro 4-8347 "retroprogesterone"

	No. of patients	Ovulation rate (%)[a]	Pregnancy rate (%)[a]
Bayer (43)	35		28.6
Bettendorf (44)	52	34.6	
Blobel (45)	14	71.4	14.3
Dapunt and Gleispach (46)	47	62.0	40.4
Ferin and Thomas (39)	10		
Hauser (47)	20	65.0	
Lauritzen (48)	11	36.4	
Lunenfeld (49)	20	40.0	20.0
Mancuso and Moneta (37)	5	60.0	20.0
Polishuk et al. (20)	82	43.9	2.4
Rauscher (50)	72	12.5	
Staemler and Jung (51)	41		21.9
Stamm et al. (36)	113	45.1	34.5
Taubert and Juergenson (52)	60	45.0	5.0

[a]Ovulation rate and pregnancy rate: numbers referring to patients and not to cycles.

no stimulatory action on LH. The discrepancy between the findings of the authors was probably due to differences in application of the drug and variations in the selection of patients.

Pregnancy rates as reported by different authors varied between zero and 40.4%. It seems that higher pregnancy rates were obtained in a selected group of patients (mild disturbances of ovarian function). The rates of conception during the treatment cycle and in the subsequent cycle were similar. Direct adverse effects either on patients or fetuses were not described. Doses of medication varied between 4 and 6 mg/day, the duration of administration being between 5 and 20 days.

Since this compound is a potent progestational agent, it might be beneficial in infertility due to corpus luteum insufficiency by supporting early pregnancy. Thus the reported pregnancy rates would be due not only to induced ovulation. It may therefore be concluded that this compound fulfills all the requirements of a potent progestational agent with the advantage that it produces no hyperthermia, practically no side effects, and, due to its lack of inhibitory action on gonadotropins, can be used on a long-term basis. It is, furthermore, a cycle regulator, inducing regular menstrual bleeding, and it possibly also stimulates ovarian function in certain ill-defined normogonadotropic patients. The types of patients with menstrual disorders who would fit into this category are young girls, unmarried women, and married women who are not overanxious to conceive. With the aquisition of further knowledge on regulatory processes and better definition of disease, defined groups of patients might be found who would respond by ovulation when given this material in the right dose, at the right time, and for a correct period.

Ever since Dodds et al. (40) discovered the strong estrogenic potency of stilbesterol, the search for new synthetic nonsteroid estrogens has been concentrated on modifications of the stilbene or dihydrostilbene configuration, as well as on derivatives of diphenylmethane, diphenylpropane, and triphenyl-ethylene. Out of those, triphenylethylene has been subject to certain attention since 1937 (41, 42) and several interesting derivatives, among them compounds of the cycloalkylidene series, have been described in the literature during recent years (53-61).

The accidental observation by Greenblatt (61) that clomiphene citrate was a potent inducer of ovulation prompted its wide clinical use. Since then an outpouring of reports corroborated the ovulatory inducing potential of clomiphene in patients with defective release of gonadotropins (Classes 2 to 4). Although a myriad of data purporting to explain the mechanism by which clomiphene brings about the release of gonadotropins has been published, its mode of action is not yet clearly understood. MacGregor et al. (62) reported computer tabulations of pooled data on 6714 anovulatory patients from individual case records accumulated during clinical investigations with clomi-phene citrate. Although the "ovulatory response" as judged by parameters such as basal body temperature records, endometrial biopsies, and pregnanediol was about 70%, the pregnancy rate was 32.7%. As discussed previously, a discrepancy between the ovulation rate (70%) and pregnancy rate of 32.7% might be attributed to the fact that in many cases the LH secretion might have occurred at an inappropriate time leading to progesterone secretion of prematurely luteinized follices. The lack of pregnancies in patients categorized as "pituitary-ovarian dysfunction" stresses the fact that in cases where FSH and LH production is impaired, clomiphene is of little use and substitutional therapy with gonadotropins is the treatment of choice. When the authors compared the short course therapy scheme, in other words, 5 days, on days 5 to 9 of the cycle, using 50 or 100 mg clomiphene/day in a total of 8996 treatment cycles, the "ovulation rate" was 55.2% and 58.2% and the pregnancy rate 8.9% and 9.1% of cycles respectively. From this data it may be concluded that the 100 mg/day schedule should be used only in those patients who failed to respond to the 50 mg/day schedule. At levels below 50 mg daily for 5 days there is a significant diminution in efficacy, while at levels above 100 mg there appeared to be an appreciable increase in the incidence of side effects. With 50 and 100 mg short course therapy, abnormal ovarian enlargement was infrequent. With higher doses or more extended treatment, ovarian enlargement and cyst formation occurred more frequently. The multiple pregnancy rate of 0.6% is significantly lower than after gonadotropic therapy (28-34%) and pregnancy wastage of 18.5% also seems lower.

Our own experience indicates that patients classified as suitable for and treated with clomiphene therapy, who either do not respond with biphasic temperature and elevated pregnanediol levels to the administration of 50 and 100 mg clomiphene/day, or do not conceive after 6 treatment courses with apparently ovulatory response, may benefit from gonadotropic therapy. Such patients should be thoroughly reinvestigated before the administration of gonadotropins in an effort to detect disturbances other than anovulation. In this group of "clomiphene failures" gonadotropic therapy resulted in a pregnancy rate of 32.9%. Only 18.9% of this group of patients succeeded in taking home a living child.

Kistner (63), Rabau et al. (64), and Greenblatt et al. (65) reported that clomiphene-resistant cases may ovulate following a combined treatment of clomiphene and gonadotropins. Since clomiphene directly or indirectly facilitates the release of both FSH and LH, the combination of clomiphene and HCG might be indicated in anovulatory patients in whom the release of FSH and production of LH is impaired (Class 7). The combination of HMG and clomiphene might be indicated in cases where production of FSH and release of LH is impaired (Class 8). In this latter group HMG might stimulate ovarian secretion of steroids which by themselves might trigger off the release of LH without any further therapy.

The successful clinical use of clomiphene citrate prompted the attempts to synthesize compounds with similar structure and action. Another compound, namely bis-(p-acetoxyphenyl)cyclohexylidenemethane (Sexovid, F-6066) seemed according to Persson (66) to modify production or release of FSH and LH. Persson (67) therefore administered this compound to 10 infertile patients in whom anovulation was assumed to be due to an unbalanced release ratio of the two gonadotropic hormones. Conception occurred in 6 of these, normal infants were delivered in 5, one aborted and no side effects of the treatment were noted in any of the patients. Schmidt-Elmendorff et al. (26) found that this compound had a similar effect on FSH secretion as clomiphene, but in contrast to the latter, it did not demonstrate any peripheral antiestrogenic activity. This quality of the compound should theoretically make it superior to clomiphene, since in some instances the latter, due to its antiestrogenic activity, causes an unsuitable environment of the cervical mucus for sperm penetration. Clinical trials with this compound were reported from several groups (68-73). Pregnancy rates as calculated from sufficiently large series varied between 32.3% (71) and 4.2% (69). Although this compound has been tested since 1965, only a few reports are available, and these do not permit any final conclusion of its stimulatory effects on ovarian function.

When one reflects on the store of knowledge accumulated on prospective fertility promoting agents developed since the use of human gonadotropins and clomiphene, one cannot help wondering about the scarcity of data available. Up to the early 1960's any compound that had any potential ovarian stimulating activity immediately attracted the attention of numerous clinical centers. The reluctance to investigate new compounds seems to stem from the fact that human gonadotropins and clomiphene have solved most of the problems in hormonal infertility. In order to interest an investigator in a clinical trial of a new compound, it would be necessary to submit convincing theoretical considerations before persuading him to change from the available drugs to the new one. Such theoretical considerations cannot be provided today, since the regulatory mechanisms of the cyclic ovarian activity are not yet fully elucidated.

The constant improvement of methodology in recent years facilitates the revaluation of (1) the regulating mechanism of normal ovarian function, (2) the understanding and location of failures leading to ovarian dysfunction; and (3) the characterization of key compounds in the regulation of reproductive processes. A multiple interdisciplinary effort is required for the final elucidation of the various aspects in reproductive processes.

ACKNOWLEDGMENT

This work was supported in part by Ford Foundation grant 670-0470 to Tel-Hashomer Government Hospital.

REFERENCES

1. Sydnor, K. L., V. C. Kelley, R. B. Raile, R. S. Ely, and G. Sayers, Proc Soc Exp Biol Med 82:695, 1953.

2. Bongiovanni, A. M., and A. W. Root, New Engl J Med 268:1283, 1963.

3. Bongiovanni, A. M., and A. W. Root, New Engl J Med 268:1342, 1963.

4. Bongiovanni, A. M., and A. W. Root, New Engl J Med 268:1391, 1963.

5. Bongiovanni, A. M., and W. R. Eberlein, A. S. Goldman, and M. New, Rec Prog Hormone Res 23:375, 1967.

6. Perloff, W. H., and B. J. Channick, Amer J Obst Gyn 77:139, 1958.

7. Perloff, W. H., K. D. Smith, and E. Steinberger, Int J Fert 10:31, 1965.

8. Mahesh, V. B., and R. B. Greenblatt, Rec Prog Hormone Res 20:341, 1964.

9. Insler, V., H. Melmed, E. Eden, D. Serr, and B. Lunenfeld, in G. Bettendorf, and V. Insler (Eds.), Clinical Application of Human Gonadotropins, George Thieme Verlag, Stuttgart, 1970, p. 87.

10. Thompson, L. R., and L. M. Hansen, Fert Steril 21:844, 1970.

11. Lunenfeld, B., V. Insler, and E. Robau, L'ovulation, Meiose, et Ouverture Folliculaire, Traitments de l'anovulation, Masson & Cie, Paris, 1969, p. 291.

12. Igarashi, M., N. Yokota, Y. Ehara, R. Mayuzumi, T. Hirano, S. Matsumoto, and M. Yamasaki, Amer J Obst Gyn 100:867, 1968.

13. Root, A. W., G. P. Smith, A. P. S. Dhariwal, and S. M. McCann, Nature 221:5180, 1969.

14. Kastin, A. J., A. V. Schally, C. Gual, A. R. jr. Midgley, C. Y. Bowers, and A. jr. Diaz-Infante, J Clin Endocrinol 29:1046, 1969.

15. McCann, S. M., J. Antumes-Rodrigues, and A. P. S. Dhariwal, Proc 23rd Int Congr Physiol Sci, Excerpta Medica, Int Congr Ser 87:292, 1965.

16. White, W. F., A. I. Cohen, R. H. Rippel, J. C. Story, and A. V. Schally, Endocrinology 82:742, 1968.

17. Schally, A. V., A. Arimura, C. Y. Bowers, A. J. Kastin, S. Sawano, and T. W. Redding, Rec Prog Hormone Res 24:497, 1968.

18. Buxton, C. L. and A. Southam, Obst and Gyn 8:135, 1956.

19. Kupperman, S. H., J. A. Epstein, H. G. Meyer, and A. Stone, Fert Steril 9:26, 1958.

20. Polishuk, Z., M. Sharf, and T. Kuzminski, Harefuah 60:4, 1961.

21. Brown, W. E., J. I. Bradbury, and E. C. Jungck, Amer J Obst Gyn 65:733, 1953.

22. Van den Drissche, Ann Endocrinol (Paris) 16:152, 1955.

23. Ferin, M., P. E. Zimmering, and R. L. Vande Wiele, Endocrinology 84:893, 1969.

24. Vande Wiele, R. L., J. Bogumil, I. Dyremfurth, M. Ferin, R. Jewelewicz, M. Warren, T. Rizkallah, and G. Mikhail, Rec Prog Hormone Res 26:63, 1970.

25. Keller, P. J., M. Ruppen, W. E. Schreimer, and H. I. Wyss, Schwz Gyn Tagung, Gastaad, 1969.

26. Schmidt-Elmendorff, H., E. Kaiser, and W. Gerteis, Proc 6th World Congr on Fert Steril, Tel-Aviv, 1968.

27. Harris, G. W., and F. Naftolin, Brit Med Bull 26:3, 1970.

28. Rust, W., Zbl Gyn 78:1363, 1956.

29. Swartz, D. P., and G. E. Seegar-Jones, Fert Steril 8:103, 1957.

30. Holmstrom, E. G., Amer J Obst Gyn 68:1321, 1954.

31. Rothschild, I., and N. H. Koh, J Clin Endocrinol 11:789, 1951.

32. Bucholz, R., L. Nocke, and W. Nocke, Int J Fert 9:231, 1964.

33. Swerdloff, R. S., and W. D. Odell, in E. Rosemberg (Ed.), Gonadotropins 1968, Geron-X, Inc., Los Altos, 1968, p. 155.

34. Keller, P. J., Bull Schweiz Akad Med Wiss 25:379, 1970.

35. Motta, M., F. Piva, and L. Martini, Bull Schweiz Akad Med Wiss 25:408, 1970.

36. Stamm, O., I. Gerhard, and D. Zarro, Bull Schweiz Akad Med Wiss 25:472, 1970.

37. Mancuso, S., and E. Moneta, Bull Schweiz Akad Med Wiss 25:441, 1970.

38. Haller, J., Bull Schweiz Akad Med Wiss 25:447, 1970.

39. Ferin, J., and K. Thomas, Bull Schweiz Akad Med Wiss 25:287, 1970.

40. Dodds, E. C., L. Goldberg, W. Lawson, and R. Robinson, Nature 141:247, 1938.

41. Dodds, E. C., M. E. H. Fitzgerald, and W. Lawson, Nature 140:772, 1937.

42. Robson, J. M., and A. Schoenberg, Nature 140:196, 1937.

43. Bayer, R., Bull Schweiz Akad Med Wiss 25:575, 1970.

44. Bettendorf, G., Bull Schweiz Akad Med Wiss 25:353, 1970.

45. Blobel, R., Bull Schweiz Akad Med Wiss 25:386, 1970.

46. Dapunt, O., and H. Gleispach, Bull Schweiz Akad Med Wiss 25:349, 1970.

47. Hauser, G. A., Bull Schweiz Akad Med Wiss 25:490, 1970.

48. Lauritzen, C. H., Bull Schweiz Akad Med Wiss 25:463, 1970.

49. Lunenfeld, B., unpublished data, 1970.

50. Rauscher, H., Bull Schweiz Akad Med Wiss 25:551, 1970.

51. Staemler, H. J., and K. Jung, Bull Schweiz Akad Med Wiss 25:560, 1970.

52. Taubert, H. D., and O. JO. Juergensen, Bull Schweiz Akad Med Wiss 25:503, 1970.

53. Robson, J. M., and A. Schoenberg, Nature 150:22, 1942.

54. Mentzer, C., and D. Xuong, Compt Rend Acad Sci 222:1004, 1946.

55. Buu-Hoi, N., L. Corre, A. Lacossagne, and S. Lecocq, Bull Soc Chim Biol Fr 29:1087, 1947.

56. Rothschild, I., and H. Keys, Proc Soc Exp Biol Med 81:539, 1952.

57. Kistner, R. W., C. J. Duncan and H. Mansell, Obst Gyn 3:351, 1954.

58. Gazave, J. M., M. A. Weill-Warlin, L. Bloncourt, and G. Dutraisse, Presse Med 64:1007, 1956.

59. Miguel, J. F., E. H. Barany, and W. Muller, Arch Int Pharmacodyn Ther 127:262, 1958.

60. Tyler, E. T., H. J. Olson, and M. H. Gotlib, Int J Fertil 5:429, 1960.

61. Greenblatt, R. B., J Amer Med Ass 178:101, 1961.

62. Macgregor, A. H., J. E. Johnson, and C. A. Bunde, Fert Steril 19:616, 1968.

63. Kistner, R. W., Fert Steril 17:569, 1966.

64. Rabau, E., S. Mashiach, D. M. Serr, and H. Melamed, Obst Gyn 31:110, 1968.

65. Greenblatt, R. B., R. D. Gumbrell, V. B. Mahesh, and H. F. L. Scholer, Nobel Symposium 15, Almqvist & Wiksell, Stockholm, 1970, p. 261.

66. Persson, B. H., Acta Soc Med Upsalien 70:1, 1965.

67. Persson, B. H., Acta Soc Med Upsalien 70:71, 1965.

68. Cohen, J., R. Merger, and D. Krulik, Gyn Obst (Paris) 66:49, 1967.

69. Neale, Ch., M. Breckwoldt, Z. Starcevic, and G. Bettendorf, Deut Gyn Kong, Travemunde, 1968.

70. Hayashi, R., E. Osawa, Y. Nishikawa, A. Maeda, M. Washio, I. Koketsu, and S. Tojo, Proc 6th World Congr on Fert Steril, Tel-Aviv, 1968.

71. Roth, F., and R. H. H. Richter, Gynecologia 167:462, 1969.

72. Schmidt-Elmendorff, H., E. Kaiser, and W. Gerteis, 37 Versammlung der Deutschen Ges Gynak, Travemunde, 1969.

73. Sato, T., Y. Ibuki, M. Hirono, M. Igarashi, and S. Matsumoto, Fert Steril 20:965, 1969.

53.　　　Induction of
Ovulation

Eugenia Rosemberg, Si G. Lee, and Philip S. Butler

Development of methods for the isolation and purification of human urinary menopausal gonadotropins (HMG) in quantities sufficient to treat substantial numbers of patients represented a milestone in gynecologic endocrinology. The delineation of the pattern of excretion of endogenous pituitary gonadotropins in various categories of anovulatory patients and the clarification of the FSH and LH excretion during the normal menstrual cycle (1, 2) greatly contributed to our rationale in the use of HMG in the treatment of specific cases of female infertility (3-8). Our studies suggested that ovarian response to HMG stimulation could be dependent upon the "total" dosages of FSH activity administered prior to the addition of HCG to the therapeutic regimen. Moreover, the amount of LH activity contained in the HMG preparations used could have influenced the response of the ovary to exogenous gonadotropin stimulation. However, the conclusions derived from our previous studies would not necessarily apply to spontaneous cycles since ovulation was induced with HCG and not with human pituitary LH.

Progress in resolution of the conflict in characterization of the pattern of secretion of pituitary gonadotropins and ovarian hormones during the normal menstrual cycle has been achieved since the advent of radioimmunoassays and variants thereof (9, 10). These analytic techniques have made it possible to follow, in the same individual, on a daily or even more frequent basis, the many changes in hormonal levels that have to be taken into account if the regulation of the normal menstrual cycle is to be understood. However, the precise physiologic role of the variations in serum FSH and LH levels during the normal menstrual cycle is not known.

In order to define experimentally the role of pituitary FSH and LH on ovarian function at least two premises should be fulfilled. One is the selection of suitable experimental subjects, and the other the availability of highly purified human pituitary FSH (HFSH) and LH (HLH) hormones. Hypophysectomized subjects are ideally suitable for such studies since only in these type of patients it is possible to rule out the synergistic effects of endogenous gonadotropins or other pituitary hormones with those of exogenous ones. Infertile patients with anovulation, associated with low or normal endogenous gonadotropins but otherwise normal pituitary function could be suitable, under strict experimental conditions, to study the effect of exogenous gonadotropins on ovarian function. These in fact, were the patients selected to conduct the present studies.

Due to the courtesy of the National Pituitary Agency, we were able to obtain the necessary quantities of purified HFSH and HLH to address ourselves to the following questions: (1) are "total" dosages of FSH activity and optimal FSH/LH ratios necessary to induce physiological follicular maturation leading to a single ovulation and (2) what is the optimal dosage of HLH necessary to trigger ovulation. The present report includes a comparison of the effect of FSH and LH derived from human pituitary and urinary sources.

SUBJECTS

A total of 10 patients were treated for one or more cycles; 4 were nulliparous subjects aged 24 to 31 years with fairly regular anovulatory cycles, normal endocrine function, and undetectable, low or normal levels of "total" urinary gonadotropins. The remaining 6 patients in this group (2 multiparous and 4 nulliparous), were subjects with anovulatory oligomenorrhea, normal endocrine function and undetectable, low or normal levels of "total" urinary gonadotropins. The husbands' semen specimens were normal. The urinary excretion of FSH and LH was studied in each patient during one cycle without medication. All patients showed absence of cyclic variations in FSH and LH excretion indicating the absence of endogenous LH discharge at midcycle. One of the patients had previously received 3 courses of HMG and HCG. She conceived during the last medication course which was given three years prior to the present studies. Two other patients had previously received one course of HMG and HCG. All other patients had never been treated with any gonadotropin preparation. The various treatment schemes used in this study are presented in Table I. Patients were treated for one or more cycles. In all 30 courses of medication were given. Pregnancy was attempted during all courses of medication.

GONADOTROPIN PREPARATIONS AND TREATMENT SCHEMES

HFSH and HLH preparations used in this study were supplied by the National Pituitary Agency, Baltimore, Maryland. The HMG preparations used were Pergonal and Ortho HMG, supplied by Cutter Laboratories, Berkeley, California,

TABLE I. Pattern of medication courses for patients in study

Course No.	Treatment	
1	Pergonal or HMG-Ortho	Followed by HCG
2	Pergonal	Followed by HLH
3	Pergonal	Followed by HLH combined with Pergonal
4	HFSH combined with HLH	Followed by HLH combined with HFSH
5	HFSH combined with HLH	Followed by HLH

TABLE II. Biologic activity of gonadotropin preparations

Preparations	IU Eq/2nd IRP-HMG/ampoule[a]		Ratio FSH/LH
	FSH	LH	
HFSH - Batch LER 862	57.0	0.27	211.0
HLH - Batch Al-LER 856-1	2.5	200.0	0.0125
Pergonal - Batch			
25 - EX - 2213	73.0	62.0	1.17
25 - EX - 2267	68.0	50.0	1.36
25 - EX - 2089	85.4	123.2	0.69
25 - EX - 2119	81.6	28.3	2.88
Ortho HMG - Batch 2010	64.3	20.2	3.2

[a]Second International Reference Preparation for Human Menopausal Gonadotropins (WHO/BS/723 Sept. 23, 1964).

and the Ortho Research Foundation, Raritan, New Jersey, respectively. HCG (Follutein) was supplied by the Squibb Institute for Medical Research, New Brunswick, New Jersey. The biologic activity of these preparations is given in Table II.

In patients with anovulatory cycles, day 1 of treatment corresponded to day 5 of their menstrual cycle; in patients with oligomenorrhea, day 1 of treatment corresponded to day 5 of their menstrual cycle or, to an arbitrary day if treatment was initiated during a period of amenorrhea. Prior to initiation of these studies, the ovulatory threshold of each individual patient was investigated using Pergonal given as a single intramuscular injection containing 500 to 900 IU

TABLE III. Scheme of treatment

Preparations	1 through 7			8 and 9			11			12			No. of courses
	IU		Ratio FSH/LH	IU		Ratio FSH/LH	IU		Ratio FSH/LH	IU		Ratio FSH/LH	
	FSH	LH		FSH	LH		FSH	LH		FSH	LH		
Pergonal HLH	730	620	1.17	171	246	0.69	38	3000	0.013	5	1000	0.005	3
Pergonal HLH + Pergonal	730	620	1.17	171	246	0.69	490	3170	0.15	245	1085	0.22	7
HFSH + HLH HLH + HFSH	798	600	1.33	171	200	0.85	228	3000	0.08	228	1000	0.23	8
HFSH + HLH HLH	798	600	1.33	171	200	0.85	38	3000	0.013	5	1000	0.005	4

Treatment days

of FSH activity on day 1 of therapy followed 6 days later by the administration of 12,000 IU of HCG.

Table III presents the details of the various treatment schemes used; the "total" FSH and LH activity administered during treatment days and the corresponding FSH/LH ratios.

Follicular maturation was induced with HMG and HFSH in combination with HLH. For the induction of ovulation, HLH was given alone or in combination with Pergonal or HFSH. The FSH/LH ratios contained in the preparations used during the proliferative and luteal phase of induced cycles followed those described by Strott et al. (11) during the follicular and midcycle phase of the normal menstrual cycle. "Total" amounts of FSH activity given on days 1 to 7 of therapy, ranged from 730 to 798 IU. In addition, the FSH/LH ratio contained in Pergonal or in the mixtures of HFSH and HLH varied from 1.17 to 1.33. An additional 171 IU of FSH activity was given on days 8 and 9 of therapy; the FSH/LH ratio ranged from 0.69 to 0.85. For the induction of ovulation, HLH was administered on days 11 and 12 of treatment. It was given alone or in combination with Pergonal or HFSH. On day 11, the dosages of HLH ranged from 3000 to 3170 IU. The FSH/LH ratios ranged from 0.013 to 0.15. On day 12, the HLH dosage ranged from 1000 to 1085; the FSH/LH ratios ranged from 0.005 to 0.23.

Pergonal was administered intramuscularly (once daily) dissolved in 1% novocaine solution; HCG was administered intramuscularly (once daily) dissolved in distilled water. Mixtures of HFSH and HLH were administered intramuscularly (once daily) during days 1 to 9 of treatment, dissolved in distilled water and 0.5% novocaine solution. The HLH and HFSH mixtures as

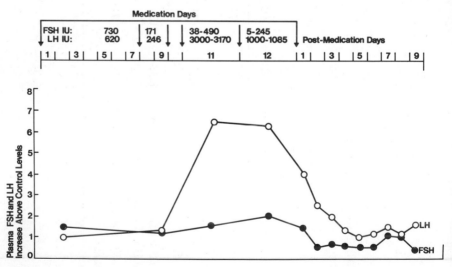

FIG. 1. Plasma FSH and LH concentrations throughout medication courses 2 and 3.

well as the HLH and Pergonal mixtures, were administered i.m. daily in three divided doses on days 11 and 12 of treatment, dissolved in distilled water and 0.5% novocaine solution; when HLH was given alone, it was administered intramuscularly daily in three divided doses on days 11 and 12 of treatment, dissolved in distilled water and 0.5% novocaine solution.

Plasma concentrations of FSH and LH were measured serially throughout each treatment cycle. Figure 1 depicts the plasma concentration of FSH and LH in patients treated during the proliferative phase of induced cycles with Pergonal alone followed by HLH for the induction of ovulation.

Figure 2 depicts the plasma concentration of FSH and LH in patients treated during the proliferative phase of induced cycles with mixtures of HFSH and HLH, followed by HLH for the induction of ovulation.

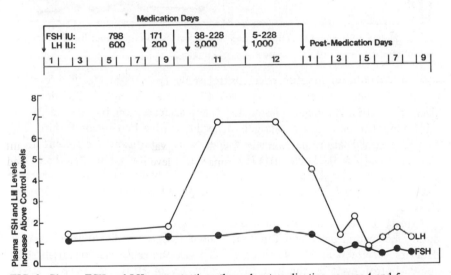

FIG. 2. Plasma FSH and LH concentrations throughout medication courses 4 and 5.

During the proliferative phase of induced cycles, the FSH/LH ratios of circulating gonadotropins followed that of the administered hormones. Moreover, a rapid increase in plasma LH concentration occurred 6 hr after the administration of the initial HLH dose. Plasma LH concentration decreased on the second day of HLH administration and continued to decrease after cessation of medication.

Figure 3 shows the mean plasma FSH and LH values corresponding to 22 courses of medication following the administration of HLH. For purpose of comparison, the circulating levels of HCG after a single shot of 10,000 IU HCG are also shown.

Six hours after the administration of the first dose of HLH, plasma LH levels

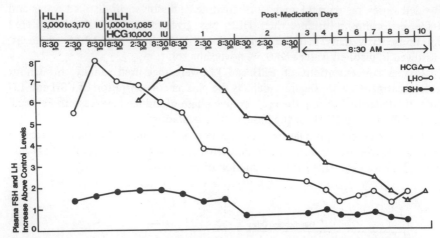

FIG. 3. Plasma FSH and LH concentrations. Mean values corresponding to 22 courses of medication.

showed a significant increase over control values (p > 0.01). Maximal levels in plasma LH concentration were observed 12 hr after the initial HLH dose was given (p > 0.01). Although, plasma LH levels decreased on the second day of HLH administration, and continued to decline on the first, second, third, and fourth postmedication days, these values were significantly different from control levels(p > 0.01).Plasma LH levels were not followed beyond the eighth postmedication day. Plasma levels of HCG were higher than those of HLH specially during postmedication days reflecting the longer circulatory half-life of HCG.

Urinary LH excretion was determined prior to the administration of HLH, during medication days, and for three consecutive postmedication days. These data are presented in Fig. 4. Urinary LH levels showed a significant increase above control levels on the first and second day of HLH therapy(p > 0.01). Although, urinary LH levels showed a steady decrease on post medication days 1 to 3, these values were significantly different from control levels (p > 0.01). Urinary LH levels were not followed beyond the third postmedication day. 3.9% of the administered HLH was excreted on the first day and 13.8% was excreted on the second day of its administration.

ASSESSMENT OF CLINICAL EFFECT AND STEROID METABOLIC EFFECT

Clinical effect was assessed on the basis of daily rectal temperatures (BBT), vaginal smears, volume of cervical mucus and arborization pattern, and pelvic examination. Plasma and urinary levels of FSH and LH were measured by

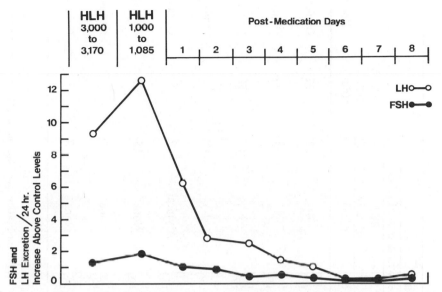

FIG. 4. Urinary FSH and LH excretion. Mean values corresponding to 22 courses of medication.

radioimmunoassay according to the method of Odell et al. (12). "Total" urinary gonadotropin levels were estimated according to the method of Rosemberg et al. (13), before and after completion of each medication course. Determination of urinary estrogen, extracted by the method of Brown (14), followed by bioassay (15) and of pregnanediol estimated by the methods of Barry et al. (16), and Goldzieher et al. (17), were carried out throughout each course of medication.

With the exception of pregnancy, the clinical confirmation of ovulation was obtained by indirect indices such as evidence of estrogenic activity judged by changes in the exfoliated cells of the vagina, appearance of ferning and volume of the cervical mucus, and increase in urinary estrogen levels. Indices of progesterone activity were considered to be rise in BBT, changes in the cervical mucus pattern, spinnbarkeit, vaginal cytology characteristic of the luteal phase of the menstrual cycle, increase in the urinary excretion of pregnanediol and estrogen, and menstruation following the shift in BBT.

RESULTS

As stated above, a first course of medication was given to establish the patient's ovulatory threshold. A single injection of Pergonal containing "total" FSH dosages ranging from 512 to 900 IU was given. The corresponding FSH/LH ratios ranged from 0.69 to 3.2. Ovulation was induced with 12,000 IU of HCG. Results are presented in Table IV.

TABLE IV. Pergonal - HCG

| Patient's diagnosis | Total activity administered[a] IU/2nd IRP-HMG | | Response | | | | | | | Remarks |
| | FSH | LH | During Pergonal administration | | After withdrawal of HCG | | | | Cycle length (day) | |
			E[b]	P[b]	E	P	BBT increase (day)	MP (day)		
Anov	680	500	28 (4)	0.3 (5)	54 (8)	1.7 (3)	4	12	27	Ovulation
Anov	544	400	24 (4)	<0.1 (5)	31 (6)	0.6 (5)	3	13	27	Ovulation
Anov	730	620	50 (2)	<0.1 (5)	13 (2)	0.7 (7)	6	17	32	Ovulation
Anov	876	744	44 (2)	0.2 (5)	30 (4)	1.4 (1)	1	10	25	Ovulation
Oligom	900	1,009	108 (4)		99 (2)	1.0 (1)	Atypical	9	c	Ovulation
Oligom	683	986	29 (2)	<0.1 (5)	27 (8)	<0.1 (9)	None	15	29	No response
Oligom	680	500	11 (3)	<0.1 (9)	35 (4)	<0.1 (5)	None	12	c	No response
Oligom	512	160	14 (5)	0.2 (8)	13 (3)	0.2 (2)	None	6	c	No response

[a] Prior to HCG administration.
[b] E (estrogen μg/24 hr) and P (pregnanediol mg/24 hr).
[c] Medication was initiated during period of amenorrhea. Numbers in parenthesis represent medication day when maximal levels were observed.

TABLE V. Pergonal-HLH[a]

Patient's diagnosis	During Pergonal administration		Response					Remarks
			After withdrawal of HLH					
	E	P	E	P	BBT increase (day)	MP (day)	Cycle length (days)	
Anov	103 (9)	0.2 (9)	36 (5)	1.0 (4)	1	12	27	Ovulation
Anov	24 (7)	0.7 (9)	11 (3)	2.0 (6)	Atypical	9	25	Ovulation
Oligom	15 (5)	0.2 (9)	77 (7)	0.5 (6)	1	16	32	Ovulation

[a]Abbreviations and symbols same as in Table IV.

Tables V and VI show the response to the administration of Perganol or of mixtures of HFSH and HLH, followed by the administration of HLH alone.

TABLE VI. HFSH and HLH - HLH[a]

| | Response | | | | | | | |
| | During HFSH and HLH administration | | After withdrawal of HLH | | | | | |
Patient's diagnosis	E	P	E	P	BBT increase (day)	MP (day)	Cycle length (day)	Remarks
Anov	132 (9)	0.4 (9)	81 (1)	1.5 (2)	Atypical	7	25	Ovulation
Anov	17 (9)	0.3 (9)	18 (2)	1.9 (6)	1	13	29	Ovulation
Oligom	47 (9)	0.3 (9)	66 (9)	2.3 (4)	1	12	30	Ovulation
Oligom	16 (9)	0.1 (9)	50 (15)		2			Pregnant

[a]Abbreviations and symbols same as in Table IV.

Estrogen and pregnanediol excretion levels never exceeded those seen in the normal menstrual cycle. Ovulation, judged by indirect indices or by pregnancy, occurred during all courses of medication. Table VII shows the response of the administration of Pergonal followed by the administration of HLH mixed with Pergonal.

Questionable ovulation occurred during one course. Ovulation judged either by indirect indices or by pregnancy occurred during six courses of medication. Steroid excretion levels followed the pattern observed during the normal menstrual cycle except in one case. This patient experienced slight ovarian enlargement which subsided in 24 hr.

Table VIII shows the response to the administration of mixtures of HFSH and HLH followed by the administration of HLH given alone or mixed with HFSH.

Ovulation judged by indirect indices occurred during three courses of medication; one patient became pregnant. Ovulation was questionable during two courses. Two patients did not respond. However, when these patients were subsequently treated with higher "total" FSH dosages, one patient ovulated and the other became pregnant. A summary of the overall results is given in Table IX.

TABLE VII. Pergonal-HLH and Pergonal[a]

| | Response | | | | | | | |
| | During Pergonal administration | | After withdrawal of HLH and Pergonal | | | | | |
Patient's diagnosis	E	P	E	P	BBT increase (day)	MP (day)	Cycle length (days)	Remarks
Anov	52 (7)	<0.1 (9)	29 (1)	0.9 (4)	atypical	10	25	Ovulation
Anov	49 (9)	0.1 (6)	18 (3)	0.6 (2)	2	8	26	Ovulation
Anov	65 (9)	<0.1 (9)	49 (3)	0.6 (2)	2	15	29	Ovulation
Anov	49 (7)	0.2 (9)	33 (3)	1.1 (2)	atypical	12	27	Ovulation
Oligom	578 (9)	0.1 (9)	985 (1)	1.1 (6)	1	16	c	Ovulation (ovarian enlargement)
Oligom	15 (7)	<0.1 (9)	25 (1)	0.7 (2)	atypical	8	24	Ovulation (?)
Oligom	9 (5)	0.1 (9)	121 (3)		15			Pregnant

[a] Abbreviations and symbols same as in Table IV.

TABLE VIII. HFSH and HLH - HLH and HFSH[a]

| | Response | | | | | | | |
| | During HFSH and HLH administration | | After withdrawal of HLH and HFSH | | | | | |
Patient's diagnosis	E	P	E	P	BBT increase (day)	MP (day)	Cycle length (days)	Remarks
Anov	44 (7)	0.3 (9)	66 (5)	0.8 (2)	Not taken	12	28	Ovulation
Anov	20 (7)	0.5 (9)	20 (1)	1.4 (2)	Atypical	11	27	Ovulation
Oligom	24 (7)	0.1 (9)	65 (1)	0.6 (4)	38	50	64	Ovulation (?)
Oligom	62 (9)	<0.1 (9)	44 (1)	0.2 (2)	None	11	27	No Response
Oligom	51 (9)	0.3 (9)	57 (5)	2.3 (6)	2			Pregnant[b]
Oligom	11 (6)	0.1 (9)	29 (2)	0.4 (5)	Atypical	8	25	Ovulation (?)
Oligom	12 (5)	<0.1 (9)	25 (2)	0.5 (4)	2	12	27	Ovulation
Oligom	22 (7)	0.1 (9)	24 (3)	0.3 (6)	None	18	34	No Response

[a] Abbreviations and symbols same as in Table IV.

716

TABLE IX.

Treatment course number	No. of courses	Pregnancy (single)	Response ovulation by indirect indices	Questionable ovulation	No response
2	3		3		
3	7	1	5	1	
4	8	1	3	2	2
5	4	1	3	—	—
Total	22	3	14	3	2
% Total		13.6	63.6	13.6	9.2

Luteal phase length (14 ovulatory cycles):   12 to 15 days (6 courses),
9 to 11 days (6 courses) and
6 to 7 days (2 courses)

Cycle Lengths (14 ovulatory cycles):   25 days (3 courses),
26 days (1 course),
27 days (4 courses),
28 days (1 course),
29 days (2 courses),
30 days (1 course),
32 days (1 course) and
not determined (1 course).

DISCUSSION

The daily fluctuations in plasma FSH and LH levels seen during the normal menstrual cycle suggest that hormonal requirements for the occurrence of ovulation could be dependent upon the relative concentrations of FSH and LH during the follicular phase of the cycle, followed by an appropriately timed pulse of LH. We have tried to analyze under strict experimental conditions, some of these aspects; specifically, dosages of FSH necessary to induce ovarian stimulation and the type of response observed in relation to predetermined FSH/LH ratios contained in the gonadotropin preparations used. Finally, the dosages of HLH necessary to induce ovulation were also investigated.

Because the evaluation of the effect of gonadotropin administration was not carried out in hypophysectomized subjects, the interpretation of the data may be somewhat limited in that results may not represent absolute effects but rather the combined effects of endogenous and exogenous gonadotropins. However, some conclusions seem to be warranted: 1) follicular maturation when "total" dosages of FSH activity ranging from 901 to 969 IU containing "fixed" FSH/LH ratios were given, followed a pattern similar to that seen during the proliferative phase of the normal menstrual cycle; 2) dosages of 3000 IU of HLH given on the first day and 1000 IU given on the second day of its administration, transformed the stimulated follicle into a normal functional corpus luteum and induced a single ovulation. The clinical findings as well as the urinary steroid excretion pattern indicated that ovarian function was stimulated to a degree similar to that observed during the normal menstrual cycle.

When HLH was given to induce ovulation, a peak in plasma LH concentration was observed 12 hours after the first HLH injection. Then, plasma LH levels decreased steadily on the second day of therapy, and continued to decrease after cessation of medication. Based solely on daily determinations of plasma LH during the menstrual cycle, a single brief discharge of this hormone at a time corresponding to the middle of the cycle is seen. Hence, the plasma LH peak observed after the administration of HLH followed closely that seen in the normal menstrual cycle.

In the present studies, elevation of the BBT occurred 3 to 4 days after the administration of the initial HLH dose. The luteal phase, calculated from the time of thermal nadir to the first day of menstrual flow, varied among patients. However, in only two patients with anovulatory cycles, short luteal phases of 6 and 7 days, respectively, were recorded. In all other subjects with anovulatory cycles, the length of the luteal phase under medication was longer than that recorded on each patient during several control cycles. Moreover, in oligomenorrheic patients, the length of the luteal phase under medication was normal.

Administration of additional HLH during the luteal phase of induced cycles was not necessary for the maintenance of the functional life of the corpus luteum. These results are not in keeping with the data reported by Vande Wiele et al. (10) who induced ovulation with HLH in hypophysectomized and amenorrheic subjects following a period during which HMG was given to induce follicular maturation. These authors reported that daily injections of 400 IU of HLH were necessary to maintain the functional life of the corpus luteum during the luteal phase of induced cycles. The difference in the conclusions arrived at by Vande Wiele et al. and us, could be ascribed to differences in the experimental design used in each case. It is also worth noting that the variation in response observed in the same patient, as well as between patients to various courses of therapy was not marked. Moreover, there was no evidence of overt ovarian overstimulation throughout these studies.

The data indicate that physiological ovarian stimulation can be achieved in most patients, with the administration during the proliferative phase of induced cycles of "total" amounts of FSH activity not exceeding 1000 IU containing defined FSH/LH ratios. Following follicular maturation, a single ovulation was triggered with the administration of HLH. With the experimental design used, a normal corpus luteum was formed requiring no additional administration of LH during the luteal phase of induced cycles.

ACKNOWLEDGMENT

This work was supported in part by grant AM-07564, USPHS, National Institutes of Health, Bethesda, Maryland, and in part by a grant from Cutter Laboratories, Berkeley, California. We are indebted to the National Pituitary Agency, Baltimore, Maryland, for the supply of purified human pituitary FSH and LH preparations and the supply of reagents used in the radioimmunoassay procedures. We are also indebted to Mr. C. R. Thompson, Cutter Laboratories, Berkeley, California, to Dr. T. C. Smith, Ortho Research Foundation, Raritan, New Jersey, and to Dr. E. C. Reifenstein, Jr., for the supply of Pergonal, Ortho HMG, and Follutein (HCG), respectively. The able technical assistance of Mr. G. Bulat, Mr. L. Fournier, Mr. R. Hanc, and Miss M. Shea is gratefully acknowledged.

REFERENCES

1. Rosemberg, E., and P. J. Keller, J Clin Endocrinol Metab 25:1262, 1965.

2. Rosemberg, E., S. R. Joshi, and T. T. Nwe, J Clin Endocrinol Metab 28:1419, 1968.

3. Rosemberg, E., J. Coleman, N. Gibree, and W. MacGillivray, Fert Steril 13:220, 1962.

4. Rosemberg, E., J. Coleman, M. Demany, and C.-R. Garcia, J Clin Endocrinol Metab 23:181, 1963.

5. Rosemberg, E., R. F. Maher, A. Stern, and M. Demany, J Clin Endocrinol Metab 24:105, 1964.

6. Rosemberg, E., in R. B. Greenblatt (Ed.), Ovulation: Stimulation, Suppression, Detection, Lippincott, Philadelphia, 1966, p. 118.

7. Rosemberg, E., and T. T. Nwe, Fert Steril 19:197, 1968.

8. Rosemberg, E., and T. T. Nwe, in E. Rosemberg (Ed.), Gonadotropins 1968, Geron-X, Inc., Los Altos, 1968, p. 471.

9. Ross, G. T., C. M. Cargille, M. B. Lipsett, P. L. Rayford, J. R. Marshall, C. A. Strott, and D. Robard, Rec Prog Hormone Res 26:1, 1970.

10. Vande Wiele, R. L., J. Bogumil, I. Dyrenfurth, M. Ferin, R. Jewelewicz, M. Warren, T. Rizkallah, and G. Mikhail, Rec Prog Hormone Res, 26:63, 1970.

11. Strott, C. A., C. M. Cargille, C. T. Ross, and M. B. Lipsett, J Clin Endocrinol Metab 30:247, 1970.

12. Odell, W. D., G. T. Ross, and P. L. Rayford, J Clin Invest 46:248, 1967.

13. Rosemberg, E., F. Smith, and R. I. Dorfman, Endocrinology 61:337, 1957.

14. Brown, J. B., Lancet 268:320, 1955.

15. Rosemberg, E., in C. A. Paulsen (Ed.), Estrogen Assays In Clinical Medicine, Univ. Washington Press, Seattle, 1965, p. 107.

16. Barry, R. D., M. Guarnieri, P. K. Besch, W. Ring, and N. S. Besh, Anal Chem 38:983, 1966.

17. Goldzieher, J. W., and Y. Nakamura, Acta Endocrinol (Kbh) 41:371, 1962.

54. Steroid-Induced Positive Feedback in the Human Female: New Aspects on the Control of Ovulation

Gerhard Leyendecker, Sharon Wardlaw, and Wolfgang Nocke

Since the emphasis in the interpretation of the endocrine regulation of ovulation has shifted from the idea of a "physiological clock" in the hypothalamus to the notion that the ovary itself might play a decisive role in the triggering of endocrine events in timing ovulation, attempts have been made to relate ovarian hormonal secretion to the midcycle LH peak. Following the first observation of Hohlweg (1) in 1934 that exogenous estrogens could cause luteinization in the immature female rat, further data have been accumulated through animal experiments demonstrating that both estrogens and gestagens cause a stimulation of the hypothalamic cyclic center (2-5). In the human female Buchholz et al. (6) first demonstrated that progesterone administered intramuscularly resulted in an immediate rise of urinary gonadotropins similar to the gonadotropin peak seen in normal midcycle. More recently a series of synthetic estrogens and gestagens (7-9) have been tested in the human female regarding feedback effect on the cyclic center. However, these results do not provide an adequate basis for understanding endocrine events of the normal menstrual cycle. Therefore, we have attempted to simulate these endocrine events with the use of naturally occurring steroids, specifically estradiol-17 β, and progesterone.

MATERIALS AND METHODS

Patients with primary ovarian insufficiency, castrate women, and postmenopausal women receiving 60 μg of ethinyl estradiol orally each day were
720

employed in the present study. Estradiol benzoate was administered intramuscularly to these patients in doses of 20 or 25 mg. Progesterone was also
administered intramuscularly as microcrystals in doses of 20, 50, or 200 mg.
Fourteen ml of blood was drawn at varying intervals from these patients and the
following determinations were made in plasma: LH and FSH by radioimmunoassay (10, 11); progesterone and 17 α-hydroxyprogesterone by a competitive
protein binding method (12); and estradiol-17β by radioimmunoassay (13).

RESULTS

Figures 1 and 2 illustrate the steroid and gonadotropin patterns in two normal
menstrual cycles. FSH shows a rise in the early proliferative phase followed by a
fall in the second half of the proliferative phase. A small midcycle elevation
concomitant with the LH surge is then seen; this is followed by low levels in the
luteal phase. LH remains low throughout the entire cycle except for the sharp
midcycle rise. LH values significantly higher than the basal values found
throughout the cycle are measured one day prior to and one day after the LH
peak value, resulting in a total LH elevation in plasma of more that 48-hr
duration. Estradiol-17β remains below 100 pg/ml in the early follicular phase;
the first sharp significant rise precedes the LH peak by three days and reaches a
concentration of 400 pg/ml one day prior to the LH peak. After the LH peak,
estradiol declines to early proliferative values followed by a second broader
luteal peak ranging from 250 to 300 pg/ml. The first significant rise of
progesterone above follicular values of 0.4 to 0.7 ng/ml coincides with the LH
peak. Progesterone then continues to rise in the luteal phase to 16 ng/ml.
17α-hydroxyprogesterone is distinctly elevated throughout the luteal phase (1.5
to 2.0 ng/ml) as compared to follicular phase values below 0.4 ng/ml; the luteal
elevation being reached on the day of the LH peak. In this cycle, a follicular
17α - hydroxyprogesterone peak (2.7 ng/ml) appears three days prior to the rise
in LH. This rise in 17α- hydroxyprogesterone did not occur in other cycles
(Fig. 2) where 17α-hydroxyprogesterone and progesterone are characterized by an
initial rise on the day of the LH peak; estradiol followed the same pattern
described in the previous cycle.

Plasma values for LH following the injection of progesterone and estradiol
benzoate are presented in Figs. 3 to 6. A rapid rise in LH seen in midcycle is
considered as a positive feedback. Figure 3 demonstrates the ability of
progesterone to elicit a positive feedback. In all three experiments there was a
significant rise in LH values 9 to 13 hr after progesterone injection. The duration
of the peak in patients receiving 20 or 50 mg of progesterone was less than 24
hr. In the patient receiving 200 mg of progesterone, however, the peak lasted
less than 8 hr. All three cases demonstrate that the LH peak following
progesterone injection is both sharp and immediate.

Figures 4 and 5 show the effect of im injection of 25 mg of estradiol
benzoate on plasma LH concentration. Estradiol benzoate was chosen because of
its rapid conversion to estradiol-17β following injection as demonstrated in

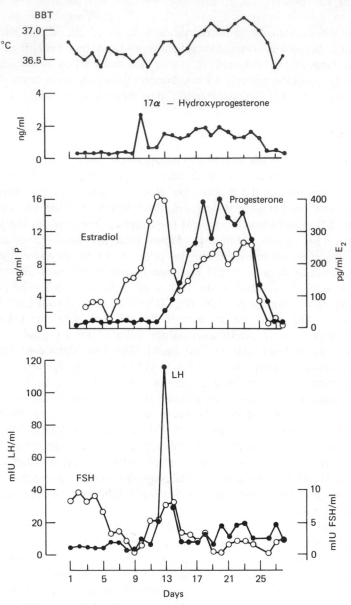

FIG. 1. 17α-hydroxyprogesterone, progesterone, estradiol-17β, FSH, and LH values in plasma determined daily throughout a normal menstrual cycle.

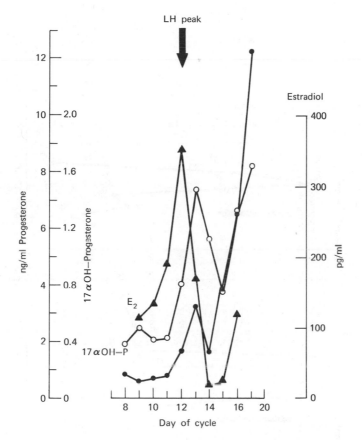

FIG. 2. The periovulatory pattern of 17α-hydroxyprogesterone, progesterone, and estradiol-17β as related to the LH peak in a cycle preceding pregnancy.

Fig. 6. In Fig. 4 the first significant LH rise is detected two days after estradiol benzoate injection with the peak being reached for days after injection. In Fig. 5 the LH peak appears two days after injection. In both patients this first positive feedback to estradiol is followed by a second LH peak four days after the first, indicating no blockage of the cyclic center by estradiol. Administration of 200 mg of progesterone (Fig. 4) coincident with the second estradiol-induced LH peak results in an abrupt termination of the LH peak comparable to the decline of the LH peak induced by progesterone alone (Fig. 3). In Fig. 5, 50 mg of progesterone was administered after the decline of the second estradiol-induced LH peak. This results in still another positive feedback.

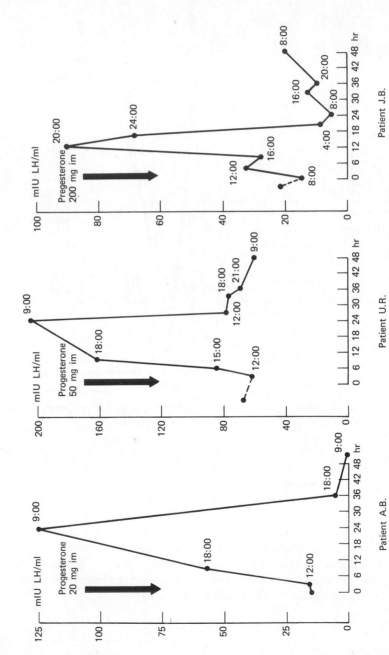

FIG. 3. The effects of 20, 50, and 200 mg of progesterone on the induction and shape of the LH peak, 60 μg ethinyl estradiol p.o.

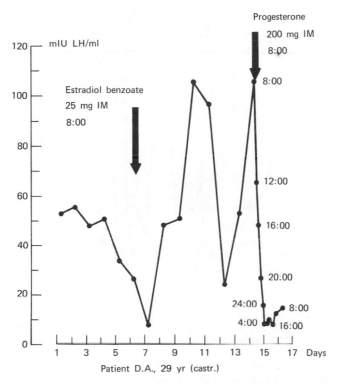

FIG. 4. The induction of two LH peaks 4 days apart following estradiol benzoate administration followed by progesterone. 60 μg ethinyl estradiol/day p.o.

When the sequence of estradiol and progesterone administration is reversed (Fig. 6), the injection of 20 mg of progesterone is followed shortly by the typical progesterone-induced LH peak. However, injection of estradiol benzoate four days after progesterone injection fails to induce a positive feedback although there is a rise of estradiol to 6.2 ng/ml.

DISCUSSION

By attempting to simulate the progesterone and estradiol patterns found in the normal menstrual cycle two distinct effects of progesterone and estradiol on the hypothalamie cyclic center were discovered by measurement of plasma LH levels. Our studies on the effect of progesterone on LH levels suggest that progesterone exerts a stimulatory as well as an inhibitory effect on the cyclic center. The stimulatory effect results in an immediate sharp rise of plasma LH shortly after administration. This release of LH seems to be dose independent once a certain

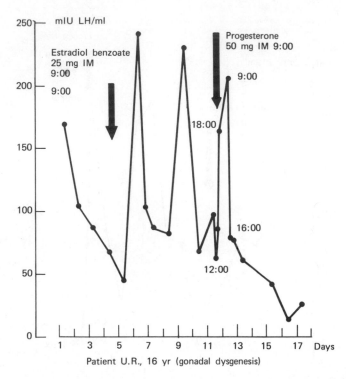

FIG. 5. The induction of two successive LH peaks 4 days apart following estradiol benzoate injection and a third LH peak following progesterone, 60 μg ethinyl estradiol/day p.o.

threshold concentration of progesterone is reached. The administration of 20, 50, or 200 mg of progesterone leads to a significant rise of LH after 9 hr in all three cases. The inhibitory effect of progesterone results in the immediate sharp decline of the induced LH peak. This inhibitory effect seems to be dose dependent. The LH peak following a dose of 20 or 50 mg of progesterone lasts from 18 to 24 hr. However, the peak lasts only 8 hr after a dose of 200 mg of progesterone. Presumably, the administration of 200 mg resulting in a faster rise of plasma progesterone, can quickly inhibit its own stimulatory effect. The inhibitory effect of progesterone is also demonstrated by the failure of estradiol benzoate to cause an LH surge after a progesterone-induced LH surge (Fig. 6). These findings are in accord with results indicating a biphasic feedback effect of progesterone in the rat (4-14). Estradiol, however, does not seem to exert an inhibitory effect. The subsequent LH surges under constantly high blood estradiol levels suggest that the cyclic center is not blocked by estradiol. Similar results have been obtained by Swerdloff and Odell (9) who demonstrated the presence of multiple LH peaks in women receiving oral sequential contraceptive therapy during the estrogenic phase of the cycle. However, when progestin was

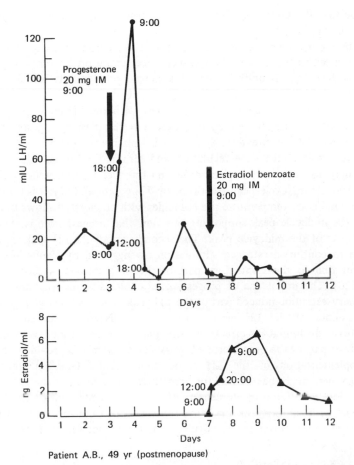

FIG. 6. The induction of an LH peak following progesterone with no significant LH rise after estradiol benzoate; estradiol-17β levels rise immediately in plasma. 60 μg ethinyl estradiol/day p.o.

administered, only one sharp LH peak was observed. Under constant administration of medroxyprogesterone acetate (8) no further LH peaks were observed after the initial LH peak.

Our findings regarding the feedback effects of estradiol and progesterone are compatible with the following endocrine events in the normal human menstrual cycle:

1. FSH-induced increase of plasma estradiol causes a significant rise in LH 24 to 48 hr after the first significant rise of plasma estradiol. From our positive feedback experiments with estradiol benzoate (Fig. 6) and from the observation of Vande Wiele (16) of a positive feedback 36 hr after i.v. Premarin, we can calculate the time interval from the LH surge in the normal cycle. We therefore

conclude that the threshold plasma estradiol concentration appears to be in the range of 150 pg/ml.

2. The inconsistency of the periovulatory 17α-hydroxyprogesterone pattern: since consistent elevation of 17α-hydroxyprogesterone prior to the LH peak has not been found, it is unlikely that this steroid provides the initial triggering stimulus.

3. The initial progesterone rise coincident with the LH peak: progesterone appears not to be the initial triggering steroid in that plasma progesterone levels are low when there is already a significant LH plasma rise (16-18). Progesterone may have a role in the dose regulation and termination of the LH peak. This steroid may also have a synergistic effect on the cyclic center which could lead to biphasic LH midcycle peaks reported by Thomas et al. (19). It is noteworthy that the basal body temperature rise coincides with or shortly follows the second part of the midcycle peak supporting our view that progesterone is responsible for this part of the midcycle peak. The second part of the LH peak is probably not due to continued estrogen stimulation as suggested by Vande Wiele et al. (15), but due to the stimulatory part of the progesterone biphasic feedback effect (20). The initial rise of progesterone in blood seems to result from the preliminary estradiol-induced part of the LH peak. The final dosage regulation in the remainder of the LH peak is then accomplished by the succession of stimulatory and inhibitory effects of rising plasma progesterone levels. While the stimulatory part of the progesterone biphasic effect seems to provide a safeguard for supplementation of the LH stimulation of the Graafian follicle, the inhibitory part might be essential for immediate termination of the LH peak and further blockage of the cyclic center. The abrupt termination of the LH peak coincident with maturity of the "first follicle" might constitute the periovulatory part of a mechanism of monoovulation in the human female (21).

ACKNOWLEDGMENT

Radioimmunoassay reagents were kindly supplied by Dr. B.B. Saxena, Cornell University Medical College, and Dr. R.W. Bates, National Institutes of Health. The skillful assistance of Miss B. Leffek and Mr. E. Jost is greatfully appreciated. Supported by Deutsche Forschungsgemeinschaft No. 67/1 and by N.V. Organon, Oss, Holland.

REFERENCES

1. Hohlweg, W., Klin Wschr 13:92, 1943.
2. Swelheim, T., Acta Endocrinol (Kbh) 49:231, 1965.
3. Everett, J. W., Physiol Rev 44:373, 1964.
4. Harris, G. W., and F. Naftolin, Brit Med Bull 26:3, 1970.
5. Martini, L., F. Riva, and M. Motta, in P. O. Hubinont, F. Leroy, C. Robyn, and P. Leleux (Eds.), Ovo-Implantation, Human Gonadotropins, and Prolactin, Karger, Basel Munchen New York, 1970, p. 170.

6. Bucholz, R., L. Nocke, and W. Nocke, Int J Fert 9:231, 1964.

7. Leyendecker, G., Dissertation, Marburg, 1968.

8. Odell, W. D., and R. S. Swerdloff, in R. L. Hayes, F. A. Goswitz, B. E. P. Murphy, and E. B. Anderson (Eds.), Radioisotopes in Medicine: in Vitro Studies, US Atomic Energy Commission, Oak Ridge, Tenn., 1968.

9. Swerdloff, R. S., and W. D. Odell, J Clin Endocrinol 29:157, 1969.

10. Thomas, K., and J. Ferin, J Clin Endocrinol 28:1667, 1968.

11. Leyendecker, G., D. M. Saunders, and B. B. Saxena, Klin Wschr 49:658, 1971.

12. Leyendecker, G., S. Wardlaw, and W. Nocke, Verlag der Wiener Medizinischen Akademie, Wien, in press, 1971.

13. Wardlaw, S., G. Leyendecker, and W. Nocke, VIII Acta Endocrinologica Congress, Copenhagen, 1971 (Abstract).

14. Rothchild, I., Vit Horm 23:209, 1965.

15. Vande Wiele, R. L., J. Bogumil, I. Dyrenfurth, M. Ferin, R. Jewelewicz, M. Warren, F. Rizkallah, and G. Mikhail, Rec Prog Hormone Res 26:63, 1970.

16. Saxena, B. B., H. Demura, H. M. Gandy, and R. E. Peterson, J Clin Endocrinol 28:519, 1968.

17. Cargille, C. M., G. T. Ross, and T. Yoshimi, J Clin Endocrinol, 29:12, 1969.

18. Ross, G. T., C. M. Cargille, M. B. Lipsett, P. L. Rayford, J. R. Marshall, C. A. Strott, and D. Rodbard, Rec Prog Hormone Res 26:1, 1970.

19. Thomas, K., R. Walchiers, and J. Ferin, J Clin Endocrinol 30:269, 1970.

20. Leyendecker, G., B. A. Barry, B. Leffek, and W. Nocke, Acta Endocrinol (Kbh) Suppl 152:5, 1971.

21. Nocke, W., and G. Leyendecker, Der Gynakologe, in press, 1971.

55. Studies on the Regulation of FSH and LH Secretion by Gonadal Steroids

Virendra B. Mahesh, T. G. Muldoon, J. C. Eldridge, and K. S. Korach

---

Studies of the secretion and regulation of pituitary gonadotropins have been greatly hampered in the past because of the absence of methods sensitive enough to measure FSH and LH in circulating blood. Studies of McCann and co-workers (1), and Schally and co-workers (2) with various hypothalamic extracts established the existence of FSH releasing factor and LH releasing factor that regulated the release of these pituitary hormones. The administration of the LH releasing factor to laboratory animals resulted in the release of some FSH along with larger quantities of LH in most experiments. Similarly some LH was released after administration of FSH releasing factor. The lack of absolute specificity of these releasing factors was attributed primarily to contaminants and possibly some inherent properties for the release of both hormones.

The existence of separate control mechanisms for the release of FSH and LH was adequately supported at that time by the classical concepts of the role of these gonadotropins during the ovulatory process. The work of Goldman and Mahesh (3) demonstrated that in the rat there was a significant depletion of both pituitary FSH and LH during the critical ovulatory period indicating secretion of both hormones. These authors further demonstrated the rupture of the mature follicle and ovulation in the hamster in the presence of liberal excess of anti-LH and the absence of such ovulations when both anti-FSH and anti-LH were present (4). The development of radioimmunoassays for the measurement of

730

serum FSH and LH enabled several investigators to measure gonadotropin secretion during the normal human menstrual cycle (5-9). The pattern of FSH and LH secretion was found to be very similar during the entire menstrual cycle and the ovulatory peak of LH was accompanied by a similar surge of FSH. Preliminary work indicates that this FSH surge in the human may be of considerable importance for normal ovulation and corpus luteum function (10, 11).

In view of the similarities in the pattern of secretion of FSH and LH during the ovulatory cycle in the human, it was of interest to us to study the secretion of these gonadotropins in the experimental animal in order to establish whether they had a common or separate mechanism for their control (12). The availability of material supplied through the National Institute of Arthritis and Metabolic Diseases for the radioimmunoassay of serum FSH, LH, and prolactin in the rat enabled us to study the secretion of these hormones during the rat ovulatory cycle. In order to obtain sufficient number of samples and avoid problems with a 4-day or a 5-day cycle, 30-day-old female rats primed with 4 IU of pregnant mare serum (PMS) were used. Indirect evidence based on injecting phenobarbital suggested that the ovulatory surge of gonadotropins occurred in these animals on the afternoon of day 32 of life (13). The results of radioimmunoassay of serum FSH, LH and prolactin are shown in Fig. 1. Duncan's multirange analysis was used to establish significance. All three hormones were significantly elevated in serum at 2 P.M. on day 32. Serum LH rose in a linear fashion after 12 noon with a peak at 4 P.M. (regression = 0.996; 3 points). A significant fall had already occurred by 6 P.M. and by 11 P.M. there was no difference from the presurge baseline levels. Serum FSH also rose in a linear fashion after 12 noon with a peak at 6 P.M. (regression 0.999; 4 points). By 11 P.M. although the levels were falling, they were significantly above the presurge baseline. Serum prolactin levels rose in a linear fashion after 12 noon of day 32 with a peak at 8 A.M. on day 33 (regression of line = 0.950; 6 points) and then started falling. The uterine weight increased significantly at 8 A.M. on day 32 with highest weights between 2 and 11 P.M. and then started falling. The ovarian weight increased linearly (regression = 0.989; 5 points) starting at 12 noon on day 32 till 11 P.M. and then remained at that level. The above experiment clearly demonstrates that the time span of secretion of FSH, LH, and prolactin differ significantly from each other, with events starting at 12 noon on day 32. This may be indicative of separate control mechanisms for the 3 hormones, although the presence of a common stimulus cannot be ruled out.

In attempts to further explore the regulation of the secretion of FSH and LH these hormones were measured in serum after castration and various substitutional therapy. Castration of 26-day-old immature male rats resulted in significant elevation of serum FSH within 8 hr and serum LH within 12 hr (Fig. 2). The levels of both hormones continued to rise with time, although the FSH rise appeared more dramatic. In immature female rats the rise in FSH became evident 24 hr after castration whereas LH started rising and was significantly

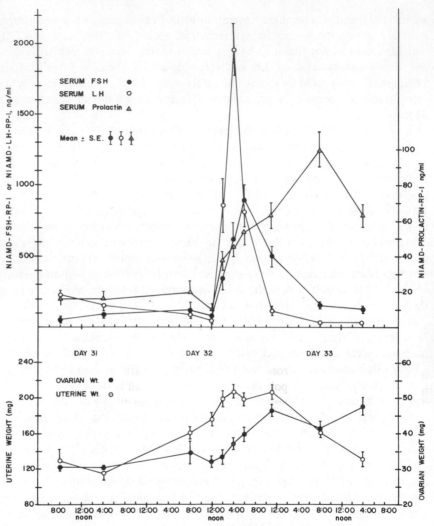

FIG. 1. Serum FSH, LH, and prolactin levels in female rats primed with PMS on day 30 along with ovarian and uterine weights. Serum LH levels starting to rise after 12 noon on day 32 of age linearly (regression = 0.996; 3 points) with a peak at 4 P.M. A significant fall occurred by 4 P.M. and by 11 P.M. the levels were comparable to the presurge levels. Serum FSH levels starting to rise after 12 noon on day 32 of age linearly (regression 0.999; 4 points) with a peak at 6 P.M. By 11 P.M. the levels were falling although still significantly above the presurge baseline. Serum prolactin rose linearly (regression 0.95; 6 points) after 12 noon on day 32 with a peak at 8 A.M. on day 33. The uterine weight increased significantly at 8 A.M. on day 32 with highest weights between 2 and 11 P.M. The ovarian weight increased linearly starting at 12 noon on day 32 till 11 P.M. and then remained constant. 17 out of 18 animals sacrificed on day 33 had fresh tubal ova.

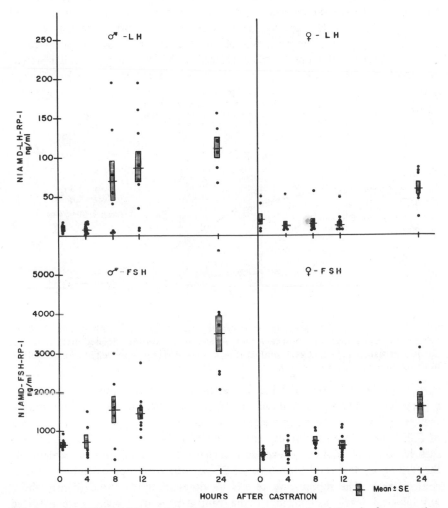

FIG. 2. Serum FSH and LH in male and female rats at various time intervals after castration on day 26 of life. In male rats, serum FSH rose significantly within 8 hr of castration (p < 0.01). Serum LH showed its first significant elevation after 12 hr of castration (p < 0.05) and showed further increase by 24 hr (p < 0.01). In female rats serum FSH rose significantly by 24 hr (p < 0.05) and LH only after 48 hr (not shown in this chart).

elevated 48 hr after castration. Once again these experiments indicate differences in the pattern of appearance of FSH and LH in serum after castration.

According to current concepts, testosterone is considered to be the main hormone responsible for the gonadal regulation of pituitary gonadotropin secretion in the male. It was therefore of interest to us to study the changes in serum gonadotropin in immature male rats castrated on day 26 of life and treated with a replacement dose of testosterone injected subcutaneously twice a day for 7 days. At the conclusion of the experiment, the animals were sacrificed and their ventral prostate and seminal vesicles compared with those of intact rats of the same age. From the mean and standard deviation of these organs weights of intact animals, the dosage of testosterone that would give similar weight ranges in the castrate animal were calculated and are shown in Fig. 3. The

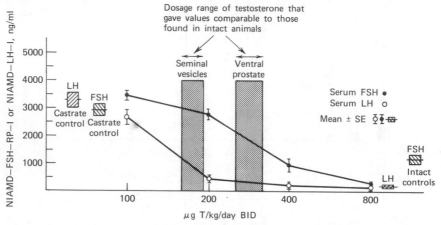

FIG. 3. Serum FSH and LH levels in castrated male rats treated with various doses of testosterone as compared to castrated controls and intact controls. Shaded areas represent the dose of testosterone that gave seminal vesicle and ventral prostate weights comparable to those found in intact controls injected with the vehicle alone.

pattern of serum FSH and LH in castrated rats clearly shows preferential suppression of LH with low doses of testosterone (even below that required for the ventral prostate to reach weights comparable to intact animals). The levels of FSH were reduced to intact control levels by the 400 μg/kg dose, which was slightly above physiological level as judged by the ventral prostate weight. At the 800 μg/kg dose level both serum FSH and LH were suppressed below intact control levels. The suppression of LH by doses of testosterone slightly above physiological levels as judged by the ventral prostate weight were reported earlier by Ramirez and McCann (14). The difference in the results of these investigators as compared to ours is probably due to lack of sensitive methods available for the measurement of serum LH at that time. Ramirez and McCann (14) did not carry out FSH studies due to the absence of a suitable method for measurement of serum FSH. The results of Swerdloff et al. (15) suggesting a relationship between serum FSH and development of mature spermatogenesis are of interest. It is reasonable to expect that this target organ should have influence on the regulation of FSH. The above studies however, show that testosterone in doses slightly above physiologic levels can also suppress serum FSH in the complete absence of spermatogenesis.

The work of several investigators during the last five years has raised the possibility that testosterone may be converted to dihydrotestosterone for manifestation of physiological activity [reviewed by Wilson et al. (16)]. The conversion of testosterone to dihydrotestosterone in the pituitary and hypothalamus of the rat has been demonstrated by Jaffe (17). It was therefore of interest to study the changes in serum FSH and LH of the male rat castrated on day 26 and treated with replacement doses of dihydrotestosterone for 7 days. Figure 4 shows suppression of serum LH from castrate levels to that comparable

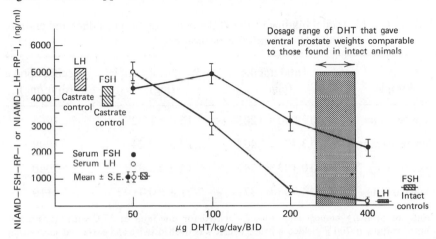

FIG. 4. Serum FSH and LH levels in castrated male rats treated with various doses of dihydrotestosterone (DHT) as compared to castrated controls and intact controls. Shaded area represents the dose of DHT that gave ventral prostate weight comparable to that found in intact controls injected with vehicle alone. The mean seminal vesicle weight of rats treated with 400 μg/kg dose of DHT approached that found in control animals.

with intact controls at a dose level judged to be physiological based on ventral prostrate weights. The serum FSH was also significantly lowered as compared to castrated controls but was nevertheless higher than the intact controls, showing only partial suppression. These results appear to be similar to the testosterone experiment with the exception that whereas the seminal vesicle weight in the testosterone experiment approached that of controls at doses far below that required for ventral prostate weight maintainence, the reverse was true for the dihydrotestosterone experiment. The seminal vesicle weight approached that found in control animals only at the 400 μg/kg level, which was higher than that required for the maintainence of ventral prostate weight.

In the regulation of gonadotropins, testosterone may act directly or by conversion to estrogens or to dihydrotestosterone or by all of these mechanisms. Therefore a study of the receptor (binding) sites for these hormones was undertaken in the rat pituitary and hypothalamus.

The demonstration of specific estradiol binding to the "nuclear" fraction of female rat anterior pituitary homogenates (18) prompted us to investigate the same phenomenon in male rats. Comparison between the uptake of ^{3}H-estradiol by the 700 g pellet of intact and castrate mature male and female anterior pituitaries is shown in Table I. For standardization among groups the uptake is expressed in milligrams of wet pituitary weight. On this basis, there was no difference in uptake among castrate females, intact females and intact males. Somewhat higher binding appeared in castrate males. It should be noted that castrate pituitaries were heavier than intact pituitaries, so that the absolute concentration of nuclear binding sites was actually higher in all castrate animals.

TABLE I. ^{3}H-Estradiol binding to the 700 g pellet fraction of intact and castrate male and female rat anterior pituitary[a]

Sample	Total uptake (cpm)	Weight of sample (mg)	Specific uptake (dpm/mg)
Female intact	12,040 ± 1205	16.0 ± 1.02	1965
Female castrate	13,475 ± 404	17.5 ± 0.24	1999
Male intact	10,103 ± 342	14.2 ± 0.31	2040
Male castrate	14,703 ± 371	21.8 ± 0.41	2110

[a]Anterior pituitary homogenates were incubated for one hour at 23 C with ^{3}H-estradiol. Centrifugation at 700 g yielded a pellet which was washed twice and extracted successively with ethanol, chloroform-ether (2 : 1) and ether. Radioactivity of the combined extracts was determined. Values reported represent the mean of 5 groups of animals (5 animals/group) ± SE.

By analogy with the extensive studies of Jensen et al. (19) and Gorski et al. (20) in the rat uterus, it appeared advisable to study the relationship of the sex of the animal to the primary uptake of estradiol by pituitary cytosol. Specific uptake of estradiol by female rat pituitary cytosol has been reported (21-23) but comparable analysis of the male rat was not performed. Using procedures including gel filtration, equilibrium dialysis, and sucrose density gradient fractionation, we have been able to demonstrate the presence of specific cytosol receptors for estradiol in the male which closely resemble those found in the female. Moreover, no specific uptake of testosterone was observed in the pituitary cytosol fraction from either sex.

The Sephadex G-200 elution patterns of ^{3}H-estradiol-incubated cytosol (i.e., 105,000 g supernatant) samples from male and female rats is shown in Fig. 5. The presence of a large peak of radioactivity immediately following void volume elution is common to both samples and represent highaffinity binding to a macromolecular species. More definitive characterization of this component is supplied by analysis of sucrose gradient centrifugation data obtained for similarly incubated samples (Fig. 6). In both males and females, a distinct peak of radioactivity is found associated with protein sedimenting in the 8S region.

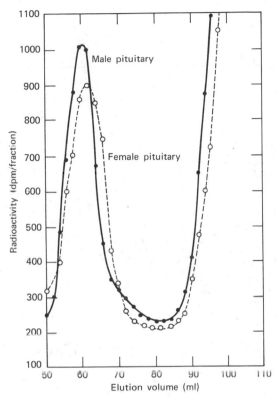

FIG. 5. Gel filtration of ³H-estradiol-treated cytosol samples of male and female rat anterior pituitaries. Samples were incubated with ³H-estradiol for 1 hr at 4 C and subjected to Sephadex G-200 filtration. Elution pattern shown is exclusive of initial void volume.

This specific binding did not occur when cytosol samples were incubated with ³H-testosterone.

For direct demonstration of specific high-affinity binding of estradiol, the method of equilibrium dialysis (24) was chosen. Cytosol samples were enclosed within cellulose dialysis bags and dialyzed to equilibrium (72 hr) against outside solutions containing radiolabeled steroid. Protein binding was assessed by specific differences (i.e., dpm/ml) between inside and outside solutions at equilibrium. The results shown in Table II demonstrate appreciable binding of ³H-estradiol, but not of ³H-testosterone, to male and female cytosol fractions. No significant difference was observed between castrate and intact animals when the results were expressed on the basis of an equal weight of cytosol protein, although, once again, the absolute concentration of binding sites was higher in the castrate animal. Binding of ³H-dihydrotestosterone occurred in both males and females at a level significantly lower than that of estradiol (Table III).

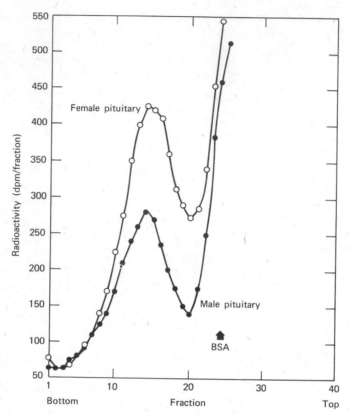

FIG. 6. Sucrose density gradient centrifugation patterns of ³H-estradiol-treated cytosol from male and female rat anterior pituitaries. Cytosol was incubated for 1 hr at 4 C with ³H-estradiol, after which 300 μl samples were layered onto a 5 to 20% sucrose gradient. Centrifugation was performed for 18 hr at 222,000 g. Sedimentation constants were determined using similtaneously centrifuged bovine serum albumin (arrow) as reference. Female animals were older than males at sacrifice and total protein content of cytosol was appreciably higher, accounting for the difference in magnitude of the 8S peaks.

Since some serum was unavoidably present in the pituitary samples, it was necessary to show that the binding which we observed was not simply nonspecific interaction with albumin. After redialysis of estradiol-equilibrated samples against buffer for 24 hr, a procedure which will disrupt low affinity steroid-albumin complexes, 37% of the estradiol remained bound to protein (Table IV). Subsequent gel filtration of this redialyzed material on Sephadex G-200 did not result in further release of free steroid. This finding was confirmatory of the presence of specific 8S binding by sucrose gradient analysis, since the 8S peak was clearly distinct from albumin which was used as a reference standard and sedimented as a 4.6S protein.

TABLE II. Binding of estradiol and testosterone to rat anterior pituitary cytosol fractions[a]

Group	Sample	Total steroid (dpm/ml)	Bound steroid (dpm/ml)	Bound (%)	Specific binding (dpm/(ml)(mg) protein)
Estradiol					
	Outside	35,626			
Female intact	Inside	69,344	33,718	48.6	11,048
Female castrate	Inside	90,794	55,168	60.8	15,414
Male intact	Inside	62,055	26,429	42.6	11,189
Male castrate	Inside	84,342	48,716	57.8	12,878
Testosterone					
	Outside	131,686			
Female intact	Inside	124,644			
Female castrate	Inside	121,928			
Male intact	Inside	120,318			
Male castrate	Inside	127,772			

[a]Multiple equilibrium dialysis of samples of cytosol from the four groups was performed for 72 hr at 4 C against a single outside solution containing either ^{3}H-estradiol or ^{3}H-testosterone. Average radioactive content of outside and various inside solutions at equilibrium are reported. The data show no specific uptake of testosterone by any of the 4 groups examined.

TABLE III. Specific uptake of dihydrotestosterone by rat anterior pituitary cytosol[a]

Group	Sample	Total steroid (dpm/ml)	Bound steroid (dpm/ml)	Bound (%)
Experiment I				
	Outside	128,400		
Female intact	Inside	142,526	14,126	9.9
Female castrate	Inside	143,474	15,074	9.5
Male intact	Inside	140,392	11,992	11.7
Male castrate	Inside	140,362	11,962	11.7
Experiment II				
	Outside	5,166		
Female intact	Inside	5,606	440	12.7
Female castrate	Inside	6,030	864	7.0
Male intact	Inside	5,896	730	8.1
Male castrate	Inside	6,172	1006	6.1

[a]Multiple equilibrium dialysis of cytosol samples from 4 groups against two different levels of ^{3}H-dihydrotestosterone. Conditions as in Table II.

TABLE IV. Extent of high-affinity binding of estradiol to female rat anterior pituitary cytosol[a]

Treatment	Sample		Total steroid (dpm/ml)	Steroid bound (dpm/ml)
Dialysis	(A)	Outside	80,524	59,301
		Inside	139,825	
	(B)	Outside	76,912	58,588
		Inside	135,500	
Redialysis		Outside	23,050	13,415
		Inside	36,465	
Gel Filtration				12,900

[a]Cytosol samples were dialyzed for 72 hr against ^{3}H-estradiol. Two ml of inside solution at equilibrium were redialyzed for 24 hr against buffer. The dialysand was then subjected to Sephadex G-200 gel filtration and total radioactivity was measured in the frontal peak eluted.

Data on hypothalamic uptake are somewhat preliminary, since the extremely low concentration of binding sites within this tissue makes it difficult to accurately reproduce values from one experiment to another. Nevertheless, both male and female hypothalami display a much more avid affinity for primary binding of estradiol than for testosterone.

It is tempting to postulate from these findings that the in vivo inhibition of gonadotropin secretion induced by testosterone may be, at least in part, mediated by the conversion of testosterone to dihydrotestoserone and/or estradiol. Further work is presently in progress to examine further this possibility.

ACKNOWLEDGMENT

This investigation was supported by a research contract 70-2149 from the Center for Population Research, National Institute of Child Health and Human Development, National Institutes of Health, USPHS. The material for the radioimmunoassay for serum gonadotropins was obtained through the National Institute of Arthritis and Metabolic Diseases, National Institutes of Health, USPHS. The antisera to ovine LH used for LH determinations was made available to us by Drs. G. D. Niswender and A. R. Midgley, Jr.

REFERENCES

1. McCann, S. M., and V. D. Ramirez, Rec Prog Hormone Res 20:131, 1964.
2. Schally, A. V., A. Arimura, C. Y. Bowers, A. J. Kastin, S. Sawano, and T. W. Redding, Rec Prog Hormone Res 24:497, 1968.
3. Goldman, B. D., and V. B. Mahesh, Endocrinology 83:97, 1968.
4. Goldman, B. D., and V. B. Mahesh, Endocrinology 84:236, 1969.
5. Faiman, C., and R. J. Ryan, J Clin Endocrinol 27:1711, 1967.
6. Odell, W. D., G. T. Ross, and P. L. Rayford, J Clin Invest 46:248, 1967.
7. Odell, W. D., A. F. Parlow, C. M. Cargille, and G. T. Ross, J Clin Invest 47:2551, 1968.
8. Saxena, B. B., H. Demura, H. M. Gandy, and R. E. Peterson, J Clin Endocrinol 28:519, 1968.
9. Midgley, A. R., and R. B. Jaffe, J Clin Endocrinol 28:1699, 1968.
10. Strott, C. A., C. M. Cargille, G. T. Ross, and M. B. Lipsett, J Clin Endocrinol 30:246, 1970.
11. Mahesh, V. B., R. B. Greenblatt, H. F. L. Scholer, and J. O. Ellegood, Proc 7th Pan American Congress of Endocrinology, Brazil, August 1970, in press.
12. Eldridge, J. C., H. F. L. Scholer, and V. B. Mahesh, Proc 52nd and 53rd Meetings of the Endocrine Society, 1970-71.
13. McCormack, E. C., and R. K. Meyer, Proc Soc Exp Biol Med 110:343, 1962.
14. Ramirez, V. D., and S. M. McCann, Endocrinology 72:452, 1963.
15. Swerdloff, R. S., P. C. Walsh, H. S. Jacobs, and W. D. Odell, Endocrinology 88:120, 1971.

16. Wilson, J. D., and R. E. Gloyna, Rec Prog Hormone Res 26:309, 1970.

17. Jaffe, R. B., Steroids 14:483, 1969.

18. Leavitt, W. W., J. P. Friend, and J. A. Robinson, Science 165:496, 1969.

19. Jensen, E. V., E. R. DeSombre, P. W. Jungblut, W. E. Stumpf, and L. J. Roth, in L. J. Roth and W. E. Stumpf (Eds.), Autoradiography of Diffusible Substances, Academic, New York, 1969, p. 81.

20. Gorski, J., D. Toft, G. Shyamala, D. Smith, and A. Notides, Rec Prog Hormone Res 24:45, 1968.

21. Kato, J., and C. A. Villee, Endocrinology 80:1133, 1967.

22. Eisenfeld, A. J., Endocrinology 86:1313, 1970.

23. Notides, A. C., Endocrinology 87:987, 1970.

24. Westphal, U., in R. B. Clayton (Ed.), Methods in Enzymology, Vol. 15, Academic, New York and London, 1969, p. 761.

DISCUSSION

M. L. TAYMOR. We, too, have had an opportunity to study the National Pituitary Agency's FSH. The first slide (Fig. 1) illustrates studies on a woman with amenorrhea, who had pituitary irradiation for a chromophobe adenoma. She was initially given a pituitary FSH preparation which contained 57 IU of FSH and 0.27 IU of LH/ampule (top panel). After giving as much as 300 IU of FSH daily, accompanied by a significant rise in serum levels of immunoreactive FSH, there was no evidence of ovarian stimulation as noted by urinary estrogen excretion and no change in the basal temperature after HCG. In a subsequent cycle, the patient was given HMG containing 75 IU of FSH and 75 IU of LH/ampule. After 7 days of treatment at a level of 150 IU/day (lower panel), a good response in urinary estrogen excretion occurred. In addition, there was evidence of ovulation after HCG was given. I believe studies such as these suggest that LH may play a role in the development of the follicle, either directly or, more likely, indirectly, by stimulation of estrogen secretion by the ovaries, which in turn, has a secondary effect upon the follicles. Further studies with additional subjects should shed more light on this proposition.

The next slide (Fig. 2) illustrates the possibility of supplementing or improving our approach to induction of ovulation. This is a patient with polycystic ovaries, post wedge resection, who did not respond to Clomid therapy, as far as conception was concerned. She was given HMG (top panel); there was a rapid increase in estrogen. The level reached 476 μg/24 hr, so HCG was not given. There was a moderate degree of ovarian enlargement. In a subsequent cycle she was given HFSH (bottom panel). She had a relatively slow and perhaps, a more physiologic rise in estrogen excretion. There was evidence of ovulation by BBT; the ovaries did not enlarge. She did not conceive in this cycle. These preliminary studies suggest that we should have various plans for therapy in terms of FSH and LH for patients with different endogenous ratios of FSH and LH. All of us who have had the opportunity and privilege of working with these medications over the past few years will always feel indebted to Dr. Gemzell and Dr. Lunenfeld for their pioneering efforts, but perhaps we are now on the threshold of an even more rational approach to the induction of ovulation.

743

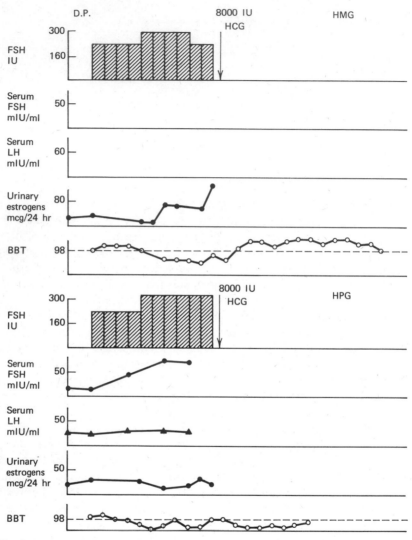

FIG. 1

P. CYZGAN. In addition to the data presented, I would like to make two comments on Dr. Rosemberg's and Dr. Leyendecker's papers. This slide (Fig. 3) demonstrates plasma FSH, LH, HCG, and placental lactogen during one of our four HMG treatment cycles following pregnancy. LH and FSH were higher during treatment than in normal cycles. The degree of increase probably depends on the different half-life of the two gonadotropins. HCG injection resulted in a sharp peak in plasma LH which is higher than the normal ovulatory LH peak.

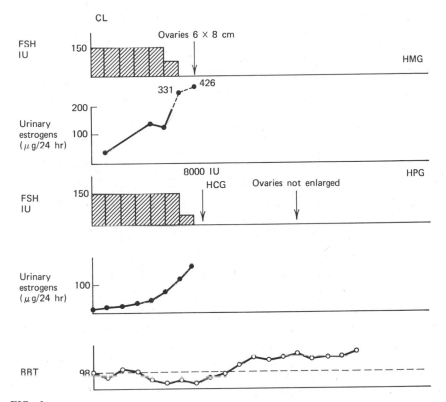

FIG. 2

The elevation of LH decreased over 3 to 5 days. These differences in plasma LH may provide an explanation for the large increase in plasma steroids 3 to 4 days after ovulation shown by Dr. Bettendorf. Surprisingly, we found elevated LH and FSH levels during the luteal phase, although additional exogenous gonadotropins were not administered. Sele and Starup noted high gonadotropic excretion in this phase. The possibility of stimulatory effects of endogenous pituitary FSH and LH secretion by exogenous treatment should be discussed. Starting on day 9 to 11 after administration of HCG, a sharp rise of HCG (probably placental) is seen; plasma FSH decreases to low or undetectable levels. This is in agreement with reports by Midgley and Parlow. High FSH occurred in one of our patients with ovarian hyperstimulation. Now in reference to Dr. Leyendecker's paper, we are doing similar studies in women with normal cycles and those with anovulatory cycles. As far as we can see from our first results, the LH surge is induced 1 to 2 days after 5 mg of estradiol. Unfortunately, we have not measured estrogen secretion in these subjects.

E. D. JOHANSSON. It should be recognized that the group of patients that are

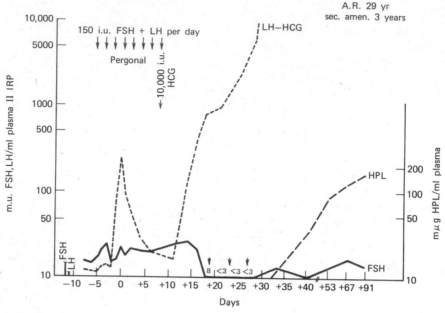

FIG. 3

given therapy, as Dr. Lunenfeld said is a very pathological and heterogeneous group. I would like to comment on what Dr. Rosemberg said regarding the normal luteal function after induction of ovulation with LH. The studies were made by Dr. Gemzell and his group. The patients were primarily amenorrheic women with low plasma levels of LH and FSH. They were given a highly purified FSH preparation made by Dr. Roos. Ovulation was induced with LH; a very short period of progesterone elevation was seen. The luteal phase could be prolonged by administration of additional LH. The peaks of LH correspond with the rise of progesterone and estradiol during the period. Immunoreactive FSH level increased and plateaued during FSH treatment but decreased when the estradiol levels began to increase.

E. ROSEMBERG. It was quite obvious that the problem of LH requirements for maintenance of luteal function was to come up. Dr. Vande Wiele reported that additional HLH is needed to maintain the functional life of the corpus luteum. We have seen other results here. However, my contention is the following: in our case and those of Dr. Vande Wiele and Dr. Johansson, the experimental designs used were quite different. If I interpret Dr. Johansson's data correctly, the amounts of HFSH given were considerably higher than the amounts we have used during the proliferative phase of induced cycles. Moreover, I don't know how much LH was contained in the preparations used in his studies; only a single injection of 10,000 IU of HLH was given. Hence, follicular stimulation was achieved in a manner different from that reported by us. Dr. Vande Wiele induced follicular stimulation with high dosages of Pergonal. We intend to repeat our experiment in hypophysectomized patients using our strict experimental design in order to confirm the data presented here today.

R. JAFFE. Dr. Rosemberg, as I understand it, there is an essential difference, beside the dosage manipulation, between your experimental design and that which Dr. Vande Wiele reported to us at the Laurentian Hormone Conference. Your patients, it seems, have endogenous LH throughout the cycle, whereas Dr. Vande Wiele's patient was hypophysectomized. Therefore, it would not be inconceivable to me that in your patient, when given only a single injection of LII, corpus luteum function was maintained since she had some endogenous LH. If LH is needed during the luteal phase of the cycle, Dr. Vande Wiele's patient would have required additional LH, since there was no endogenous LH.

E. ROSEMBERG. As Dr. Jaffe pointed out, our patients elicited endogenous gonadotropin function. The levels of immunoreactive plasma LH increased immediately after the first injection of HLH given on day 11 of the induced cycles when 3,000 to 3,170 IU of HLH were administered, then decreased on the second day of its administration, when about 1,000 IU were given. Thereafter, the levels of plasma LH were indicative of the endogenous circulating hormone. I would agree that the difference between our data and that reported by Dr. Vande Wiele is related not only to the experimental design used, but also to the difference in types of patients. However, the continuous administration of 400 IU of HLH/day for maintenance of corpus luteum function, as reported by Vande Wiele, should have resulted in levels of immunoreactive plasma LH much higher than those recorded for endogenous LH.

G. BETTENDORF. Dr. Rosemberg, I think you showed very clearly that you can mimic the FSH and LH patterns during the cycle. I would be interested in hearing something about the steroid patterns. Were these similar to those seen in the normal cycle?

E. ROSEMBERG. Yes. At least the urinary pattern of estrogen and pregnanediol was similar to that seen in the normal menstrual cycle. We did not measure plasma levels of these hormones.

L. MARTINI. I wish to make a brief comment on what Dr. Weisz presented to us. We have done the same sort of experiment in vivo. We obtained practically the same results when intravenous injections of LH-RF were given to the rat; every injection is followed by an increase in plasma LH. The interesting thing is that the same phenomenon does not occur if you consider another hormone, in other words, growth hormone. This probably explains why one does not find any activity in growth hormone releasing factor preparations when a radio-immunoassay is used for estimation of growth hormone. One injection of a growth hormone releasing factor preparation does not liberate growth hormones into the circulation. Only a second injection given 1 hr later will produce a large increase in plasma growth hormone levels. Thus it appears that the first stimulus must do something to the pituitary; for instance, increase the concentration of growth hormone in the gland or prepare a pool which is more easily released.

C. A. GEMZELL. I fully agree with Dr. Rosemberg that it is very important to try to obtain an ovarian response which is as similar as possible to events in a normal spontaneous menstrual cycle. However, one should not forget that ovaries are very different in sensitivity. As Dr. Taymor showed in his slide, there was one woman who had a very high plasma level of FSH and did not respond at all. We have found that some women need very high doses of FSH in order to respond. Actually, we had one woman who did not respond until she obtained 600 U of FSH/day, and the increase in FSH levels in urine was considerable. We feel that it is much more important to obtain a steroid pattern in plasma or urine that is as normal as possible. That is, after the first estrogen peak you should have a drop and then a second peak. The plasma progesterone and 17a-hydroxy-progesterone should also be similar to what one finds during a normal menstrual cycle. Therefore, when treating a woman, we are very careful not to stimulate her above a level of 50 to 60 μg/24 hr or to a level corresponding to that at the time of ovulation in a spontaneous menstrual cycle.

R. VANDE WIELE. It is not necessarily true that in treating patients with infertility, we have to imitate the events of the normal cycle. Whatever scheme yields a large number of pregnancies is the one desired, provided major side effects are avoided. There was only a 13% incidence of pregnancies in Dr. Rosemberg's series, which I consider unsatisfactory.

C. A. GEMZELL. We have a good correlation between the pregnancy rate and the normal pattern of plasma steroids. In other words, when we obtain a normal plasma steroid pattern, the percentage of pregnancies is high; in the absence of a normal steroid pattern, the rate of pregnancy is low.

J. WEISZ. I wonder whether some observations from animal experiments might be relevant to the human. In the rat, we find that only a small portion of the preovulatory LH peak is required for ovulation per se. This does not necessarily mean, however, that the rest of the peak is redundant. If we combine the earlier observations of Everett with what we now know about the timing of the LH surge, we may conclude that if the surge is short, ovulation can still take place, but the histological appearance of the corpora lutea formed is not normal. Could similar dissociation occur in the human? Is ovulation itself enough or might there be something more needed to make a really good corpus luteum?

56. Plasma Steroid Pattern During Gonadotropin Stimulation

Gerhard Bettendorf, Frank Lehmann, Ch. Neale, and M. Breckwoldt

During gonadotropin therapy, as the most effective treatment of anovulation, we face three major problems: 1) evaluation of the endocrine status before treatment; 2) optimal treatment schedule; and 3) monitoring of the ovarian response during therapy. Induction of ovulation with human hypophyseal gonadotropins (HHG) or HMG preparations (Humegon and Pergonal) is justified only in women with infertility problems associated with anovulation due to one of the following diagnosis: Group I, primary or secondary amenorrhea with no detectable gonadotropin excretion; Group II, primary or secondary amenorrhea with normal gonadotropin excretion without response to clomiphene; and Group IIa, anovulatory cycles without response to clomiphene.

As indicated in Table I, the pregnancy rate was high in Group I and lowest in the group of patients with anovulatory cycles, Group IIa. The three preparations (HHG, Pergonal, and Humegon) tested were equally effective in inducing ovulation and pregnancy rate. Initially, gonadotropin was administered over a period of 10 to 12 days. Later on, individualized treatment schedules were preferred. The dose of gonadotropin and the duration of therapy were monitored by ovarian response as indicated by daily vaginal smears and cervical mucus. Vaginal cytology proved to be of little value in evaluating response to therapy; examination of cervical mucus, however, was a more reliable parameter. During the last two years treatment was monitored by daily total urinary estrogens. Comparing the results obtained with different types of parameters for monitoring response, there was no difference in ovulation and pregnancy rates.

749

TABLE I. Results of treatment with HHG and HMG

	No. of patients	No. of courses	Ovulation	Pregnancy	Ovarian enlargement	Intensity	Efficiency	Pregnancy rate
HHG								
Iᵃ	18	36	26	8	14	2.0	4.5	44%
IIᵇ	24	52	41	6	22	2.2	8.6	25%
IIaᶜ	8	10	10	1	3	1.2	10	12%
Pergonal								
I	8	15	9	3	2	1,9	5	40%
II	24	39	32	11	11	1,6	3,5	45%
IIa	11	19	15	2	3	1,7	3,5	18%
Humegon								
I	9	10	8	5		1,1	2	56%
II	52	87	67	12	18	1,7	7,2	23%
IIa	31	45	42	8	7	1.5	5,6	26%

ᵃI = patients with nonmeasurable gonadotropin excretion and hypophysectomized patients.

ᵇII = patients with normal gonadotropin excretion.

ᶜIIa = patients with anovulatory cycles.

In order to get better parameters for endocrine activity of ovaries before and during treatment, daily plasma steroid patterns were investigated and results compared to those obtained during normal menstrual cycles.

METHODS

Total plasma estrogens were determined by radioimmunoassay (1), plasma progesterone (P), and 17α-hydroxyprogesterone (17-OHP) were quantitated by competitive protein binding method (2-5) and total urinary estrogens were measured by the rapid method of Brown (6).

Usually treatment was started with 1 or 2 ampules daily for a period of 4 to 5 days. If there was no effect on the cervical mucus or an elevation of estrogen excretion, the dosage was increased by adding one ampule for the same period. When more than one ampule was administered, injections were given twice a day. HCG was injected when estrogen excretion reached levels between 70 and 100 $\mu g/24$ hr. Three groups of patients were studied: 1) normal menstrual cycles (7 patients); 2) HMG treatment followed by pregnancy (8 patients); and 3) HMG treatment resulting in an ovulation but without subsequent pregnancy (13 patients).

We tried to compare the patterns of urinary estrogen excretion and plasma estrogens, 17-OHP, and P in each of the three groups. The patterns of the individual cycles were arranged according to day 0, the day before the rise of the basal body temperature. Day 0 in the treatment cycles, represents the day of HCG injection. The geometrical means of the values of the individual curves are presented in Figs. 1 to 4. Some individual patterns have been published elsewhere (7).

RESULTS

Total Estrogens

The urinary output of total estrogens was significantly higher in patients treated with HMG than in women during normal cycles. In Group 2, estrogen excretion started to rise between day 5 and 6; in Group 3, this elevation occurred one day earlier. In the normal cycles, excretion of estrogens started to rise between day 2 and 3. The first estrogen peak which occurred in normal ovarian cycles at day 0 was noted in Group 2 on day 1 and in Group 3 on day 0. In the luteal phase, the values were definitely higher during treatment cycles than in the normal control cycles. In the pregnancy group (Group 2), values decreased after ovulation. This decrease was followed by a subsequent increase to values higher than those of the ovulatory peak. In Group 3, the postovulatory decrease was absent and mean values were even higher than in Group 2.

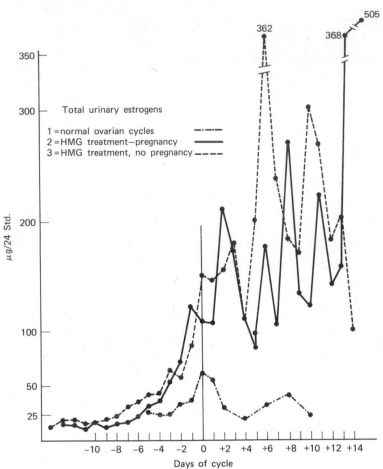

FIG. 1. Total urinary estrogen excretion. Group 1: n = 7, Group 2: n = 8, and Group 3: n = 13.

Plasma Estrogens

Plasma estrogen patterns were quite similar to those of urinary estrogens. The increase started earlier in treatment cycles compared to normal cycles. In all three groups, a definite peak at day 0 was found. The subsequent decrease was strongly pronounced in Groups 1 and 2, but not in Group 3. The luteal peak in the normal cycle was found to be lower than the ovulation peak in the group of treated patients that became pregnant; the estrogen levels during the luteal phase were just as high as the ovulation peak. In the group of treated patients who did not become pregnant, luteal estrogen levels were even higher.

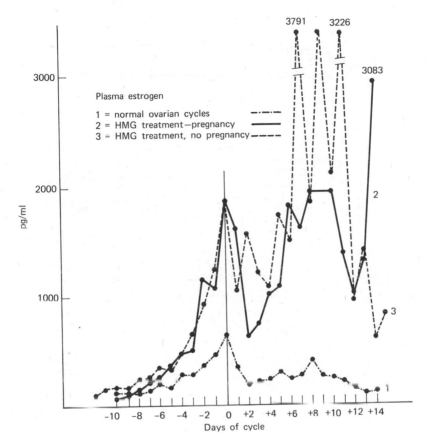

FIG. 2.

Plasma 17α-Hydroxyprogesterone

Increased levels of 17-OHP could be observed 2 to 3 days earlier than in normal cycles. In Group 2, on day 0, the values were elevated more than twofold higher than in Groups 1 and 3. During the luteal phase, both treatment groups showed higher values of 17-OHP; highest levels were found in Group 2. Levels of 17-OHP were about ten times higher in Group 2 and fivefold higher in Group 3 than in normal cycles.

We noted significant differences in P during HMG treatment in patients who became pregnant and those who did not. In Group 3, P was already 3 times higher at days 0 and 1 as compared to levels during the follicular phase. At that time no increase was found in Group 1 or 2; a significant rise was noted on days 1 and 2. In the first two days after ovulation, the increase in P was most pronounced in Group 3, but not in Groups 1 and 2 until day 3. Starting at day

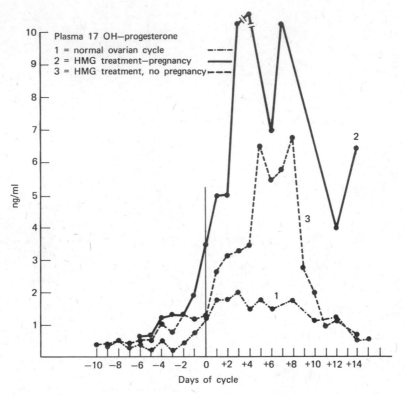

FIG. 3.

4, there was no real difference between Groups 2 and 3, but both had much higher values than Group 1. On days 8 and 9 of the luteal phase, P levels showed a slight decrease and a subsequent sharp rise in the group of treated patients who became pregnant.

DISCUSSION

Based on estrogen levels in urine and in plasma, it can be concluded that estrogen production in stimulated follicles was higher than in normal cycles. In normal cycles, increasing follicular activity, as measured by estrogen levels, occurred 2 to 3 days prior to ovulation. In the stimulated patients, however, increased follicular activity was observed at least 5 to 6 days before ovulation. This prolonged period of increased estrogen production was followed by even higher levels of estrogen at the time of ovulation. Since exogenous stimulation was not continued in the luteal phase, higher estrogen production has to be regarded as a reaction to nonphysiological stimulation during follicular matura-

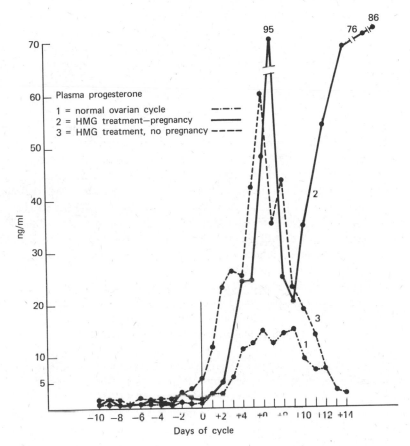

FIG. 4.

tion. In addition, elevated levels of 17-OHP and P in the luteal phase of treatment cycles clearly demonstrate that corpus luteum function after exogenous stimulation is different from that in normal cycles. This may possibly indicate the function of multiple corpora lutea. The only difference between the two HMG-treated groups is the minimal decrease of estrogens after ovulation in Group 3 and higher levels in the middle of the luteal phase. No pregnancies occurred in this group. It is unlikely that these higher levels exclusively represent multiple corpora lutea, otherwise a higher rate of pregnancy would be expected. Determination of plasma estrogens seems to be no better index of follicular maturation than urinary estrogens.

Plasma 17-OHP values are comparable to estrogen values. Here again we have a 3 to 4 day longer period of elevated levels prior to day 0. There is evidence that theca interna cells are the most active follicular compartment in the synthesis of estrogens and 17-OHP. Therefore, the period of theca interna cell function is supposedly prolonged during stimulation with exogenous gonadotropins. In those patients who became pregnant, this function was very active as reflected by the high 17-OHP levels. It is assumed that theca interna cells persist in the corpus luteum and can be regarded as the source of estrogens and 17-OHP during the luteal phase. Based on this assumption, different 17-OHP levels in Groups 2 and 3 could possibly be explained. In Group 2 in which pregnancy occurred, 17-OHP levels were higher than in Group 3 in which the patients did not become pregnant. In Group 2, 17-OHP levels are highest, while the estrogens are relatively low. In Group 3 this phenomenon is reversed. This indicates a different enzymatic activity of the ovaries in these two groups.

Plasma levels of P serve as an index of corpus luteum function. Levels begin to increase after ovulation in the normal menstrual cycle. Levels in the treatment cycles were markedly different in the two stimulated groups. On the day before assumed ovulation, an elevation of P was found in women receiving HMG. This elevation was maintained until the second or third day after ovulation. It might be speculated that the stimulated growing follicle is luteinized before reaching full maturity either by nonphysiological exogenous stimulation or by superimposing endogenous gonadotropins. This preceding luteinization could explain the fact that conception did not occur in this group of patients. The determination of plasma progesterone during follicular stimulation could give further information on the status of follicular maturity in order to determine the proper time for administration of HCG.

Discussion of steroid patterns clearly demonstrates that ovarian stimulation with exogenous gonadotropin is nonphysiological. As a result of our studies, we conclude that measurement of plasma estrogens and 17-OHP are of questionable value in monitoring ovarian response to gonadotropin treatment. These studies, however, present valuable information on ovarian physiology and are helpful in explaining the discrepancy in the rate of ovulations and pregnancies achieved. The determination of plasma progesterone and simultaneous determination of urinary estrogen output are certainly an improvement in monitoring gonadotropin treatment.

ACKNOWLEDGMENT

This work was supported by a grant from Deutsche Forschungsgemeinschaft (SFB 34).

REFERENCES

1. Abraham, G. E., J Clin Endocrinol 29:866, 1969.
2. Yoshimi, T., and M. B. Lippsett, Steroids 11:527, 1968.
3. Johannsson, E. D. B., Acta Endocrinol 61:592, 1969.
4. Murphy, B. E. P., J Clin Endocrinol 27:973, 1967.

5. Strott, C. A., and M. B. Lippsett, J Clin Endocrinol 28:1426, 1968.

6. Brown, J. B., S. C. McLeod, C. Macnaughtan, and M. A. Smith, J Endocrinol 5:42, 1968.

7. Lehmann, F., C. Neale, and G. Bettendorf in G. Bettendorf and V. Insler (Eds.), Clinical Application of Human Gonadotropins, Thieme, Stuttgart, 1970, p. 113.

57. Plasma Levels of Estradiol and Estrone during Treatment with Ovulation Inhibiting Compounds

Elof D. B. Johansson, Britt Boilert, and Carl A. Gemzell

The oral contraceptives of the combined type inhibit ovulation in most cases (1). Even if elevated plasma levels of progesterone have been found in a few cycles, normal luteal phase pattern of plasma progesterone is rarely seen (2, 3). The present trend in the development of oral contraceptives is based on the finding that the estrogen content of the tablet can give serious side effects and thus should be reduced. The estrogenic effect on the target organ will be a summation of the estrogen in the tablet and the endogenous production in the ovary. Previous studies have generally concluded that the estrogen levels found in urine or plasma during oral contraceptive therapy are similar to those found prior to the ovulatory estrogen peak in the normal menstrual cycle (4-6).

This is a preliminary report of decreased plasma levels of estradiol and estrone in women treated with five different ovulation inhibiting estrogen-progestin combinations as compared to the levels found prior to the ovulatory estrogen peak during the normal menstrual cycle. However, the estrogen levels were significantly higher than those found in women after the menopause.

MATERIALS AND METHODS

Blood samples for normal menstrual cycle studies were obtained from healthy women who participated in our earlier studies of the menstrual cycle (7). Samples from postmenopausal women were obtained from patients admitted to

758

the hospital for nonovarian diseases. Five different combinations of oral contraceptives were used. 1) Tablets containing 100 μg mestranol and 1 mg of norethindrone. This combination is one of the most common contraceptives used in Sweden. 2) Tablets containing 80 μg mestranol and 0.5 mg of norethindrone. This combination was for investigational use only (5). 3) Tablets containing 50 μg of ethinyl estradiol and 0.5 mg of norethindrone. This combination was for investigational use only. 4) Tablets containing 37.5 μg of ethinyl estradiol and 1 mg of lynestrenol. The complete report of the effect on the ovarian function of this combination will be published elsewhere. 5) Tablets containing 30 μg ethinyl estradiol and 5 mg of medroxyprogesterone acetate. A complete report of the effect on the ovarian function of this combination will be published elsewhere. The women that took part in the study were instructed to take one tablet a day for 21 days with 7-day tablet-free intervals.

Assay Methods

Estradiol and estrone were assayed using radioimmunoassay following ether extraction and separation on a Sephadex LH-20 column (8). The antiserum, a gift from Dr. Vande Wiele, New York (9), was used in a dilution of 1 : 150,000 (8). The radioimmunoassay procedure adhered very closely to that of Hotchkiss et al. (10). Two milliliters of plasma was extracted once with 5 volumes of ether. The samples were evaporated to dryness and transferred to a Sephadex LH-20 column (0.5 × 30 cm) in the eluent benzene-methanol 85 : 15. Ten columns could easily be operated simultaneously by one technician.

The separation of estrogens on the Sephadex column yielded a distinct estrone fraction thus far found free from other steroids that could interfere in the radioimmunoassay system used. Estradiol-17β was collected in a distinct fraction but separation from estradiol-17α or ethinyl estradiol was not obtained. Estradiol-17α has about one-third the affinity of estradiol-17β to the antibody. Dilution studies of the estradiol fraction indicate that estradiol-17β is the major estrogen in the fraction collected from human plasma in this study. Ethinyl estradiol was also partly collected in the estradiol fraction, but since its affinity to the antibody is only 0.5% of estradiol-17β its influence on the measurements was regarded as minimal.

The detection limit was 5 pg for estradiol and 10 pg for estrone. Since 2 ml of plasma was extracted throughout the study and more than 95% of estradiol and estrone was extracted, all values, except for estradiol levels in the postmenopause samples, were above the detection limit. Precision was calculated from duplicate determinations according to Snedecor (11). The coefficient of variation was 14.3% in the range of 5 to 25 pg of estradiol and 19.0% in the range of 10 to 30 pg of estrone.

RESULTS

The estradiol and estrone levels during the follicular phase of the menstrual cycles were measured in plasma pools containing plasma samples from the same woman from day 1 of her menstrual cycle up to 3 days prior to the midcycle rise of estrogens. During treatment with the five different combinations of estrogens and progestins the plasma levels of progesterone were measured to rule out ovulation. Pools were made from plasma that contained less than 0.5 ng/ml of progesterone. Levels after the menopause were measured in single blood samples from individual women. The levels of estradiol and estrone found are shown in Fig. 1. The levels of estradiol in the postmenopausal women were below the

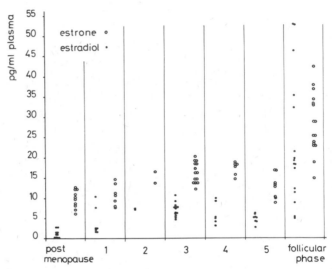

FIG. 1. Levels of estrone and estradiol in plasma from women after menopause, women in the early follicular phase of the cycles and women during treatment with 5 different oral contraceptives: 1) 100 μg of mestranol and 1 mg of norethindrone, 2) 80 μg of mestranol and 0.5 mg of norethindrone, 3) 50 μg of ethinyl estradiol and 0.5 mg of norethindrone, 4) 37.5 μg of ethinyl estradiol and 1 mg of lynestrenol, and 5) 30 μg of ethinyl estradiol and 5 mg of medroxyprogesterone acetate.

detection limit of the method but an average level of 9.5 pg/ml of estrone was found. During the early follicular phase a mean of 23.3 pg of estradiol and 27.9 pg/ml of estrone was found. During the treatment with the five different oral contraceptives very low levels of estradiol were found while the estrone levels were less reduced. No clear differences were seen in estradiol or estrone levels during treatment with the different combinations but the number of the measurements in each group was too small to allow statistical evaluation. If the values found during treatment were regarded as one group, both the estradiol and estrone levels found during treatment were significantly lower than those found during the early follicular phase but higher than the levels found after the menopause.

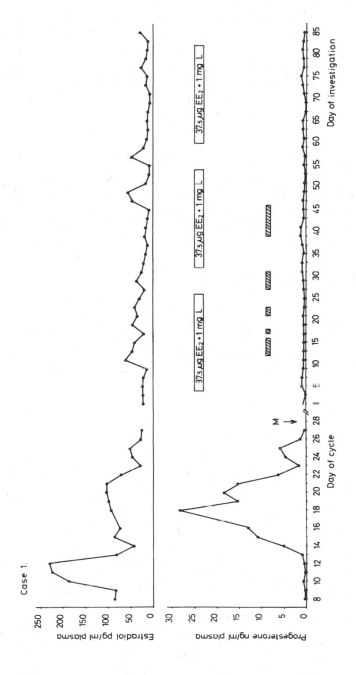

FIG. 2. Plasma levels of progesterone and estradiol, during one control cycle followed by three treatment periods with 37.5 μg of ethinyl estradiol (EE₂) and 1 mg of lynestrenol (L). M indicates the first day of bleeding after the control cycle. The shadowed areas indicate vaginal bleedings during treatment.

761

Three women have been investigated during their normal untreated menstrual cycle and also during treatment with two or three of the combinations investigated. The level of estrone during treatment was reduced to one-half the levels during the early follicular phase, while the levels of estradiol were reduced to one-fourth the levels during the early period of the normal menstrual cycle. Thus the ratio between estradiol and estrone changed from approximately 1 : 1 during the early follicular phase to 1 : 2 during the treatment with the ovulation inhibiting combinations of estrogens and progestins.

The effect of the treatment with combinations 3 to 5 was studied during 8 to 12 cycles for each combination with measurements of progesterone and estrogens every other day. During the treatment with combination 3 (50 μg of ethinyl estradiol and 0.5 mg of norethindrone) one normal luteal phase pattern of progesterone was found together with three cycles of subnormal rise of progesterone during the 12 cycles investigated. During the treatment with the other combination no ovarian steroid production indicating ovulation was found. A typical result during treatment is illustrated in Fig. 2.

DISCUSSION

Recent methodological progress of the assay methods have enabled daily determinations of estradiol and estrone during the normal menstrual cycle of women (4, 5, 9, 10, 12-14). The improvement of the radioimmunoassay technique for estradiol made by Hotchkiss et al. (10) has reduced the detection limit and improved the precision. This technical improvement, combined with purification of the ether extract on small Sephadex columns, has made possible precise and accurate measurements of the levels of estrone and estradiol during the treatment with combined oral contraceptives and during the postmenopausal period.

The levels of estradiol reported in this study are generally lower than those reported by other workers. The best agreement is found between the values reported by Baird and Guevara (13) for estrone and estradiol during the early follicular phase. These workers also reported a ratio of estradiol to estrone of about 1 : 1 during this period of the cycle. Their measurements were obtained by use of a double-isotope derivative method. The difference in values between the present studies and previous work may, however, be more apparent than real, as large individual variation seems to occur and the number of individuals investigated are small. The finding of decreased levels of both estrone and estradiol in women treated with combined oral contraceptives as compared to the early part of their normal follicular phase is at variance with previous reports (4, 5). Previous studies were done with less sensitive methods and with some blank problems, which might have obscured the difference.

In the five different combinations tested in this study, the estrogen content varied between 100 μg of mestranol to 30 μg of ethinyl estradiol. As long as no ovulation occurred during the treatment, the estrone and estradiol levels were low. This would mean that the women treated with combinations containing low levels of estrogens were submitted to less estrogenic activity than those who received a higher dose of estrogen as no increase of their endogenous levels of estrogens were found.

The levels of progestins may also be of importance for the evaluation of estrogen production in the ovary. In pills containing low levels of estrogens, the ovulation inhibiting effect was mainly dependent on the progestin component of the tablet. It is possible that progestins have a negative feedback effect on the production of estradiol in the human ovary either directly or via the hypothalamus-pituitary system. All progestins used in the combinations studied when given after ovulation have been found to produce a decrease in both progesterone and estradiol synthesis in the human corpus luteum (15).

ACKNOWLEDGMENT

The study was supported by the Ford Foundation and the Population Council, New York. The authors are indebted to the women that endured all the venipunctures necessary to make this study possible.

REFERENCES

1. Diczfalusy, E., Preventive Medicine and Family Planning, Proc 5th Conference of the Europe and Near East Region of the IPPF, 1967, pp. 27-32.

2. Larsson-Cohn, U., and E. D. B. Johansson, Lancet 1:160, 1969.

3. Erb, H., and K. S. Ludwig, Gynaecologia (Basel) 159:309, 1965.

4. Shutt, D. A., Steroids 13:69, 1969.

5. Dufau, M., K. J. Catt, A. Dulmanis, M. Fullerton, B. Hudson, and H. G. Burger, Lancet 1:271, 1970.

6. Larsson-Cohn, U., E. D. B. Johansson, and C. Gemzell, Schweiz Z Gynäk Geburtsh 1:463, 1970.

7. Johansson, E. D. B., L. Wide, and C. Gemzell, Acta Endocrinol (Kbh), in press, 1971.

8. Mikhail, G., C. H. Wu, M. Ferin, and R. L. Vande Wiele, Steroids 15:333, 1970.

9. Ferin, M., P. E. Zimmering, S. Lieberman, and R. L. Vande Wiele, Endocrinology 83:565, 1968.

10. Hotchkiss, J., L. E. Atkinsson, and E. Knobil, Endocrinology, in press, 1971.

11. Snedecor, G. W., Statistical Methods, 5th ed. Iowa State College Press, Ames, 1956.

12. Corker, C. S., and D. Exley, Steroids 15:469, 1970.

13. Korenman, S. G., L. E. Perrin, and T. P. McCallum, J Clin Endocrinol 29:879, 1969.

14. Baird, D. T., and A. Guevara, J Clin Endocrinol 29:149, 1969.

15. Johansson, E. D. B., Acta Obst Gyn Scand 50:75, 1971.

DISCUSSION

F. LEHMANN. In addition to the paper given by Dr. Bettendorf in which he summarized our results of ovarian response to exogenous gonadotropins in 21 treatments, I would like to support the discussion by showing our findings in some individual treatment courses.

Figure 1 shows two steroid patterns which we would like to achieve in every

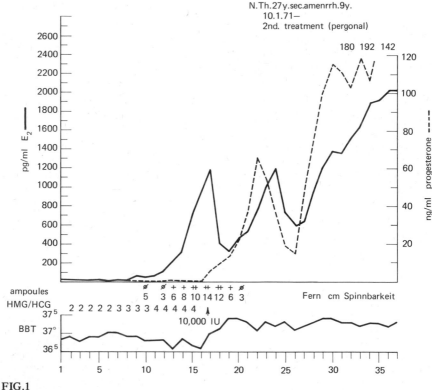

FIG.1

patient treated with HMG. Prior to HMG, plasma estrogens were less than 0.2 ng/ml. During HMG treatment, estrogens show a biphasic pattern with peaks of about 1000 pg/ml. Progesterone increased after the HCG injection. This treatment cycle resulted in pregnancy.

Figure 2 shows a treatment pattern which we often find in that group of patients who do not become pregnant. Treatment with HMG was started when plasma estrogens were 300 pg/ml. Progesterone was between 0.5 and 1 ng/ml. During treatment with the HMG preparation, estrogens increased to values of 1200 pg/ml. The level of progesterone increased before the first HCG injection. Following HCG, the estrogen level continued to be elevated and progesterone increased slowly to values comparable to those found in a spontaneous menstrual cycle. In this patient the basal body temperature does not reflect an early rise in progesterone.

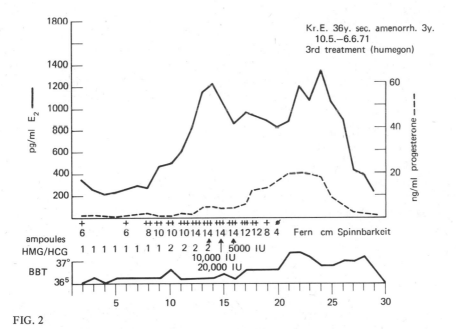

FIG. 2

R. M. NAKAMURA. We would like to show a slide (Fig. 3) that verifies the data presented by Dr. Johansson. The shaded area represents the mean estradiol levels ± 2 SE of a group of 10 normal women during ovulatory cycles. The three patterns below the shaded area represent estradiol levels during cycles for 3 women treated with a combination oral steroid contraceptive. A question was raised earlier as to the possible action of contraceptives on the gonadotropin pattern. FSH levels are relatively constant with values slightly lower than in the

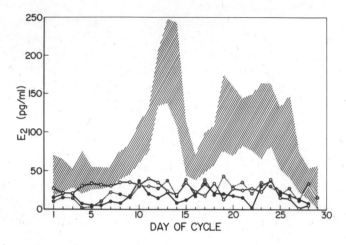

FIG. 3

normal luteal phase. The immunoreactive LH in our system shows considerable daily fluctuation initially but with continual treatment, LH levels stabilize at low luteal phase levels. Therefore, together with the drop in estradiol and progesterone levels there is a concomitant fall in both gonadotropins to low luteal-phase levels.

A. JACOBSON. Another manifestation of abnormal steroid levels in gonadotropin stimulated ovulatory cycles, using a variety of injection schedules, is the absence of a spontaneous preovulatory LH peak when no HCG is given following follicular gonadotropin stimulation. The absence of a spontaneous preovulatory LH peak is noted in individuals who have a spontaneous LH peak following clomiphene stimulation. The missing LH peak is probably not due to excessive estradiol, progesterone, or 17α-hydroxyprogesterone, as all of these steroids have been shown to cause a positive feedback on the hypothalamus resulting in a midcycle-like LH peak. So one wonders whether there are some other steroids that we have not measured or a gross asynchrony of steroids that may be inhibiting a spontaneous LH peak.

DR. F. FUCHS. There are many topics that we have neglected in these three days of discussion of gonadotropins. I alluded to it yesterday and perhaps now that we are reaching the end of the proceedings I may be permitted to show three slides. The period of lactation is a period of female life which really has been neglected. Here we have a period of spontaneous inhibition of ovulation with high levels of gonadotropin secretion (Fig. 4) in a patient who lactated for 45 weeks postpartum, which is much longer than in the average patient, even in

Denmark. She did not resume menstruation until around 40 weeks. The question is: what is it that inhibits ovulation during this long period of lactation and what is it that permits the resumption of the menstrual cycle during continuous

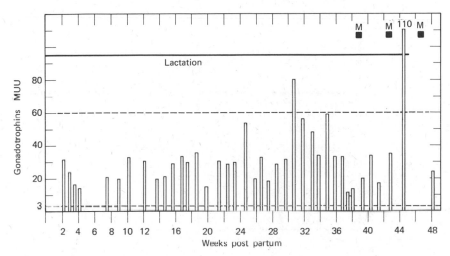

FIG. 4. Urinary total gonadotropins during lactation. (Johnsen, S. and F. Fuchs, unpublished.)

lactation? We have recently looked further into this. We have not come to any conclusions, although we have done better hormone profiles than in the early studies.

The next slide (Fig. 5) illustrates a patient who lactated for about 5 weeks. The FSH levels were higher than the LH levels. The progesterone values indicate that the first bleeding was anovulatory and the next one ovulatory. There is a progressive rise in estrogen excretion following parturition. In the next slide (Fig. 6) again, the FSH values are higher than the LH values; the first menstruation is anovulatory and the second ovulatory. In view of the discussion of prolactin yesterday, one might speculate about a role of prolactin in inhibiting ovulation.

S. MARCUS. I would like to present some data regarding levels of pituitary gonadotropins and progesterone in plasma during the administration of chlormadinone acetate. Martinez-Manautou and his group (Fert Steril 17:49, 1966) first reported the use of a microdose (500 µg daily) of an acetoxyprogestin, chlormadinone acetate, for conception control. In their study, 73% of endometrial biopsies revealed secretory changes suggestive of ovulation during chlormadinone treatment. Subsequent studies have reported that 64 to 78% of cycles in patients taking clormadinone were considered to be ovulatory. It has therefore been suggested in the literature that clormadinone may be contraceptive, not by altering hypothalamic-pituitary function, but by an effect on other functions such as capacitation of spermatozoa, ovum transport, cervical mucus

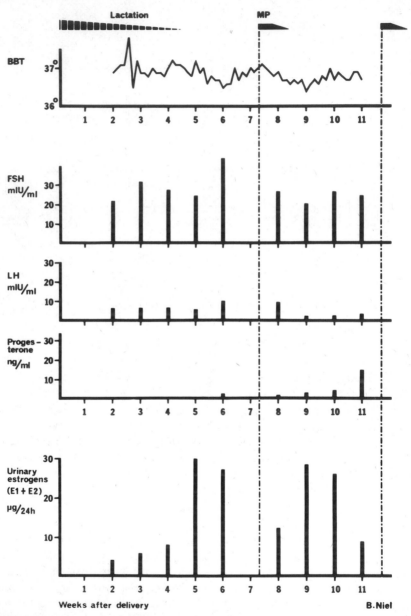

FIG. 5. Plasma levels of FSH, LH, and progesterone and urinary estrogens in a 26-year-old primipara. (Fuchs, F., C. G. Beling, V. A. Frandsen, J. B. Josimovich, K.J.A. Moller, D. M. Saunders, and B. B. Saxena, unpublished.)

physiology, or the process of implantation. However, the recent availability of
specific and sensitive assays for FSH, LH, and progesterone have allowed us to

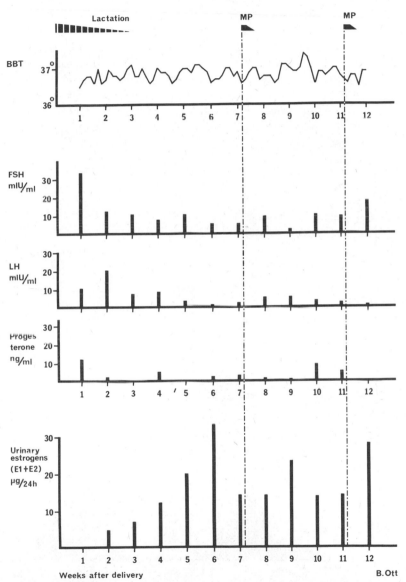

FIG. 6. Plasma levels of FSH, LH, and progesterone and urinary estrogens in a 28-year-old
woman who lactated for 3 weeks only. (Fuchs, F., C. G. Beling, V. A. Frandsen, J. B.
Josimovich, K.J.A. Moller, D. M. Saunders, and B. B. Saxena, unpublished.)

study further the effects of chlormadinone on the hypothalamic-pituitary system.

We have studied 9 healthy women with regular menstrual cycles for two consecutive cycles, the first one being a control cycle and the second being the treatment cycle in which chlormadinone acetate was administered daily at a dose level of 500 μg. Daily levels of plasma FSH, LH, and progesterone were studied.

I will present data from only 3 of the patients. In Fig. 7, it is evident that both in the control and treatment cycles, the basal body temperature (BBT) recordings were biphasic and that there were significant LH peaks and luteal levels of progesterone to suggest that ovulation occurred in both cycles. Figure 8 represents another patient in whom the control cycle appeared to be ovulatory according to the same parameters. In the treatment cycle, however, the BBT pattern was atypical. Interestingly, there were two LH peaks, but rather low

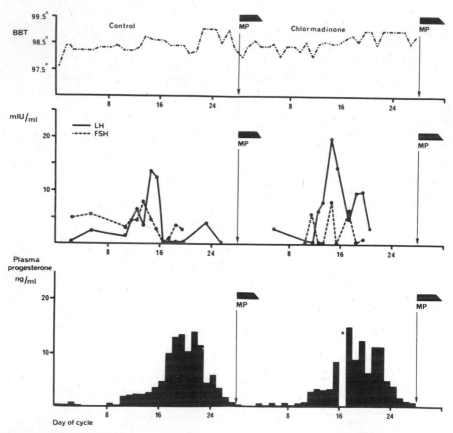

FIG. 7. 35-year-old, para 3, with regular 28-day cycles and an average menstrual flow of 3 days. (*)Represents days when plasma sample for progesterone determinations were not available; (MP) menstrual period. Reproduced by permission of Williams & Wilkins Company.

levels of progesterone. Figure 9 represents the third patient in whom the control cycle revealed a biphasic temperature chart, an early LH peak on about the eighth day corresponding to a rise in body temperature at about the same time, and an elevation in progesterone level on about the ninth day. In the treatment cycle, although there was a biphasic temperature pattern, there was an absence of an LH peak and there were low levels of progesterone suggesting that ovulation probably did not occur. Figure 10 depicts the mean FSH and LH values with SD in the 9 patients as well as the range of progesterone levels. The mean LH peak is reduced in chlormadinone-treated cycles compared to the control cycles, and although there is a considerable range, there appears to be a trend towards suppression of progesterone levels during chlormadinone treatment.

Using the parameters of BBT, LH peak, and progesterone levels, 8 of the 9

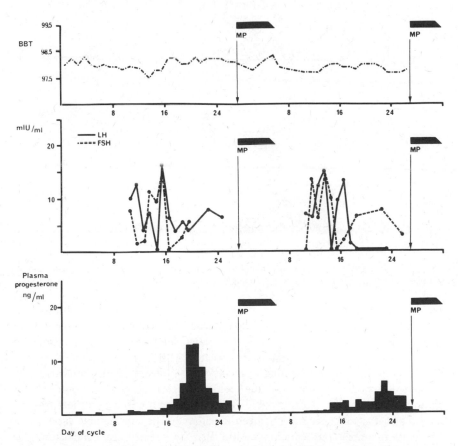

FIG. 8. 35-year-old, para 3, with a history of regular 28-day cycles and an average menstrual flow of 5 days. Reproduced by permission of Williams & Wilkins Company.

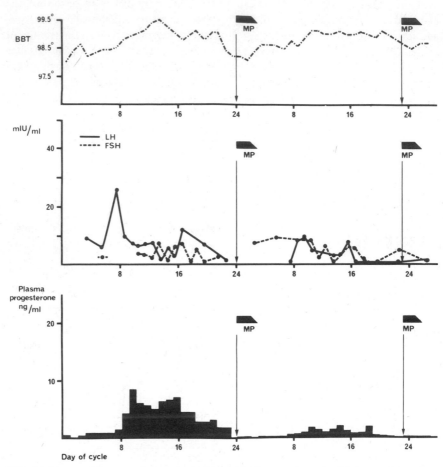

FIG. 9. 36-year-old, no previous pregnancies, with history of regular 28-day cycles and an average menstrual flow of 7 days. Reproduced by permission of Williams & Wilkins Company.

patients in our study appeared to ovulate in the control cycle. However, only 3 of the 9 patients appeared to ovulate during chlormadinone treatment. The study illustrated the difficulty in determining whether or not ovulation has occurred using individual parameters such as BBT, LH peak, and plasma progesterone level. An interesting observation was the appearance of two clearly defined LH peaks in some of the control cycles as well as some of the chlormadinone cycles. These double peaks have been noted by others but the physiological significance has not been elucidated. The considerable variation in LH pattern among our patients should also be stressed. In conclusion, our findings, which were published just a month ago (Saunders, D. M., S. L. Marcus, B. B. Saxena, C. G. Beling, and E. B. Connell, Fert Steril 22:332, 1971), suggest

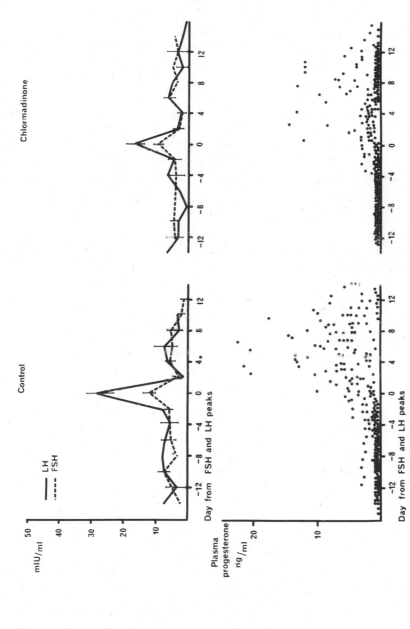

FIG. 10. Composite of FSH, LH, and progesterone values during control and chlormadinone cycles in the nine women studied. Mean values ± SE of FSH and LH are shown. Reproduced by permission of Williams & Wilkins Company.

that the continuous administration of a microdose of a progestin such as 500 μg of chlormadinone acetate daily, may alter the hypothalamic-pituitary axis to a greater degree than has heretofore been believed. Our findings are similar to those reported by Taymor and Levesque (Fert Steril 22:1, 1971).

DR. LLOYD. I would like to confirm a couple of things that Dr. Johansson has said and add a little to his remarks. The first point is that we can confirm Dr. Johansson as far as methods are concerned. We have done a similar study in collaboration with the group at the University of Chile (Professor Puga and Drs. Pupkin and Zanartu). This was a companion study to the one that Dr. Weisz mentioned earlier in which plasma from the ovarian vein and peripheral blood were collected during operation for elective tubal ligation. She mentioned the normal subjects. This study was on a number of women receiving contraceptives. The operations were carried out in Chile and various studies on histochemistry of the ovary were done there. The hormone analyses were done at the Worcester

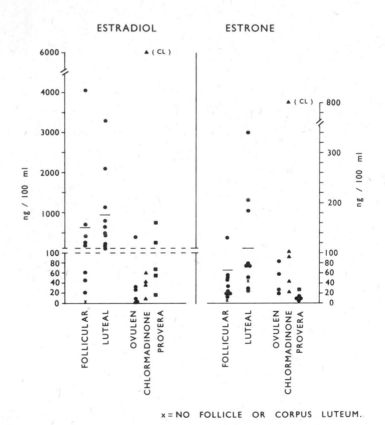

FIG. 11. Concentration of estrogens in ovarian venous plasma of normal women and women receiving contraceptives. Reproduced by permission of J. B. Lippincott Company.

Foundation. There are several slides which illustrate these data. Estradiol and estrone levels in the ovarian and peripheral venous plasma are shown in the next 2 slides (Figs. 11 and 12). As we have reported before, there tend to be fairly wide ranges of ovarian venous estradiol with somewhat higher ranges in the luteal phase. In all the contraceptors, (Ovulen, Chlormadinone, and Depo-Provera) estradiol is down and estrone tends to be somewhat decreased. To reinforce what Dr. Marcus has just said, 6 of the women receiving Chlorma-dinone did not ovulate. In the peripheral blood, estradiol is clearly suppressed in all of the contraceptors, whereas the estrone is not suppressed as much. This then confirms what Dr. Johansson has just shown us. It also confirms his method because these were measured by the double isotope derivative dilution procedure. Our measurements, using the immunoassay, give us the same general levels.

In the normal woman, the ratios of estradiol to estrone and of androstene-dione to testosterone are high (Fig. 13). A high androstenedione in plasma is as

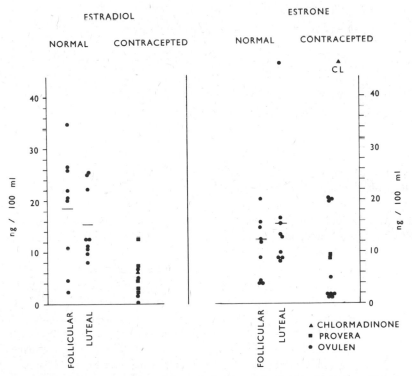

FIG. 12. Concentrations of estrogens in peripheral venous plasma of women with normal cycles and women receiving contraceptives. Reproduced by permission of J. B. Lippincott Company.

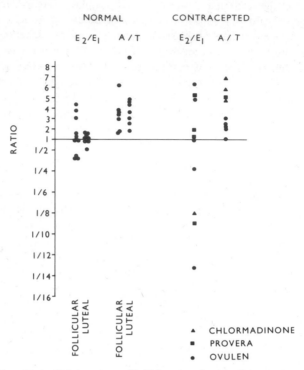

FIG. 13. Ratios of estradiol to estrone (E_2/E_1) and androstenedione to testosterone (A/T) on peripheral venous blood of normal women and women receiving contraceptives. Reproduced by permission of J. B. Lippincott Company.

characteristic of the normal female as is a high estradiol. The estradiol to estrone and androstenedione to testosterone ratios in plasma are considerably decreased in women receiving contraceptives (Fig. 14). This is presumably because ovarian secretion of estradiol and androstenedione are markedly suppressed, whereas secretion of estrone and testosterone, much of which come from the adrenals, is less suppressed.

Finally, I would like to make a comment about plasma gonadotropin levels of women receiving contraceptives. In the normal woman, there is a significantly lower level of LH in plasma coming from the ovary than in peripheral blood. In other words, passage through the ovary alters gonadotropin which results in a lower level of LH as measured by radioimmunoassay. This difference is not present in patients who have received ovulation inhibiting contraceptives. The ovary that has been inhibited for a long time seems to have lost the ability to metabolize gonadotropins.

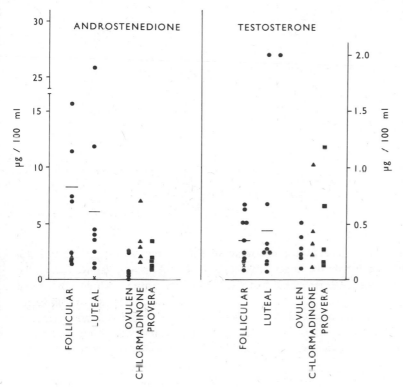

FIG. 14. Concentrations of androstenedione and testosterone in ovarian venous plasma of normal women and women receiving contraceptives. Reproduced by permission of J. B. Lippincott Company.

58.   Closing Remarks

Bruno Lunenfeld

It is usually the duty of the chairman of the closing session of a successful symposium to thank the organizing committee, the secretarial staff, and the sponsors for their efforts which had made this symposium both an intellectual and a pleasant experience. It would be an almost impossible task to summarize the wealth of experimental data which has been presented and critically evaluated during the symposium. With your permission, therefore, I intend to restrict my concluding remarks to the historical perspectives in gonadotropic research.

The gonadotropic era started in 1910 with Crowe's discovery of a relationship between the pituitary gland and the gonads (1). In 1926, the pituitary-gonadal (2, 3, 21) and placental-gonadal relationships (4) were established. Between 1927 and 1934, the gonad-stimulating principles were shown to be circulating hormones secreted by the pituitary gland and placental tissue (5-10). The existence of FSH, LH, PMSG, and HCG was demonstrated and the effect of HCG on animal gonads was exploited as a pregnancy test (7-23). Collip (24) demonstrated the antigenic nature of gonadotropic hormones in 1934. Attempts to use these hormones as therapeutic agents were made as early as 1930 (25, 26). The period between 1934 and 1953 was essentially devoted to the development of extraction and purification procedures for gonadotropins (27-36) as well as specific assay methods for FSH (37, 38) and LH (37, 39, 40). The antigenic nature of gonadotropins was further investigated during the initial part of this period (41, 42). International standards for HCG and PMSG were established by the League of Nations in 1939 (43), however, no reference preparations of human pituitary gonadotropins existed.

In 1953, de Watteville, Borth, and myself invited a number of scientists to Geneva to coordinate and boost research efforts in the gonadotropic field. At this first G-Club meeting, there were only ten representatives from five centers. At this symposium today, 150 participants from 50 centers are present and represent a cross-section of scientists interested in the anatomy, biochemistry, and physiology of the hypothalamic-pituitary-gonadal axis. It was only by the most rigorous selection on the part of the organizing committee that the total number has been kept to a manageable size. Discussions were held during the 1953 Geneva Meeting on the development of statistically valid bioassay procedures (44). Collaborative assays of gonadotropic extracts were planned (45), leading to the establishment of international reference preparations. Studies were initiated on urinary patterns of gonadotropins and steroids during the menstrual cycle (46, 47) and in men (48). The problem of international standards was not resolved.

Data accumulated by an increasing number of investigators culminated in a meeting in Gatlinburg in 1959 (49). Investigators at this meeting reported that ovaries of amenorrheic women could be stimulated by HPG and HMG. By the 10th anniversary of the G-Club in Tel-Aviv, progress in gonadotropic research had proceeded in three areas: (1) the antigenic nature of gonadotropins (50-52) and its application in the development of immunoassay procedures (51, 51, 53); (2) purification of gonadotropic hormones (54-57); and (3) the use of gonadotropins in the induction of ovulation. Numerous pregnancies resulting from induction of ovulation by HMG were reported at the second international congress of endocrinology held in London in 1964 (58).

The chemical nature of both pituitary and urinary gonadotropins was poorly understood until 1953. The Ciba Foundation study group meeting in 1965 was devoted to physicochemical and immunological properties of gonadotropins. Labeling of HCG with radioactive iodine and its use for radioimmunoassay was discussed for the first time (59).

Data on the reliability and sensitivity of extraction procedures were presented at the meeting held in Edinburgh in 1966. Specific bioassay methods which had been exploited for the determination of FSH and LH patterns in relationship to urinary steroids at the various stages of the normal menstrual cycle were also discussed. The therapeutic use of gonadotropic preparations received wide consideration. It seemed to be apparent that even with the partial knowledge on the endocrine mechanisms governing the menstrual cycle, ovulation could be inhibited or induced. Moreover, these possibilities served as tools in a better understanding of the control of ovarian and testicular function. Data on specific ovarian receptors binding HCG was presented by Eshkol (60). The availability of highly purified FSH, LH, and HCG, and the perfection of labeling techniques has had a tremendous impact on progress in development of radioimmunoassays for these hormones. The Ciba meeting in 1965 and the Edinburgh meeting in 1966 shifted their interests to physicochemical properties and mechanism of action of gonadotropins.

At the next meeting held in 1968 in Vista Hermosa, the major topics discussed were biological and immunological assays, therapeutic use of gonado-tropins and the problem of standards (61). Further consideration was also given to the mechanism of action of gonadotropins as well as their action at the genetic level. The existence of organ-specific receptor sites for HCG was substantiated. Possible implications of prostaglandins as regulatory agents in release or action of gonadotropins were reported. The ultrastructure of the pituitary was described for the first time in this meeting.

By 1969 research on gonadotropins had expanded in many directions. There were three independent workshop meetings in 1969-70 devoted to three specific aspects of the field. The Birmingham meeting was devoted to the chemistry of gonadotropins (62). Bahl (63, 64) determined the number and size of carbohydrate units of HCG and reported their tentative monosaccharide sequence. He postulated that HCG was composed of two identical subunits (62). Canfield and co-workers confirmed the existence of subunits in HCG but presented conclusive evidence of their nonidentity (62). The postulated existence of subunits of ovine LH (65) was confirmed and their terminal sequences were reported (66). Physicochemical and immunological properties of the two subunits of human LH were reported (67). The second meeting was held in Stockholm and was concerned with the immunoassays of gonadotropins. This meeting assembled expert knowledge of the leading scientists in the field such as Midgley, Odell, Saxena, Catt, and others. The rapid publication of the proceeding (68) and their wide distribution introduced immunoassay procedures to every corner of the world. The third meeting held in Hamburg in 1970 was devoted to the clinical application of human gonadotropins (69). One of the main topics of this workshop was a progress report on the retrospective analysis of gonadotropic therapy. This report as well as that by Thompson and Hansen (70) demonstrated that there were more than 750 pregnancies in 10 years as the result of induction of ovulation with human gonadotropins.

It was with this background that Fritz Fuchs, Ralph Peterson, Brij Saxena, Carl Beling, and Hortense Gandy set out in organizing this international symposium on gonadotropins as part of the celebration of the bicentennial anniversary of the New York Hospital. The names of those present as well as the content of the lectures and discussions during these past few days are testimony that the current state of knowledge on the hypothalamic-hypophyseal-gonadal axis has been comprehensively evaluated. This meeting was highlighted by presentation of contributions on the isolation and chemistry of subunits and receptor site mechanisms of human pituitary gonadotropins as well as induction of ovulation and regulation of gonadotropin secretion. This symposium will be remembered by participating biochemists, biologists, and clinicians as a cornerstone in scientific cross-fertilization and will stimulate all of us to continue to strive for the final elucidation of the blueprint which governs the regulation of reproductive processes.

I hope no one will consider this talk as a historical document on gonadotropic research. A rigorous literature review was not attempted; many important and excellent contributions may have been omitted. I only tried, looking back over the past 18 years, to revive the pleasant memories from a number of meetings and to note how such research changed its course, direction, and scope. As some problems have been solved, new ones have appeared on the horizon. I confidently predict that the 20th anniversary meeting of the G-Club, which we hope to hold in Tel-Aviv, will be as lively and stimulating as this symposium which we are now closing.

REFERENCES

1. Crowe, S. J., H. Cushing, and J. Homans, Johns Hopk Hosp Bull 21:169, 1910.
2. Evans, II. M., and J. A. Long, Anat Rec 21:62, 1921.
3. Zondek, B., and S. Aschheim, Dtsch Med Wschr 52:343, 1926.
4. Hirose, T., J Kinki Gynec Soc 16: (Cit. Murata, M. and K. Adachi, q.v.) 1920.
5. Murata, M., and K. Adachi, Z Gerburtsh Gynak 92:45, 1927.
6. Aschheim, S., and B. Zondek, Klin Wschr 6:1322, 1927.
7. Aschheim, S., Lecture to Beilinger gyn. Gesellschaft, December 14, 1928.
8. Fluhmann, C. F., J Amer Med Assoc 93:672, 1929.
9. Engle, E. T., J Amer Med Assoc 93:276, 1929.
10. Evans, H. M., and M. E. Simpson, Amer J Physiol 89:381, 1929.
11. Friedman, M. H., Amer J Physiol 90:617, 1929.
12. Brouha, L., and H. Simonnet, C R Soc Biol (Paris), 101:368, 1929.
13. Hamburger, C, Ugeskr Laeg 93:27, 1931.
14. Fevold, H. L., and S. L. Leonard, Amer J Physiol 97:291, 1931.
15. Collip, J. B., H. Selye, and D. L. Thomson, Nature 131:56, 1933.
16. Evans, H. M., M. E. Simpson, and P. R. Austin, J Exp Med 57:897, 1933.
17. Freud, J., and S. E. de Jongh, Acta Brev Neerl Physiol 3:57, 1933.
18. Hamburger, C., Thesis, Copenhagen, Levin and Munksgaard, 1933.
19. Reiss, M., R. Pick, and K. A. Winter, Endokrinologie, 12:18, 1933.
20. Schockaert, J., Amer J Physiol 105:497, 1933.
21. Smith, P. E., Proc Soc Exp Biol (NY), 24:131, 1926.
22. Cole, H. H., and G. H. Hart, Amer J Physiol 93:57, 1930.
23. Reichert, F. L., R. I. Pencharz, M. E. Simpson, K. Meyer, and H. M. Evans, Amer J Physiol 100:157, 1932.
24. Collip, J. B., J Mt. Sinai Hosp 1:28, 1934.
25. Schapiro, B., Dtsch Med Wschr 56:1605, 1930.
26. Wiesner, B. P., and F. A. E. Crew, Proc Roy Soc Edinb 50:79, 1930.
27. Katzman, P. A., and E. A. Doisy, J Biol Chem 106:125, 1934.
28. Levin, L., and H. H. Tyndale, Proc Soc Exp Biol (NY) 34:516, 1936.
29. Scott, L. D., Brit J Exp Pathol 21:320, 1941.
30. Katzman, P. A., M. Godfrid, C. K. Cain, and E. A. Doisy, J Biol Chem 148:501, 1943.
31. Gorbman, A., Endocrinology 37:177, 1945.
32. Crooke, A. C., and W. R. Butt, Proc Roy Soc Med 45:805, 1952.
33. Li, C. H., M. E. Simpson, and H. M. Evans, Endocrinology 27:803, 1940.

34. Greep, R. O., H. B. Van Dyke, and B. F. Chow, J Biol Chem 133:289, 1940.
35. Gurin, S., G. Bachman, and D. W. Wilson, J Biol Chem 133:467, 477, 1940.
36. Li, C. H., M. E. Simpson, and H. M. Evans, Science, 109:445, 1949.
37. Evans, H. M., M. E. Simpson, S. Tolksdorf, and H. Jensen, Endocrinology 25:205, 1939.
38. Steelman, S. L., and F. M. Pohley, Endocrinology 53:604, 1953.
39. Frank, R. T., and R. L. Berman, Amer J Obstet Gynec 42:492, 1941.
40. Greep, R. O., H. B. Van Dyke, and B. F. Chow, Endocrinology 30:635, 1942.
41. Zondek, B., and F. Sulman, The Antigonadotropic Factor, Williams & Wilkins, Baltimore, Maryland, 1942, p. 25.
42. Ostergaard, E., Antigonadotrophic Substances, Ejnas Munksgaard, Copenhagen, 1942, pp. 110 and 130.
43. League of Nations, Bull Health Org 8:884, 898, 1939.
44. Borth, R., E. Diczfalusy, and H. D. Heinrichs, Arch Gynak 188:497, 1957.
45. Benz, F., R. Borth, P. S. Brown, A. C. Crooke, J. B. Dekanski, E. Diczfalusy, J. A. Loraine, B. Lunenfeld, and W. Schuler, Endocrinology 19:158, 1959.
46. Loraine, J. A., and J. B. Brown, J Clin Endocrinol 16:1180, 1956.
47. Borth, R., B. Lunenfeld, and H. de Watteville, Fert Steril 8:233, 1957.
48. Johnsen, S. G., Acta Endocrinol (Kbh) 28:69, 1958.
49. Albert, A. (Ed.), Human Pituitary Gonadotropins, Charles C Thomas, Springfield, Ill., 1961.
50. Brody, S., and G. Carlstrom, Lancet 2:99, 1960.
51. Wide, L., and C. Gemzell, Acta Endocrinol (Kbh) 35:261, 1960.
52. Lunenfeld, B., D. Givol, and M. Sela, J Clin Endocrinol 21:474, 1961.
53. Wide, L., and C. Gemzell, Acta Endocrinol (Kbh) 39:539, 1962.
54. Legault-Demare, J., H. Clauser, and M. Jutisz, Bull Soc Chem Biol (Paris) 43:897, 1961.
55. Squire, P. G., C. H. Li, and R. N. Andersen, Biochemistry 1:412, 1962.
56. Reichert, L. E., Jr., Endocrinology 71:729, 1962.
57. Donini, P., D. Puzzuoli, and I. D'Alessio, Acta Endocrinol (Kbh) 45:329, 1964.
58. Lunenfeld, B., Excerpta Med Internat Congr Sr No. 83:814, 1964.
59. Wolstenholme, G. E. W., and J. Knight (Eds.), Gonadotropins: Physicochemical and Immunological Properties, J. and A. Churchill, London, 1965, Wilde, C. E., p. 58; and Lunenfeld, B., p. 60.
60. Bell, T., and J. A. Loraine (Eds.), Recent Research on Gonadotrophic Hormones: Proceedings of Fifth Gonadotrophin Club Meeting Edinburgh, 1966, E. & S. Livingstone, Edinburgh, 1967, Eshkio, A., p. 202.
61. Rosemberg, E., (Ed.), Gonadotropins 1968, Proceedings of the Workshop Conference Vista Hermosa, Geron-X Inc., Los Altos, 1968.
62. Butt, W. R., A. C. Crooke, and M. Ryle (Eds.), Gonadotrophins and Ovarian Development, E. & S. Livingstone, Edinburgh, 1971.
63. Bahl, O. P., J Biol Chem 244:507, 1969.
64. Bahl, O. P., J Biol Chem 244:575, 1969.
65. De La Llosa, P., C. Courte, and M. Jutisz, Biochem Biophys Res Commun 26:411, 1967.
66. Papkoff, H., and C. H. Li, in W. R. Butt, A. C. Crooke, and M. Ryle (Eds.), Gonadotrophins and Ovarian Development, E. & S. Livingstone, Edinburgh, 1971, p. 138.

67. Reichert, L. E., Jr., D. N. Ward, G. D. Niswender, and A. R. Midgley, Jr., in W. R. Butt, A. C. Crooke, and M. Ryle (Eds.), Gonadotrophins and Ovarian Development, E. & S. Livingstone, Edinburgh, 1971, p. 149.

68. Karolinska Symposia on Research Methods in Reproductive Endocrinology; 1st Symposium: Immunoassay of Gonadotrophins, in Acta Endocrinol (Kbh), Supp. 142, 1969.

69. Bettendorf, G., and V. Insler (Eds.), Clinical Application of Human Gonadotropins: Proceedings of a Workshop Conference—Hamburg, 1970, Georg Thieme Verlag, Stuttgart, 1970.

70. Thompson, L. R., and L. M. Hansen, Fert Steril 21:844, 1970.

Abbreviations and Symbols

adrenocorticotrophin (or tropin)	ACTH
Ångstrom	Å
centigrade	C
centimeter(s)	cm
chorionic gonadotropin (or tropin), human	HCG
counts per minute	cpm
cubic centimeter(s)	cc or cm³
curie(s)	Ci
diphosphopyridine nucleotide	DPN or NAD
diphosphopyridine nucleotide, reduced form of	DPNH or NADH
disintegrations per minute	dpm
equivalent (equivalent wt per liter)	Eq
extinction (molar extinction coefficient)	E (s)
follicle stimulating hormone	FSH
gram(s)	g
gravity	g
growth hormone	GH
hour(s)	hr
international unit	IU
interperitoneal	ip
intramuscular(ly)	im
intravenous(ly)	iv
liter(s)	l
kilogram	k
luteinizing hormone	LH
melanocyte stimulating hormone	MSH
meter(s)	m
micro (10^{-6})	μ
microgram(s)	μg

microliter(s)	μl
micron(s)	μ
milli (10^{-3})	m
minute(s)	min
molar (mole per liter)	M
mole(s)	mole(s)
molecular weight	mol wt
nano (10^{-9})	n
normal (concentration)	N
not significant	NS
number	no.
optical density	OD
osmole(s)	Osm
parts per million	ppm
pico (10^{-12})	p
per cent	%
precipitate	ppt
pregnant mare's serum	PMS
probability	p
releasing factor	RF (preceded by symbol for hormone released)
revolutions per minute	rpm
second	sec
specific activity	SA
square centimeter	cm²
standard deviation	DS
standard error	SE
subcutaneous(ly)	sc
"t" test	t
thyroid-stimulating hormone	TSH
thyrotrophin(or tropin)	TSH
tris (hydroxymethyl) amino-methane	Tris
ultraviolet	UV
unit(s)	U
volt(s)	V
volume	vol
volume/volume (concentration)	v/v
wavelength	λ
weight	wt
weight/volume (concentration)	w/v

Index